## PDxMD
# Gastroenterology

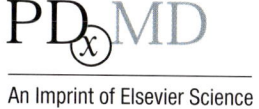

An Imprint of Elsevier Science

Philadelphia ■ St Louis ■ London ■ Sydney ■ New York ■ Toronto

*PDxMD Medical Conditions Series is dedicated to health and healing professionals everywhere. We are privileged to be in your service and hope our efforts help you in your quest for better quality-of-life and optimized outcomes for all your patients.*

PDxMD
An imprint of Elsevier Science

| | |
|---|---|
| Publisher: | Steven Merahn, MD |
| Project Managers: | Caroline Barnett, Lucy Hamilton, Zak Knowles |
| Programmer: | Narinder Chandi |
| Production: | Aoibhe O'Shea – GMS UK, Alan Palfreyman – PTU |
| Designer: | Jayne Jones |
| Layout: | Jane Tozer |

Copyright © 2003 PDxMD

All rights reserved. No part of this publication may be reproduced, stored in a retrieval system, or transmitted, in any form or by any means, electronic, mechanical, photocopying, recording, or otherwise, without written permission of the publisher.

NOTICE
Medicine is an ever-changing field. Standard safety precautions must be followed, but as new research and clinical experience broaden our knowledge, changes in treatment and drug therapy may become necessary or appropriate. Readers are advised to check the most current product information provided by the manufacturer of each drug to be administered to verify the recommended dose, the method and duration of administration, and contraindications. It is the responsibility of the licensed prescriber, relying on experience and knowledge of the patient, to determine dosages and the best treatment for each individual patient. Neither the publisher nor the editor assumes any liability for any injury and/or damage to persons or property arising from this publication.

All PDxMD contributors are participating in the activities of PDxMD in an individual capacity, and not as representatives of or on behalf of their individual affiliated hospitals, associations or institutions (where indicated herein), and their participation should not be taken as an endorsement of PDxMD by their individual affiliated hospitals, associations or institutions. Individual affiliated hospitals, associations or institutions are not responsible for the accuracy or availability of information on the product.

Permission to photocopy or reproduce solely for internal or personal use is permitted for libraries or other users registered with the Copyright Clearance Center, provided that the base fee of $4.00 per chapter plus $.10 per page is paid directly to the Copyright Clearance Center, 222 Rosewood Drive, Danvers, MA 01923. This consent does not extend to other kinds of copying, such as copying for general distribution, for advertising or promotional purposes, for creating new collected works, or for resale.

Printed in China by RDC Group

PDxMD
Elsevier Science
The Curtis Center
625 Walnut Street,
Philadelphia, PA 19106

The Publisher's policy is to use **paper manufactured from sustainable forests**

ISBN 1-932141-04-9

# Contents

## Introduction
| | |
|---|---|
| What is PDxMD? | v |
| About this book | v |
| How to use this book | v |
| How is PDxMD created? | vi |
| Continuous Product Improvement | vi |
| Evidence-Based Medicine Policies | vii |

## Editorial Faculty and Staff
## MediFiles

**Acute appendicitis** — **1**
- Summary Information — 2
- Background — 3
- Diagnosis — 5
- Treatment — 11
- Outcomes — 12
- Prevention — 13
- Resources — 14

**Budd-Chiari syndrome** — **15**
- Summary Information — 16
- Background — 17
- Diagnosis — 19
- Treatment — 32
- Outcomes — 39
- Prevention — 40
- Resources — 41

**Celiac disease** — **43**
- Summary Information — 44
- Background — 45
- Diagnosis — 47
- Treatment — 57
- Outcomes — 67
- Prevention — 69
- Resources — 70

**Cholecystitis** — **73**
- Summary Information — 74
- Background — 75
- Diagnosis — 77
- Treatment — 88
- Outcomes — 95
- Prevention — 97
- Resources — 99

**Cirrhosis** — **101**
- Summary Information — 102
- Background — 103
- Diagnosis — 105
- Treatment — 117
- Outcomes — 125
- Prevention — 127
- Resources — 128

**Crohn's disease** — **131**
- Summary Information — 132
- Background — 133
- Diagnosis — 135
- Treatment — 148
- Outcomes — 161
- Prevention — 163
- Resources — 164

**Diverticular disease** — **167**
- Summary Information — 168
- Background — 169
- Diagnosis — 171
- Treatment — 179
- Outcomes — 186
- Prevention — 188
- Resources — 189

**Gastroesophageal reflux disease in adults** — **193**
- Summary Information — 194
- Background — 195
- Diagnosis — 198
- Treatment — 208
- Outcomes — 221
- Prevention — 223
- Resources — 224

**Hemorrhoids** — **229**
- Summary Information — 230
- Background — 231
- Diagnosis — 233
- Treatment — 238
- Outcomes — 253
- Prevention — 255
- Resources — 256

**Alcoholic hepatitis** — **257**
- Summary Information — 258
- Background — 259
- Diagnosis — 261
- Treatment — 276
- Outcomes — 288
- Prevention — 290
- Resources — 292

**Viral hepatitis** — **295**
- Summary Information — 296
- Background — 297
- Diagnosis — 299
- Treatment — 310
- Outcomes — 314
- Prevention — 316
- Resources — 318

**Femoral and inguinal hernia** — **321**
- Summary Information — 322
- Background — 323
- Diagnosis — 325
- Treatment — 329
- Outcomes — 334
- Prevention — 335
- Resources — 337

**Irritable bowel syndrome** — **339**
- Summary Information — 340
- Background — 341
- Diagnosis — 343
- Treatment — 352
- Outcomes — 364
- Prevention — 365
- Resources — 366

# Contents

| | | |
|---|---|---|
| **Lactose intolerance** | **369** | |
| ■ Summary Information | 370 | |
| ■ Background | 371 | |
| ■ Diagnosis | 373 | |
| ■ Treatment | 379 | |
| ■ Outcomes | 383 | |
| ■ Prevention | 384 | |
| ■ Resources | 385 | |
| | | |
| **Mallory-Weiss syndrome** | **387** | |
| ■ Summary Information | 388 | |
| ■ Background | 389 | |
| ■ Diagnosis | 391 | |
| ■ Treatment | 397 | |
| ■ Outcomes | 402 | |
| ■ Prevention | 404 | |
| ■ Resources | 405 | |
| | | |
| **Pancreatitis** | **407** | |
| ■ Summary Information | 408 | |
| ■ Background | 409 | |
| ■ Diagnosis | 411 | |
| ■ Treatment | 422 | |
| ■ Outcomes | 426 | |
| ■ Prevention | 428 | |
| ■ Resources | 430 | |
| | | |
| **Peptic ulcer** | **433** | |
| ■ Summary Information | 434 | |
| ■ Background | 435 | |
| ■ Diagnosis | 438 | |
| ■ Treatment | 447 | |
| ■ Outcomes | 458 | |
| ■ Prevention | 460 | |
| ■ Resources | 462 | |

| | | |
|---|---|---|
| **Acute peritonitis** | **465** | |
| ■ Summary Information | 466 | |
| ■ Background | 467 | |
| ■ Diagnosis | 468 | |
| ■ Treatment | 477 | |
| ■ Outcomes | 486 | |
| ■ Prevention | 487 | |
| ■ Resources | 488 | |
| | | |
| **Proctitis** | **489** | |
| ■ Summary Information | 490 | |
| ■ Background | 491 | |
| ■ Diagnosis | 493 | |
| ■ Treatment | 498 | |
| ■ Outcomes | 505 | |
| ■ Prevention | 506 | |
| ■ Resources | 507 | |
| | | |
| **Pseudomembranous colitis** | **509** | |
| ■ Summary Information | 510 | |
| ■ Background | 511 | |
| ■ Diagnosis | 512 | |
| ■ Treatment | 518 | |
| ■ Outcomes | 525 | |
| ■ Prevention | 527 | |
| ■ Resources | 528 | |
| | | |
| **Pyloric stenosis** | **529** | |
| ■ Summary Information | 530 | |
| ■ Background | 531 | |
| ■ Diagnosis | 533 | |
| ■ Treatment | 539 | |
| ■ Outcomes | 548 | |
| ■ Prevention | 549 | |
| ■ Resources | 550 | |

| | | |
|---|---|---|
| **Rectal malignancy** | **553** | |
| ■ Summary Information | 554 | |
| ■ Background | 555 | |
| ■ Diagnosis | 558 | |
| ■ Treatment | 572 | |
| ■ Outcomes | 581 | |
| ■ Prevention | 584 | |
| ■ Resources | 587 | |
| | | |
| **Ulcerative colitis** | **591** | |
| ■ Summary Information | 592 | |
| ■ Background | 593 | |
| ■ Diagnosis | 595 | |
| ■ Treatment | 608 | |
| ■ Outcomes | 619 | |
| ■ Prevention | 621 | |
| ■ Resources | 622 | |
| | | |
| **Ulcerative colitis** | **591** | |
| ■ Summary Information | 592 | |
| ■ Background | 593 | |
| ■ Diagnosis | 595 | |
| ■ Treatment | 608 | |
| ■ Outcomes | 619 | |
| ■ Prevention | 621 | |
| ■ Resources | 622 | |
| | | |
| **MediFile Index** | | |
| | | |
| **Road Map** | | |

# Introduction

## What is PDxMD?
PDxMD is a new, evidence-based primary care clinical information system designed to support your judgment with practical clinical information. The content is continuously updated by expert contributors with the latest on evaluation, diagnosis, management, outcomes and prevention – all designed for use at the point and time of care.

First and foremost, PDxMD is an electronic resource. This book gives you access to just a fraction of the content available on-line. At www.pdxmd.com, you will find:

- Over 1400 differential diagnoses for you to search for information according to your patient's chief complaint via a unique signs and symptoms matrix
- Information on more than 450 medical conditions and more than 750 drugs and other therapies, organised in condition-specific 'MediFiles'
- Patient information sheets on 300 topics for you to customize and hand to your patient during consultation

## About This Book
The PDxMD Medical Conditions Series is a print version of the comprehensive approach offered on line. Concise information on medical conditions is systematically organized in a consistent MediFile format, our electronic equivalent of chapters.

Each MediFile covers summary information and background on each condition, and comprehensive information on diagnosis, treatment, outcomes, and prevention, and other resources, especially written and designed for use in practice. Each MediFile is organized identically to allow you to find information consistently and reliably for every condition. See the MediFile 'Road Map' inside the back cover for more information.

Ranging from epidemiology to risk assessment and reduction, from diagnostic evaluation and testing to therapeutic options, prognosis and outcomes - you'll find the information that you need is easier to locate with this methodical approach.

## How to Use This Book
Find the MediFile for any specific medical condition in the Contents list. Familiarize yourself with the MediFile Road Map (see inside back cover) to rapidly find the precise information you require.

Information on drugs and tests are found within the MediFiles for the specific conditions. For an overview, see the 'Summary of options' sections under DIAGNOSIS and under TREATMENT in the relevant MediFile. Details of tests, drugs and other therapies then follow.

PDxMD believes that physician clinical judgment is central to appropriate diagnostic and therapeutic decision-making. The information is designed to support professional judgment and, accounting for individual patient differences, does not provide direct answers or force specific practices or policies.

## Introduction

### How is PDxMD created?

PDxMD is created through Collaborative Authoring. This process allows medical information to be reviewed and synthesized from multiple sources – including but not limited to peer-reviewed articles, evidence databases, guidelines and position papers – and by multiple individuals. The information is organized around and integrated into a template that matches the needs of primary care physicians in practice.

Professional medical writers begin the process of reviewing and synthesizing information for PDxMD, working from core evidence databases and other expert resources and with the guidance of Editorial Advisory Board (EAB) members. This first draft is sent to a physician 'clinical reviewer', who works with the writer to make sure the information is accurate and properly organized. A second review by the physician clinical reviewer ensures that appropriate changes are in place.

After these first two levels of clinical review, the files are reviewed and edited by the relevant specialist member of the Editorial Advisory Board. A primary care member of the EAB, who has final sign-off authority, then conducts the final review and edit. Editorial checks are conducted between all review stages and, after primary care sign-off, a pharmacist double checks the drug recommendations prior to a final editorial review.

There are a minimum of three and as many as five physicians involved in each MediFile, and additional clinical reviewers and/or EAB members are added when appropriate (e.g., alternative/complementary medicine experts, or conditions requiring multi-disciplinary approaches). The contributor team for each MediFile is listed in the Resources section.

A complete list of Editorial Faculty and staff of PDxMD is provided below. All Editorial Faculty, and specifically the Editorial Advisory Board members, participate in PDxMD as individuals and not as representatives of, or on behalf of, their affiliated institutions or associations and any indication of their affiliation with a specific institution or association should not be taken as an endorsement of PDxMD or any participation of their institution or association with PDxMD.

### Continuous Product Improvement

PDxMD is committed to continuous quality improvement and welcomes any comments, suggestions and feedback from the professional community. Please send any ideas or considerations regarding this volume or any other volume in the PDxMD series via e-mail to feedback.pdxmd@elsevier.com or to PDxMD, Elsevier Science, The Curtis Center, 625 Walnut Street, Philadelphia, PA 19106.

# Introduction

## Evidence-Based Medicine Policies
PDxMD is committed to providing available and up-to-date evidence for the diagnostic and therapeutic recommendations provided in our knowledge base. All MediFiles begin with a core set of evidence-based references from recognized sources. These are supplemented with extensive searches of the literature and reviews of reference books, peer-reviewed journals, association guidelines and position papers, among others.

## Criteria for Evidence-Based Medicine
### Evidence Sources
PDxMD has taken the best evidence currently available from the following:

*Published Critically Evaluated Evidence*
- Cochrane Systematic Reviews – respected throughout the world as one of the most rigorous searches of medical journals with highly structured systematic reviews and use of meta-analysis to produce reliable evidence
- Clinical Evidence – produced jointly by the British Medical Journal Publishing Group and the American College of Physicians–American Society of Internal Medicine. Clinical Evidence provides a concise account of the current state of knowledge on the treatment and prevention of many clinical conditions based on the search and appraisal of the available literature
- The National Guideline Clearinghouse – a comprehensive database of evidence-based clinical practice guidelines and related documents produced by the Agency for Healthcare Research and Quality in partnership with the American Medical Association and the American Association of Health Plans

*Evidence Published in Peer-Reviewed Journals*
- Association Guidelines and Position Papers

Where evidence exists that has not yet been critically reviewed by one of the sources listed above, for example randomized controlled trials and clinical cohort studies, the evidence is summarized briefly, categorized, and fully referenced.

## Clinical Experience
While recognizing the importance of these evidence-based resources, PDxMD also highlights the importance of experience in clinical practice. Therefore, our Editorial Advisory Board also provide advice from their own clinical experience, within Clinical Pearl sections of the MediFiles and elsewhere. Contributing expert physicians are identified in the Resources section of every MediFile.

# Introduction

**Evaluation of Evidence**
PDxMD evaluates all cited evidence according to the AAFP Recommended Basic Model for Evaluating and Categorizing the Clinical Content of CME, based on the model used by the University of Michigan:

Level M   Evidence from either:
          Meta-analysis or
          Multiple randomized controlled trials

Level P   Evidence from either:
          A well-designed prospective clinical trial or
          Several prospective clinical cohort studies with consistent findings (without randomization)

Level S   Evidence from studies other than clinical trials, such as:
          Epidemiological studies
          Physiological studies

**References**
The information provided by PDxMD is concise and action-oriented. As a result, our editorial policy is to cite only essential reference sources. References and evidence summaries are provided in four areas:
1.   In the Diagnostic Decision section under Diagnosis
2.   In the Guidelines and Evidence sections under Treatment
3.   In the Outcomes section under Evidence
4.   In the Key Reference Section under Resources

Where on-line references to the Cochrane Abstracts, BMJ Clinical Evidence and National Guideline Clearinghouse are cited in the text, the internet addresses of the home pages are given. The internet addresses of individual reports are not given.

When references are to association guidelines and position papers, the internet address of the association home page is generally provided. When possible, the internet address of the specific report is provided.

# Editorial Faculty and Staff

## Executive Committee

**Fred F Ferri, MD, FACP**
*Editorial Board & Medical Chair, Executive Committee Family Medicine*
Clinical Professor
Brown University of Medicine, Chief
Division of Internal Medicine
Fatima Hospital, St Joseph's Health Services
Providence, RI

**George T Danakas, MD, FACOG**
*Editorial Board & Executive Committee*
*Obstetrics, Gynecology*
Clinical Assistant Professor
SUNY at Buffalo
Williamsville, NY

**David G Fairchild, MD, MPH**
*Editorial Board & Executive Committee*
*Primary Care, Signs & Symptoms*
Brigham and Women's Hospital
Boston, MA

**Russell C Jones, MD, MPH**
*Editorial Board & Executive Committee*
*Family Medicine*
Dartmouth Medical School
New London, NH

**Kathleen M O'Hanlon, MD**
*Editorial Board & Executive Committee*
*Primary Care*
Professor, Marshall University School of Medicine
Department of Family & Community Health
Huntington, WV

**John L Pfenninger, MD, FAAFP**
*Editorial Board & Executive Committee*
*Primary Care, Procedures*
President and Director
The National Procedures Institute
Director, The Medical Procedures Center, PC
Clinical Professor of Family Medicine
Michigan State University
Midland, MI

**Joseph E Scherger, MD, MPH**
*Editorial Board & Executive Committee*
*Primary Care, Site Search*
Dean, College of Medicine
Florida State University
Tallahassee, FL

**Myron Yanoff, MD**
*Editorial Board & Executive Committee*
*Ophthalmology, Otolaryngology*
Professor & Chair, Department of Ophthalmology
MCP Hahnemann University
Philadelphia, PA

## Editorial Board

**Philip J Aliotta, MD, MHA, FACS**
*Editorial Board, Urology*
Attending Urologist and Clinical Research Director Center for Urologic Research of Western New York
Main Urology Associates, PC
Williamsville, NY

**Gordon H Baustian, MD**
*Editorial Board, Family Medicine*
Director of Medical Education and Residency
Cedar Rapids Medical Education Foundation
Cedar Rapids, IA

# Editorial Faculty and Staff

**Diane M Birnbaumer, MD, FACEP**
*Editorial Board, Emergency Medicine*
Associate Residency Director
Department of Emergency Medicine
Harbor-UCLA Medical Center
Torrance, CA

**Richard Brasington Jr, MD, FACP**
*Editorial Board, Rheumatology*
Director of Clinical Rheumatology
Department of Internal Medicine/Rheumatology
Washington University School of Medicine
St Louis, MO

**Christopher P Cannon, MD**
*Editorial Board, 2000-2001 Cardiology*
Cardiovascular Division
Brigham and Women's Hospital
Boston, MA

**Daniel J Derksen, MD**
*Editorial Board, 2000-2001 Primary Care*
Associate Professor
Department of Family & Community Medicine
Executive Director
University Physician Associates
University of New Mexico School of Medicine
Albuquerque, NM

**Benjamin Djulbegovic, MD, PhD**
*Editorial Board, Oncology, Hematology*
Associate Professor of Oncology and Medicine
H Lee Moffitt Cancer Center & Research
Institute at the University of South Florida
Interdisciplinary Oncology Program
Division of Blood and Bone Marrow Transplant
Tampa, FL

**Martin Goldberg, MD, FACP**
*Editorial Board, Nephrology*
Professor Emeritus (Medicine and Physiology)
Temple University School of Medicine
Philadelphia, PA

**John McB Hodgson, MD, FACC, FSCAI**
*Editorial Board, Cardiology*
Associate Professor of Medicine and Director of
Invasive Cardiology
Health and Vascular Center, Metrohealth
Medical Center
Case Western Reserve University
Cleveland, OH

**Robert Iannone MD**
*Editorial Board, 2000-2001 Pediatrics*
Department of Pediatric Oncology
Johns Hopkins Hospital
Baltimore, MD

**Martin L Kabongo, MD, PhD**
*Editorial Board, Family Medicine*
Associate Clinical Professor
Division of Family Medicine, Department of
Family and Preventive Medicine
University of California, San Diego
San Diego, CA

**Robert W Lash, MD**
*Editorial Board, 2000-2001 Endocrinology*
University of Michigan Medical Center
Ann Arbor, MI

**Sara C McIntire, MD**
*Editorial Board, Pediatrics*
Associate Professor of Pediatrics
Children's Hospital of Pittsburgh
University of Pittsburgh School of Medicine
Pittsburgh, PA

**Karl E Misulis, MD, PhD**
*Editorial Board, Neurology*
Clinical Professor of Neurology
Vanderbilt University
Chairman, Department of Medicine
Jackson General Hospital
Jackson, TN

# Editorial Faculty and Staff

**Jane L Murray, MD**
*Editorial Board, Alternative Medicine*
Medical Director
Sastun Center of Integrative Health Care
Mission, KS

**Steven M Opal, MD**
*Editorial Board, Infectious Diseases*
Professor of Medicine, Infectious Disease Division, Brown University School of Medicine
Pawtucket, RI

**Randolph L Pearson, MD**
*Editorial Board, Primary Care*
Associate Professor
Department of Family Practice
Michigan State University
East Lansing, MI

**Eric F Pollak, MD, MPH**
*Editorial Board, Family Medicine*
Concord Family Medicine
Concord, NH

**Dennis F Saver, MD**
*Editorial Board, Primary Care, Clinical Pictures*
Primary Care of the Treasure Coast
Vero Beach, FL

**Jeffrey L Saver, MD**
*Editorial Board, 2000 Neurology*
UCLA Reed Neurologic Research Center
Los Angeles, CA

**Raymond G Slavin, MD**
*Editorial Board, 2000 Allergy*
Chief, Division of Allergy
St Louis University Hospital
St Louis, MO

**Andrew H Soll, MD**
*Editorial Board, Gastroenterology*
Professor, UCLA School of Medicine
Los Angeles, CA

**Ronnie S Stangler, MD**
*Editorial Board, Psychiatry*
Clinical Professor
Department of Psychiatry and Behavioural Sciences, University of Washington
Seattle, WA

**Seth R Stevens, MD**
*Editorial Board, Dermatology*
Assistant Professor of Dermatology
University Hospitals of Cleveland
Department of Dermatology
University Hospitals of Cleveland, Case Western Reserves University
Cleveland, OH

**Mark B Stockman, MD**
*Editorial Board, 2000 Cardiology*
Department of Cardiology, Harvard Vanguard Medical Associates, Boston, MA

**Austin B Thompson, MD**
*Editorial Board, Pulmonology*
Associate Professor of Medicine
University of Nebraska Medical Center
Omaha, NE

**David W Toth, MD**
*Editorial Board, Endocrinology*
Clinical Assistant Professor
Endocrine and Diabetes Center
St Luke's Medical Center
Medical College of Wisconsin
Milwaukee, WI

**Ron M Walls, MD**
*Editorial Board, 2000-2001*
*Emergency Medicine*
Chair, Department of Emergency Medicine
Brigham and Women's Hospital
Associate Professor of Medicine
(Emergency Medicine)
Harvard Medical School
Boston, MA

# Editorial Faculty and Staff

**Gary M White, MD**
*Editorial Board, Dermatology Illustration*
Associate Clinical Professor
Dept of Dermatology
University of California, San Diego
San Diego, CA

**Basil J Zitelli, MD**
*Editorial Board, Pediatrics Illustration*
Professor of Pediatrics
University of Pittsburgh School of Medicine
Children's Hospital of Pittsburgh
Pittsburgh PA

## Clinical Reviewers

**Rudolph A Bedford, MD**
*Gastroenterology*
Department of Gastroenterology
UCLA
Los Angeles, CA

**Lawrence S Friedman, MD**
*Gastroenterology*
Professor of Medicine
Harvard Medical School
Physician, Gastrointestinal Unit
Massachusetts General Hospital
Boston, MA

**Andrew F Ippoliti, MD**
*Gastroenterology*
Clinical Professor in Medicine/Gastroenterology
UCLA
Los Angeles, CA

**Hetal A Karsan, MD**
*Gastroenterology*
Senior Gastroenterology and Hepatology Fellow
Division of Digestive Diseases
UCLA Medical Center
Los Angeles, CA

**Braden Kuo, MD**
*Gastroenterology*
Assistant Physician in Medicine
Gastrointestinal Unit
Massachusetts General Hospital
Boston, MA

**J Adrian Lunn, MD**
*Gastroenterology*
Gastroenterology Fellow
Department of Medicine
Division of Digestive Diseases
UCLA
Los Angeles, CA

**Jaime Oviedo, MD**
*Gastroenterology*
Senior Fellow
Section of Gastroenterology
Boston University Medical Center
Boston, MA

**Brennan Spiegel, MD**
*Gastroenterology*
Fellow in Gastroenterology
Division of Digestive Diseases
UCLA
Los Angeles, CA

**Laura Targownik, MD, FRCP(C)**
*Gastroenterology*
Division of Digestive Diseases
University of California, Los Angeles
Los Angeles, CA

**Vijay Yajnik, MD**
*Gastroenterology*
Gastrointestinal Unit
Massachusetts General Hospital
Boston, MA

# Editorial Faculty and Staff

## Writers

Thomas A Adamec, MD, FCAP
Anjan K Banerjee, MSc, MS (Lond), DM
Jon M Berkowitz, MD
Kim S Berman
Elly C Blake
Michele Campbell
Rosalyn S Carson-DeWitt, MD
Simon J Cathcart, MB ChB
Patricia M Clark, MSN, RN, CS

Tony C Fisher, MD
Jacqueline Furnace, BSc MBChB Med
Scott Gottlieb, MD
Kelly D Karpa, RPh, PhD, BSPharm
Andy R Oppenheimer
Colin R Tidy, MBBS, MRCGP, MRCP
Robert Whittle, MB BS (NSW)
Everetta M Woods

## Staff

**Management Team**
Fiona Foley, Steven Merahn, MD, Daniel Pollock, Zak Knowles, Howard Croft, Tanya Thomas, Lucy Hamilton, Julie Volck, Bill Bruggemeyer, Andrea Ford

**Editorial Team**
Anne Dyson, Sadaf Hashmi, Debbie Goring, Louise Morrison, Ellen Haigh, Robert Whittle, Claire Champion, Caroline Barnett, Laurie Smith, Li Wan, Paul Mayhew, Carmen Jones, Fi Ward

**Technical Team**
Martin Miller, Narinder Chandi, Roy Patterson, Aaron McGrath, John Wylie, Sarah Craze, Cameron Sangster

We would also like to acknowledge the extraordinary contributions of the following individuals to the conceptualization and realization of PDxMD over the initial years of its growth and development:

Tim Hailstone, Jonathan Black, Alison Whitehouse, Jayne Harris, Angela Baggi, Sharon Bambaji, Sam Bedser, Layla van den Bergh, Stuart Boffey, Siobhan Egan, Helen Elder, Mark Mitchenall, Chris Moodie, Tony Pollard, Simon Seljeflot, Liz Southey, Tim Stentiford, Matthew Whyte

# ACUTE APPENDICITIS

| | | |
|---|---|---|
| ■ | Summary Information | 2 |
| ■ | Background | 3 |
| ■ | Diagnosis | 5 |
| ■ | Treatment | 11 |
| ■ | Outcomes | 12 |
| ■ | Prevention | 13 |
| ■ | Resources | 14 |

## SUMMARY INFORMATION

### DESCRIPTION
- Abdominal pain, progressing from diffuse central or periumbilical pain to very localized right lower quadrant pain occurring at McBurney's point, one-third of the way up the oblique line that joins the right anterior superior iliac spine to umbilicus
- Frequent anorexia, nausea, vomiting
- Delayed diagnosis may result in perforation, peritonitis, greatly increased morbidity and mortality

### URGENT ACTION
- Patients with the typical signs and symptoms of acute appendicitis should receive prompt surgical referral
- Be alert for signs of peritonitis

### KEY! DON'T MISS!
Be aware that occasionally brief cessation of pain may occur just as the appendix perforates; threshold of suspicion for appendicitis should remain high, and patient closely monitored, until reasonable length of time has passed with negative abdominal examination.

# BACKGROUND

## ICD9 CODE
540.9 Appendicitis, unspecified

## CARDINAL FEATURES
- Diffuse periumbilical or central abdominal pain usually lasting several hours, with brief cessation, followed by migration of pain to the right lower quadrant in a more constant, more localized form (this is the classic progression of appendicitis; absence of this exact progression does not rule out appendicitis)
- Tenderness to palpation of right lower quadrant
- Rebound tenderness
- Anorexia is invariably present
- Nausea, vomiting, and constipation may occur after right lower quadrant pain is established
- Fever around 37.8°C is common
- Leukocytosis, neutrophilia is common

## CAUSES
### Common causes
- Thought to be initiated by luminal obstruction (secondary to lymphoid hyperplasia, fecalith, or less commonly by calculus, tumor, foreign body, parasites)
- Secondary infectious processes (following obstruction) may involve bacteria, viruses, or parasites
- Mucoid secretions result in organ distension, increased intraluminal pressures, decreased venous drainage with venous engorgement, and arterial compromise leading to ischemia
- With diagnostic delay, increase in intraluminal pressures can ultimately result in gangrene leading to perforation, contamination of abdominal cavity with fecal contents, and development of peritonitis

### Rare causes
May rarely be caused by barium inspissation after diagnostic examination.

### Serious causes
- As all appendicitis requires surgery, all causes are serious
- Obstruction of appendiceal lumen owing to tumor (mucinous cystadenoma or mucinous cystadenocarcinoma)

## EPIDEMIOLOGY
### Incidence and prevalence
INCIDENCE
1.1/1000 per year, overall; 2.3/1000 between ages 10–20.

### Demographics
AGE
Peak incidence among teenagers.

GENDER
- Male:female, 3:2, between 10 and 30 years
- Male = female, >30 years

RACE
Caucasian:noncaucasian, 1.5:1.

GENETICS
Some research suggests familial predisposition.

GEOGRAPHY
Suspected, not well established.

SOCIOECONOMIC STATUS
Increased risk of morbidity, mortality associated with underinsured population.

# DIAGNOSIS

## DIFFERENTIAL DIAGNOSIS
Differential diagnosis varies depending on patient's gender and age.

### Mesenteric lymphadenitis
FEATURES
- Inflammation of lymph nodes at base/root of mesenteric root and appendix
- May cause right lower quadrant pain, fever
- Rebound tenderness, rigidity usually absent
- May follow a viral upper respiratory infection
- May be because of infection with *Yersinia, Shigella, Mycobacterium tuberculosis*, actinomycosis

### Pelvic inflammatory disease
FEATURES
- Duration is frequently days or weeks before medical care is sought
- Frequent history of previous pelvic/venereal infections
- Abdominal pain less localized to right lower quadrant
- Nausea and vomiting less prominent features
- Unique features include cervical motion tenderness, vaginal discharge, bilateral tenderness of adnexae on vaginal examination
- Transvaginal ultrasonography may aid diagnosis

### Ruptured graafian follicle or corpus luteum cyst
FEATURES
- Ruptured graafian follicle usually occurs mid-menses
- Ruptured corpus luteum cyst usually occurs at onset of menses
- Fever and leukocytosis are usually absent
- May involve vaginal bleeding

### Acute gastroenteritis
FEATURES
- Diarrhea and vomiting
- Colicky abdominal pain
- No peritonism
- Leukocytosis and fever less common

### Acute cholecystitis
FEATURES
- Commonly causes epigastric or right upper quadrant pain, frequently with right scapular radiation
- Patients tend to move around, in an effort to find a position of comfort, in contrast with appendicitis patients with peritoneal signs who tend to lie very still
- May demonstrate positive Murphy sign
- Fever less common

### Diverticular disease
FEATURES
- Pain generally located in left lower quadrant
- Previous history of episodic diffuse abdominal pain, flatulence, distension, and bowel habit changes, especially diarrhea
- May have nausea and vomiting

### Crohn's terminal ileitis
FEATURES
- Subacute onset
- Diarrhea with blood and mucus
- Weight loss
- Anemia

### Pyelonephritis
FEATURES
- Dysuria and frequency
- Fever with rigors
- Urinalysis positive for leukocytes, nitrite, protein, and blood

### Ectopic pregnancy
FEATURES
- Positive pregnancy test
- Severe abdominal pain, may be colicky initially
- Tenderness and fullness in fornices

### Psoas abscess
(Particularly if immunocompromised, from the Asian subcontinent or diabetic/steroids.)

FEATURES
- Abdominal pain with fever
- Pain on flexion of the hip

### Cecal tumor with localized perforation
FEATURES
- Acute abdomen
- Toxic appearance
- Generally: elderly patient with long history of bowel symptoms

### Renal colic
FEATURES
- Sudden onset
- Severe colicky right or left flank pain
- Frank or microscopic hematuria

### Perforated Meckel's diverticulum
FEATURES
- Central or lower abdominal pain
- Often indistinguishable clinically from appendicitis

## SIGNS & SYMPTOMS
### Signs
- Fever
- Tachycardia
- Abdominal tenderness and rebound tenderness, referred to right lower quadrant
- Cough tenderness
- May have positive psoas sign (pain with right thigh extension), obturator sign (pain with internal rotation of the flexed right thigh), Rovsing's sign (right lower quadrant pain on palpation of the left lower quadrant pain)

- May demonstrate cutaneous hyperesthesia between T10 and T12
- May demonstrate both voluntary and involuntary guarding, abdominal muscle rigidity
- Patient often lies still, in right lateral decubitus position, slightly flexing hip

## Symptoms
- Diffuse periumbilical abdominal pain, ultimately localizing to the right lower quadrant, approximately at McBurney's point
- Anorexia
- Nausea
- Vomiting
- Occasional diarrhea or constipation
- Atypical presentation common in the elderly, poorly localized pain

## KEY! DON'T MISS!
Be aware that occasionally brief cessation of pain may occur just as the appendix perforates; threshold of suspicion for appendicitis should remain high, and patient closely monitored, until reasonable length of time has passed with negative abdominal examination.

## CONSIDER CONSULT
Peritonitis or signs of peritonism require immediate referral regardless of the underlying diagnosis.

## INVESTIGATION OF THE PATIENT
### Direct questions to patient
**Q** When did your pain begin? Typically the history of appendicitis is short – less than 48h
**Q** Have you ever had episodes of this kind of pain before? 'Grumbling appendix' is no longer a widely accepted diagnosis; consider an alternative diagnosis in patients with recurrent symptoms
**Q** Where is your pain located? Initially generalized, the pain localizes to the right lower quadrant. Unilateral left lower quadrant pain is compatible with appendicitis but uncommon
**Q** Please describe the pain; has it changed at all over time? Colicky pain may be an early feature of appendicitis
**Q** When did you last have anything to eat or drink? A necessary question prior to anesthesia, may be useful in determining if the patient has had anorexia
**Q** Have you had any nausea, vomiting, diarrhea? These are nonspecific symptoms
**Q** Have you had your appendix removed?
**Q** Do you have any other medical conditions?
**Q** For women: When was your last menstrual period? Are you sexually active? What form of contraception/protection do you use? Have you ever had a pelvic infection in the past? Is there any chance you are pregnant? Are you experiencing any vaginal discharge? Always consider ectopic pregnancy in a woman of child-bearing age

## Examination
- Take temperature, pulse rate, blood pressure: temperature and pulse rate are usually elevated in appendicitis
- Does patient appear toxic, dehydrated? Consider perforation, gastroenteritis and diabetic ketoacidosis
- Auscultate abdomen. If bowel sounds silent, consider perforation
- Perform abdominal examination
- Observe for cough tenderness, rebound tenderness, guarding (both voluntary and involuntary), these are signs of peritonism
- Check for psoas sign, obturator sign, Rovsing's sign
- Perform rectal examination: tenderness on the right hand side is suggestive of appendicitis

## Summary of investigative tests
Occasionally there are circumstances in which blood tests prior to transfer to surgical care are appropriate. However, they are not normally required.
- Serum pregnancy test: consider ectopic pregnancy in women of child-bearing age
- Complete blood count with differential: leukocytosis with left shift is present in 90% of patients with appendicitis
- Urinalysis: hematuria and pyuria occur in <20% of patients and their presence may suggest other diagnosis
- Appendiceal computed tomography (CT) scan has an accuracy of >90%. Its use improves patient care and reduces the use of hospital resources
- Ultrasound is useful in women of child-bearing age when diagnosis is unclear

## THE TESTS
### Body fluids
COMPLETE BLOOD COUNT WITH DIFFERENTIAL
*Description*
Blood sample.

*Advantages/Disadvantages*
- Simple, standard, may be ordered stat for immediate results
- Nonspecific; indicates presence of infection but not source

*Normal*
Leukocyte profile:
- Total: $3.9–9.8 \times 10^3$/mcL
- Lymphocytes: $1.2–3.3 \times 10^3$/mcL
- Mononuclear cells: $0.2–0.7 \times 10^3$/mcL
- Granulocytes: $1.8–6.6 \times 10^3$/mcL

*Abnormal*
- Leukocytosis: 10,000–20,000 cells/mm$^3$, with left shift
- Keep in mind the possibility of a false-positive result

*Cause of abnormal result*
May be abnormal in infection or owing to a blood disorder.

*Drugs, disorders and other factors that may alter results*
Steroid usage may cause artifact, by causing leukocyte demargination.

SERUM PREGNANCY TEST
*Description*
Blood test, performed stat, should be done on all female patients of reproductive age.

*Advantages/Disadvantages*
Quick, inexpensive.

*Normal*
Normal depends on patient's indication of likelihood of pregnancy.

*Abnormal*
Keep in mind the possibility of a falsely abnormal result.

*Drugs, disorders and other factors that may alter results*
- A positive pregnancy test in a patient with abdominal pain should raise the possibility of ectopic pregnancy, a surgical emergency, the diagnosis of which must not be delayed
- In the absence of ectopic pregnancy, a positive pregnancy test may require that other special measures be taken during diagnosis and treatment, so as not to endanger the fetus

URINALYSIS
*Description*
Clean-catch urine specimen.

*Advantages/Disadvantages*
Simple, easily obtained, can be performed stat.

*Normal*
- Sample should be negative for red blood cells, significant pyuria, bacteriuria
- A mild degree of pyuria in a sterile urine sample devoid of erythrocytes may be seen in appendicitis

*Abnormal*
- Any significant degree of hematuria, pyuria or bacteriuria should raise suspicion of a urinary problem as a source for the patient's symptoms
- Keep in mind the possibility of a falsely abnormal result

*Cause of abnormal result*
- Slight pyuria may accompany appendicitis
- More severe pyuria with hematuria and/or bacteriuria indicate that urinary disease should move ahead of appendicitis on the differential

## Imaging
GRADED COMPRESSION ULTRASONOGRAPHY
*Description*
Abnormal:
- Appendiceal diameter >6mm
- Noncompressibility of appendix
- Absent peristalsis
- Collection of fluid surrounding the appendix
- Keep in mind the possibility of a falsely abnormal result

*Cause of abnormal result*
Abnormal results have 85–90% sensitivity and 92–96% specificity for the diagnosis of appendicitis.

CT SCAN
*Normal*
Normal abdomen visualized.

*Abnormal*
- Any number of abdominal processes may be visualized during CT, particularly with contrast or using a helical technique
- Keep in mind the possibility of a falsely abnormal result

*Cause of abnormal result*
Abnormal abdominal processes visualized with CT may include:
- Appendicitis
- Diverticulitis
- Nephrolithiasis
- Ovarian disease processes
- Tumors
- Hernias of the small intestine
- Bowel ischemia
- Crohn's ileitis/cecum

## TREATMENT

### CONSIDER CONSULT
Refer to surgeon as soon as typical symptoms/signs of appendicitis are confirmed, or if any other question remains as to presence of acute surgical abdomen.

### IMMEDIATE ACTION
Consider analgesia if patient is distressed.

### MANAGEMENT ISSUES
**Goals**
- Obtain prompt surgical consult if appendicitis appears likely, or to evaluate other causes of acute abdomen
- Treat/avoid dehydration in a patient unable to eat or vomiting

### SUMMARY OF THERAPEUTIC OPTIONS
**Choices**
Appendectomy is the only course of treatment.

### DRUGS AND OTHER THERAPIES: DETAILS
**Surgical therapy**
APPENDECTOMY
*Efficacy*
Curative.

*Risks/benefits*
- Risks include high chance (10–15%) for removal of benign appendix
- Benefits include curative nature of appendectomy in cases of appendicitis, chance to make alternative diagnosis through laparascopy/laparatomy if appendix is benign, avoidance of perforation and subsequent complications if appendectomy is performed promptly

*Patient and caregiver information*
Patient should receive informed consent, including information on risk of benign abdomen found during surgery.

## OUTCOMES

### EFFICACY OF THERAPIES
Appendectomy has been the undisputed treatment of choice for 100 years.

### PROGNOSIS
Prognosis is excellent with prompt surgical treatment to avoid danger of perforation and subsequent complications.

#### Recurrence
Rarely, inflammation of overly-long appendiceal stump or regrowth of appendix may require reoperation.

### COMPLICATIONS
Complications are rare if appendectomy occurs prior to perforation but may include:
- Wound abscess formation
- Deep vein thrombosis and other operative complications
- Untreated perforation may result in septic shock and death. Other complications of perforation include adhesion formation with consequent risk of reduction of fertility in women

## PREVENTION

Appendicitis is not specifically preventable in the general population

# RESOURCES

## ASSOCIATIONS
**American Gastroenterological Association**
National Office
7910 Woodmont Avenue, Suite 700
Bethesda, MD 20814
Tel: (301) 654-2055
Fax: (301) 654-5920
E-mail: member@gastro.org
http://www.gastro.org

## KEY REFERENCES
- Crawford JM. Appendix. In: Cotran RS, ed. Robbins pathologic basis of disease. Philadelphia: W.B. Saunders, 1999
- Graffeo C, Counselman FL. Gastrointestinal emergencies, Part II. In: Emergency medicine clinics of North America, Vol 14, No 4. Philadelphia: W.B. Saunders, 1996
- Greenfield RH, Henneman PL. Appendicitis. In: Rosen P, ed. Emergency medicine: concepts and clinical practice. St Louis: Mosby,1998
- Sabiston DC. Appendicitis. In: Sabiston DC, Coston D, eds. Textbook of surgery. Philadelphia: W.B. Saunders, 1997
- Schrock TR. Appendicitis. In: Feldman M. et al, eds. Sleisenger & Fordtran's gastrointestinal and liver disease. Philadelphia: W.B. Saunders, 1998
- Silen W. Acute Appendicitis. In: Fauci AS, ed.: Harrison's principles of internal medicine. New York: McGraw-Hill, 1998
- Wilcox CM. Miscellaneous inflammatory diseases of the intestine. In: Goldman L, Bennett JC, eds. Cecil's textbook of medicine. Philadelphia: W.B. Saunders, 2000
- Feldman M, et al, eds. Sleisenger and Fordtran's gastrointestinal and liver disease. Philadelphia: W.B. Saunders, 1998

## CONTRIBUTORS
Fred F Ferri, MD, FACP
Andrew H Soll, MD
J Adrian Lunn, MD

# BUDD–CHIARI SYNDROME

| | | |
|---|---|---|
| ■ | Summary Information | 16 |
| ■ | Background | 17 |
| ■ | Diagnosis | 19 |
| ■ | Treatment | 32 |
| ■ | Outcomes | 39 |
| ■ | Prevention | 40 |
| ■ | Resources | 41 |

## SUMMARY INFORMATION

### DESCRIPTION
- Impediment of venous blood flow from the liver
- May occur at any level in the liver from the deep, small lobar veins to the proximal inferior vena cava
- May be caused by thrombosis, external compression, or venous malformation
- End result of this syndrome may be portal hypertension, cirrhosis, and/or liver failure
- Treatment includes thrombolytic therapy, re-establishing venous flow by shunting or stenting, and in fulminant cases, orthotopic liver transplantation

### URGENT ACTION
- Fulminant Budd–Chiari syndrome (more common in pregnant women) is fatal without treatment. Early recognition and treatment are key to survival. Severe pain, hepatomegaly, jaundice, acuities, and rapid deterioration of liver function and encephalopathy mark fulminant Budd–Chiari syndrome
- Referral for orthotopic liver transplantation should happen immediately when this diagnosis is suspected – transfer the patient to a transplantation center under the care of a transplantation hepatologist and liver transplantation surgical team
- Early surgical intervention with creation of a portosystemic venous shunt allows reverse flow through the portal vein and may improve prognosis. Angiography may allow for direct opening of the caval obstruction

### KEY! DON'T MISS!
- In pregnant women, the more common possibility of pre-eclampsia should not be missed. Likewise the HELLP syndrome (hemolysis, elevated liver enzymes, low platelets), and the syndrome of acute fatty liver of pregnancy should also not be missed by primary care physicians
- The far more rare fulminant Budd–Chiari syndrome may mimic the subcapsular hepatic hemorrhage associated with eclamptic liver disease and should always be kept in mind because, unlike the above-mentioned disorders, Budd–Chiari syndrome will not resolve with delivery

# BACKGROUND

## ICD9 CODE
453.0 Budd–Chiari syndrome

## SYNONYMS
- Hepatic vein thrombosis
- Postsinusoidal obstruction
- Hepatic venous outflow obstruction

## CARDINAL FEATURES
Features vary with the origin, extent, and speed of onset.

Fulminant Budd–Chiari:
- Jaundice
- Hepatomegaly
- Ascites
- Acute liver failure
- Encephalopathy

Acute Budd–Chiari:
- Abdominal pain
- Hepatomegaly
- Progressive liver failure

Chronic Budd–Chiari is related to chronic portal hypertension:
- Ascites
- Esophageal varices
- Splenomegaly
- Coagulopathy
- Encephalopathy

## CAUSES
### Common causes
- In Western countries, 30–40% of cases are idiopathic in origin
- Membranous obstruction of the vena cava accounts for 40% of cases in Asia and Africa
- Hematologic abnormalities account for 25% – the most commonly noted hypercoagulable states include polycythemia vera, essential thrombocytosis, deficits in protein C and/or protein S, activated protein C resistance, antiphospholipid syndrome, antithrombin III deficiency, factor V Leiden, lupus anticoagulant, paroxysmal nocturnal hemoglobinuria, postpartum thrombocytopenic purpura, and sickle cell anemia
- Pregnancy (10% of cases) and the postpartum state
- Oral contraceptives
- Cancers (10% of cases), including adrenal, bronchogenic, fibrolamellar hepatocellular carcinoma, renal, and leiomyosarcoma
- Infections (10% of cases), including liver abscess, aspergillosis, filariasis, schistosomiasis, hydatid cysts, pelvic cellulitis, syphilis, and tuberculosis
- Treatment for cancer, including total body irradiation with or without cytotoxic chemotherapy
- Hepatocellular carcinoma is a special case – it may be both the cause and a complication of Budd–Chiari
- Trauma

### Contributory or predisposing factors
- Cirrhosis
- Coagulopathy
- Hepatocellular carcinoma
- Any carcinoma causing procoagulable state leading to inferior vena cava clot formation

## EPIDEMIOLOGY
### Incidence and prevalence
Budd–Chiari syndrome is very rare.

### Demographics
AGE
Rare in infants and young children except in Africa and Asia, where the incidence of membranous obstruction of the vena cava is more common (however, even in India and Africa the incidence is low).

GENDER
More common in pregnant women but still very rare.

GEOGRAPHY
More common in Africa and Asia, where the incidence of membranous obstruction of the vena cava is more common.

# DIAGNOSIS

## DIFFERENTIAL DIAGNOSIS
### Cholecystitis
FEATURES
- Right upper quadrant pain; pain may radiate to the infrascapular region
- Positive Murphy's sign: with palpation of the right upper quadrant, there is marked tenderness and halting of inspired breath
- Palpable gallbladder
- Fever, chills, vomiting
- Jaundice
- History of recently ingested large, fatty meal prior to onset of pain

### Peptic ulcer disease
FEATURES
- Physical examination may be normal
- Epigastric tenderness
- Tachycardia
- Pallor
- Hypotension
- Nausea, vomiting
- With perforated ulcer: boardlike abdomen, rebound tenderness; with bleeding ulcer: hematemesis, melena

### Cirrhosis
Cirrhosis may be of viral (e.g. chronic hepatitis B or C), alcoholic, or cardiac etiology or have other etiologies such as Wilson's disease, hemachromatosis, alpha-1-antitrypsin deficiency, or an autoimmune basis.

FEATURES
- Skin changes, including jaundice, palmar erythema, spider angiomata, ecchymosis, increased pigmentation
- Kayser–Fleischer rings, scleral icterus on eye examination (this is only true for Wilson's disease)
- Fetor hepaticus

Abdominal examination:
- Hepatomegaly with tenderness; small, nodular liver, palpable gallbladder and spleen, ascites
- Hemorrhoids, guaiac-positive stools
- Testicular atrophy
- Pedal edema, arthropathy
- Neuroexamination: asterixis, dysarthria, encephalopathy

Laboratory abnormalities:
- Decreased hemoglobin and hematocrit, increased blood urea nitrogen and creatinine; liver function tests may be slightly to severely elevated depending upon presence or absence of obstruction

### Hepatitis
Hepatitis of viral, toxic, or alcoholic etiology.

## FEATURES
- Symptoms may be nonspecific
- Anorexia, malaise
- Hepatomegaly and right upper quadrant tenderness
- Jaundice and dark urine in hepatitis A and B; rare in hepatitis C
- Fever preceding jaundice in hepatitis A and B
- Aspartate aminotransaminase (AST), alanine aminotransaminase (ALT) elevated to at least eight times normal
- Bilirubin elevated 5–15 times normal

## Pancreatitis
### FEATURES
- Sudden epigastric tenderness with guarding
- Hypoactive bowel sounds
- Tachycardia
- Confusion
- Jaundice
- Ascites
- Palpable abdominal mass

## Shock liver
Liver involvement in shock.

### FEATURES
- Most common: mild elevation in ALT, AST, and lactate dehydrogenase
- With severe hypoperfusion of liver: significant elevation in ALT and AST accompanied by hepatocellular damage
- Transaminase levels peak in 1–3 days and resolve by 10 days
- In septic shock, greatly increased bilirubin may occur

## SIGNS & SYMPTOMS
### Signs
Fulminant Budd–Chiari syndrome:
- Jaundice
- Hepatomegaly
- Ascites
- Encephalopathy

Acute Budd–Chiari syndrome:
- Hepatomegaly

Chronic Budd–Chiari syndrome:
- Ascites
- Splenomegaly
- Encephalopathy

### Symptoms
Fulminant Budd-Chiari syndrome:
- Severe abdominal pain
- Confusion

Acute Budd–Chiari syndrome:
- Right upper quadrant abdominal pain

Chronic Budd–Chiari syndrome:
- Right upper quadrant tenderness

## ASSOCIATED DISORDERS
Liver cirrhosis.

## KEY! DON'T MISS!
- In pregnant women, the more common possibility of pre-eclampsia should not be missed. Likewise the HELLP syndrome (hemolysis, elevated liver enzymes, low platelets), and the syndrome of acute fatty liver of pregnancy should also not be missed by primary care physicians
- The far more rare fulminant Budd–Chiari syndrome may mimic the subcapsular hepatic hemorrhage associated with eclamptic liver disease and should always be kept in mind because, unlike the above-mentioned disorders, Budd–Chiari syndrome will not resolve with delivery

## CONSIDER CONSULT
Fulminant Budd–Chiari syndrome requires immediate referral to a liver transplantation center.

## INVESTIGATION OF THE PATIENT
### Direct questions to patient
Q How severe is the abdominal pain? Severe abdominal pain is associated with fulminant disease. Mild pain or hepatic tenderness is associated with acute and chronic disease, respectively

Q Do you have any history of cancer? Many cancers may lead to hypercoagulable state

Q Have you ever been diagnosed with a clotting disorder, polycythemia vera, thrombocytosis, or sickle cell anemia? Myeloproliferative diseases and protein C, protein S, and antithrombin III deficiencies are all possible causes of Budd–Chiari

Q Do you take oral contraceptives? Oral contraceptives are associated with hypercoagulable conditions

### Family history
There is no genetic predisposition to this disease, so family history is irrelevant.

### Examination
- Does the patient have severe right upper quadrant tenderness with jaundice, hepatomegaly, ascites and asterixis, mental confusion? These findings on examination are suggestive of fulminant Budd–Chiari and prompt referral to liver transplantation center
- Is the patient pregnant? Associated conditions in pregnant women that should not be missed include pre-eclampsia and the HELLP syndrome
- Does the patient have esophageal varices and splenomegaly in addition to abdominal pain? This is suggestive of chronic Budd–Chiari syndrome
- Check mental status examination for signs of encephalopathy

### Summary of investigative tests
- Liver function tests: AST, ALT, alkaline phosphatase, prothrombin time, albumin, bilirubin, platelet count. Determination of liver function is key to differentiating between fulminant, acute, and chronic Budd–Chiari. Fulminant disease is characterized by rapid deterioration of liver function
- Other useful tests are serum iron, transferrin saturation
- Liver biopsy: when considering treatment option for chronic Budd–Chiari syndrome, refer to a hepatologist or radiologist for liver biopsy to evaluate the state of the liver parenchyma. This will help define treatment plan (transplantation work-up vs shunt operation)

- Alpha-1-antitrypsin, ceruloplasmin, antismooth muscle antibody, antimitochondrial antibody, double-stranded DNA antibody: these tests may further define the underlying cause of Budd–Chiari (normally performed by a specialist)

Radiographic studies:
- Doppler ultrasound is the diagnostic procedure of choice
- Magnetic resonance imaging (MRI) and computed tomography (CT) may be used if Doppler ultrasound does not yield satisfactory information

## DIAGNOSTIC DECISION
Clinical suspicion may be confirmed with a Doppler ultrasound, which is the diagnostic procedure of choice.

## CLINICAL PEARLS
Diagnosis and treatment of the underlying cause of Budd–Chiari syndrome are paramount to successful transplantation.

## THE TESTS
### Tests of function
ASPARTATE AMINOTRANSFERASE
*Description*
Venous blood sample.

*Advantages/Disadvantages*
- Advantage: easy to obtain
- Disadvantage: not specific to Budd–Chiari syndrome

*Normal*
- Adult males: 15–45U/L
- Adult females: 5–30U/L

*Abnormal*
- Adult males: <15 or >45U/L
- Adult females: <5 or >30U/L
- Keep in mind the possibility of a false-positive result

*Cause of abnormal result*
Increased levels:
- Liver diseases: active necrosis of liver parenchymal cells, acute viral hepatitis, extrahepatic biliary disease, hepatotoxic drugs and chemicals, cirrhosis, biliary obstruction, primary or metastatic cancer, hepatic ischemia
- Eclampsia
- Musculoskeletal disorders: trauma, surgery, intramuscular injections, rhabdomyolysis
- Acute myocardial infarction
- Acute pancreatitis
- Intestinal injury
- Pulmonary infarction
- Cerebral infarction or neoplasm
- Renal infarction
- Burns
- Heat exhaustion
- Mushroom poisoning

- Lead poisoning
- Hemolytic anemia

Decreased levels:
- Azotemia
- Chronic renal dialysis
- Malnutrition
- Pregnancy
- Alcoholic liver disease

*Drugs, disorders and other factors that may alter results*
- Opioids, salicylates, tetracycline, chlorpromazine, isoniazid
- Heat exhaustion
- Alcoholic liver disease
- Burns
- Chronic hemodialysis

## ALANINE AMINOTRANSFERASE
*Description*
Venous blood.

*Advantages/Disadvantages*
- Advantage: easily obtainable
- Disadvantage: not specific for Budd–Chiari syndrome

*Normal*
- Male: 10–40U/L
- Female: 5–35U/L

*Abnormal*
- Male: <10 or >40U/L
- Female: <5 or >35U/L
- Keep in mind the possibility of a false-positive result

*Cause of abnormal result*
Increased levels:
- Liver diseases: active necrosis of liver parenchymal cells, acute viral hepatitis, extrahepatic biliary disease, hepatotoxic drugs and chemicals, cirrhosis, biliary obstruction, primary or metastatic cancer, hepatic ischemia
- Severe pre-eclampsia
- Obesity
- Rapidly progressing acute lymphoblastic leukemia
- Musculoskeletal disorders: trauma, surgery, intramuscular injections, rhabdomyolysis
- Acute myocardial infarction
- Acute pancreatitis
- Intestinal injury
- Pulmonary infarction
- Cerebral infarction or neoplasm
- Renal infarction
- Burns
- Heat exhaustion
- Mushroom poisoning

- Lead poisoning
- Hemolytic anemia

Decreased levels:
- Genitourinary tract infection
- Cancer
- Malnutrition
- Pregnancy
- Alcoholic liver disease

*Drugs, disorders and other factors that may alter results*
- Inadequate food intake (extreme dieting or malnutrition)
- Obesity
- Ingestion of opioids, salicylates, tetracycline, chlorpromazine, isoniazid
- Heat exhaustion
- Alcoholic liver disease
- Burns
- Chronic hemodialysis

ALKALINE PHOSPHATASE
*Description*
Venous blood.

*Advantages/Disadvantages*
Advantage: easy to collect.

Disadvantages:
- Nonspecific
- Multiple sites of origin including bone, liver, placenta, intestinal, vascular endothelium

*Normal*
- Male: 65–260U/L
- Female: 50–130U/L

*Abnormal*
- Male: <65 or >260U/L
- Female: <50 or >130U/L
- Keep in mind the possibility of a false-positive result

*Cause of abnormal result*
Alkaline phosphatase of bone origin is elevated with increased deposition of calcium, including the following disorders (this occurs mostly in children; increases in adults over 50 years of age):
- Hyperparathyroidism
- Paget's disease
- Osteoblastic bone tumors (primary or metastatic)
- Osteogenesis imperfecta
- Familial osteoectasia
- Osteomalacia
- Osteomyelitis
- Hyperthyroidism

Alkaline phosphatase of liver origin is elevated in the following disorders (mostly in adults):
- Any obstruction of the biliary system

- Nodules in liver
- Liver infiltrates
- Cholangiolar obstruction in hepatitis
- Hepatic congestion due to heart disease
- Adverse reaction to therapeutic drug
- Diabetes mellitus
- Hodgkin's disease

Liver diseases with increased alkaline phosphatase:
- Two times normal: acute hepatitis, acute fatty liver, cirrhosis
- Five times normal: infectious mononucleosis, postnecrotic cirrhosis
- 10 times normal: carcinoma of head of pancreas, choledocholithiasis, drug-induced cholestatic hepatitis
- 15–20 times normal: primary biliary cirrhosis, primary or metastatic carcinoma

Decreased levels:
- Excess vitamin D ingestion
- Congenital hypophosphatasia
- Achondroplasia
- Hypothyroidism, cretinism
- Pernicious anemia
- Celiac disease
- Malnutrition
- Scurvy
- Zinc, magnesium deficiency
- Postmenopausal women with osteoporosis who are taking estrogen replacement therapy
- Cardiac surgery with cardiopulmonary bypass pump
- Medications: corticosteroids, trifluoperazine, antilipemic agents, hyperalimentation

*Drugs, disorders and other factors that may alter results*
- May be decreased in malnutrition
- May be decreased in women with osteoporosis who are taking estrogen replacement therapy

PROTHROMBIN TIME
*Description*
Venous blood.

*Advantages/Disadvantages*
Advantage: specimen easy to obtain.

Disadvantages:
- May be affected by drug intake
- Not specific to Budd–Chiari syndrome

*Normal*
- +/- 2s of control
- Control should be 11–16s

*Abnormal*
- >18s
- <9s
- Keep in mind the possibility of a false-positive result

*Cause of abnormal result*
- Prolonged due to decrease in vitamin K absorption if obstruction or lack of synthesis in hepatocellular disease
- Markedly prolonged prothrombin time indicates hepatic cell damage in hepatitis and cirrhosis; it may be an indicator of fulminant hepatic necrosis

*Drugs, disorders and other factors that may alter results*
- Malnutrition with inadequate vitamin K in diet
- Heavy alcohol intake with cirrhosis
- Ingestion of warfarin

## BILIRUBIN
*Description*
Venous blood.

*Advantages/Disadvantages*
- Advantage: easy to obtain
- Disadvantage: not very sensitive; may not reflect the degree of liver dysfunction

*Normal*
- Total: <1.0mg/dL (17.1mcmol/L)
- Direct: <0.6mg/dL (10.26mcmol/L)

*Abnormal*
- Total: >1.0mg/dL (17.1mcmol/L); >40mg/dL (684mcmol/L) indicative of hepatocellular rather than extrahepatic obstruction
- Direct: >0.6mg/dL (10.26mcmol/L)
- Keep in mind the possibility of a false-positive result

*Cause of abnormal result*
Increased direct levels:
- Hereditary disorders such as Dubin–Johnson syndrome, Rotor's syndrome
- Hepatic cellular damage caused by viral-, toxic-, alcohol-, or drug-related causes
- Extrahepatic or intrahepatic biliary duct obstruction
- Space-occupying lesions such as primary or metastatic tumor, abscess, granuloma, amyloidosis

Increased indirect levels:
- Hemolytic disorders: hemoglobinopathies, red blood cell (RBC) enzyme deficiencies, disseminated intravascular coagulation, autoimmune hemolysis
- Pernicious anemia
- Blood transfusion
- Hematoma
- Hereditary disorders: Gilbert's syndrome, Crigler–Najjar syndrome
- Drugs that cause hemolysis

Decreased direct or indirect:
- Ingestion of barbiturates

*Drugs, disorders and other factors that may alter results*
- Exposure to white or ultraviolet light decreases total and indirect bilirubin
- Fasting for 48h causes at least a doubling of bilirubin in otherwise healthy persons
- Renal disease may cause increased levels of serum bilirubin

- Acute alcoholic hepatitis
- Viral hepatitis

## ALBUMIN
*Description*
Venous blood.

*Advantages/Disadvantages*
Advantage: specimen is easy to obtain.

Disadvantages
- Slow to reflect liver damage
- Nonspecific

*Normal*
3.7–5.6g/dL (536.1–811.4mcmol/L).

*Abnormal*
- <3.7g/dL (536.1mcmol/L)
- >5.6g/dL (811.4mcmol/L)
- Keep in mind the possibility of a false-positive result

*Cause of abnormal result*
Increased levels:
- Dehydration
- Intravenous albumin administration

Decreased levels:
- Malnutrition (decreased intake, dieting)
- Malabsorption syndromes
- Abnormal synthesis (liver disease, chronic infection)
- Increased need (hyperthyroidism, pregnancy)
- Increased breakdown (cancer, infection, trauma)
- Increased loss (edema, ascites, burns, hemorrhage, nephrotic syndrome)
- Dilution (intravenous fluids, syndrome of inappropriate antidiuretic hormone secretion (SIADH), water intoxication)
- Congenital deficiency

*Drugs, disorders and other factors that may alter results*
- Dehydration increases albumin
- Malnutrition
- Water intoxication

## SERUM IRON
*Description*
Venous blood.

*Advantages/Disadvantages*
Advantages:
- Specimen easily obtained
- Degree of increase parallels the amount of liver necrosis

Disadvantage: nonspecific for liver function.

*Normal*
- Male: 65–175mcg/dL (11.6–31.3mcmol/L)
- Female: 50–170mcg/dL (8.95–30.4mcmol/L)

*Abnormal*
- Male: <65 or >175mcg/dL (<11.6 or >31.3mcmol/L)
- Female: <50 or >170mcg/dL (<8.95 or >30.4mcmol/L)
- Keep in mind the possibility of a false-positive result

*Cause of abnormal result*
Increased levels:
- False increase from hemolysis, iron contamination of glassware
- Iron dextran administration causes increased levels for several weeks
- Idiopathic hemochromatosis
- Repeated blood transfusions
- Iron therapy, iron-containing vitamins
- Thalassemia
- Pyridoxine-deficiency anemia
- Pernicious anemia in relapse
- Hemolytic anemias
- Acute liver damage
- Chronic liver disease
- Progesterone birth control pills
- Premenstrual period

Decreased levels:
- Iron-deficiency anemia
- Anemia of chronic disease and infection
- Nephrosis
- Pernicious anemia
- Menstruation

*Drugs, disorders and other factors that may alter results*
- Excessive iron intake
- Ingestion of progesterone birth control pills
- Pregnancy
- Menstruation
- Iron-deficiency anemia
- Pernicious anemia
- Diurnal variation: normal midmorning values, low midafternoon values, and very low values near midnight

## TRANSFERRIN SATURATION
*Description*
- Specimen is venous blood
- Result obtained by dividing the total iron-binding capacity by the serum iron level

*Advantages/Disadvantages*
Advantage: specimen easy to obtain.

Disadvantages:
- Indirect measurement
- Not specific for liver disease

*Normal*
16% or more.

*Abnormal*
- <16%
- Keep in mind the possibility of a false-positive result

*Cause of abnormal result*
Increased levels:
- Hemochromatosis
- Hemosiderosis
- Thalassemia
- Progesterone birth control pills
- Ingestion of iron
- Iron dextran causes increase for several weeks

Decreased levels:
- Iron-deficiency anemia
- Anemia of chronic disease and/or infection

*Drugs, disorders and other factors that may alter results*
- Progesterone birth control pills
- Ingestion of iron

## PLATELET COUNT
*Description*
Venous blood.

*Advantages/Disadvantages*
- Advantage: specimen easy to obtain
- Disadvantage: nonspecific for Budd–Chiari syndrome

*Normal*
- 140,000–340,000/mm$^3$ (Rees-Ecker)
- 150,000–350,000/mm$^3$ (Coulter counter)

*Abnormal*
- <40,000/mm$^3$
- >1,000,000/mm$^3$
- Keep in mind the possibility of a false-positive result

*Cause of abnormal result*
Increased levels:
- Myeloproliferative diseases such as polycythemia vera, chronic myelogenous leukemia, agnogenic myeloid metaplasia, essential thrombocythemia
- Cancer
- Surgery, especially splenectomy
- Severe trauma
- Infection
- Chronic inflammation such as inflammatory bowel disease, collagen diseases, rheumatoid arthritis
- Iron-deficiency anemia
- Other diseases such as cardiac disease, cirrhosis of liver, chronic pancreatitis, burns, hypothermia, pre-eclampsia, ethanol withdrawal, renal failure

Decreased levels:
- Disorders such as aplastic anemia, myelophthisis
- Exposure to ionizing radiation
- Infections
- Presence of antiplatelet antibodies
- Hypersplenism
- Inherited platelet disorders

*Drugs, disorders and other factors that may alter results*
- Ingestion of quinidine, quinine, gold, sulfonamides, penicillins, or heparin
- Ingestion of alcohol
- Malnutrition (decreased folate, vitamin B12)

## Biopsy
LIVER BIOPSY
*Description*
Liver tissue.

*Advantages/Disadvantages*
Advantage: specific changes associated with Budd–Chiari are identifiable.

Disadvantages:
- Painful
- May cause hemorrhage
- Serial biopsies may be needed to evaluate treatment

*Abnormal*
- Zonal necrosis
- Centrilobular areas necrotic with evidence of hemorrhage and pale in appearance
- Expanded sinusoids filled with RBCs
- Centrilobular fibrosis when thrombosis develops slowly, such as in chronic disease

*Cause of abnormal result*
Hepatic congestion, cirrhosis (many of the underlying causes of cirrhosis have specific findings on biopsy).

*Drugs, disorders and other factors that may alter results*
Cirrhosis.

## Imaging
DOPPLER ULTRASOUND
*Description*
Imaging method of choice for assessment of the hepatic venous system and the inferior vena cava.

*Advantages/Disadvantages*
Advantages:
- Venous flow can be directly visualized
- Noninvasive
- Widely available

Disadvantages:
- Equipment expensive
- Accuracy requires an experienced sonographer

*Normal*
- Hepatic venous connections to inferior vena cava are visible
- Intrahepatic, comma shaped, vessels are visible
- Wave form visible in hepatic veins

*Abnormal*
- No visible connection between hepatic veins and inferior vena cava
- Intrahepatic vessels not visible
- No discernible wave form in hepatic veins
- Keep in mind the possibility of a false-positive result

*Cause of abnormal result*
- Membranous obstruction of the inferior vena cava
- Thrombus at the hepatic veins at the opening to the inferior vena cava
- Obstruction of the intrahepatic veins caused by thrombus or cirrhosis

# TREATMENT

## CONSIDER CONSULT
Refer to hepatobiliary surgeon because most cases require surgical intervention.

## IMMEDIATE ACTION
If liver enzymes are greatly increased, decompression of the liver should be undertaken immediately to relieve hepatic congestion.

## PATIENT AND CAREGIVER ISSUES
### Health-seeking behavior
- Fulminant Budd–Chiari syndrome will be brought to medical attention because patients are severely ill, complete with encephalopathy
- Acute Budd–Chiari is associated with significant abdominal pain; patients are likely to seek help. However, in the case of chronic Budd–Chiari, patients may have a remitting course that would allow them to delay seeking therapy
- Has patient visited emergency department? Budd–Chiari may be mistaken for simple cirrhosis because this is one of its signs. Without Doppler sonography to confirm diagnosis, this could lead to a delay in treatment

## MANAGEMENT ISSUES
### Goals
- To refer patient to liver transplantation center
- Re-establish venous blood flow from the liver
- Decrease liver congestion, and establish normal liver function

### Management in special circumstances
- Fulminant Budd–Chiari syndrome requires prompt treatment for survival, usually liver transplantation
- When paroxysmal nocturnal hematuria is the cause, thrombolytic therapy may be used alone
- When local disease is thought to be the cause, balloon angioplasty or metallic stents have been used for treatment
- When tumor or membranous obstruction are thought to be the cause, tumor may be resected and webs removed with transcardiac membranectomy
- For patients with chronic Budd–Chiari syndrome, a shunt may be placed (type depends upon extent of thrombus)

### COEXISTING DISEASE
Many patients with chronic Budd–Chiari have liver cirrhosis with or without ascites and esophageal varices. Collateral circulation may allow these patients to live longer without treatment than those with acute or fulminant disease.

### COEXISTING MEDICATION
Salicylates used for abdominal pain will contribute to bleeding with surgical intervention.

### SPECIAL PATIENT GROUPS
Pregnancy: early delivery by cesarean section and treatment with orthotopic liver transplantation may be required in fulminant Budd–Chiari. Nonsurgical approaches using antibiotics, antidiuretics, and anticoagulants have been successful in some case reports.

### PATIENT SATISFACTION/LIFESTYLE PRIORITIES
- If treatment is orthotopic liver transplantation, it is necessary to remain on immunosuppressive therapy indefinitely. This may affect lifestyle choices due to increased risk of infection

- Anticoagulation therapy may be necessary indefinitely to prevent recurrent disease. This may affect lifestyle choices due to increased risk of bleeding
- Elderly are probably not candidates for orthotopic liver transplantation but may benefit from shunt or stent placement with anticoagulant therapy or from supportive measures

## SUMMARY OF THERAPEUTIC OPTIONS
### Choices
- Fulminant Budd–Chiari may require orthotopic liver transplantation
- Shunting with transjugular intrahepatic portosystemic shunt (TIPS)
- Stenting with expandable metallic stents to maintain hepatic vein patency
- Streptokinase: off-label medication
- Urokinase: off-label medication
- Tissue plasminogen activator: off-label medication

### Clinical pearls
- Treatment selection is based on the severity of liver disease and the patency of the inferior vena cava and portal vein
- Care must be taken in order not to decrease chances of successful transplantation in the future with the temporizing shunt procedures
- Diagnosis and treatment of the underlying cause of Budd–Chiari syndrome are paramount to successful transplantation

## FOLLOW UP
Follow up is dependent upon underlying condition and treatment selected.

### Plan for review
- Patients receiving orthotopic liver transplantation will require careful follow up for compliance with immunosuppression, rejection
- Patients on anticoagulant therapy will require follow up for compliance with therapy and prothrombin times
- Repeat liver biopsies will be required to assess for recurrent Budd–Chiari syndrome
- Repeat Doppler ultrasound will be required for assessment of recurrent thrombosis

### Information for patient or caregiver
Patients receiving orthotopic liver transplantation will require immunosuppressive therapy indefinitely. Failure to comply with this therapy will lead to rejection of liver and failure of treatment.

## DRUGS AND OTHER THERAPIES: DETAILS
### Drugs
STREPTOKINASE

*Dose*
250,000 IU given intravenously over 30min, then 100,000 IU/h for 24–72h.

*Efficacy*
Resolution of thrombus and recurrent thrombus shown in published case reports.

*Risks/benefits*
Risks:
- Use caution with recent surgery, obstetric delivery, and trauma
- Use caution with subacute bacterial endocarditis, recent streptococcal infection, diabetic hemorrhagic retinopathy, and bleeding disorders
- Use caution with the elderly

Benefits:
- Less expensive than liver transplantation or shunt placement
- May be repeated for recurrent thrombus

*Side effects and adverse reactions*
- Cardiovascular system: hypotension, reperfusion dysrhythmias
- Central nervous system: fever, headache
- Eyes, ears, nose, and throat: periorbital edema
- Gastrointestinal: nausea
- Hematologic: hemorrhage, anemia
- Respiratory: bronchospasm, dyspnea, pulmonary edema
- Skin: flushing, irritation, phlebitis at injection site, urticaria

*Interactions (other drugs)*
**Anticoagulants (may cause bleeding complications).**

*Contraindications*
- **Active bleeding** ■ **Cerebral vascular accident within 2 months** ■ **Intracranial or intraspinal surgery** ■ **Intracranial neoplasm** ■ **Severe uncontrolled hypertension**

*Acceptability to patient*
Medium acceptability:
- Intravenous administration may be difficult in chronically ill patients
- Requires follow-up clotting studies several times weekly

*Follow up plan*
- Measure prothrombin time daily during administration; at least weekly after administration
- May require long-term anticoagulant therapy

*Patient and caregiver information*
- Report bleeding immediately to healthcare provider
- Avoid any sharp tools or instruments while on this therapy, e.g. use electric razor

## UROKINASE
*Dose*
4400 IU/kg intravenously over 10min followed by 4400 IU/kg/h intravenously for 12h; after thrombin time has decreased to less than twice normal, begin heparin

*Efficacy*
Resolution of thrombus and recurrent thrombus shown in published case reports.

*Risks/benefits*
Risks:
- Fast acting
- Use caution with recent surgery, obstetric delivery, and trauma
- Use caution with subacute bacterial endocarditis, streptococcal infection, diabetic hemorrhagic retinopathy, bleeding disorders, and hypertension
- Use caution with the elderly

Benefits:
- Onset of action is rapid
- Less expensive than liver transplantation or shunt placement
- May be repeated for recurrent thrombus

*Side effects and adverse reactions*
- Cardiovascular system: hypotension, hypertension, myocardial infarction, reperfusion dysrhythmias
- Gastrointestinal: nausea
- Hematologic: hemorrhage, surface bleeding
- Metabolism: acidosis
- Respiratory: bronchospasm, dyspnea
- Skin: rash

*Interactions (other drugs)*
- Anticoagulants
- Antiplatelet agents

*Contraindications*
- Active bleeding
- Intraspinal surgery
- Intracranial tumor
- Ulcerative colitis
- Enteritis
- Coagulation defects
- Rheumatic valvular heart disease
- Cerebral embolism
- Thrombosis or hemorrhage within 2 months
- Intra-arterial diagnostic procedure
- Surgery or trauma within 10 days
- Severe hypertension

*Acceptability to patient*
Medium acceptability:
- Intravenous administration may be difficult in chronically ill patients
- Requires follow-up clotting studies several times weekly

*Follow up plan*
- Measure prothrombin time daily during administration; at least weekly after administration
- May require long-term anticoagulant therapy

*Patient and caregiver information*
- Report bleeding immediately to healthcare provider
- Avoid any sharp tools or instruments while on this therapy, e.g. use electric razor

TISSUE PLASMINOGEN ACTIVATOR
Alteplase.

*Dose*
100mg alteplase by intravenous infusion over 30min.

*Efficacy*
Resolution of thrombus and recurrent thrombus shown in published case reports.

*Risks/benefits*
Risks:
- Use caution in recent major surgery
- Most common complication is bleeding: internal bleeding, involving intracranial and retroperitoneal sites or the gastrointestinal, genitourinary, or respiratory tracts; and superficial bleeding, mainly at invaded or disturbed sites (e.g. venous cutdowns, arterial punctures, sites of recent surgical intervention)
- Avoid noncompressible arterial puncture
- Avoid internal jugular and subclavian venous punctures
- Minimize arterial and venous punctures

Benefits:
- Onset of action is rapid
- Less expensive than liver transplantation or shunt placement
- May be repeated for recurrent thrombus
- Associated with fewer hemorrhagic events

*Side effects and adverse reactions*
- Cardiovascular system: cardiac arrhythmias, tachycardia
- Hematologic: intracranial, retroperitoneal, surface, gastrointestinal, genitourinary bleeding, increased prothrombin time, partial prothrombin time
- Skin: rash, urticaria

*Interactions (other drugs)*
- Heparin (increased bleeding) - Acetylsalicylic acid (increased bleeding) - Dipyridamole (increased bleeding)

*Contraindications*
- Active bleeding - Hemorrhagic stroke - Severe uncontrolled hypertension
- Intracranial/intraspinal surgery - Trauma - Aneurysm - Arteriovenous malformation
- Brain tumor - Known bleeding disorder

*Acceptability to patient*
Medium acceptability:
- Requires intravenous administration, which may be difficult in chronically ill person
- Requires follow-up blood work to assess bleeding time

*Follow up plan*
Requires at least weekly monitoring of prothrombin time.

*Patient and caregiver information*
- Report bleeding to healthcare provider immediately
- Avoid use of sharp objects that may cause injury and bleeding, e.g. use electric razor while on this therapy

## Surgical therapy
- Surgical therapy may be contraindicated in pregnant women, and orthotopic liver transplantation may be impractical in the elderly
- Stent and shunt placement will correct hepatic vein outflow problems but not the underlying cause of disease
- Orthotopic liver transplantation may correct underlying cause of disease and is the treatment of choice in fulminant Budd–Chiari. If disability prevents patient from complying with immunosuppression protocol, then orthotopic liver transplantation would be contraindicated

### ORTHOTOPIC LIVER TRANSPLANTATION
*Efficacy*
5-year survival rates of 45–80%. Prevention of recurrent thrombosis is key to successful treatment.

*Risks/benefits*
Risks:
- Rejection of organ
- Chronic immunosuppression makes patient more susceptible to infection
- Chronic anticoagulant therapy puts patient at risk for hemorrhage
- Risk of secondary malignancy (lymphoma)

Benefits:
- Treats underlying cause of coagulopathy by replacing liver
- Provides alternative to shunt in case of shunt failure
- Acute or chronic liver failure patients benefit the most from this procedure

*Acceptability to patient*
Medium acceptability:
- Requires patience to stay on waiting list for organ
- Requires lifestyle changes due to chronic immunosuppressive and anticoagulant therapy
- Requires close follow-up to monitor for rejection
- May require painful procedures in clinic, such as liver biopsies

*Follow up plan*
- Frequent clinic visits to monitor immunosuppression therapy
- Weekly evaluation of prothrombin time, liver function studies
- Ultrasound at intervals to evaluate patency of hepatic vessels

*Patient and caregiver information*
- Requires careful follow up and lifelong immunosuppression
- Report signs and symptoms of infections to healthcare provider immediately
- Report bleeding to healthcare provider immediately
- Clinic follow up is extensive and necessary to carefully monitor for organ rejection

## TRANSJUGULAR INTRAHEPATIC PORTOSYSTEMIC SHUNT
*Efficacy*
Patency of TIPS can be maintained in 90% of patients for 2 years. Efficacy in Budd–Chiari syndrome has been reported in case studies only.

*Risks/benefits*
Risks:
- Increases right-sided cardiac pressure – should not be performed in patients with right-sided cardiac failure or primary pulmonary hypertension
- Recurrent thrombosis
- Renal failure caused by contrast material
- Stent migration
- Infection
- Puncture of gallbladder or other organs

Benefits:
- No general anesthesia
- Decreased morbidity/mortality rate
- No surgery in the hepatic hilum – important for liver transplantation candidates

*Acceptability to patient*
High acceptability:
- Avoids surgery
- Procedural complications infrequent
- Requires repeat sonography to determine patency of shunt

*Follow up plan*
- Follow-up sonography every 3 months to monitor patency of shunt
- Weekly coagulation studies to monitor prothrombin time

*Patient and caregiver information*
- Report bleeding to healthcare provider immediately
- Report abdominal pain to healthcare provider immediately because this could indicate blockage of shunt or infection
- Report signs and symptoms of infection to healthcare provider (fever, chills)

## STENT PLACEMENT
*Efficacy*
Efficacy has been reported in case studies with resolution of ascites in 3–4 weeks and duration of symptom-free interval reported to be 3 years.

*Risks/benefits*
Risks:
- Bleeding
- Infection
- Stent migration
- Pulmonary embolus

Benefits:
- Avoids lengthy surgery and anesthesia
- May be a 'bridge' to transplantation for selected patients
- Symptoms alleviated within weeks

*Acceptability to patient*
High acceptability:
- Avoids surgery and anesthesia
- Requires follow-up appointments for ultrasound and coagulation studies, but this can be accomplished as an outpatient
- Relieves discomfort of ascites
- May act as 'bridge' to liver transplantation, allowing more time to find donor

*Follow up plan*
- Ultrasound every 3 months and as necessary to determine patency of stent
- Weekly prothrombin time to monitor anticoagulant therapy

*Patient and caregiver information*
- Report increase in abdominal girth (possible reaccumulation of ascites) to healthcare provider
- Report fever, chills to healthcare provider
- Report bleeding to healthcare provider
- Repeat ultrasound necessary to monitor patency of stent
- Anticoagulant therapy is needed indefinitely to decrease incidence of thrombus
- Does not treat underlying cause of coagulopathy

# OUTCOMES

## EFFICACY OF THERAPIES
- Use of transjugular intrahepatic portosystemic shunt (TIPS) or stent placement may act as a bridge to orthotopic liver transplantation. Avoidance of hepatic hilar surgery is important for liver transplantation candidates
- Stent placement has been reported to provide symptom relief for 3 years; TIPS have efficacy as reported in case studies
- With orthotopic liver transplantation, 45–80% of patients are alive at 5 years post-transplantation

### Review period
- Ultrasound every 3 months to assess patency of hepatic vein
- Prothrombin time weekly to assess anticoagulant therapy

## PROGNOSIS
- Prognosis with liver transplantation: 45–80% alive 5 years post-transplantation
- Those who fail stent or shunt placement may go on to have liver transplantation
- Recurrent thrombosis is most common cause of treatment failure in all forms of treatment
- Prognosis is highly dependent upon time to recognition of condition, etiology, acuity, and type of intervention

### Clinical pearls
- Care must be taken in order not to decrease chances of successful transplantation in the future with the temporizing shunt procedures
- Diagnosis and treatment of the underlying cause of Budd–Chiari syndrome are paramount to successful transplantation

### Terminal illness
- Failure of liver transplantation and stent and shunt placement in Budd–Chiari syndrome are all most likely to be caused by recurrent thrombosis
- Liver failure may be associated with ascites, coagulopathy, and encephalopathy in addition to abdominal pain

## COMPLICATIONS
- Bleeding: anticoagulant therapy is required as part of treatment for Budd–Chiari syndrome
- Infection with stent or shunt placement after liver transplantation due to chronic immunosuppressive therapy
- Organ rejection after liver transplantation
- Thrombosis of stent or shunt, or of hepatic vein post-transplantation

## PREVENTION

Budd–Chiari syndrome is not specifically preventable in the general population.

## PREVENT RECURRENCE
Preventing recurrent thrombosis is key to preventing recurrent Budd–Chiari syndrome. This means chronic anticoagulant therapy.

### Reassess coexisting disease
- Weekly monitoring of prothrombin time to monitor anticoagulant therapy
- Ultrasound every 3 months to monitor hepatic veins for thrombosis

# RESOURCES

## ASSOCIATIONS

**American Gastroenterological Association**
7910 Woodmont Ave, 7th Floor
Bethesda, MD 20814
Tel: (301) 654-2055
Fax: (301) 652-3890
http://www.gastro.org

**American Association for the Study of Liver Diseases**
1729 King Street, Suite 100
Alexandria, VA 22314
Tel: (703) 299-9766
http://www.aasld.org

**American Society of Transplantation**
17000 Commerce Parkway, Suite C
Mt. Laurel, NJ 08054
Tel: (856) 439-9986
Fax: (856) 439-9982
http://www.a-s-t.org

## KEY REFERENCES

- Schafer DF, Sorrell MF. Vascular diseases of the liver. In: Feldman M, Friedman LS, Sleisenger MH, eds. Sleisenger & Fordtran's gastrointestinal and liver disease, 6th edn. Philadelphia, PA: WB Saunders, 1998, p1188–90
- Borum ML. Hepatobiliary diseases in women. Med Clin North Am 1998:82:51–75
- Shrestha R, Durham JD, Wachs M, et al. Use of transjugular intrahepatic portosystemic shunt as a bridge to transplantation in fulminant hepatic failure due to Budd-Chiari syndrome. Am J Gastroenterol 1997:92:2304–6
- Michl P, Bilzer M, Waggerhauser T, et al. Successful treatment of chronic Budd-Chiari syndrome with a transjugular intrahepatic portosystemic shunt. J Hepatol 2000:32:516–20
- Raju GS. Thrombolysis for acute Budd-Chiari syndrome: case report and literature review. Am J Gastroenterol 1996;91:1262–3

## FAQS

**Question 1**
When hepatic vein thrombosis is suspected, what is the sequence of tests?

ANSWER 1
Doppler ultrasound. If no flow, perform hepatic venography.

**Question 2**
Do all patients with Budd-Chiari syndrome require anticoagulation?

ANSWER 2
Yes. All patients usually require anticoagulation no matter what the cause or form of treatment they have received.

## CONTRIBUTORS

Fred F Ferri, MD, FACP
Rudolph A Bedford, MD
J Adrian Lunn, MD

# CELIAC DISEASE

| | |
|---|---|
| ■ Summary Information | 44 |
| ■ Background | 45 |
| ■ Diagnosis | 47 |
| ■ Treatment | 57 |
| ■ Outcomes | 67 |
| ■ Prevention | 69 |
| ■ Resources | 70 |

## SUMMARY INFORMATION

### DESCRIPTION
- An inflammatory condition of the small intestine that is characterized by malabsorption and is precipitated by the ingestion of gluten-containing foods such as wheat, rye, and barley in individuals with a genetic predisposition
- Clinical manifestations are protean and the disease often remains unrecognized for many years
- Affects the mucosa of the small intestine. The characteristic lesion is a flat mucosa with loss of villi and increased intraepithelial lymphocytes. The abnormality is most marked proximally and decreases in severity with distal progression through the small intestine. In severe cases the entire small intestine may be affected, and there may even be involvement of the stomach and colon
- In 70% of celiac patients clinical improvement is observed within 2 weeks following withdrawal of gluten-containing food from the diet

### KEY! DON'T MISS!
- Because celiac disease is a preventable condition, the diagnosis should not be missed and the primary care physician should remember that celiac disease is the 'great imitator' of today
- Bone mineral density should be obtained in all patients with celiac disease because osteopenia is a complication of chronic malabsorption that should not be missed

# BACKGROUND

## ICD9 CODE
579.0 Celiac disease; celiac sprue

## SYNONYMS
- Gluten-sensitive enteropathy
- Celiac sprue
- Nontropical sprue
- Previously called idiopathic steatorrhea and primary malabsorption

## CARDINAL FEATURES
- A chronic diarrheal condition characterized by malabsorption of most nutrients and precipitated by the ingestion of gluten-containing foods
- Caused by sensitivity to the alcohol-soluble protein components (prolamins) of grains, known as gliadin in wheat, secalin in rye, and hordeins in barley
- Causes mucosal abnormalities of the small intestine, which vary considerably in severity and extent; submucosa, muscularis, and serosa are usually unaffected
- In 70% of patients, clinical improvement in symptoms can be observed following withdrawal of gluten-containing food from the diet within 2 weeks
- In patients with refractory sprue, oral prednisone may be effective
- A small percentage of patients with severe disease refractory to a gluten-free diet develop deposition of collagen in the lamina propria (collagenous sprue), which has a poor prognosis

## CAUSES
### Common causes
Sensitivity to the alcohol-soluble protein components (prolamins) of grains, known as gliadin in wheat, secalin in rye, and hordeins in barley.

### Rare causes
Oat grains appear to be less toxic than wheat, barley, and rye. Toxicity attributable to oat grains is probably due to small quantities of wheat, which contaminate oats as they are harvested (usually harvested using the same combines).

## EPIDEMIOLOGY
### Incidence and prevalence
PREVALENCE
- Estimates in the US range from 5 per 100,000 to 500 per 100,000
- In the UK, celiac disease affects about 40 per 100,000 people
- Prevalence is higher among people of northern European ancestry; in the West of Ireland the prevalence is 300 per 100,000

FREQUENCY
Frequency has been estimated at 0.05–0.2% of the general population in Europe.

### Demographics
AGE
- Incidence is highest during infancy and the first 3 years when gluten-containing foods are introduced into the diet
- May recur during the third or fourth decades of adult life; frequently associated with pregnancy and severe anemia during pregnancy
- May occur in the seventh decade as digestive properties begin to wane with age

## GENDER
Slight female predominance (female:male = 3:2).

## RACE
- Highest incidence in Caucasians of northern European ancestry (1 in 300)
- Rare in African and Asian (Chinese, Japanese) populations

## GENETICS
- Approximately 10–15% of first-degree relatives of affected individuals have celiac disease
- Concordance for celiac disease in HLA identical siblings is approximately 30%, whereas that for identical twins is about 70%
- Predisposition to gluten sensitivity has been mapped to the HLA-D region on chromosome 6
- 90–95% of celiac patients have the DQ2 heterodimer coded by allele DQA1*0501 and DQB1*0201
- Other genetic markers such as alloantigens on the surface of B cells and Gm allotype markers on the IgG heavy chain have been identified

## GEOGRAPHY
- High prevalence in northern and western Ireland, where prevalence is 300 per 100,000
- Data indicate a prevalence of 0.35% in Sweden and 0.5% in Italy among schoolchildren
- Data from Denmark indicate a prevalence significantly lower than that in Sweden and Italy

# DIAGNOSIS

## DIFFERENTIAL DIAGNOSIS
### Lactose intolerance
Lactose intolerance is a malabsorption syndrome, also known as lactase deficiency, that is characterized by insufficient concentration of lactase, leading to fermentation of malabsorbed lactose by intestinal flora and resulting in production of intestinal gas and acids.

FEATURES
- Patients have an inability to digest foods that are high in lactose, such as milk, ice cream, and other dairy products
- Symptoms include diarrhea, abdominal tenderness, cramping, bloating, and flatulence
- May be caused by congenital lactase deficiency or secondary intolerance as a result of injury to the intestinal mucosa by Whipple's disease, AIDS enteropathy, Crohn's disease, viral gastroenteritis, or celiac disease
- The diagnosis of lactose intolerance can be confirmed by positive hydrogen breath test

### Crohn's disease
Crohn's disease is an inflammatory disease of the bowel, most commonly involving the terminal ileum, colon, or both.

FEATURES
- Main symptoms include diarrhea, abdominal pain, weight loss, and fatigue
- There may be abdominal tenderness, mass, or distension at examination
- There may be hyperactive bowel sounds in patients with partial obstruction and bloody diarrhea
- Laboratory findings include reduced hemoglobin and hematocrit due to blood loss
- Barium imaging studies reveal deep ulcerations and segmental lesions with 'skip' (uninvolved) areas
- Extraintestinal manifestations include arthralgias, arthritis, hepatosplenomegaly due to liver diseases (especially sclerosing cholangitis), sacroiliitis, erythema nodosum, and other skin lesions

### Whipple's disease
Whipple's disease is a multisystem illness that is characterized by malabsorption and caused by the Gram-positive bacillus *Tropheryma whippelii*.

FEATURES
- Peak age for the condition is 30–60 years and is more frequent in men than in women
- Disease may present with extraintestinal symptoms, including arthralgia and neurologic abnormalities
- There may be abdominal distension, often with tenderness, and less commonly with mass or bloating
- Gastrointestinal symptoms include diarrhea, steatorrhea, abdominal bloating and cramps, and anorexia
- Other symptoms include weight loss, anemia, fatigue, edema and ascites, bleeding diathesis, and osteomalacia

### Tropical sprue
Tropical sprue is a malabsorption syndrome of unknown etiology, which is endemic in tropical regions such as the Middle East, the Far East, India, and the Caribbean.

FEATURES
- Symptoms include diffuse, nonspecific abdominal tenderness and distension, low-grade fever, glossitis, cheilosis, hyperkeratosis, and hyperpigmentation

- There may be a possible link to infection and an initial response to antibiotics and folate supplementation
- Imaging of the small bowel may reveal coarsening of the jejunal folds
- With appropriate antibiotic therapy, complete recovery often ensues

### Zollinger–Ellison syndrome

Zollinger–Ellison syndrome is a hypergastrinemic state caused by pancreatic or extrapancreatic nonbeta-islet-cell tumor, resulting in peptic acid disease.

FFATURES

- Disease occurs equally in both sexes and at any age, being most common in those aged 30–50 years
- The majority of patients have symptoms similar to those of peptic ulcer; one-third of patients have diarrhea and steatorrhea

### Giardiasis

Giardiasis is an intestinal tract infection caused by the protozoon *Giardia lamblia* and acquired by ingestion of viable cysts of the organism, typically in contaminated food or by fecal-oral contact.

FEATURES

- Common in preschool children (especially those in day care), people returning from summer camps, and sexually active, homosexual men
- Patients with common variable immunodeficiency or X-linked agammaglobulinemia are at increased risk of infection
- The majority of patients have diarrhea, flatulence, cramps, bloating, and nausea
- Often there is chronic diarrhea with malabsorption, and weight loss is common, although gastrointestinal bleeding is unusual
- There may be transient secondary lactase deficiency
- Stool specimen or duodenal aspirate establishes diagnosis and excludes other pathogens

### Irritable bowel syndrome

Irritable bowel syndrome is a chronic functional disorder of the intestine of unknown etiology, occurring in approximately 20% of the population of industrialized countries and manifested by an alteration in bowel habits and recurrent abdominal pain and bloating.

FEATURES

- Nearly half of patients presenting to a physician have psychiatric abnormalities such as anxiety disorders
- There may be nonspecific abdominal tenderness and distension, whereas physical examination is generally normal
- Small-bowel series and barium enema are normal

### Chronic pancreatitis

Chronic pancreatitis is a recurrent or persistent inflammation of the pancreas, most commonly found in alcoholic males and characterized by chronic pain and by endocrine or exocrine insufficiency.

FEATURES

- Symptoms include bulky, foul-smelling and greasy stools, weight loss, tenderness over the pancreas, and persistent or recurrent epigastric pain
- Serum lipase and amylase may be elevated and hyperglycemia, hyperbilirubinemia, glycosuria, and elevated serum alkaline phosphatase may also occur

### AIDS enteropathy

AIDS enteropathy is caused by infection with HIV and is characterized by a progressive deterioration of the cellular immune system.

FEATURES
- Symptoms such as diarrhea, weight loss, and malabsorption syndromes may mimic the nonspecific manifestations of AIDS
- Positive HIV antibody test confirms diagnosis of AIDS

### Cystic fibrosis

Cystic fibrosis is an autosomal recessive disorder that is characterized by dysfunction of exocrine glands.

FEATURES
- Physical findings include failure to thrive in children, abdominal distension, and greasy, foul-smelling feces; these features may resemble those of celiac disease
- Other symptoms include increased chest diameter, basilar crackles and hyper-resonance to percussion, chronic cough, and digital clubbing
- Diagnosis of cystic fibrosis includes a positive quantitative pilocarpine iontophoresis and genetic testing of patients with one or more phenotypic features of the disease, or documented disease in a sibling

### Bacterial overgrowth

Bacterial overgrowth of the small intestine resulting from a condition that causes intestinal stasis (e.g. pseudo-obstruction, jejunal diverticulosis) or partial small-bowel obstruction may result in malabsorption resembling celiac disease.

FEATURES
- The intestinal flora may have a direct toxic effect on the mucosa and may lead to megaloblastic anemia
- Radiography may show anatomic abnormalities which may assist in diagnosis. Treatment with courses of oral broad-spectrum antibiotics is useful

### Eosinophilic gastroenteritis

Eosinophilic gastroenteritis is a gastrointestinal disorder that is commonly associated with intolerance to specific foods, characterized by intestinal inflammatory cell infiltrates with a predominance of eosinophils, and edema.

FEATURES
- Any area of the gastrointestinal tract can be affected, but disorder most commonly affects the stomach or small bowel
- The most common form of the disorder affects the mucosal (and sometimes submucosal) layer; less commonly the muscularis is primarily involved; a rare form affects the serosal layer and presents with eosinophilic ascites
- Symptoms include diarrhea, nausea, abdominal pain, and malabsorption

### Short bowel syndrome

Short bowel syndrome is a malabsorption syndrome that results from extensive small intestinal resection.

FEATURES
Symptoms include diarrhea, steatorrhea, weight loss, anemia, bleeding diasthesis related to vitamin K malabsorption, osteoporosis related to calcium malabsorption, hyponatremia, hypokalemia, and other macronutrient and micronutrient deficiencies.

## SIGNS & SYMPTOMS
### Signs
- Personality: affected children are usually irritable, unhappy, and miserable. Adults may present with depression, Korsakoff syndrome, neurasthenia, or frank schizophrenia
- Height: celiac patients are frequently shortest in their families, and children are often shorter than their same sex parents
- Malabsorption of fat, carbohydrate, protein, electrolytes, and all nutrients
- Pallor may occur as a result of iron deficiency, and anemia is common
- Vitamin K deficiency resulting in coagulopathy
- Female infertility
- Calcium deficiency may be present with resulting tetany, muscle cramps, and/or seizures; these can be exacerbated by concomitant magnesium deficiency
- Severe hypokalemia as a result of excess potassium loss; may result in weakness
- Hyposplenism and splenic atrophy
- Osteopenia may occur
- Secondary hyperparathyroidism may develop in patients with severely impaired calcium absorption

### Symptoms
Patients often have chronic, mild symptoms for most of their lives, but never significant enough to warrant medical attention.
- Diarrhea, which varies from patient to patient; stools may be watery or semisolid, light tan or gray, oily or frothy, and often foul-smelling
- Flatulence
- Weight loss
- Failure to thrive in children and infants
- Increased appetite without weight gain in adults
- Abdominal distension
- Fatigue
- Severe abdominal pain, nausea, and vomiting are rare in uncomplicated celiac disease but can occur, particularly in children
- Aphthous ulcers, atopic dermatitis, dermatitis herpetiformis, and angular cheilitis frequently associated with the disorder
- Clubbing of nails is often seen in severe disease
- Temporal lobe epilepsy

## ASSOCIATED DISORDERS
A number of diseases are associated with celiac disease. Some of the most important ones are as follows:
- Dermatitis herpetiformis: 10% of patients with celiac disease have dermatitis herpetiformis. Gluten withdrawal reverses the intestinal and skin manifestations. Of patients with dermatitis herpetiformis, 80% have celiac disease or latent celiac disease that will manifest with exposure to gluten
- Lactose intolerance: a lactose-free diet should be implemented alongside a gluten-free diet until symptoms improve
- Diabetes mellitus type 1: frequency is increased in patients with celiac disease. In one study, the frequency of celiac disease was 4.1% in 195 type 1 diabetic people. Diabetic people have an increased frequency of the DQ alleles that are associated with celiac disease
- Autoimmune thyroid disease: there is an increased frequency in celiac disease patients, with hypothyroidism being more common than hyperthyroidism
- Osteoporosis or osteopenia
- IgA deficiency: a frequent finding in celiac patients; occurs in approximately 20% of patients with celiac disease

## KEY! DON'T MISS!
- Because celiac disease is a preventable condition, the diagnosis should not be missed and the primary care physician should remember that celiac disease is the 'great imitator' of today
- Bone mineral density should be obtained in all patients with celiac disease because osteopenia is a complication of chronic malabsorption that should not be missed

## CONSIDER CONSULT
Refer to a gastroenterologist for definitive diagnosis, as the 'gold standard' for diagnosis is small-bowel biopsy. However, patients can first undergo serologic testing for antigliadin, antiendomysial, and antitransglutaminase antibodies. The primary care physician should refer those patients with refractory and/or unclassified sprue to rule out small-bowel lymphoma, which is a not infrequent association in refractory sprue.

## INVESTIGATION OF THE PATIENT
### Direct questions to patient
General:

**Q** Do you have anemia or a history of anemia? This is often mistakenly attributed to heavy menses in young women, but is probably the most common sign of celiac disease. It is obviously not specific, however

**Q** Do you have diarrhea? The most common symptoms are diarrhea and flatulence, with diarrhea varying from patient to patient, but stool mass being increased in all patients

**Q** What is the appearance of your stools? Stools may be fatty/oily

**Q** Are you intolerant to foods that contain milk and/or other dairy products? Patients with celiac disease commonly have secondary lactase deficiency

**Q** (In women) Have you had frequent miscarriages and/or difficulty becoming pregnant?

**Q** Are you tired? Do you feel generally weak? Fatigue is among the recognized symptoms of celiac disease

In infants/children:

**Q** Is your child failing to thrive or losing weight? Failure to gain weight and slow growth may be the primary manifestations of celiac disease

**Q** Have wheat or wheat products recently been introduced into you child's diet? Celiac disease usually manifests in infancy following introduction of gluten-containing foods into the diet

In adults:

**Q** Has your appetite increased with no apparent gain in weight? Some celiac patients do not lose weight, but develop enormous appetites to compensate for the malabsorption. Daily calorie intakes may be well in excess of normal, despite lack of weight gain

**Q** Have you recently been taking laxatives? Laxative abuse is a cause of chronic diarrhea and malabsorption

### Contributory or predisposing factors

**Q** Do you have/have you ever had dermatitis? Try to ascertain whether the patient has a history of dermatitis herpetiformis. Celiac disease is often associated with dermatitis herpetiformis (10%). Conversely, of patients with dermatitis herpetiformis, 80% have celiac disease or latent celiac disease

**Q** Do you have type 1 diabetes mellitus? People with diabetes have an increased frequency of DQ alleles associated with celiac disease

**Q** Have wheat or wheat products recently been introduced into your/your child's diet? Latent celiac disease will manifest on exposure to gluten

## Family history

Do you have a family history of this problem? Approximately 10–15% of first-degree relatives of affected individuals have celiac disease. Concordance for celiac disease in HLA-identical siblings is approximately 30%, whereas that for identical twins is 70%.

## Examination

- **Is the patient well/unwell?** If the patient is systemically unwell, consider intestinal parasitic infestation/infection, such as giardiasis
- **Does the patient have an elevated temperature?** Fever suggests infection
- **Has the patient suffered significant weight loss?** May be a symptom of celiac disease
- **Is the patient's appetite large without significant weight gain?** In adults with celiac disease, appetite often increases to compensate for the malabsorption, but there is no weight gain
- **Is there abdominal distension?**
- **Is there a rash?** Dermatitis herpetiformis is often associated with celiac disease
- **Is there abdominal pain?** This is rare in celiac disease
- **Is the patient pale?** Pallor associated with anemia may be a result of iron deficiency in celiac disease

## Summary of investigative tests

- Serum carotene: a very quick and easy screen for malabsorption. A very low serum carotene is highly suggestive of malabsorption or malnutrition
- Fecal fat estimation: qualitative 72h fecal fat microscopic examination of stool suspension stained with Sudan black
- D-xylose absorption test: reveals malabsorption of sugar
- Serological markers: for celiac disease: antigliadin IgG and IgA antibodies. IgA endomysial antibodies and antitissue transglutaminase are the best screening tests for celiac disease
- Biopsy of the small bowel: reveals absence or flattening of villi and other histological manifestations of celiac disease; essential for confirming diagnosis; abnormalities should reverse on a gluten-free diet. This test would normally be done by a specialist
- Blood chemistry: check levels of serum iron, calcium, potassium, magnesium, liver enzymes (alanine and aspartate aminotransferase), zinc, cholesterol, vitamins, and proteins
- Hematologic tests: hematocrit, prothrombin time
- X-ray: small-bowel follow-through (if done) reveals edema and flattening of mucosal folds

## DIAGNOSTIC DECISION

- Initial evaluation consists of laboratory tests followed by upper gastrointestinal endoscopy with biopsy of duodenum or proximal jejunum
- Repeat biopsy of the duodenum, demonstrating reversal of the histologic abnormality on a gluten-free diet (usually after one year), is necessary before a firm diagnosis can be made
- Diagnosis of celiac disease is confirmed by demonstrating impairment of small-intestinal mucosal function, the presence of typical mucosal lesion, and observation of prompt clinical response and improvement in mucosal histology following withdrawal of gluten from the diet

## CLINICAL PEARLS

- Age may affect the clinical presentation because the classical symptoms of diarrhea, steatorrhea, and weight loss on wheat products are more commonly seen earlier in life rather than later. If patient is older in age, look for iron deficiency, coagulopathy, hypocalcemia, nonspecific serum aminotransferase elevations, and symptoms of chronic illness
- The sensitivity of the serologic tests for celiac disease is highest if the patient is on a diet that contains wheat. A common mistake is to place the patient on a gluten-free diet and then to obtain serologies. Also, beware of the frequent IgA deficiency in celiac patients; an antiendomysial antibody negative IgA may be falsely negative because of IgA deficiency

# THE TESTS
## Body fluids
### FECAL FAT ESTIMATION
*Description*
Qualitative stool fat determination by Sudan black III or IV staining, confirmed by quantitative 72h fecal fat determination.

*Advantages/Disadvantages*
Advantage: steatorrhea is present in many patients with celiac disease and its severity correlates with the severity of the intestinal lesion.

Disadvantages:
- Steatorrhea may be absent in patients with disease limited to the proximal small intestine
- Not specific for celiac disease
- More importantly, it is an unwieldy test, with sample collection and the test itself often not performed well

*Normal*
2–6g/24h.

*Abnormal*
>7% fecal fat malabsorption.

*Cause of abnormal result*
Elevated in celiac disease and any other cause of steatorrhea.

### SERUM CAROTENE
*Description*
Carotene is released from dietary proteins in the stomach. It then joins lipid micelles and bile salts in the small bowel for absorption. Serum carotene is therefore a marker for fat absorption. In cases of steatorrhea, serum carotene will be low.

*Advantages/Disadvantages*
Advantages:
- Rapid method to diagnose malabsorption because quantitative fecal fat is a cumbersome test to perform. It presumes that patients are on a normal diet, and therefore is not applicable to those from underdeveloped countries because the major cause of low serum carotene in such countries is nutritional deficiency
- The serum carotene test can be modified to overcome variation in dietary intake. Carotene tolerance test is a measure of serum carotene after daily oral loading of serum carotene

Disadvantage: the test is not specific for celiac disease or any other small-bowel disease.

*Normal*
- >60mcg/dL
- In carotene tolerance test an increase in serum carotene >35mcg/dL is normal

*Abnormal*
- <60mcg/dL
- In carotene tolerance test an increase in serum carotene <35mcg/dL is diagnostic for steatorrhea

*Cause of abnormal result*
- All causes of malabsorption or maldigestion, such as cystic fibrosis, pancreatic insufficiency, cholestatic liver diseases, and diseases of the small bowel such as Crohn's disease and celiac disease, will cause abnormal serum carotene
- Low intake of carotene or fat may cause low levels of serum carotene

*Drugs, disorders and other factors that may alter results*
- Patients on a fat-free diet will have low absorption of carotene, and therefore low serum levels
- It takes a while for serum carotene to return to normal, even when celiac disease is in remission

## D-XYLOSE ABSORPTION TEST
*Description*
D-xylose absorption and measurement of xylose excretion in the urine, and peak xylose blood levels to indicate absorption of this sugar.

*Normal*
21–31% excreted in urine within 5h.

*Abnormal*
Reduced excretion of D-xylose in urine and reduced peak serum blood levels.

*Cause of abnormal result*
Proximal intestine, where D-xylose absorption occurs, is affected.

## SEROLOGIC EXAMINATION
*Description*
Serum antibodies useful in supporting the diagnosis of celiac disease.

*Advantages/Disadvantages*
Advantages:
- Useful for noninvasive screening of celiac disease
- Antiendomysial IgA and antitissue transglutaminase antibodies are more specific for celiac disease than antigliadin, and are the best screening tests for the disorder
- Sensitivity of antiendomysial IgA antibodies is >90% in patients with untreated celiac disease, and specificity ranges from 90–100%
- Can be used to monitor dietary compliance

Disadvantages:
- Although antigliadin IgA and IgG are sensitive, they are not specific
- Antiendomysial and antigliadin IgA antibodies are not detected in patients with IgA deficiency (common in patients with celiac disease)
- Antitissue transglutaminase is highly specific for celiac disease
- Antiendomysial and antitissue transglutaminase antibodies often become undetectable when celiac disease is in remission

*Abnormal*
Antigliadin IgA and IgG antibodies are elevated in 90% of patients who are on wheat-containing diets.

*Cause of abnormal result*
Sensitivity to gliadin.

*Drugs, disorders and other factors that may alter results*
Antiendomysial and antigliadin IgA antibodies are not detected in patients with IgA deficiency.

## BLOOD CHEMISTRY
*Description*
Serum levels of calcium, iron, magnesium, potassium, vitamins, and cholesterol may all be reduced in celiac disease.

*Advantages/Disadvantages*
Advantages:
- Simple, cheap, and noninvasive test
- Results available rapidly

Disadvantage: not specific for celiac disease.

*Normal*
- Normal serum levels of iron, calcium, potassium, magnesium, alanine aminotransferase (ALT), aspartate aminotransferase (AST), serum zinc, serum cholesterol, vitamins, folic acid, and protein
- Note that reference ranges will vary, and the individual laboratory should be consulted

*Abnormal*
- Calcium, cholesterol, vitamin A, vitamin B12, vitamin C, folic acid, iron, and proteins may all be reduced in celiac disease
- Keep in mind the possibility of falsely abnormal results

*Cause of abnormal result*
Malabsorption of fat-soluble vitamin D is the main cause of calcium deficiency.

## Tests of function
### HEMATOLOGIC FUNCTION
*Description*
Blood function.

*Normal*
- Prothrombin time: 10–12s
- Hemoglobin: male 13.6–17.7g/dL (136–177g/L); female 12.0–15.0g/dL (120–150g/L)
- Hematocrit: male 39–49%; female 33–43%
- Normal red blood cell morphology

*Abnormal*
- Prothrombin time is prolonged
- Anemia is frequently present (hemoglobin and hematocrit below normal range)
- Red blood cell morphology may be altered secondary to hyposplenism
- Leukopenia and thrombocytopenia may occur, but are less common

*Cause of abnormal result*
- Prothrombin time prolonged due to malabsorption of vitamin K
- Anemia in celiac disease commonly due to iron deficiency, folate deficiency or, rarely, vitamin B12 deficiency
- Red blood cell morphology altered depending on the cause of anemia
- Leukopenia and thrombocytopenia occur if there is severe folate or vitamin B12 deficiency

## Biopsy
SMALL-BOWEL BIOPSY
*Description*
Small-bowel biopsy specimen obtained by endoscopy or suction biopsy tube, and is the standard diagnostic technique for celiac disease.

*Advantages/Disadvantages*
Disadvantage: several biopsy specimens must be obtained for proper diagnosis. Ideally, the correct orientation of the biopsy sample before sampling should be achieved.

*Abnormal*
Findings that indicate the presence of celiac disease:
- Absent, shortened, or flattened villi; hyperplasia and lengthening of crypts; infiltration of plasma cells and lymphocytes in the lamina propria
- Resolution of changes within one year on a strict gluten-free diet
- Scalloping of duodenal folds has been observed on endoscopy in some patients with celiac disease

## Imaging
X-RAY
*Advantages/Disadvantages*
- Advantage: radiographic examination after a barium meal reveals abnormal findings such as dilation of lumen, edema, and flattening of mucosal folds
- Disadvantage: radiography not as sensitive as intestinal biopsy; patients with mild celiac disease often have normal barium contrast studies of the small intestine

*Abnormal*
- Dilation of small intestine and altered mucosal folds
- In patients with mild to moderate disease, the mucosal pattern is distorted in the proximal small intestine, but the ileal region is normal
- In severe disease, the mucosal pattern is abnormal throughout the small intestine

## TREATMENT

### CONSIDER CONSULT
- Refer to a gastroenterologist for endoscopy/biopsy if other intestinal disorders are suspected
- Refer to a dietitian/nutritionist for counseling on a gluten-free diet
- Refer to a celiac support group for help/advice in maintaining adherence to a gluten-free diet
- Refer for screening for vitamin and mineral deficiencies

### IMMEDIATE ACTION
Withdrawal of gluten-containing foods from the diet.

### PATIENT AND CAREGIVER ISSUES
#### Health-seeking behavior
**Has the patient been self-medicating?** Patients may self-medicate with antidiarrheals to treat the diarrhea, not realizing the underlying problem is a food intolerance, so they do not often consult a doctor in the early stages.

### MANAGEMENT ISSUES
#### Goals
- To alleviate the symptoms of celiac disease
- To prevent recurrences of the disease

#### Management in special circumstances
COEXISTING DISEASE
- Because many patients with celiac disease have secondary lactase deficiency, these patients must be on a lactose-free diet in addition to a gluten-free diet. Such eating restrictions may result in noncompliance
- There is an increased frequency of celiac disease in patients with diabetes mellitus type 1: management choices must be consistent with diabetic therapy

COEXISTING MEDICATION
Caution should be exercised in management of refractory celiac disease, because prednisone may interact with antidiabetic agents and increase blood sugar in those patients with concomitant diabetes mellitus type 1.

SPECIAL PATIENT GROUPS
Infants/children:
- Nutritional deficiencies must be corrected as needed to ensure continued growth and development of the child
- Children reaching adolescence may outgrow intolerance to wheat but should be cautioned to be aware of signs of recurrence in later life

PATIENT SATISFACTION/LIFESTYLE PRIORITIES
- General fatigue and weakness associated with celiac disease may prevent patients from carrying out normal activities of daily living
- Chronic diarrhea will impair quality of life and may result in psychological symptoms, such as depression
- Gluten-free (and lactose-free) diets may be difficult to adhere to

### SUMMARY OF THERAPEUTIC OPTIONS
#### Choices
- In patients with celiac disease immediate initiation of a gluten-free diet (avoidance of wheat, barley, and rye) is indicated (lifestyle). The patient will need expert dietitian counseling because

- gluten is ubiquitous in modern Western diets (e.g. it may be assumed that 'hydrolyzed vegetable protein' contains gluten). Hence, this diet is very difficult to adhere to
- A lactose-free diet should be initiated because of secondary lactase deficiency. Lactose may be reintroduced once the mucosa has had time to heal on a gluten-free diet
- Supplemental calcium carbonate and vitamin D (ergocalciferol) should be administered to patients with calcium deficiency who are at risk of developing osteopenia
- Supplemental iron, potassium, and folate should be given as needed to correct nutritional deficiencies. Note it may be necessary to replenish a patient's iron stores with intravenous iron. Clearly, this should be done under medical supervision with the newer preparations that have become available
- Parenteral potassium chloride corrects hypokalemia
- In cases of tetany, intravenous calcium gluconate should be administered; hypomagnesemia should be corrected before hypocalcemia is treated
- For patients with refractory disease, oral prednisone is useful; such patients should be managed by a specialist
- Some reports suggest that immunosuppressive therapy with azathioprine or cyclosporine may be useful in refractory cases; these patients should be managed by a specialist. Immunosuppressive drug therapy is rarely necessary

### Clinical pearls
- Think of this diagnosis in seniors, who may develop this digestive deficiency as part of aging
- Removal of gluten from the diet almost always leads to clinical improvement
- Secondary lactase deficiency takes 1–2 months to resolve
- Small-bowel biopsy should be repeated, particularly if the patient does not improve on a gluten-free diet, to reconfirm the diagnosis of celiac disease and to rule out lymphoma or malignancy
- Dermatitis herpetiformis should improve on gluten withdrawal

### Never
Do not attribute anemia in a young woman to heavy menses without considering celiac disease.

## FOLLOW UP
### Plan for review
- Initiate gluten-free diet
- If the patient has failed to respond symptomatically to a gluten-free diet after 6–8 weeks, then the patient's dietary intake must be meticulously monitored for noncompliance
- If the patient is still not responding to a gluten-free diet after strict adherence to it, monitor for causative agents other than gluten products
- Those patients who do not respond should be referred to a specialist
- Monitor periodically for nutritional deficiencies and correct with supplements, as needed
- It is customary to repeat endoscopy/biopsy after one year on a gluten-free diet (histologic resolution lags behind clinical improvement)

### Information for patient or caregiver
- Patients must be instructed on how to follow a gluten-free diet and that lifelong adherence to the diet is necessary to prevent recurrence
- Self-help and support groups are available
- Prognosis is good with adherence to a gluten-free diet
- Children reaching adolescence may outgrow intolerance to gluten; caution should be taken to maintain gluten-free diet to prevent recurrences later in life

# DRUGS AND OTHER THERAPIES: DETAILS
## Drugs
PREDNISONE

*Dose*
- 40–60mg/day, orally, gradually tapered
- The dose should be individualized

*Efficacy*
Long-term treatment is helpful to some patients with refractory celiac disease. Should be managed by a specialist to ensure that lymphoma is not missed. May also be necessary for emergent treatment of the rare gliadin shock, which is occasionally observed when treated patients are given a gluten challenge.

*Risks/benefits*
Risks:
- Use caution when administering to patients with congestive heart failure, diabetes mellitus, glaucoma, renal disease, ulcerative colitis, peptic ulcer
- Use caution when administering to the elderly
- Prednisone taken in doses higher than 7.5mg for a period of 3 weeks or longer may lead to clinically relevant suppression of the pituitary-adrenal axis

*Side effects and adverse reactions*
- Side effects are minimized by short duration of therapy
- Cardiovascular system: hypertension, thromboembolism
- Central nervous system: insomnia, euphoria, depression, psychosis, seizures
- Endocrine: adrenal suppression, impaired glucose tolerance, growth suppression in children
- Eyes, ears, nose, and throat: cataract, glaucoma, blurred vision
- Gastrointestinal: dyspepsia, peptic ulceration, esophagitis, oral candidiasis
- Musculoskeletal: proximal myopathy, osteoporosis
- Skin: delayed healing, acne, striae, fragile skin

*Interactions (other drugs)*
- Aminoglutethimide (increased clearance of prednisone) - Antidiabetics (hypoglycemic effect inhibited) - Antihypertensives (effects inhibited) - Barbiturates (increased clearance of prednisone) - Cardiac glycosides (toxicity increased) - Cholestyramine, colestipol (may reduce absorption of corticosteroids) - Clarithromycin, erythromycin, troleandomycin (may enhance steroid effect) - Cyclosporine (may increase levels of both drugs; may cause seizures) - Diuretics (effects inhibited) - Isoniazid (reduced plasma levels of isoniazid) - Ketoconazole - Nonsteroidal anti-inflammatory drugs (increased risks of bleeding) - Oral contraceptives (enhanced effects of corticosteroids) - Rifampin (may inhibit hepatic clearance of prednisone) - Salicylates (increased clearance of salicylates) - Warfarin (alters clotting time)

*Contraindications*
- Systemic infection - Avoid live virus vaccines in those receiving immunosuppressive doses
- History of tuberculosis - Cushing's syndrome - Recent myocardial infarction

*Acceptability to patient*
High.

*Follow up plan*
Taper dose and follow-up to monitor response. If the patient fails to respond, then consider whether a toxin other than gluten is responsible for the disorder or another disorder, and refer to a gastroenterologist for re-evaluation.

## CYCLOSPORINE
This is an off-label indication.

*Dose*
Adults and children: initial oral dose of 1.25mg/kg twice daily, titrated very gradually to a maximum dose of 4mg/kg/day.

*Efficacy*
There are anecdotal reports that it is effective in the treatment of refractory celiac disease.

*Risks/benefits*
Risks:
- Increased susceptibility to infection and possible development of neoplasia
- Bacterial, fungal, viral, and protozoal infections often occur and can be fatal
- Avoid excessive sunlight
- Use caution in hypertension, and hepatic or biliary tract disease
- Use caution in children and the elderly
- Recent vaccinations will be rendered ineffective

Benefits: has no depressant effects on bone marrow.

*Side effects and adverse reactions*
- Cardiovascular system: hypertension
- Central nervous system: tremors, seizures, encephalopathy, confusion, depression, headache, dizziness, insomnia, paresthesias, fever
- Eyes, ears, nose, and throat: gingival hyperplasia
- Gastrointestinal: nausea, vomiting, diarrhea, elevated hepatic enzymes, hepatotoxicity, abdominal pain, gingivitis, stomatitis, anorexia, dyspepsia, flatulence
- Genitourinary: nephrotoxicity, hyperuricemia, menstrual irregularity, spermatogenesis inhibition, gynecomastia
- Hematologic: thrombotic thrombocytopenic purpura, leukopenia
- Metabolic: hyperkalemia, hypercholesterolemia, hypomagnesemia, hyperglycemia
- Musculoskeletal: arthralgia, fatigue, weakness, dysarthria, myalgia
- Skin: hirsutism, acne, alopecia, rash, skin ulcers, flushing

*Interactions (other drugs)*
- Drugs utilizing cytochrome P-450 to be metabolized ■ Allopurinol, colchicine ■ Antidysrhythmics (amiodarone, calcium channel blockers, digoxin) ■ Antihypertensives (angiotensin-converting enzyme [ACE] inhibitors, acetazolamide, carvedilol, clonidine, potassium sparing diuretics) ■ Antivirals (acyclovir, ganciclovir, antiretroviral protease inhibitors, foscarnet, nevirapine, delavirdine) ■ Antibiotics (aminoglycosides, ceftriaxone, ciprofloxacin, clarithromycin, clindamycin, erythromycin, dalfopristin, quinupristin, imipenem; cilastatin, nafcillin, norfloxacin, polymyxin B, sulfamethoxazole; trimethoprim, troleandomycin, vancomycin, sulfonamides) ■ Antifungals (amphotericin B, bacitracin, fluconazole, itraconazole, ketoconazole, griseofulvin) ■ Anticonvulsants (carbamazepine, fosphenytoin, phenobarbital, phenytoin, primidone) ■ Antineoplastics (daunorubicin, doxorubicin, epirubicin, docetaxel, etoposide (VP-16), melphalan, mitoxantrone, paclitaxel) ■ Antilipemics (fenofibrate, statins, probucol) ■ Antidiabetics (glipizide, glyburide, pioglitazone, troglitazone)
- Antidepressants (fluoxetine, fluvoxamine, nefazodone, St John's Wort) ■ Androgens
- Bromocriptine ■ Cisplatin ■ Corticosteroids ■ Creatine ■ Danazol ■ Estrogens
- Immunosuppressives ■ Methotrexate ■ Metoclopramide ■ Misoprostol ■ Modafinil
- Mycophenolate ■ Neuromuscular blockers ■ Nonsteroidal anti-inflammatory drugs (NSAIDs)

- Omeprazole, rabeprazole ■ Orlistat ■ Rifampin ■ Sirolimus ■ Tacrolimus ■ Vinca alkaloids
- Warfarin

Other:
- Food (decreases cyclosporine levels) ■ Grapefruit juice (increases cyclosporine levels)

*Contraindications*
- PUVA (psoriasis patients are at increased risk of developing skin cancer with this treatment)
- Rheumatoid arthritis ■ Renal impairment ■ Known polyoxyethylated castor oil hypersensitivity ■ Pregnancy and breast-feeding

*Acceptability to patient*
High.

## CALCIUM SUPPLEMENTATION
Calcium carbonate or calcium gluconate.

*Dose*
- Calcium carbonate: usual adult dose 2–3g/day (of elemental calcium) in two divided doses
- Calcium gluconate: dose dependent on individual requirements; usual adult dose 500mg–2g intravenously (slowly); usual pediatric dose 500mg/kg/day or $12g/m^2$/day, well diluted and given very slowly in divided doses

*Efficacy*
- Calcium carbonate is effective in treating calcium deficiency associated with celiac disease, and in preventing osteopenia
- Calcium gluconate is effective in treating tetany caused by severe hypocalcemia in celiac disease

*Risks/benefits*
Risks:
- Use caution when administering to patients with mild hypercalciuria or renal disease
- Use caution when administering to the elderly
- Risk of overcorrection resulting in hypercalcemia

*Side effects and adverse reactions*
Calcium carbonate:
- Cardiovascular system: dysrhythmias, hypotension, bradycardia, cardiac arrest
- Gastrointestinal: anorexia, constipation, nausea, vomiting
- Genitourinary: renal dysfunction and failure
- Metabolic: hypercalcemia

Calcium gluconate:
- Cardiovascular: bradycardia, cardiac arrest, dysrhythmias, heart block, hemorrhage, hypotension, rebound hypertension, shortened Q-T
- Gastrointestinal: anorexia, constipation, diarrhea, eructation, flatulence, nausea, obstruction, rebound hyperacidity, vomiting
- Genitourinary: renal dysfunction, renal failure, renal stones
- Metabolic: hypercalcemia (drowsiness, lethargy, muscle weakness, headache, constipation, coma, anorexia, nausea, vomiting, polyuria, thirst), metabolic alkalosis, milk-alkali syndrome (nausea, vomiting, disorientation, headache)
- Other: burning at intravenous site, extravasation, necrosis, pain, severe venous thrombosis

*Interactions (other drugs)*
- ACE inhibitors ■ Antacids ■ Antibiotics (azithromycin, fluoroquinolone derivatives, tetracyclines) ■ Anticonvulsants (gabapentin, phenytoin) ■ Antidysrhythmics (cardiac glycosides, quinidine, calcium channel blockers) ■ Antifungals ■ Antituberculosis drugs (isoniazid, rifampin) ■ Bisphosphonates ■ Chloroquine ■ Cholestyramine ■ Colestipol ■ Diuretics, thiazide ■ Fexofenadine ■ Orlistat ■ Phenothiazines ■ NSAIDs (aspirin, diflunisal) ■ Zalcitabine

*Contraindications*
- Hypercalcemia ■ Severe hypercalciuria ■ Renal calculi ■ Hyperparathyroidism ■ Metatastic calcification ■ Digitalis therapy ■ Ventricular fibrillation ■ Sarcoidosis ■ Hypervitaminosis D ■ Hyperphosphatemia

*Acceptability to patient*
High.

*Follow up plan*
Serum calcium levels need to be monitored to prevent hypercalcemia.

## AZATHIOPRINE
This is an off-label indication.

*Dose*
- Initial dose of 1mg/kg/day in one dose or two equally divided doses
- Dose may be titrated very slowly (e.g. dose increments or reductions of 0.5mg/kg/day)
- Maximum dose 2.5mg/kg/day
- Off-label indication; doses should be individualized

*Efficacy*
Effective in refractory celiac disease.

*Risks/benefits*
Risks:
- Use caution when administering to patients with bone marrow depression and infection, or renal or hepatic impairment
- Severe blood cell disorders may occur
- May increase risk of neoplasia

*Side effects and adverse reactions*
- Gastrointestinal: nausea, vomiting, diarrhea, abdominal pain, hepatic failure, jaundice
- Genitourinary: depression of spermatogenensis
- Hematologic: anemia, leukopenia, pancytopenia, thrombocytopenia
- Musculoskeletal: arthralgia, myalgia, malaise
- Skin: rash, alopecia
- Other: fungal, bacterial, protozoal, and viral infections may increase risk of neoplasm (skin cancer, reticulocyte, or lymphomatous tumors)

*Interactions (other drugs)*
- ACE inhibitors ■ Allopurinol ■ Anticoagulants ■ Carbamazepine ■ Clozapine ■ Co-trimoxazole (trimethoprim and sulfamethoxazole) ■ Cyclosporine ■ Methotrexate ■ Nondepolarizing muscle blockers ■ Vaccines ■ Warfarin

*Contraindications*
- Intramuscular injections ■ Pregnancy or breast-feeding ■ Vaccines

*Acceptability to patient*
High.

## VITAMIN D (ERGOCALCIFEROL)
This is an off-label indication.

*Dose*
- Dosage must be individualized
- 10–100mcg/day orally; up to 2.5mg/day in severe malabsorption

*Efficacy*
Effective in treating vitamin D deficiency caused by celiac disease, and in prevention of osteopenia.

*Risks/benefits*
Risks:
- Overtreatment may be harmful, and serum calcium levels must be monitored to prevent hypercalcemia
- The therapeutic range is narrow
- Use caution in cardiac disease, arteriosclerosis, renal disease, kidney stones, sarcoidosis and other granulomatous diseases, hypoparathyroidism
- Use caution in pregnancy and breast-feeding

*Side effects and adverse reactions*
- Cardiovascular system: dysrhythmias, hypertension
- Central nervous system: anorexia, overt psychosis, headache, hyperthermia
- Gastrointestinal: nausea, vomiting, pancreatitis, constipation, dry mouth
- Genitourinary: decreased libido, nocturia, and polyuria
- Metabolic: hypercholesterolemia, mild acidosis, hyperphosphatemia, vitaminosis D, hypercalcemia
- Musculoskeletal: muscle and bone pain

*Interactions (other drugs)*
- Antacids, magnesium, calcium salts - Anticonvulsants (phenobarbital, phenytoin, primidone, carbamazepine, barbiturates) - Cardiac glycosides - Cholestyramine, colestipol, mineral oil, orlistat - Phosphorus salts - Thiazide diuretics - Vitamin D analogs

*Contraindications*
- Hypercalcemia - Hypervitaminosis D - Hyperphosphatemia - Metastatic calcification

*Acceptability to patient*
High.

*Follow up plan*
Monitor for serum calcium levels, because hypercalcemia may occur.

## POTASSIUM SUPPLEMENTS
Potassium chloride or other potassium salts.

*Dose*
- Parenteral potassium chloride used in severe hypokalemia; salts such as gluconate, acetate, or bicarbonate used in less severe hypokalemia
- Oral potassium for prevention of hypokalemia: usual adult dose 20mEq/day
- Oral potassium for potassium depletion: usual adult dose 40–100mEq/day (although more may be required), given in divided doses not to exceed 20mEq/dose

- Intravenous potassium: if serum potassium is >2.5mEq/L, potassium should be given at a rate not to exceed 10mEq/h in a concentration <30mEq/L. In cases of severe potassium deficiency faster rates and greater concentrations (usually up to 40mEq/L) may be indicated

*Efficacy*
Used for treatment of hypokalemia due to celiac disease.

*Risks/benefits*
Risks:
- Use caution when administering to patients with cardiac disease, renal impairment, systemic acidosis, adrenal insufficiency
- Use caution when administering to patients using concurrent treatment with potassium-sparing diuretics, or to patients with acute dehydration or diarrhea, severe burns, heat or muscle cramps
- Use caution when administering to the elderly

*Side effects and adverse reactions*
- Cardiovascular system: ECG changes, arrhythmias, hypotension, atrioventricular block, cardiac arrest
- Central nervous system: paresthesias, confusion, shock
- Gastrointestinal: nausea, vomiting, abdominal pain, diarrhea, gastrointestinal bleeding, esophageal/small-bowel ulceration
- Metabolic: hyperkalemia, metabolic acidosis
- Musculoskeletal: weakness

*Interactions (other drugs)*
- ACE inhibitors - Aluminum-containing antacids - Amphotericin B - Angiotensin II receptor antagonists - Antimuscarinics - Beta-blockers - Cardiac glycosides - Cyclosporine - Disopyramide - Diuretics (potassium sparing, loop, thiazide) - H1 antagonists - Heparin - Hypoglycemics - Loperamide - NSAIDs - Opiate agonists - Penicillins - Phenothiazines - Quinidine - Sodium polystyrene sulfonate - Tricyclic antidepressants

*Contraindications*
- Aluminum toxicity - Heart failure - Severe renal disease - Hyperkalemia - Dehydration - Peptic ulcer disease - Concentrated potassium solution given intravenously is fatal, always dilute - Gastrointestinal/esophageal obstruction - Sodium polystyrene sulfonate - Severe hemolytic reactions

*Acceptability to patient*
High.

## IRON SALT SUPPLEMENTS
*Dose*
- Adults: the equivalent of 50–200mg elemental iron per day
- Children: the equivalent of 50mg elemental iron per day

*Efficacy*
May be effective in the treatment of iron-deficiency anemia caused by celiac disease; patients who do not adhere to a gluten-free diet may not respond to oral iron.

*Risks/benefits*
Risks:
- The treatment of any anemic condition should be under the advice and supervision of a physician

- As oral iron products interfere with absorption of oral tetracycline antibiotics, these products should not be taken within 2h of each other
- Accidental overdose of iron-containing products is a leading cause of fatal poisoning in children under 6

Benefits:
- Oral medication that is usually tolerated with food
- Subjective improvement in symptoms may occur within days

*Side effects and adverse reactions*
Gastrointestinal: nausea, vomiting, bloating, abdominal discomfort, black stools, diarrhea, constipation (leading to colic), anorexia.

*Interactions (other drugs)*
- Alkalinizers ■ Antacids ■ Calcium carbonate ■ Chloramphenicol ■ Cimetidine
- Doxycycline ■ Famotidine ■ Levodopa ■ Methyldopa ■ Nizatidine ■ Quinolones
- Pancreatic enzymes ■ Penicillamine ■ Ranitidine ■ Tetracycline ■ Vitamin E

*Contraindications*
- Hypersensitivity to iron or any component of treatment ■ Ulcerative colitis ■ Regional enteritis ■ Hemosiderosis ■ Hemochromatosis ■ Hemolytic anemia

*Acceptability to patient*
High.

## FOLATE SUPPLEMENTS
*Dose*
- Usual therapeutic dose for folic acid deficiency: up to 1mg/day for adults and children (regardless of age); resistant cases may require larger doses
- Once deficiency has subsided, usual maintenance doses are: 0.1mg/day for infants, 0.3mg/day for children aged 4 and under, 0.4mg/day for adults and children aged over 4 years, 0.8mg/day for pregnant and breast-feeding women
- Intravenous, intramuscular, or subcutaneous therapy can be used in very severe or resistant cases

*Efficacy*
May be effective in the treatment of folic acid deficiency in patients with celiac disease; patients who do not adhere to a gluten-free diet may not respond to oral folate.

*Risks/benefits*
Risks: use caution when administering to patients with undiagnosed anemia.

*Side effects and adverse reactions*
- Respiratory: bronchospasm (rare)
- Skin: itching and rash

*Interactions (other drugs)*
- Anticonvulsants ■ Cholestyramine ■ Colestipol ■ Colchicine ■ Fluoxetine ■ Lithium
- Lometrexol ■ Metformin ■ Methotrexate ■ NSAIDs ■ Phenobarbital ■ Phenytoin
- Pyrimethamine ■ Sulfasalazine

*Contraindications*
Hypersensitivity to folic acid.

*Acceptability to patient*
High.

*Follow up plan*
Monitor serum folate concentrations; concentrations less than 0.002mcg/mL usually result in megaloblastic anemia.

## LIFESTYLE
Diet.

### RISKS/BENEFITS
- Risks: continuation of a diet of gluten-containing foods will lead to persistent symptoms and nutritional deficiencies
- Benefits: removal of toxic gluten is absolutely essential to the treatment of celiac disease

### ACCEPTABILITY TO PATIENT
Poor. Compliance with a gluten-free diet is difficult to achieve and maintain due to the vast number of foods containing gluten. Many celiac patients have secondary lactase deficiency and must follow a lactose-free diet in addition to a gluten-free diet, thus limiting their choice of foods further.

### FOLLOW UP PLAN
- Monitor patients after initiation of gluten-free (and lactose-free) diet
- By definition, celiac patients should respond to gluten withdrawal. If there is no symptomatic response to withdrawal of gluten after 6–8 weeks, the dietary intake must be meticulously monitored for any trace amounts of gluten
- Truly refractory celiac disease is uncommon but may respond to treatment with prednisone or immunosuppressive therapy with azathioprine and/or cyclosporine
- Celiac disease that becomes refractory years after initiation of a gluten-free diet raises concern that a complication has developed (e.g. collagenous sprue, refractory sprue, ulcerative jejunoileitis, or enteropathy-associated T-cell lymphoma)
- If there is no response after absolute gluten withdrawal, refer to gastroenterologist for the possibility of overlooked intestinal infection, other food intolerances, or an alternative diagnosis

### PATIENT AND CAREGIVER INFORMATION
Lifelong adherence to a gluten-free diet is necessary to treat and prevent recurrences of celiac disease.

## OUTCOMES

### EFFICACY OF THERAPIES
Withdrawal of gluten from the diet usually results in clinical improvement within 2 weeks.

### Review period
Initial review following institution of gluten-free diet is 6–8 weeks.

### PROGNOSIS
- Prognosis of correctly diagnosed celiac disease is good with strict adherence to a gluten-free diet. However, the prognosis for patients with refractory sprue is poorer (Robert ME, Ament ME, Weinstein WM. The histologic spectrum and clinical outcome of refractory and unclassified sprue. Am J Surg Pathol 2000;24:676–87)
- Absorptive defects disappear promptly in infants and children following institution of a gluten-free diet

### Clinical pearls
- Regular nutritional evaluation and membership of support groups affects prognosis in a positive way because symptoms and nutritional deficiencies are largely reversible
- Patients need to be reminded of the importance of lifelong gluten abstinence. This is because they tend to believe that they do not have the disease when most symptoms disappear on appropriate therapy
- A decrease in titer of antiendomysial IgA antibody is an indicator that the patient is adherent to the gluten-free diet and that the disease is in remission
- Lymphoma is a complication of long-standing celiac disease and should be kept in mind when symptoms recur despite strict adherence to a gluten-free diet

### Therapeutic failure
- Oral prednisone or immunosuppressive therapy with azathioprine and/or cyclosporine may be effective in the treatment of celiac disease not responding to gluten withdrawal
- Removal of oats and proteins (egg, soy, poultry, and fish) sequentially in the diet may help

### Recurrence
- Lifelong avoidance of all gluten-containing products prevents recurrence
- Celiac disease may diminish as the affected child approaches adolescence, with the result that adherence to gluten-free diet wanes without ill-effects, initially. These patients remain intolerant to gluten, however, and most patients will develop recurrent celiac disease in later life if gluten consumption continues

### Deterioration
If not recognized and treated, celiac patients will develop severe malnutrition and debilitation.

### Terminal illness
Advanced malnutrition and debilitation as a result of untreated celiac disease may result in hemorrhage and intercurrent infections with fatal results.

### COMPLICATIONS
- Refractory celiac disease: disease becomes refractory to gluten withdrawal. Some of these patients respond to prednisone or immunosuppressives, whereas others develop progressive malabsorption. A small number of patients develop collagenous sprue, in which collagen deposits underneath the surface epithelium
- Malignancy: celiac patients are at an increased risk for intestinal T-cell lymphomas and some carcinomas (e.g. esophageal cancer). Some reports indicate that malignant disease develops in

10–13% of celiac patients; strict adherence to a gluten-free diet may lessen the risk of malignancy
- Ulceration of the small intestine (ulcerative jejunoileitis)
- Osteoporosis secondary to reduced calcium and vitamin D absorption
- Reproductive disorders such as infertility, amenorrhea, spontaneous abortions
- Hemorrhages

## CONSIDER CONSULT

Patients with celiac disease who are unresponsive to gluten withdrawal and corticosteroid or immunosuppressive treatment should be referred for re-evaluation to establish whether there is a complication, such as malignancy.

# PREVENTION

Celiac disease in susceptible individuals can only be successfully prevented by strict avoidance of all gluten-containing foods.

## RISK FACTORS

- **Diet**: celiac disease results from sensitivity to alcohol-soluble prolamins found in wheat, barley, and rye
- **Family history**: predisposition to gluten sensitivity has been mapped to HLA-D region on chromosome 6

## MODIFY RISK FACTORS
### Lifestyle and wellness
DIET
Avoidance of all gluten-containing products necessary to prevent celiac disease in susceptible individuals.

FAMILY HISTORY
Individuals with family members affected by celiac disease should be serologically screened to assess whether disease is present.

## SCREENING
SEROLOGIC SCREENING
Serologic screening for antibodies reactive to gliadin, endomysium, and tissue transglutaminase may be used to select for individuals who may require small-bowel histologic investigations.

HISTOLOGY
- For diagnosis of celiac disease and before a prescription for a gluten-free diet can be issued, clear histologic changes in the small bowel must be demonstrated
- Histologic examination of the small intestine must be performed in addition to serologic screening
- A diagnosis of celiac disease is confirmed when symptoms and small-bowel histology improve when gluten is withdrawn

## PREVENT RECURRENCE
Strict adherence to gluten-free diet prevents recurrence.

### Reassess coexisting disease
In patients with secondary lactose deficiency, lactose intolerance may be reassessed once symptoms disappear after gluten and lactose withdrawal. Lactose intolerance can be confirmed by the hydrogen breath test.

PATIENT SATISFACTION/LIFESTYLE PRIORITIES
Adherence and compliance to a gluten-free diet is difficult but must be maintained if the patient is to remain symptom-free.

# RESOURCES

## ASSOCIATIONS

**Gluten Intolerance Group of North America**
15110 10th Ave S.W.
Suite A
Seattle, WA 98166
Tel: (206) 246-6652
Fax: (206) 246-6531
http://www.gluten.net/

**Celiac Sprue Association**
CSA/USA
PO Box 31700
Omaha, NE 68131-0700
Tel: (402) 558-0600
Fax: (402) 558-1347
http://www.csaceliacs.org

**Celiac Disease Foundation**
13251 Ventura Boulevard
Suite 1
Studio City, CA 91604
Tel: (818) 990-2354
Fax: (818) 990-2379
http://www.celiac.org

**American Celiac Society-Dietary Support Coalition**
59 Crystal Avenue
West Orange, NJ 07052
Tel: (973) 325-8837
Fax: (973) 669-8808
E-mail: bentleac@umdnj.edu

## KEY REFERENCES

- Bernstein EF, Whitington PF. Successful treatment of atypical sprue in an infant with cyclosporine. Gastroenterology 1988;95:199–204
- Ciacci C, Maurelli L, Klain M, et al. Effects of dietary treatment on bone mineral density in adults with celiac disease: factors predicting response. Am J Gastroenterol 1997;92:992–6
- Farrell RJ, Kelly CP. Celiac sprue. N Engl J Med 2002;346:180–8
- Farrell RJ, Kelly CP. Celiac sprue and refractory sprue. In: Feldman M, Friedman LS, Sleisenger MH, eds. Sleisenger & Fordtran's gastrointestinal and liver disease, 7th edn. Philadelphia: WB Saunders, 2002
- Mautalen C, Gonzalez D, Mazure R, et al. Effect of treatment on bone mass, mineral metabolism, and body composition in untreated celiac disease patients. Am J Gastroenterol 1997;92:313–8
- Trier JS, Falchuk ZM, Carey MC, Schreiber DS. Celiac sprue and refractory sprue. Gastroenterology 1978;75:307–16
- Vaidya A, Bolanos J, Berkelhammer C. Azathioprine in refractory sprue. Am J Gastroenterol 1999;94:1967–9

## FAQS

### Question 1
Does a patient have to have diarrhea to have celiac disease?

ANSWER 1
Absolutely not. It is quite common for patients to present with several nonspecific complaints, including fatigue, and have a long history of anemia only.

## Question 2
What is tissue transglutaminase and how is it connected to celiac disease?

### ANSWER 2
The antigen to which endomysial antibodies are directed is an enzyme called tissue transglutaminase. Tissue transglutaminase crosslinks gliadin peptides to itself, and it is to this modified enzyme that patients develop antibodies.

## Question 3
Why do patients with celiac disease have to adhere to their strict gluten-free diet?

### ANSWER 3
Reasons include better levels of iron, vitamins D, E, A, K, calcium absorption, resolution of diarrhea, decreased risk of seizure, among other factors. There is a controversy as to whether a gluten-free diet decreases the risk for intestinal lymphoma (and other malignancies); one prospective cohort study demonstrated that it does.

## CONTRIBUTORS
Joseph E Scherger, MD, MPH
Lawrence S Friedman, MD
Vijay Yajnik, MD
J Adrian Lunn, MD

# CHOLECYSTITIS

| | |
|---|---|
| ■ Summary Information | 74 |
| ■ Background | 75 |
| ■ Diagnosis | 77 |
| ■ Treatment | 88 |
| ■ Outcomes | 95 |
| ■ Prevention | 97 |
| ■ Resources | 99 |

## SUMMARY INFORMATION

### DESCRIPTION
Calculous cholecystitis:
- Persistent steady pain for more than one day in the epigastrium or right upper quadrant
- Fever and chills
- Nausea and/or vomiting (>70%)
- Murphy's sign
- Palpable gallbladder (20%)

Acalculous cholecystitis:
- Unexplained fever
- Leukocytosis
- Initial signs or symptoms referable to the right upper quadrant are typically missing (these patients often have vague abdominal pain)
- Thickened gallbladder wall with pericholecystic fluid in the absence of ascites or hypoalbuminemia at ultrasound or computed tomography scan
- Acute acalculous cholecystitis can be more fulminant than stone-related cholecystitis

### URGENT ACTION
- Immediate surgery is indicated if patient presents with suspected gangrenous cholecystitis, perforation with peritonitis, or pericholecystic abscess
- Complications in acute acalculous cholecystitis develop rapidly and early diagnosis is critical. High suspicion of biliary tract sepsis should be kept in mind for early treatment
- Intravenous fluids with broad-spectrum antibiotics may be indicated if patient appears to be dehydrated, has fever, appears to have acalculous cholecystitis, or there is suspicion of sepsis

### KEY! DON'T MISS!
- Patients can experience postcholecystectomy cholecystitis pain syndrome due to dysfunction of the sphincter of Oddi
- Complications of acute untreated cholecystitis include gallbladder empyema and perforation, which can be fatal
- Acute myocardial infarction can present with epigastric pain. All patients presenting with epigastric pain should be investigated with an ECG
- Ascending cholangitis should be differentiated from cholecystitis

# BACKGROUND

## ICD9 CODE
- 575.0 Acute cholecystitis
- 574.0 Calculus of the gallbladder with acute cholecystitis
- 575.1 Cholecystitis without mention of calculus

## SYNONYMS
Gallbladder attack.

## CARDINAL FEATURES
Calculous cholecystitis:
- Defined as acute or chronic inflammation of the gallbladder due to cystic duct obstruction secondary to the presence of gallstones (bile duct stricture or neoplasm may also be causative)
- Occurs most frequently in women over the age of 50 years
- Typical signs are prolonged right upper quadrant or epigastric pain with fever and leukocytosis
- Most frequently diagnosed on the basis of clinical manifestations, combined with imaging studies (usually right upper quadrant ultrasound)
- Optimal treatment typically involves removal of the gallbladder by cholecystectomy

Acalculous cholecystitis:
- Defined as acute inflammation of the gallbladder in the absence of gallstones
- Occurs most frequently in critically ill patients and the bedridden elderly
- Typical physical findings include unexplained fever, leukocytosis, or vague abdominal discomfort
- Symptoms or signs referable directly to the right upper quadrant are initially absent in 75% of cases
- Most frequently diagnosed by ultrasound or computed tomography scans of the right upper quadrant
- Definitive treatment is cholecystectomy with drainage of any associated abscess; if the patient is unstable, then percutaneous cholecystostomy may be indicated

## CAUSES
Common causes
- Gallstones (calculous cholecystitis), which are cholesterol stones, mixed stones, or pigment stones (the first two account for 80% of the total)
- Ischemic damage to gallbladder (acalculous cholecystitis): seen most frequently in critically ill patients
- Pigment stones secondary to hemolytic conditions (e.g. sickle cell anemia)

Rare causes
- Neoplasms, primary or metastatic in classification
- Infectious agents (cytomegalovirus, *Cryptosporidium* spp.) causing acalculous cholecystitis, seen most frequently in immunocompromised patients (e.g. AIDS). *Campylobacter jejuni*, *Clostridium perfringens*, *Vibrio cholerae*, leptospirosis, and typhoid fever can cause acalculous cholecystitis in immunocompetent individuals
- Xanthogranulomatous cholecystitis: destructive, inflammatory disease of the gallbladder characterized by either a diffuse or a focal inflammatory process with lipid-laden macrophages, inflammatory cells, and fibrous tissue (diagnosed by pathology after cholecystectomy)

Contributory or predisposing factors
- Hemolytic disease may cause pigment stones

- Birth control pill or other estrogen use predisposes to gallstone formation by causing gallbladder hypomotility and by affecting cholesterol and bile-salt metabolism
- Alcoholic liver disease is associated with an increased incidence of pigment stones
- Cirrhosis decreases bile acid secretion and thus increases gallstone formation
- Total parenteral nutrition causes stones by inducing gallbladder hypomotility
- Prolonged starvation/fasting causes gallbladder hypomotility
- Obesity and rapid weight loss predispose to stone formation
- Terminal ileal disease leads to decreased reabsorption of bile acids and increased gallstone production
- Pregnancy is a risk factor for gallstone formation
- Elevated triglycerides and pancreatitis predispose to cholelithiasis

## EPIDEMIOLOGY
### Incidence and prevalence
FREQUENCY
- Calculous cholecystitis: 0.6% of general population
- Acalculous cholecystitis: 0.03–0.06% of general population (5–10% of cholecystitis population)

### Demographics
AGE
- Calculous cholecystitis: most common in those over age 50 years
- Acalculous cholecystitis: most common in those over age 50 years

GENDER
- Calculous cholecystitis: greater prevalence in females
- Acalculous cholecystitis: greater prevalence in males

RACE
Calculous cholecystitis is more prevalent among Native Americans (Pima Indians) and Caucasians (Scandinavians), and less prevalent among African-Americans and Asians.

GENETICS
- Calculous cholecystitis: apolipoprotein E4 genotype is linked with an increase in intestinal absorption of cholesterol and development of gallstones
- Acalculous cholecystitis: there may be a familial component to the occurrence of this condition

# DIAGNOSIS

## DIFFERENTIAL DIAGNOSIS
Conditions that may mimic acute cholecystitis are those that cause significant abdominal pain, upper gastrointestinal symptoms, and fever.

### Acute hepatitis
Acute hepatitis of any etiology (including viral or alcoholic hepatitis) may be mistaken for cholecystitis.

FEATURES
- Profound malaise
- Hepatomegaly with right upper quadrant tenderness
- Jaundice
- Variable fever
- Elevated alanine and aspartate aminotransferases, bilirubin, alkaline phosphatase
- Positive viral hepatitis screen in acute viral hepatitis

### Complicated peptic ulcer disease
Peptic ulcer that perforates may be mistaken for cholecystitis.

FEATURES
- Epigastric tenderness
- Gastrointestinal bleeding
- Nausea and vomiting
- Board-like abdomen and rebound tenderness

### Biliary colic
Biliary colic is often the predecessor of acute cholecystitis, lasting from 30min to 3h.

FEATURES
- Right upper quadrant or epigastric pain
- Nausea and vomiting
- Fever may be present

### Ascending cholangitis
Partial or complete bile duct obstruction can subsequently lead to infection. Suspected diagnosis of ascending cholangitis requires immediate referral to hospital for emergency treatment.

FEATURES
- Charcot's triad: fever, right upper quadrant abdominal pain, jaundice
- Reynold's pentad: Charcot's triad plus hypotension and altered mental state

### Acute pancreatitis
Pancreatitis is frequently associated with excessive alcohol consumption or gallstones.

FEATURES
- Epigastric tenderness and guarding
- Nausea and vomiting
- Hypoactive bowel sounds
- Tachycardia
- Palpable abdominal mass

- Fever
- Typical findings on abdominal computed tomography (CT) scan include varying degrees of a pancreatic inflammatory process

## Pyelonephritis

Pyelonephritis is usually bacterial in origin.

FEATURES
- Fever, chills
- Flank pain
- Dysuria, hematuria
- Nausea and vomiting
- Typically diagnosed by clinical scenario, and urine and serum showing bacteria and increased white blood cells

## Right basal pneumonia

Right basal pneumonia may cause pain in the same area as in cholecystitis.

FEATURES
- Fever, chills
- Cough, sputum production
- Pleurisy
- Dyspnea
- Typically diagnosed by clinical scenario and characteristic chest X-ray findings

## Acute myocardial infarction

Acute myocardial infarction is caused by occlusive coronary thrombus.

FEATURES
- Chest pain, which may radiate to the epigastrium or shoulder, similar to cholecystitis
- Dyspnea
- Nausea and vomiting
- Diaphoresis
- Palpitations
- Typically diagnosed by clinical scenario and characteristic ECG findings

## Abdominal aortic aneurysm

A ruptured abdominal aortic aneurysm must be ruled out in any patient presenting with acute abdominal pain.

FEATURES
- Sudden onset of severe abdominal pain, which may radiate to the back
- Expansile abdominal mass
- Nausea and vomiting may be present
- Hypotension and tachycardia
- Typically diagnosed by clinical scenario and characteristic abdominal ultrasound findings

## Hepatic abscesses

FEATURES
- Right upper quadrant pain
- Fever, leukocytosis
- Usually differentiated on basis of ultrasound findings

### Perforated viscus
FEATURES
- Abdominal pain usually diffuse
- Fever, leukocytosis, possible elevated amylase
- Usually associated with some from of instrumentation
- Abdominal X-ray or CT of the abdomen are useful diagnostic tools

### Gonococcal perihepatitis (Fitz-Hugh-Curtis syndrome)
FEATURES
- Right upper quadrant pain and tenderness
- Leukocytosis
- Pelvic complaints may be overshadowed by right upper quadrant symptoms
- Adnexal tenderness is present on physical examination
- Gram stain of cervical smear should show gonococci

## SIGNS & SYMPTOMS
### Signs
- Right upper quadrant pain, localized tenderness overlying gallbladder, fever, and leukocytosis are typical signs of cholecystitis
- Right subcostal tenderness with inspiratory arrest (Murphy's sign)
- Palpable gallbladder
- Guarding due to local peritonitis
- Mild jaundice may occur secondary to edema of the bile ducts and surrounding lymph nodes
- Fever: unexplained fever or hyperamylasemia with vague abdominal pain are sometimes the only clues in elderly, postoperative patients with acalculous cholecystitis

### Symptoms
- Cholecystitis may be preceded by attacks of biliary colic
- Epigastric pain in right upper quadrant, back, shoulder, or chest (rare) lasting >6h
- Pain may be exacerbated by deep inspiration or movement
- Fever and chills
- Nausea and vomiting

## ASSOCIATED DISORDERS
- Pancreatitis and cholangitis are other conditions that are also caused by gallstones
- Infection or systemic illness is associated with acalculous cholecystitis
- Bacterial infection (streptococci, *Leptospira interrogans*, *Salmonella* spp., *Shigella* spp., *Escherichia coli*, *Campylobacter jejuni*, *Clostridia perfringens*, *Vibrio cholerae*, typhoid) and parasitic infection (*Ascaris* spp., *Giardia lamblia*) may be associated with the development of pigment stones
- In immunocompromised patients, bacterial or fungal infections (cytomegalovirus, *Iaspora belli*, *Cryptosporidium* spp., *Aspergillus* spp., *Candida* spp.)
- Polyarteritis nodosa and Kawasaki disease may present with acute cholecystitis
- Congenital narrowing or inflammation of the cystic duct or external compression from enlarged lymph nodes is associated with this disorder in children

## KEY! DON'T MISS!
- Patients can experience postcholecystectomy cholecystitis pain syndrome due to dysfunction of the sphincter of Oddi
- Complications of acute untreated cholecystitis include gallbladder empyema and perforation, which can be fatal

- Acute myocardial infarction can present with epigastric pain. All patients presenting with epigastric pain should be investigated with an ECG
- Ascending cholangitis should be differentiated from cholecystitis

## CONSIDER CONSULT
- Suspected diagnosis of any of the following requires immediate referral: sepsis or evidence of infection, duct blockage, evidence of acute fulminant cholecystitis, ascending cholangitis, and suspected cancer
- All patients with symptoms and signs consistent with cholecystitis should be referred for immediate ultrasound

## INVESTIGATION OF THE PATIENT
### Direct questions to patient
**Q** Can you describe your pain? Constant right upper quadrant or epigastric pain is typical of cholecystitis

**Q** Have you had similar but less severe attacks before (these may have been associated with food intake)? Intense epigastric or right upper quadrant pain beginning suddenly and rising in intensity over a 15min period, continuing for several hours then slowly subsiding, describes biliary colic. Pain attacks are frequently precipitated by a fat-rich meal and are sometimes accompanied by restlessness and vomiting. Between attacks, physical examination is usually normal with possible exception of residual upper abdominal tenderness

**Q** Have you had any nausea and vomiting? Nausea and vomiting are commonly associated with acute cholecystitis, but may also be present with biliary colic

**Q** Have you experienced any chills, rigors, or fevers? The main difference between biliary colic and cholecystitis is the inflammatory involvement. Elderly patients with acalculous cholecystitis may not have pain or fever, or fever may be the only evidence of acalculous cholecystitis

### Contributory or predisposing factors
**Q** Are you taking any prescription medications? Chronic thiazide treatment, birth control pills, or other estrogen-based medications may contribute to gallstone formation

**Q** Are you on a diet or fasting to lose weight? Obesity, prolonged fasting, or extreme dieting leading to rapid weight loss may contribute to cholecystitis

**Q** Do you drink large amounts of alcohol on a regular basis? Alcoholism and cirrhosis of the liver are predisposing factors

**Q** Are you receiving total parenteral nutrition? This contributes to the formation of gallstones

**Q** Have you had abdominal surgery in the past? Surgically related strictures and narrowing of vessels often impede movement of bile through the bile duct, leading to possible cystic duct obstruction and cholecystitis

**Q** Do you have HIV or AIDS? These conditions, with their accompanying predisposition to bacterial and fungal infections, often present with associated cholecystitis

**Q** Do you have a vasculitis or hemolytic anemia? Polyarteritis nodosa may cause cholecystitis; hemolysis causes pigment stones

### Family history
Does any other immediate family member have a history of gallstones or gallbladder diseases? There appears to be some genetic component to this condition.

### Examination
- Is the patient febrile? Inflammation causes fever, which is commonly seen with cholecystitis
- Does the patient have right subcostal tenderness with inspiratory arrest on palpation (Murphy's sign)? This is typical for patients experiencing acute cholecystitis
- Does the patient have a palpable gallbladder? This is seen with 20% of patients with cholecystitis

- **Is the patient displaying abdominal guarding during examination?** Abdominal pain is typical of cholecystitis
- **Does the patient appear jaundiced?** Mild jaundice is seen in 25–50% of patients with cholecystitis. Serum bilirubin, transaminase, and alkaline phosphatase values may be elevated

## Summary of investigative tests
- White blood cell (WBC) count: leukocytosis (12,000–20,000cells/mm$^3$) is present in >70% of patients with cholecystitis
- Liver function tests, including serum bilirubin, serum alkaline phosphatase, serum alanine aminotransferase (ALT), serum aspartate aminotransferase (AST), and serum amylase. Mildly elevated values for these serum tests may be indicative of cholecystitis
- Ultrasound of the gallbladder demonstrates the presence or absence of stones, as well as typical features of gallbladder inflammation
- Computed tomography (CT) of the abdomen is useful in cases of suspected abscess or neoplasm
- Biliary scintigraphy: many gallbladder-related conditions are clearly identified or ruled out using one scintigraphy scan. In the case of cholecystitis, it is best at excluding this condition
- Nuclear imaging (HIDA scan) is highly sensitive and specific for detection of cystic duct obstruction (normally performed by a specialist)
- Endoscopic retrograde cholangiopancreatography (ERCP) may be useful in cases in which ultrasonography or scintiscanning has not established a diagnosis, or when there is common bile duct obstruction from a gallstone (choledocholithiasis)

## DIAGNOSTIC DECISION
Formal diagnosis is made through laboratory tests and imaging studies:
- Leukocytosis (present in >70% of cases)
- Positive symptom screen (inclusive of, but not limited to fever, right upper quadrant or epigastric pain for >6h, nausea, vomiting, signs of localized peritonitis; older patients may have altered mental status and sepsis) followed by abdominal ultrasound to confirm presence of stones or dilated gallbladder with thickened walls and surrounding edema is the basis for the diagnosis of cholecystitis
- Patients in whom stones are not apparent on ultrasound may have acalculous cholecystitis

## THE TESTS
### Body fluids
WHITE BLOOD CELL COUNT
*Description*
5mL anticoagulated sample (sodium EDTA) should be obtained and time of collection recorded. If sample cannot be analyzed immediately, then refrigeration is indicated.

*Advantages/Disadvantages*
Advantages:
- Blood sampling is a relatively simple procedure
- Results are easily and quickly obtained using standard laboratory procedures

Disadvantage: changes in WBC count are not clearly indicative of diagnosis.

*Normal*
5000–10,000 cells/mm$^3$.

*Abnormal*
- <5000 or >10,000 cells/mm$^3$ with increased neutrophils and/or band forms (left shift)
- Keep in mind possibility of a falsely elevated or suppressed value

*Cause of abnormal result*
- Elevated WBC count in cholecystitis indicates inflammation of the gallbladder with or without sepsis
- Decreased WBC count can be due to viral infection or overwhelming bacterial infection

*Drugs, disorders and other factors that may alter results*
- Stressful situations or other infectious or noninfectious inflammatory conditions may increase WBC count
- Elderly patients with sepsis may not have a raised WBC count

## SERUM BILIRUBIN
*Description*
5mL nonhemolyzed sample should be obtained from a fasting patient. Protect sample from sunlight, and avoid air bubbles and unnecessary shaking during blood collection. If sample cannot be analyzed immediately, then refrigeration is indicated. Serum is isolated via centrifugation.

*Advantages/Disadvantages*
Advantages:
- Blood sampling is relatively simple
- Results are easily and quickly obtained using standard laboratory procedures

Disadvantage: elevated serum bilirubin is not clearly indicative of diagnosis.

*Normal*
- Total bilirubin: 0.2–1.3mg/dL (3.4–17.1mcmol/L)
- Conjugated (direct) bilirubin: 0.0-0.2mg/dL (0.0–3.4mcmol/L)

*Abnormal*
- Total bilirubin: >1.3mg/dL (>17.1mcmol/L)
- Conjugated bilirubin: >0.2mg/dL (>3.4mcmol/L)
- Keep in mind the possibility of a falsely elevated or suppressed value

*Cause of abnormal result*
- Total bilirubin can be elevated due to liver disease or obstructive jaundice (cholecystitis, choledocholithiasis, neoplasm)
- In acute cholecystitis, edema of the gallbladder wall may cause mild jaundice

*Drugs, disorders and other factors that may alter results*
- Many drugs (e.g. chlorpromazine) can elevate total bilirubin levels
- A high-fat meal before blood sampling decreases bilirubin level
- Certain foods and drugs increase the yellow color of serum and may falsely increase bilirubin levels when tests are performed spectrophotometrically
- Prolonged fasting and anorexia raise serum bilirubin levels
- Certain genetic conditions (Gilbert's disease, Dubin–Johnson syndrome) raise bilirubin levels

## SERUM ALKALINE PHOSPHATASE
*Description*
Obtain a 5mL fasting venous blood sample. Do not use anticoagulants in sample collection. Refrigerate sample as soon as possible.

*Advantages/Disadvantages*
Advantages:
- Blood sampling is relatively simple
- Results are easily and quickly obtained using standard laboratory procedures

Disadvantage: elevated serum alkaline phosphatase results alone are not completely decisive regarding diagnosis.

*Normal*
30–120 IU/L.

*Abnormal*
- Results outside the normal reference range
- Keep in mind the possibility of a falsely elevated or suppressed value

*Cause of abnormal result*
Alkaline phosphatase is elevated by:
- Obstructive jaundice (gallstones)
- Intra- and extrahepatic cholestasis

*Drugs, disorders and other factors that may alter results*
- Many drugs alter alkaline phosphatase levels. For example, levels are increased by antibiotics, anticonvulsants, antineoplastics, fluconazole, fluvastatin, indomethacin, methyldopa, oral contraceptives, phenobarbital, phenothiazines, probenecid, and verapamil. Levels are decreased by calcitriol, clofibrate, cyanides, fluorides, nitrofurantoin, oxalates, and zinc salts
- Young children, those experiencing rapid growth, pregnant women, and postmenopausal women have physiologically high levels of alkaline phosphatase

## SERUM ALANINE AMINOTRANSFERASE
*Description*
Obtain a 5mL fasting venous blood sample.

*Advantages/Disadvantages*
Advantages:
- Blood sampling is relatively simple
- Results are easily and quickly obtained using standard laboratory procedures

Disadvantage: elevated ALT results are not completely decisive regarding diagnosis.

*Normal*
- Adult: 10–60U/L
- Child: 5–30U/L

*Abnormal*
- Adult: <10 or >60U/L
- Child: <5 or >30U/L
- Keep in mind the possibility of a falsely elevated or suppressed value

*Cause of abnormal result*
Serum ALT is elevated by:
- Liver disease
- Obstructive jaundice or biliary obstruction
- Coexistent pancreatitis

*Drugs, disorders and other factors that may alter results*
- Salicylates may increase or decrease ALT levels
- Many drugs may alter ALT levels. For example, levels are increased by acetaminophen, anabolic steroids, antibiotics, antifungals, antineoplastic agents, aspirin, barbiturates,

benzodiazepines, beta-blockers, bismuth subsalicylate, cimetidine, clonidine, codeine, cortisone, dantrolene, dapsone, iron, levodopa/methyldopa, monoamine oxidase inhibitors, nonsteroidal anti-inflammatory drugs, oral contraceptives, phenothiazines, progesterone, simvastatin, sulfasalazine, verapamil, and warfarin. Levels are decreased by ibuprofen, interferon, cyclosporine, metronidazole, and phenothiazines

### SERUM ASPARTATE AMINOTRANSAMINASE
*Description*
Obtain a 5mL fasting venous blood sample. Avoid hemolysis during collection.

*Advantages/Disadvantages*
Advantages:
- Blood sampling is relatively simple
- Results are easily and quickly obtained using standard laboratory procedures

Disadvantage: elevated AST results are not completely decisive regarding diagnosis.

*Normal*
Adult (>18 years): 5–40U/L.

*Abnormal*
- <5 or >40U/L
- Keep in mind the possibility of a falsely elevated or suppressed value

*Cause of abnormal result*
Serum AST is elevated by:
- Acute pancreatitis
- Cholecystitis
- Liver disease
- Muscular disorders

*Drugs, disorders and other factors that may alter results*
- Slight decrease occurs during pregnancy
- False decrease occurs in diabetic ketoacidosis, severe liver disease, and uremia
- Many drugs alter AST values
- Alcohol ingestion affects results

### SERUM AMYLASE
*Description*
Obtain a 5mL venous blood sample. Do not use EDTA anticoagulants in sample collection.

*Advantages/Disadvantages*
Advantages:
- Blood sampling is relatively simple
- Results are easily and quickly obtained using standard laboratory procedures

Disadvantage: elevated amylase results are not completely decisive regarding diagnosis.

*Normal*
- Adult: 25–125U/L
- Elderly: 21–160U/L

*Abnormal*
- Adult: <25 or >125U/L
- Elderly: <21 or >160U/L
- Keep in mind the possibility of a falsely elevated or suppressed value

*Cause of abnormal result*
Serum amylase is elevated by:
- Coexistent pancreatitis
- Obstruction of pancreatic duct
- Acute cholecystitis

*Drugs, disorders and other factors that may alter results*
- Anticoagulated blood gives lower results
- Lipemic serum interferes with test
- Increased levels are found in alcoholics, pregnant women, and in diabetic ketoacidosis
- Many drugs interfere with this test
- Perforated viscus, salivary disease, macroamylasemia, and renal failure cause elevated serum amylase levels

## Imaging

COMPUTED TOMOGRAPHY
*Advantages/Disadvantages*
Advantage: imaging the abdomen can rule out suspected abscess, neoplasm, perforation, or pancreatitis.

Disadvantages:
- Expensive
- May require specialist interpretation of results

*Abnormal*
Acute acalculous cholecystitis:
- Thickened gallbladder wall, defined as >4mm thickness in the absence of ascites or hypoalbuminemia
- Pericholecystic fluid, subserosal edema (in the absence of ascites), intramural gas, or sloughed mucosa

*Cause of abnormal result*
Acute acalculous cholecystitis.

*Drugs, disorders and other factors that may alter results*
- Biliary, pancreatic neoplasm
- Abscesses
- Pancreatitis

BILIARY SCINTIGRAPHY
*Advantages/Disadvantages*
Advantage: many gallbladder-related conditions are clearly identified or ruled out using one scan.

Disadvantages:
- Requires referral to hospital or specialist
- Better at excluding acute cholecystitis than confirming it, as it does not demonstrate presence of stones

*Normal*
Normal visualization of gallbladder.

*Abnormal*
- Cystic duct obstruction reveals nonvisualization of gallbladder with visualization of bile excretion into the duodenum
- Common bile duct obstruction reveals nonvisualization of the ampulla and/or small intestine

*Cause of abnormal result*
- Cystic duct obstruction
- Common bile duct obstruction

*Drugs, disorders and other factors that may alter results*
- High bilirubin may decrease sensitivity (test is only reliable when serum bilirubin is <5mg/dL)
- Fasting patients on total parenteral nutrition have a full gallbladder because it is not stimulated; thus, it does not take up the tracer and this may affect results
- Critically ill, immobilized patients may have false-positive scans because of viscous bile
- Severe liver disease may lead to abnormal uptake and excretion of the contrast
- Previous biliary sphincterotomy may lower resistance to bile flow, leading to increased excretion of the tracer into the duodenum without filling the gallbladder

## ULTRASONOGRAPHY
*Advantages/Disadvantages*
Advantages:
- Ultrasound of the gallbladder is test of choice for evaluation of patients with biliary colic pain and suspected acute cholecystitis
- Test takes 15min
- Adequate images are obtained in the majority of cases
- Confirms presence of sludge and identifies complications (perforation, empyema, abscess)
- Dilated common bile duct and intrahepatic ducts may be seen, which indicate choledocholithiasis
- High sensitivity and specificity (90%)

Disadvantages:
- May not be immediately available
- Small gallstones can be missed

*Abnormal*
- Thickened gallbladder wall defined as >4mm thickness in the absence of ascites or hypoalbuminemia
- Sonographic Murphy's sign. This is more accurate than Murphy's sign demonstrated by hand palpation because it can confirm that the gallbladder is being pressed by the transducer when the patient has inspiratory arrest
- Pericholecystic fluid collection
- Distended gallbladder
- Gallbladder sludge in lumen

*Cause of abnormal result*
Acute cholecystitis.

*Drugs, disorders and other factors that may alter results*
- Obesity can reduce visualization
- Hypoalbuminemia, ascites, and congestive cardiac failure may cause a false-positive result

## Special tests
ENDOSCOPIC RETROGRADE CHOLANGIOPANCREATOGRAPHY
*Advantages/Disadvantages*
Advantages:
- Useful where diagnosis has not been established by ultrasound, CT, or cholescintigraphy
- May be therapeutic if common bile duct stones are found and removed

Disadvantages:
- Requires referral to hospital or specialist
- Risk of complications, including pancreatitis, cholangitis, perforation, bleeding, and cardiopulmonary complications secondary to sedation

*Normal*
Normal visualization of biliary system.

*Abnormal*
- Cystic duct obstruction revealed
- Common bile duct obstruction revealed

*Drugs, disorders and other factors that may alter results*
Mirizzi's syndrome: impacted distal cystic duct gallstone causing extrinsic compression of the common bile duct.

# TREATMENT

## CONSIDER CONSULT
- Refer for surgery
- Referral to a gastroenterologist if endoscopic retrograde cholangiopancreatography (ERCP) is indicated for sphincterotomy or for stone removal in patients with cholecystitis and ultrasound evidence of common bile duct stones

## IMMEDIATE ACTION
- If patient presents with acute severe cholecystitis, refer immediately for inpatient surgical consultation
- If patient displays features defined as Charcot's triad (right upper quadrant pain, fever, jaundice) or progresses to Reynold's pentad (Charcot's triad plus hypotension and altered mental state), possible ascending cholangitis should be evaluated immediately. This is a surgical and medical emergency requiring prompt treatment

## PATIENT AND CAREGIVER ISSUES
### Impact on career, dependants, family, friends
- Frequent visits to the physician are needed, especially in the 'watchful waiting' phase of the condition
- Time off work may be necessary if sick or to visit the primary care physician (PCP)
- In acute cholecystitis, the symptoms of the illness will likely require bed rest, necessitating caregiver support

### Patient or caregiver request
Q I seem to have a flare-up of pain after eating fatty meals. If I discontinue this type of diet, will the problem go away? No. If gallstones are causing this problem, only their removal will resolve the immediate problem. Changes in diet do not guarantee that stones will not recur, because there are many contributing factors in gallstone formation, biliary colic, and cholecystitis

Q Will removal of the gallstones solve the problem forever? No. Removal of stones does not guarantee that they will not recur in the bile ducts

Q I've heard that you can dissolve gallstones without any surgery being necessary. Will this work for me? Some drugs have been used to dissolve certain types of gallstones, but the procedure takes several months and side effects of drug treatment are possible

Q I know that you can break up kidney stones with a 'shock wave' device. Can you do this to gallstones? Lithotripsy is used to fragment kidney stones, but this procedure has not been approved by the FDA for use in the removal of gallstones in the US

Q How can I be having this problem if I don't have gallstones? Inflammation of the gallbladder is not always due to the presence of stones in the organ or the bile ducts. The condition can be caused by a gallbladder that is not emptying bile, causing injury to the cells of the gallbladder and leading to possible bacterial infection

### Health-seeking behavior
Have you taken any herbs or supplements for previous attacks of pain? Biliary colic may be experienced before an episode of acute cholecystitis, and the patients may have taken medication for suspected indigestion.

## MANAGEMENT ISSUES
### Goals
- Pain relief
- Treatment of any underlying condition
- Treatment of infection with antibiotics
- Treatment of cholelithiasis

## Management in special circumstances
### COEXISTING DISEASE
- Alcoholism and cirrhosis: severity of pre-existing cirrhosis and associated conditions may warrant extra caution when selecting medical treatment options. Referral for surgery may be indicated earlier than typical for patient without coexisting morbidity
- Obesity, fasting, or prolonged starvation: severity of dehydration, anorexia, or obesity may warrant extra caution when selecting medical treatment options. Referral for surgery may be indicated later than typical for patient with coexisting morbidity, allowing PCP to confirm that the patient is in best possible health for the surgical procedure
- Other severe illness: severely ill patients who are not surgical candidates may be able to undergo drainage by percutaneous cholecystostomy

### COEXISTING MEDICATION
Total parenteral nutrition: if the patient is receiving this type of nutritional support, the likelihood of recurrence of gallstones is high. Referral for surgery may be warranted for certain patients.

### SPECIAL PATIENT GROUPS
- Pregnant women: cholecystitis occurs in 3.5% of pregnancies. Most cases can be managed with abstinence from oral intake and nasogastric suction, pain control, and antibiotics. Failure to respond to conservative treatment, systemic toxicity, and recalcitrant pancreatitis may warrant referral for surgery
- Elderly patients: treat early for infection and surgery is indicated when patient does not respond to conservative treatment. A deceptively benign presentation does not indicate that the patient does not need aggressive treatment; this asymptomatic scenario may mask complications and cause an inappropriate delay in surgery
- Children (uncommon, more likely to have pigment stones): treat early for infection. Surgery is indicated when patient does not respond to conservative treatment

### PATIENT SATISFACTION/LIFESTYLE PRIORITIES
- Laparoscopic cholecystectomy has minimal impact on lifestyle because the patient can return to normal activities within 10 days
- Delayed cholecystectomy may be less favorable because further attacks may occur in the meantime

## SUMMARY OF THERAPEUTIC OPTIONS
### Choices
Cholecystitis:
- First and optimal treatment for acute cholecystitis is early cholecystectomy (laparoscopic cholecystectomy is preferred over conventional open cholecystectomy for patient recovery)
- If symptoms are mild or resolving, surgical referral may be appropriate within a few weeks rather than the same day for acute presentation
- High-risk patients may require inpatient conservative management with intravenous fluids and antibiotics
- If patient also has pancreatitis or evidence of choledocholithiasis, endoscopic retrograde cholangiopancreatography (ERCP) may be indicated to treat both conditions. Urgent ERCP is indicated in selected patients with severe gallstone pancreatitis and suspected biliary obstruction, and to prevent biliary sepsis

Gallstones:
- First-choice treatment is surgery (cholecystectomy) for removal of gallstones (if present) or gallbladder
- Second-choice treatment for stones is nonsurgical drug therapy, ursodiol (ursodeoxycholic acid) or chenodiol (chenodeoxycholic acid)

Comments regarding surgical therapies:
- Surgical treatment typically involves removal of gallstones and gallbladder through conventional open cholecystectomy or laparoscopic cholecystectomy
- Initial conservative treatment of acute cholecystitis with antibiotics followed by elective surgery several weeks after inflammation has subsided, contrary to what was believed in the past, does not reduce morbidity or conversion rate (from laparoscopic to open procedure)
- Optimal timing of laparoscopic cholecystectomy for treatment of acute cholecystitis is as soon after diagnosis as possible (within 72h of diagnosis during the hospital stay)

## FOLLOW UP
### Plan for review
- Monitor patient periodically for evaluation of gallstone development or worsening of condition
- If patient worsens, consider referral for surgery or percutaneous cholecystostomy (if not candidate for surgery)
- If patient presents with acute severe cholecystitis, refer immediately for inpatient surgical consultation

### Information for patient or caregiver
- Patient should follow all treatments prescribed by the PCP
- If patient is overweight, they should talk with physician about how best to lose weight. This must be done without fasting, which can encourage further gallstone development
- Patient should be encouraged to take plenty of exercise and enough rest

## DRUGS AND OTHER THERAPIES: DETAILS
### Drugs
URSODIOL (URSODEOXYCHOLIC ACID )
*Dose*
Radiolucent gallstones:
- Adult initial dose: 8–10mg/kg/day in 2–3 divided doses
- Adult maintenance therapy: 250mg/day for 6–12 months

*Efficacy*
- Effective for dissolution of radiolucent cholesterol gallstones
- Overall stone dissolution rate is just under 50%; higher for those with pure cholesterol stones
- Best results are obtained in patients with a few small stones
- Stones recur in 50% of patients within 5 years
- Larger or calcified stones fail to achieve complete dissolution

*Risks/benefits*
Risks:
- Use caution when administering to patients with liver disease
- Patients should be given dietary advice (including avoidance of excessive cholesterol and calories)

Benefits:
- Gallstone dissolution is achieved for small (2cm) cholesterol stones
- Many patients are pain-free before full dissolution

*Side effects and adverse reactions*
- Gastrointestinal: nausea, vomiting, diarrhea
- Skin: pruritus
- Other: gallstone calcification

*Interactions (other drugs)*
Bile acid sequestering agents such as cholestyramine and colestipol (may interfere with ursodiol action).

*Contraindications*
- Will not dissolve calcified cholesterol stones, radiopaque stones, or radiolucent bile pigment stones. Hence, patients with such stones are not candidates for ursodiol therapy
- Patients with unremitting acute cholecystitis, cholangitis, biliary obstruction, gallstone pancreatitis, or biliary-gastrointestinal fistula are not candidates for ursodiol therapy
- Allergy to bile acids - Pregnancy and breast-feeding - Safety and efficacy in children have not been established

*Acceptability to patient*
Acceptable: side effects are minor.

*Follow up plan*
- Perform gallbladder ultrasound at 6 months to determine whether stones have dissolved. If so, continue therapy at maintenance dose and repeat ultrasound within 1–3 months
- Note that use of this drug beyond 24 months is not established

*Patient and caregiver information*
Recommend that patient or caregiver administer drug with food to facilitate drug dissolution in intestine.

CHENODIOL (CHENODEOXYCHOLIC ACID)
*Dose*
250mg twice a day for 2 weeks, then increased by 250mg/day, but not exceeding 16mg/kg/day.

*Efficacy*
Dissolves radiolucent gallstones in well-opacifying gallbladders, but has no effect on radiopaque (calcified) gallstones or radiolucent bile pigment stones.

*Risks/benefits*
Risks:
- Chenodiol is not appropriate treatment for many patients with gallstones
- Should be reserved for carefully selected patients
- Systemic monitering of liver function changes required
- Epidemiologic studies suggest that bile acids might contribute to human colon cancer

Benefit: beneficial for patients in whom surgical risk is excessive (e.g. because of systemic disease or age).

*Side effects and adverse reactions*
- Gastrointestinal: dose-related diarrhea
- Other: dose-related serum aminotransferase (mainly serum glutamic pyruvic transaminase) elevations, higher cholecystectomy rates

*Interactions (other drugs)*
- Bile acid sequestering agents, such as cholestyramine and colestipol (may interfere with the action of chenodiol by reducing its absorption) - Aluminum-based antacids (may adsorb bile acids in vitro and may be expected to interfere with chenodiol) - Estrogens, oral contraceptives, and clofibrate (may increase biliary cholesterol secretion)

*Contraindications*
- Known hepatocyte dysfunction or bile ductal abnormalities ■ Radiopaque stones
- Gallstone complications or compelling reasons for gallbladder surgery including unremitting acute cholecystitis, cholangitis, biliary obstruction, gallstone pancreatitis, or biliary gastrointestinal fistula ■ Pregnancy category X ■ Breast-feeding ■ Safety and efficacy of chenodiol in children have not been established

*Acceptability to patient*
Acceptable: side effects may be a problem for some.

*Follow up plan*
- Perform monthly aminotransferase level testing for 3 months, then every 3 months thereafter
- Serum cholesterol should be monitored
- Cholecystogram or ultrasonogram should be performed to monitor stone size and location

*Patient and caregiver information*
- Patient should take medication per physician instructions
- Patient should report any side effects or adverse reactions noted during treatment

## Surgical therapy
CONVENTIONAL OPEN CHOLECYSTECTOMY
For the past century, open cholecystectomy has been the 'gold standard' for the treatment of patients with symptomatic gallstones.

*Efficacy*
Most commonly performed of all surgical procedures for the treatment of cholecystitis.

*Risks/benefits*
Risks:
- Mortality rates are 0.3–0.5% in patients under 50 and 0.4–2.7% in those over 70 years
- Problems are retained common bile duct stones, iatrogenic bile duct injuries, and infection

*Acceptability to patient*
- Patients may have concern about undergoing surgery
- Risk of duct injury

*Follow up plan*
- PCP should follow up patient after release from hospital
- Postcholecystectomy syndrome should be evaluated periodically following surgery

*Patient and caregiver information*
Patient should be told to follow up with PCP if any symptoms of infection or gastrointestinal disorder occur during the postoperative period.

LAPAROSCOPIC CHOLECYSTECTOMY
Guidelines have been provided by the Society of American Gastrointestinal Endoscopic Surgeons. Guidelines for the clinical application of laparoscopic biliary tract surgery. Surg Endosc 2000;14:771–2.

*Efficacy*
Highly effective in cases of noncomplicated cholecystitis, where strictures and adhesions from prior abdominal surgery are not a hazard.

*Risks/benefits*
Risks:
- Reported complication rate is 1% (hemorrhage and bile leak)
- Overall rate of bile duct injury is 0.5%
- Superficial infection possible at site of scope insertion

Benefits:
- Significantly less invasive than open surgery: shorter hospital stay, faster return to work (within 10 days) and minimal abdominal scarring
- Serious complications reduced

*Acceptability to patient*
Highly acceptable to patients who fear open procedures or for those with a less complicated condition.

*Follow up plan*
- PCP should follow up patient after release from hospital
- Postcholecystectomy syndrome should be evaluated periodically following surgery

*Patient and caregiver information*
Patient should be told to follow up with PCP if any symptoms of infection or gastrointestinal disorder occur during the postoperative period.

## Endoscopic therapy
ENDOSCOPIC RETROGRADE CHOLANGIOPANCREATOGRAPHY
*Efficacy*
- Highly effective in cases of noncomplicated choledocholithiasis where endoscopic sphincterotomy and stone extraction are needed
- Often used in treatment of coexisting common bile duct stones, which occur in 10% of patients with cholecystitis
- Used as an alternative to surgery for stricture dilation and in sphincterotomy for sphincter of Oddi dysfunction
- Urgent ERCP for sphincterotomy and stone removal is indicated in selected patients with ascending cholangitis secondary to choledocholithiasis or severe gallstone pancreatitis

*Risks/benefits*
Risks:
- ERCP without sphincterotomy: complication rate is 3%
- ERCP with sphincterotomy: complication rate is 8%, mortality rate is 0.4%
- Major complications include pancreatitis, cholangitis, perforation, infection, and bleeding. Cardiopulmonary complications secondary to sedation are also possible

Benefits:
- Significantly less invasive than open surgery
- Obstruction may be relieved rapidly without the need for urgent surgery. Elective cholecystectomy may be performed in the near future

*Acceptability to patient*
Generally acceptable.

*Follow up plan*
- PCP should follow up with patient after release from hospital
- Monitor patient for possible postsphincterotomy complications

*Patient and caregiver information*
Patient should be told to follow up with PCP if any symptoms of infection or gastrointestinal disorder occur after the procedure.

# OUTCOMES

## EFFICACY OF THERAPIES
- Most patients with acute cholecystitis treated with pain relief and antibiotics have a complete remission within 1–4 days
- 25–30% of patients do not respond to these measures or develop complications and require immediate surgery
- Medication is less effective than surgery and is not indicated in the setting of acute cholecystitis
- Medical treatment may be effective when used to dissolve cholesterol gallstones in patients with recurrent stones after cholecystectomy

### Review period
- After cholecystectomy, patient requires follow up if pain persists or patient develops fever and/or jaundice
- With dissolution therapy, liver profile should be checked occasionally to ascertain possible delivery of gallstones into common bile duct. Additionally, sonography should be performed periodically to document effect of therapy

## PROGNOSIS
- Elective laparoscopic cholecystectomy may require only an overnight hospital stay; complication rate is approx. 1%
- Open cholecystectomy can require 4–7 days in hospital after surgery; complication rate is <0.5%
- After cholecystectomy, gallstones may recur in bile ducts

### Therapeutic failure
If nonsurgical treatment fails, then patient may need referral for surgery to remove gallbladder.

### Recurrence
If nonsurgical treatment fails to prevent recurrence, then patient may need to be referred for surgery to remove gallbladder.

### Deterioration
- If patient's condition worsens during nonsurgical treatment, then surgery may be needed to remove gallbladder
- If patient starts to display the features defined as Charcot's triad (right upper quadrant pain, fever, jaundice) or progresses to Reynold's pentad (Charcot's triad plus hypotension and altered mental state), possible ascending cholangitis should be evaluated immediately. This is a surgical and medical emergency requiring prompt treatment

### Terminal illness
- Patients with biliary or pancreatic neoplasms (primary or metastatic) should be referred to specialist for additional evaluation or treatment
- Patients with HIV or AIDS should be followed by their specialist for additional evaluation or treatment

## COMPLICATIONS
Complications in acute acalculous cholecystitis develop rapidly and early diagnosis is critical:
- Acute pancreatitis may require additional surgical intervention
- Ascending cholangitis requires hospitalization to treat
- Carcinoma of the gallbladder is a rare complication of cholelithiasis

- Gangrene results from further deterioration of gallbladder tissue following acute attack: often seen in diabetic patients
- Confined perforation of the gallbladder
- Fistulas secondary to inflammation may form with adjacent structures, including the duodenum, colon, or abdominal wall
- Empyema occurs when superinfection of the bile with a pus-forming organism occurs in an obstructed gallbladder
- Gallstone ileus may occur when a fistula forms with the bowel and a stone is passed into the bowel lumen; bowel obstruction may result from obstruction at the ileocecal valve
- Urgent surgery is required for acute complications such as perforation, emphysematous cholecystitis, and empyema: cholecystectomy or cholecystostomy should be considered

## CONSIDER CONSULT
- Immediate referral is indicated if complications occur that the primary care physician does not feel comfortable treating
- If patient has ongoing concomitant illnesses that make determination of next steps in therapy difficult, referral to specialists is indicated
- If patient also has a terminal illness that influences anticipated additional treatment for cholecystitis, then referral to the physician treating the terminal illness may be warranted

# PREVENTION

## RISK FACTORS
- **High saturated fat intake, low fiber intake, and high sugar intake:** linked to increased risk of gallbladder disease
- **Vitamin C deficiencies and total parenteral nutrition:** also linked to increased risk
- **Obesity and caloric excess are major risk factors for gallstone formation:** number of calories consumed rather than the proportion of calories coming from saturated fat or cholesterol intake appears to correlate best with risk
- **Fasting and starvation diets:** cause bile to become very lithogenic
- **Excessive alcohol intake**
- **Clofibrate and thiazides:** associated with gallstone formation
- **Estrogen intake** (for birth control or postmenopausal hormone replacement)
- **Low level of physical activity**

## MODIFY RISK FACTORS
### Lifestyle and wellness
TOBACCO
Smoking appears to reduce risk in women, probably due to its adverse effects on estrogen production and degradation, but it is not recommended that women start smoking.

ALCOHOL AND DRUGS
- Instruct patient as to what volume of alcohol is acceptable (daily small amounts – 1oz – correlate with a 20% reduction in risk of symptomatic gallstone disease in women, but excessive consumption is contraindicated)
- Discontinue use of clofibrate and thiazides if possible
- If taking estrogens (for birth control or postmenopausal hormone replacement), individual should be watchful for possible biliary tract disorder symptoms

DIET
- Decrease saturated fat and sugar intake and increase fiber intake
- Increase consumption of vegetable protein
- Obese individuals should lose weight gradually and slowly with emphasis on exercise, and not through fasting or starvation diets

PHYSICAL ACTIVITY
Regular exercise helps to maintain blood sugar and insulin levels, along with controlling weight.

FAMILY HISTORY
Individuals with a family history of gallstones, gallbladder disease, or other biliary tract disorders should be especially aware of the possibility that they may experience these conditions.

## SCREENING
Two-thirds of gallstones are asymptomatic and are managed conservatively with no medical or surgical intervention. As patients with silent stones have only a 1–2% chance per year of developing biliary pain, screening would not be cost beneficial.

## PREVENT RECURRENCE
- Discontinue offending medications (e.g. estrogen, thiazide) if possible
- Gradual, slow weight reduction with emphasis on exercise in obese individuals
- Enteral feeding in patients who are on total parenteral nutrition or fasting

**Reassess coexisting disease**
- Treat underlying ileal disease (e.g. Crohn's disease)
- Treat underlying liver disease
- Treat infectious processes (bacterial, viral, or parasitic)

# RESOURCES

## ASSOCIATIONS

National Digestive Diseases Information Clearinghouse
2 Information Way
Bethesda, MD 20892-3570
Tel: (301) 654-3810
http://www.niddk.nih.gov

American Gastroenterological Association, American Digestive Health Foundation
7910 Woodmont Avenue, 7th Floor
Bethesda, MD 20814
Tel: (301) 654-2055
Fax: (301) 652-3890
http://www.gastro.org

American Society for Gastrointestinal Endoscopy
13 Elm Street
Manchester, MA 01944
Tel: (978) 526-8330
Fax: (978) 526-4018
http://www.asge.org

American College of Gastroenterology
4900 B South 31st Street
Arlington, VA 22206
Tel: (703) 820-7400
http://www.acg.gi.org

## KEY REFERENCES

- Lo C-M, Liu CL, Fan ST, et al. Prospective randomized study of early versus delayed laparoscopic cholecystectomy for acute cholecystitis. Ann Surg 1998;227:461–7
- Howard DE, Fromm H. Bile salts: metabolic, pathologic, and therapeutic considerations. Nonsurgical management of gallstone disease. Gastroenterol Clin 1999;28:133–44
- Leitzmann MF, Rimm EB, Willett WC, et al. Recreational physical activity and the risk of cholecystectomy in women. N Engl J Med 1999;341:777–84
- Leitzmann MF, Giovannucci EL, Rimm EB, et al. The relation of physical activity to risk for symptomatic gallstone disease in men. Ann Intern Med 1998;128:417–25
- Leitzmann MF, Giovannucci EL, Stampfer MJ, et al. Prospective study of alcohol consumption patterns in relation to symptomatic gallstone disease in men. Alcohol Clin Exp Res 1999;23:835–41
- Fisher MM, Roberts EA, Rosen IE, et al. The Sunnybrook Gallstone Study: a double-blind controlled trial of chenodeoxycholic acid for gallstone dissolution. Hepatology 1985;5:102–7
- Schoenfield LJ, Lachin JM. Chenodiol for dissolution of gallstones: the National Cooperative Gallstone Study. A controlled trial of efficacy and safety. Ann Intern Med 1981;95:257–82
- Fromm H, Roat JW, Gonzalez V, et al. Comparative efficacy and side-effects of ursodeoxycholic and chenodeoxycholic acids in dissolving gallstones. A double-blind controlled study. Gastroenterology 1983;85:1257–64
- Sawyers JL. Current status of conventional cholecystectomy versus laparoscopic cholecystectomy. Ann Surg 1996;223:P1–P3
- May GR, Sutherland LR, Shaffer EA. Efficacy of bile acid therapy for gallstone dissolution: a meta-analysis of randomized trials. Aliment Pharmacol Ther 1993;7:139–48
- Petroni ML, Jazrawi RP, Pazzi P, et al. Ursodeoxycholic acid alone or with chenodeoxycholic acid for dissolution of cholesterol gallstones: a randomized multicentre trial. The British-Italian Gallstone Study group. Aliment Pharmacol Ther 2001;15:123–8

- Tomida S, Abei M, Yamaguchi T, et al. Long-term ursodeoxycholic acid therapy is associated with reduced risk of biliary pain and acute cholecystitis in patients with gallbladder stones: a cohort analysis. Hepatology 1999;30:6–13
- Moscati RM. Cholelithiasis, cholecystitis, and pancreatitis. Emerg Med Clin North Am 1996;14(4):719–37
- ASGE guidelines for clinical application. The role of ERCP in diseases of the biliary tract and pancreas. American Society for Gastrointestinal Endoscopy. Gastrointest Endosc 1999;50:915–20
- Moscati RM. Cholelithiasis, cholecystitis, and pancreatitis. Emerg Med Clin North Am 1996;14:719–37
- Treatment of gallstone and gallbladder disease. Manchester, MA: Society for Surgery of the Alimentary Tract; 2000, p5
- Procedure guideline for hepatobiliary scintigraphy. Reston: Society of Nuclear Medicine; 1999 Feb, p16 (Society of Nuclear Medicine Procedure Guidelines; version 2)
- Guidelines for the clinical application of laparoscopic biliary tract surgery. Surg Endosc 2000;14(8):771–2. Society of American Gastrointestinal Endoscopic Surgeons (SAGES)

## FAQS
### Question 1
What are the most common symptoms of cholecystitis?

ANSWER 1
Right upper quadrant pain, fever, and leukocytosis.

### Question 2
Are there any recognized risk factors for developing cholecystitis?

ANSWER 2
- Age, female sex, obesity
- Weight loss, total parenteral nutrition
- Pregnancy
- Drugs (clofibrate, estrogens, ceftriaxone, and octreotide, among others)
- Native Americans, Scandinavians
- Decreased high-density lipoprotein, increased triglycerides

### Question 3
What kinds of medical tests are used to establish the diagnosis of cholecystitis?

ANSWER 3
- Sonography: sensitivity of 95% for stones >2mm
- Oral cholecystography: sensitivity and specificity exceeds 90% when gallbladder is opacified
- Cholescintigraphy assesses patency of the cystic duct, and nothing more
- Endoscopic retrograde cholangiopancreatography (ERCP) is the 'gold standard' for common bile duct stones
- Computed tomography and magnetic resonance imaging may prove useful as a noninvasive means of excluding common bile duct stones

## CONTRIBUTORS
Randolph L Pearson, MD
Rudolph A Bedford, MD
Hetal A Karsan, MD

# CIRRHOSIS

| | | |
|---|---|---|
| ■ | Summary Information | 102 |
| ■ | Background | 103 |
| ■ | Diagnosis | 105 |
| ■ | Treatment | 117 |
| ■ | Outcomes | 125 |
| ■ | Prevention | 127 |
| ■ | Resources | 128 |

## SUMMARY INFORMATION

### DESCRIPTION
- Chronic disease of the liver
- Cirrhosis is a pathologic diagnosis characterized by fibrosis, disorganization of the lobular and vascular architecture, and regenerating nodules of hepatocytes
- Liver biopsy is the gold standard in diagnosis
- Specific treatment depends on the cause and presence of complications
- Prognosis is very variable and depends on the cause, stage of disease, and patient's adherence to alcohol abstinence, medical compliance, and nutritional advice

### URGENT ACTION
Urgent hospital admission may be necessary for:
- Bleeding esophageal varices
- Hepatic encephalopathy
- Spontaneous bacterial peritonitis

### KEY! DON'T MISS!
Do not miss clinical signs of the disease, e.g. palmar erythema, firm nodular liver, or splenomegaly – the earlier the clinical suspicion and confirmation of cirrhosis, the better the prognosis.

## BACKGROUND

### ICD9 CODE
- 571.2 Alcoholic cirrhosis of liver
- 571.5 Cirrhosis of liver without mention of alcohol

### CARDINAL FEATURES
- Cirrhosis has traditionally been classified as either macronodular (>3mm nodules) or micronodular (<3mm) but there is no etiologic, functional, or prognostic value to the nodule size
- Compensated cirrhosis can lead to hepatomegaly (but liver is small and hard in advanced cirrhosis), palmar erythema, Dupuytren's contracture, gynecomastia, testicular atrophy, clubbing, and spider naevi
- Decompensated cirrhosis is defined by the clinical manifestations of portal hypertension such as persistent jaundice, hepatic encephalopathy, ascites, bleeding gastroesophageal varices, and hepatorenal syndrome
- Abstinence of alcohol and appropriate medical nutritional therapy are crucial for effective management
- Specific treatment depends on the cause and presence of complications
- Prognosis is very variable and depends on the cause, stage of disease, and patient's adherence to alcohol abstinence, medical compliance, and nutritional advice

### CAUSES
#### Common causes
- Large majority have either alcoholic liver disease or chronic viral infection
- In the US, obesity and its associated fatty liver might become the most frequent cause of cirrhosis if the general trend of increasing obesity continues
- Alcohol
- Viral hepatitis (B, C, D)
- Secondary biliary cirrhosis: obstruction of the common bile duct by stone, stricture, pancreatitis, neoplasm
- Hepatic congestion, e.g. congestive heart failure, constrictive pericarditis, hepatic vein thrombosis, vena cava obstruction
- Drugs, e.g. methotrexate, methyldopa (other drugs such as acetaminophen and isoniazid cause acute liver failure, not cirrhosis)

#### Rare causes
- Primary biliary cirrhosis
- Hemochromatosis
- Wilson's disease
- Alpha-1-antitrypsin deficiency
- Budd–Chiari syndrome
- Schistosomiasis
- Cystic fibrosis
- Autoimmune chronic hepatitis with cirrhosis
- Primary sclerosing cholangitis
- Nonalcoholic steatohepatitis (NASH)
- Inherited causes that may present in infancy and childhood: glycogen storage disease, galactosemia, fructose intolerance, tyrosinemia, acid cholesterol ester hydrolase deficiency

#### Contributory or predisposing factors
- Alcohol abuse

- Injectable (venous and subcutaneous ('skin popping')) drug abuse – shared needles
- Cocaine snorting – blood contamination of shared equipment
- Hemodialysis – up to 10% of patients on hemodialysis are infected with hepatitis C
- Sexual promiscuity – greater risk factor in hepatitis B than hepatitis C
- Risk of perinatal transmission with hepatitis B is high and much lower with hepatitis C

## EPIDEMIOLOGY
### Incidence and prevalence
INCIDENCE
US: estimated at 3.6/1000.

FREQUENCY
- Eleventh leading cause of death in the US, but 25% decline since 1980, possibly due to reduced alcohol consumption, hepatitis B vaccination, improved supportive care, and liver transplantation
- Accounts for over 30,000 deaths/year in the US
- Cirrhosis is one of the leading causes of death for people over age 65

### Demographics
AGE
- Incidence increases with age
- Etiology dependent

GENDER
- Etiology dependent
- In females there is greater likelihood of progression to cirrhosis than in males ingesting the same relative amount of alcohol

RACE
People from Asia and sub-Saharan Africa have high rates of chronic hepatitis B and C infection.

GENETICS
Genetics of some etiologies are known, e.g. hemochromatosis, Wilson's disease, alpha-1-antitrypsin deficiency.

GEOGRAPHY
People from Asia and sub-Saharan Africa have high rates of chronic hepatitis B and C infection.

# DIAGNOSIS

## DIFFERENTIAL DIAGNOSIS
- The differential diagnosis depends on presentation, as cirrhosis can present clinically with portal hypertension, hepatic encephalopathy, and variceal bleeding
- The diagnosis requires a careful history of drug use and exposure to hepatitis viruses; evaluation of the results of laboratory tests such as those for hepatitis B surface antigen, hepatitis C antibodies, autoantibodies, serum ceruloplasmin, copper, and iron, and measurement of the metal content of the liver biopsy specimen
- The clinician should also be alert for disease processes that mimic cirrhosis, like constrictive pericarditis, Budd–Chiari syndrome, veno-occlusive disease, idiopathic portal hypertension, portal vein thrombosis, and myeloid metaplasia

### Other causes of ascites
- Malignancy: usually occurs in the setting of weight loss; sometimes, but not always, a primary tumor is obvious, and ascites may be the presenting feature; other features of cirrhosis are absent and the patient usually lacks risk factors for cirrhosis
- Low albumin, e.g. nephrotic syndrome, malabsorption; usually occurs in the context of renal failure
- Congestive cardiac failure: patients not always symptomatic with heart disease. Requires a high index of suspicion
- Pericarditis: may be late manifestation of viral pericarditis
- Infection, especially tuberculosis, usually associated with fever and weight loss
- Hypothyroidism: patients are clinically hypothyroid with hoarse voice and hypoactive reflexes. Can be associated with heart disease
- With portal hypertension consider Budd–Chiari syndrome due to inferior vena cava thrombosis or portal vein thrombosis

### Other causes of upper gastrointestinal bleeding
Most importantly, these other forms of bleeding lack clinical evidence of cirrhosis and all of the associated complications that confound management of gastrointestinal bleeding.
- Peptic ulcer: there are two major causes of peptic ulcer bleeding, aspirin and other nonsteroidal anti-inflammatory drugs (NSAIDs), and *Helicobacter pylori*. Half of those with NSAIDs and 75% without NSAIDs have associated abdominal pain or dyspeptic symptoms
- Mallory–Weiss tear: usually the only preceding symptom is vomiting, which causes the tear. Of course, patients with other gastrointestinal disorders can develop a tear if they vomit
- Arterial-venous malformation (AVM): AVMs cause gastrointestinal bleeding more frequently in older patients and in those with end-stage liver disease. Associations with von Willebrand's disease and aortic stenosis have been reported, but the latter is controversial

### Other causes of encephalopathy
Infection, generalized or encephalitis:
- Usually infection is straightforward, associated with elevated white blood cell count and fever

Central nervous system malignancy:
- Prior history of malignancy with the potential for metastasis to the brain
- Focal neural defects consistent with a space-occupying lesion
- A space-occupying lesion in the brain on imaging studies
- Patients may have focal neurologic signs

Hypoxia due to severe cardiac or respiratory disease or arrest:
- Profound hypoxia due to respiratory or cardiovascular compromise
- A short-term, profound cardiac or respiratory arrest

Renal failure:
- Blood urea nitrogen (BUN) usually markedly elevated and patients may have metabolic acidosis
- Patients tend to respond to dialysis

Drugs, e.g. barbiturates, benzodiazepines:
- A careful history of medication use may reveal factors that have caused or precipitated encephalopathy

Metabolic abnormalities:
- Diabetic coma – associated with elevated glucose and ketones

## SIGNS & SYMPTOMS
### Signs
- Variable, depending on stage of the disease – may be entirely normal in the early stages
- Most signs are nonspecific and do not reflect the underlying etiology

Skin and nails:
- Jaundice
- Palmar erythema (alcohol abuse)
- Spider telangiectases
- Ecchymosis (thrombocytopenia, coagulation factor deficiency)
- Caput medusae (dilated superficial periumbilical vein)
- Increased pigmentation – bronze appearance (hemochromatosis)
- Xanthomas (primary biliary cirrhosis)
- Needle tracks (viral hepatitis)
- Clubbing
- Nail changes (Muehrcke lines, Terry's nails)

Eyes:
- Kayser–Fleischer rings (corneal copper deposition in Wilson's disease)
- Sunflower cataracts (less commonly seen in Wilson's disease than Kayser-Fleisher rings; central greenish disk in anterior portion of lens with appearance like petals radiating outwards from the posterior capsule)

Abdomen:
- Small nodular liver
- Tender hepatomegaly in congestive hepatomegaly
- Palpable nontender gallbladder in neoplastic extrahepatic biliary obstruction
- Palpable spleen (portal hypertension)
- Venous hum over periumbilical veins in portal hypertension
- Ascites (portal hypertension, hypoalbuminemia)
- Testicular atrophy – hypogonadism is particularly prominent in male patients with cirrhosis due to alcoholism or hemochromatosis

Neurologic:
- Flapping tremor
- Choreoathetosis, dysarthria (Wilson's disease)

Other signs:
- Gynecomastia – feminization is particularly prominent in male patients with cirrhosis due to alcoholism or hemochromatosis
- Dupuytren's contracture
- Peripheral edema (right heart failure or hypoalbuminemia)
- Arthropathy (hemochromatosis)

## Symptoms
- Well compensated cirrhotics are asymptomatic (40–60% of patients)
- Anorexia, nausea, vomiting, diarrhea
- Fatigue, weakness
- Fever
- Yellowing of skin or sclera
- Pale stools and dark urine occur with obstructive or cholestatic jaundice as urobilinogen is unable to reach the intestine
- Itch

## KEY! DON'T MISS!
Do not miss clinical signs of the disease, e.g. palmar erythema, firm nodular liver, or splenomegaly – the earlier the clinical suspicion and confirmation of cirrhosis, the better the prognosis.

## CONSIDER CONSULT
- Definitive diagnosis of cirrhosis needs liver biopsy
- Evaluation of etiology is essential for appropriate management

## INVESTIGATION OF THE PATIENT
### Direct questions to patient
**Q** Have you had any episodes of abdominal pain? Recurrent right upper quadrant abdominal pain may indicate biliary tract disease

**Q** Have you ever had persistent pale stools and/or dark urine? Both pale stools and dark urine may be associated with cholestatic obstructive jaundice

**Q** Have you ever been told you have a disease such as idiopathic thrombocytopenia purpura, myasthenia gravis, thyroiditis, or any autoimmune connective tissue diseases? Other diseases with immune or autoimmune features may be associated with autoimmune chronic hepatitis with cirrhosis

**Q** Have you ever had inflammatory bowel disease? This may be associated with primary sclerosing cholangitis

**Q** Do you itch a lot? Pruritus may be caused by cholestasis secondary to primary biliary cirrhosis

**Q** Have you ever been told that you have hyperlipoproteinemia or xanthomas? These conditions in a middle-aged or elderly woman may be associated with primary biliary cirrhosis

**Q** Have you had any trouble with impotence, diabetes mellitus, hyperpigmentation, or arthritis? These conditions may be associated with hemochromatosis

**Q** Have you ever had any neurologic problems? Neurologic disturbances may be associated with Wilson's disease

### Contributory or predisposing factors
**Q** How much alcohol do you drink? Alcohol abuse is a common etiologic factor in liver disease

**Q** Have you had hepatitis B or C, a blood transfusion, injectable drugs, or intranasal cocaine? All of these are risk factors for viral hepatitis. Infection may predispose to liver disease and cirrhosis

**Q** What medications do you take or have you taken in the past? A history of exposure to hepatotoxic drugs should be sought. This should include a complete list of any herbal or over-the-counter (OTC) medications

### Family history
Do you have a family history of liver disease? Hemochromatosis (positive family history in 25% of patients) and alpha-1-antitrypsin deficiency have a hereditary etiology.

### Examination
Examine the skin and nails:
- Increased pigmentation: bronze appearance – hemochromatosis
- Hands: leukonychia, clubbing, palmar erythema, bruising – signs of chronic liver disease

- Face: jaundice, scratch marks, spider nevi – signs of chronic liver disease
- Legs: bruising, edema, muscle wasting – signs of chronic liver disease
- Xanthomas – primary biliary cirrhosis
- Needle tracks – viral hepatitis

Examine the eyes:
- Kayser–Fleischer rings or sunflower cataracts – signs of Wilson's disease

Examine the abdomen:
- Caput medusae: dilated superficial periumbilical vein in portal hypertension
- Liver: small nodular liver of cirrhosis; tender hepatomegaly in congestive hepatomegaly
- Gallbladder: palpable nontender gallbladder in neoplastic extrahepatic biliary obstruction
- Spleen: often palpable due to portal hypertension
- Ascites: portal hypertension, hypoalbuminemia
- Scrotum: testicular atrophy due to hypogonadism is particularly prominent in male patients with cirrhosis due to alcoholism or hemochromatosis
- Auscultation of periumbilical veins: venous hum in portal hypertension

Neurologic examination:
- Flapping tremor, choreoathetosis, dysarthria: Wilson's disease

Other signs:
- Gynecomastia: feminization is particularly prominent in male patients with cirrhosis due to alcoholism or hemochromatosis
- Peripheral edema: right heart failure, hypoalbuminemia
- Arthropathy: hemochromatosis

## Summary of investigative tests

Assessment of liver function:
- Complete blood count
- Liver function tests – serum albumin concentration and prothrombin time (PT) or international normalization ratio (INR). The PT or INR is the first to become abnormal and serves as a good marker of liver function
- Renal function and electrolytes

Assessment of the cause:
- Hepatitis virology – hepatitis B surface antigen (HBsAg), anti-HBc, anti-HBs, anti-HCV (hepatitis C virus), anti-HDV (hepatitis D virus)
- Autoantibodies – antimitochondrial antibody (AMA), smooth muscle antibody (SMA), anti-KLM antibody (ANA); antimitochondrial antibodies (anti-M2) in those with primary biliary cirrhosis
- Alpha-1-antitrypsin (and protease inhibitor typing) – protease inhibitor, produced by the liver, that inactivates trypsin. It can be detected by protein electrophoresis revealing the absence of alpha-1-globulin peak. More specific testing is necessary to confirm the diagnosis and establish the genotype
- Serum ferritin
- Serum copper and ceruloplasmin
- Alpha fetoprotein (AFP) – elevated in primary liver cell carcinoma

Imaging:
- Ultrasonography – good for detecting bile duct dilation and space-occupying lesions but cirrhosis cannot be diagnosed by ultrasound alone; Doppler ultrasound is useful for indicating direction of flow in and patency of portal and hepatic veins
- Computed tomography (CT) – if ultrasound is technically inadequate. May show changes consistent with a cirrhotic liver, splenomegaly, collaterals, venous thrombosis

Investigations normally performed by a specialist:
- Technetium-99m sulfur colloidal scan – useful in diagnosis of cirrhosis, detection of hepatic adenomas and diagnosis of Budd–Chiari syndrome
- Endoscopic retrograde cholangiopancreatography (ERCP) – useful in diagnosis of periampullary carcinoma, common duct stones, and primary sclerosing cholangitis
- Percutaneous transhepatic cholangiography – useful in ruling out common duct obstruction and recognizing sclerosing cholangitis; most often used when ERCP is not possible
- Visceral angiography to determine vascular anatomy, patency, and collaterals
- Esophagogastroduodenoscopy to assess varices
- Portal venography
- Wedged hepatic vein pressure measurement
- Liver biopsy is the gold standard for diagnosis and is always performed by a specialist

## CLINICAL PEARLS
- 80% of ascites are caused by hepatic cirrhosis
- Patients with viral hepatitis should be counseled on recommendations by the Centers for Disease Control and Prevention to avoid household transmission of hepatitis B and C
- Patients with decompensated hepatic cirrhosis may be candidates for referral to a transplant center
- The etiologies of most causes of hepatic cirrhosis can be identified by history and results of blood tests
- Most causes of hepatic cirrhosis are preventable or available treatment can reduce the risk of cirrhosis, including alcohol, hepatitis B and C, hemochromatosis, and Wilson's disease

## THE TESTS
### Body fluids
COMPLETE BLOOD COUNT
*Description*
Venous blood test.

*Advantages/Disadvantages*
- Advantage: inexpensive, simple to perform
- Disadvantage: nonspecific abnormalities

*Normal*
- Hemoglobin: male 13.6–17.7g/dL (136–177g/L); female 12–15g/dL (120–150g/L)
- Hematocrit: male 39–49%; female 33–43%
- Mean corpuscular volume (MCV): 76–100mcm$^3$ (76–100fL)

*Abnormal*
- Hemoglobin reduced
- Hematocrit reduced
- MCV elevated

*Cause of abnormal result*
- Anemia of chronic disease
- Malabsorption
- Folate deficiency in alcoholism

*Drugs, disorders and other factors that may alter results*
Macrocytic anemia is also found in:
- Folic acid or vitamin B12 deficiency
- Hypothyroidism
- Reticulocytosis

- Neoplasms, monocytic leukemia, lymphomas, myeloma, sarcoidosis
- Inflammatory bowel disease

## LIVER FUNCTION TESTS
*Description*
Venous blood test.

*Advantages/Disadvantages*
Advantages: inexpensive, simple to perform.

Disadvantages:
- Nonspecific abnormalities
- Alanine aminotransferase (ALT, SGPT) and aspartate aminotransferase (AST, SGOT) may be normal even with significant cirrhosis, especially in patients with jejunoileal bypass operations, hemochromatosis, or after methotrexate

*Normal*
- ALT: 0–35U/L (0–0.58mckat/L)
- AST: 0–35U/L (0–0.58mckat/L)
- Bilirubin, total: 0–1.0mg/dL (2–18mcmol/L)
- Serum gammaglutamyl transferase (GGT): 0–30U/L (0.050mckat/L)
- Alkaline phosphatase: 30–120U/L (0.5–2.0mckat/L)
- Albumin: 4–6g/dL (40–60g/L)
- Note: upper limit of normal depends on laboratory

*Abnormal*
- Alcoholic hepatitis and cirrhosis: mild elevation of ALT and AST; AST > ALT (>2:1)
- Extrahepatic obstruction: moderate elevation of ALT and AST (but <500 IU)
- Viral, toxic, or ischemic hepatitis: ALT and AST >500 IU
- Extrahepatic biliary obstruction, primary biliary cirrhosis, and primary sclerosing cholangitis: elevated alkaline phosphatase
- Alcoholic liver disease and possibly cholestasis: raised GGT
- Significant liver disease: hypoalbuminemia

*Cause of abnormal result*
- Plasma conjugated bilirubin is elevated in liver disease due to reflux from liver cells. The level cannot differentiate parenchymal from obstructive causes
- Hepatocellular damage leads to the release of transaminases into the bloodstream
- The liver excretes alkaline phosphatase into the bile and its serum level is considerably increased in intra- or extrahepatic obstructive biliary disease
- GGT is present in many body tissues and is increased in the bloodstream in biliary obstruction
- Albumin is reduced in liver disease from impaired manufacture in the liver and associated malnutrition and malabsorption

*Drugs, disorders and other factors that may alter results*
Raised serum bilirubin:
- Usually elevated in significant liver disease
- Gilbert's syndrome
- Hemolysis – chronic hemolysis does not produce bilirubin levels >5mg/dL (50mg/L) in the absence of liver disease
- Ineffective erythropoiesis
- Inherited disorders of bilirubin transport and metabolism

Raised transaminases (ALT is more specific to liver disease than AST)
- Post myocardial infarction
- Post cardiac surgery
- Malignancy
- Hepatitis – alcoholic, viral
- Hemolytic and obstructive jaundice
- Mononucleosis; cytomegalovirus, Epstein–Barr virus infections
- Drugs, e.g. halothane, isoniazid, acetaminophen excess
- AST is also increased in trauma and some skeletal muscle disease

Raised serum GGT:
- Alcohol abuse, biliary obstruction, liver cell damage, hepatic malignancies
- Myocardial infarction
- Cerebrovascular accident
- Diabetes mellitus
- Chronic lung disease

Raised alkaline phosphatase:
- Bone disease: osteomalacia, rickets, primary or secondary hyperparathyroidism, Paget's disease of bone, secondary bone carcinoma, myositis ossificans
- Liver disease: intra- or extrahepatic cholestasis, hepatocellular disease, space-occupying lesions

Reduced albumin:
- Nephrotic syndrome
- Malnutrition and malabsorption
- Most forms of chronic liver disease but especially cirrhosis
- Chronic infection
- Loss from bloodstream: hemorrhage, burns, exudates
- Gastrointestinal loss – protein-losing enteropathies

PROTHROMBIN TIME
*Description*
Venous blood test.

*Advantages/Disadvantages*
Advantage: good measure of hepatocellular function.

*Normal*
- PT: 10–12s
- INR: 1.0

*Abnormal*
Prolonged PT or INR.

*Cause of abnormal result*
Reductions in vitamin K-dependent clotting factors (II, VII, IX, and X) secondary to decreased hepatic protein synthesis and increased plasma proteolytic activity.

*Drugs, disorders and other factors that may alter results*
PT or INR is prolonged in liver failure or if patient is taking oral anticoagulants.

## RENAL FUNCTION AND ELECTROLYTES
*Description*
Venous blood test.

*Advantages/Disadvantages*
- Advantage: inexpensive, simple to perform
- Disadvantage: nonspecific abnormalities

*Normal*
- Serum creatinine: 0.6–1.2mg/dL (50–110mcmol/L)
- BUN: 8–18mg/dL (3–6.5mmol/L)
- Serum sodium: 135–147mEq/L (135–147mmol/L)
- Serum potassium: 3.5–5.0mEq/L (3.5–5.0mmol/L)

*Abnormal*
Both creatinine and BUN may be increased but BUN may be normal or reduced in severe liver dysfunction.

*Cause of abnormal result*
- Hepatorenal syndrome: acute and progressive reduction in renal blood flow and glomerular filtration rate secondary to intense renal cortical vasoconstriction due to decompensated cirrhosis. Risk factors include reduction of effective blood volume in cirrhosis, e.g. excessive diuresis and gastrointestinal blood loss; excessive diarrhea (lactulose-induced); bacteremia; and malnutrition (especially with alcoholic cirrhosis)
- Sodium may be reduced due to hemodilution
- Potassium may be decreased due to secondary aldosteronism or urinary losses

*Drugs, disorders and other factors that may alter results*
- Reduced BUN can occur in pregnancy, nephrosis, and diabetes insipidus
- Raised creatinine occurs in obstruction of the urinary tract
- Decreased potassium can occur in diarrhea and vomiting and with some drugs, e.g. steroids, thiazide diuretics
- Decreased sodium may be found in diarrhea, vomiting, heart failure, renal failure and inappropriate antidiuretic hormone secretion

## HEPATITIS VIROLOGY
*Description*
- Serum hepatitis B surface antigen (HBsAg)
- Immunoglobulin M (IgM) anti-HBc (indicates acute or recent infection)
- Serum anti-HCV (hepatitis C virus)
- Serum anti-HDV (hepatitis D virus)

*Advantages/Disadvantages*
Disadvantage: immunoenzymatic assay takes up to 6 months (average 3 months) to become positive.

*Abnormal*
Hepatitis B:
- HBsAg implies active infection
- Anti-HBs implies recovery and immunity
- HBeAg implies infectivity to others
- Anti-HBe usually, but not always, implies loss of infectivity
- High titer IgM anti-HBc implies acute severe hepatitis B

- Persistence of IgG anti-HBc implies chronic hepatitis B virus if HBsAg is also positive, or recovery if anti-HBs is present

Hepatitis C:
- Immunoenzymatic (enzyme-linked immunosorbent assay (ELISA)-3) assay is 99% specific

*Cause of abnormal result*
Hepatitis B or C infection.

## AUTOANTIBODIES
*Description*
- Antimitochondrial antibodies (AMAs) are found in 80–100% of patients with primary biliary cirrhosis
- M2 subgroup of AMAs is claimed to be specific for primary biliary cirrhosis
- Anti-smooth muscle antibodies (SMAs) have been found in 40–70% of patients with chronic active hepatitis and also in patients with biliary cirrhosis and other liver diseases, but not in alcoholic cirrhosis

*Advantages/Disadvantages*
- Advantage: simple to perform
- Disadvantage: patient may still need specialist referral for further evaluation, including liver biopsy

*Drugs, disorders and other factors that may alter results*
- False-positive results with AMAs have been found in patients with drug-induced cholestasis, chronic active hepatitis, extrahepatic obstruction, acute infectious hepatitis, and rheumatoid arthritis
- Positive SMAs suggest liver disease (chronic active hepatitis), transient viral infection, drug-induced hepatitis, or cryptogenic cirrhosis

## SERUM FERRITIN
*Description*
- Iron protein complex that plays a part in absorption, transport, and storage of iron
- For detection of hemochromatosis
- Venous blood test

*Advantages/Disadvantages*
- Advantage: best screening test for idiopathic hemochromatosis
- Disadvanatage: result may be affected by recent dietary iron and oral iron therapy but this will not be significant in high levels found in alcoholic liver disease and hemochromatosis

*Normal*
<30mcg/dL (<300mcg/L).

*Abnormal*
- >100mcg/dL (>1000mcg/L) in genetic hemochromatosis
- Often 30–100mcg/dL (300–1000mcg/L) in alcoholic liver disease

*Drugs, disorders and other factors that may alter results*
Ferritin may be raised in malignancy or chronic inflammation, e.g. rheumatoid arthritis.

## SERUM COPPER AND CERULOPLASMIN
*Description*
- For detection of Wilson's disease – an autosomal recessive inherited disorder of copper metabolism

- Ceruloplasmin, an alpha-2-globulin that transports copper, is reduced. Copper not bound to ceruloplasmin may be normal or increased but total copper is reduced

*Advantages/Disadvantages*
Disadvantage: 5% of normal individuals have a ceruloplasmin level below the 'normal' range.

*Normal*
- Serum copper: 70–140mcg/dL (11–22mcmol/L)
- Ceruloplasmin: 20–35mg/dL (200–350mg/L)

*Abnormal*
- Serum copper: 19–64mcg/dL (3–10mcmol/L)
- Serum ceruloplasmin: 0–20mg/dL (0–200mg/L)
- A normal ceruloplasmin usually, but not always, excludes Wilson's disease

*Cause of abnormal result*
Wilson's disease is characterized by the inability of the liver to produce ceruloplasmin, which transports copper. Excess copper is deposited in various tissues, eventually damaging the basal ganglia of the brain, liver, eyes, and kidneys.

*Drugs, disorders and other factors that may alter results*
- Ceruloplasmin and copper levels are also reduced in malnutrition, nephrotic syndrome, and protein-losing enteropathy
- Smoking can increase ceruloplasmin by 15–30%
- As ceruloplasmin is an 'acute reaction protein', it can be increased in acute inflammation

## PROTEIN ELECTROPHORESIS
*Description*
- Venous blood sample
- Patient should not eat for at least 8h before the test
- High-fat diet should be avoided for at least 24h before the sample is taken

*Advantages/Disadvantages*
Disadvantages:
- Not specific to liver disease and not very sensitive
- Because of the lack of specificity and sensitivity, its utility as a definitive diagnostic tool in cirrhosis is questionable

*Normal*
Serum protein electrophoresis identifies five main protein groups:
albumin, alpha-1, alpha-2, beta- and gamma-globulins.

*Abnormal*
- Alpha-1-globulin is almost 90% alpha-1-antitrypsin. Protein electrophoresis detects homozygotes but heterozygotes often show normal alpha-1-globulin peaks
- Alpha-2-globulins include ceruloplasmin but reduction in one component of the alpha-2-globulins is usually masked by one of the other components
- 90% of patients with well established cirrhosis show variable elevation of gamma-globulins. Most suggestive pattern is broad-based globulin elevation plus fusion of beta- and gamma-globulin

*Drugs, disorders and other factors that may alter results*
- Albumin may be reduced in: nephrotic syndrome, malnutrition, malabsorption, chronic infection, loss from bloodstream (hemorrhage, burns, exudates), and gastrointestinal loss (protein-losing enteropathies)

- Beta-globulin zone also increased in hypothyroidism, biliary cirrhosis, nephrosis, and some cases of diabetes
- Gamma-globulin levels may be increased in some patients with Hodgkin's disease, lymphoma, and chronic lymphocytic leukemia

### ALPHA FETOPROTEIN
*Description*
Marker for primary liver carcinoma and non-neoplastic liver disease.

*Advantages/Disadvantages*
Advantage: modern radioimmunoassay has greatly improved sensitivity.

*Normal*
0–20ng/mL (0–20mcg/L).

*Abnormal*
AFP of 500ng/mL has been suggested as a cutoff point in differentiating hepatoma from non-neoplastic liver disease.

*Drugs, disorders and other factors that may alter results*
- Most frequent non-neoplastic AFP elevations in liver disease occur in conditions associated with active necrosis of liver cells, e.g. hepatitis and alcoholic cirrhosis
- AFP can be elevated in cancer of the gastrointestinal tract, ovaries, or testicles

## Biopsy
### LIVER BIOPSY
*Advantages/Disadvantages*
Advantages:
- Gold standard for diagnosis
- Definitive diagnosis often depends on liver biopsy (percutaneous, transjugular, open)
- Patterns of injury as well as special stains may identify a precise etiology such as alcoholic liver disease, hemochromatosis, alpha-1-antitrypsin deficiency, hepatitis B, primary biliary cirrhosis

Disadvantages:
- Mortality is a risk, although the rate is low (0.01–0.1%); laparoscopic liver biopsy does not influence mortality from the procedure, although it does reduce the sampling error
- Transcutaneous liver biopsy is not safe if the PT is prolonged but transjugular biopsy provides an option

*Normal*
Normal liver architecture only.

*Abnormal*
- Depends on underlying etiology
- Nodular disorganized cirrhotic pattern

## Imaging
### ULTRASONOGRAPHY
*Advantages/Disadvantages*
Advantages:
- Sensitivity for detection of gallbladder stones is >90%
- Allows quick differentiation of obstruction of the intrahepatic and extrahepatic bile ducts from other causes of jaundice, such as hepatitis

- Excellent imaging tool for the evaluation of the hepatic parenchyma
- Allows detection of fatty liver as well as textural changes of cirrhosis and has a sensitivity of 80–90% for detection of hepatic neoplasms
- Cystic lesions within the liver and hepatic abscesses are readily detected
- Spleen is readily imaged to determine its size as well as to visualize intrasplenic or perisplenic fluid collections or mass lesions
- Doppler and color Doppler studies can evaluate portal venous flow in patients with portal hypertension before and after placement of a transjugular intrahepatic portosystemic shunt (TIPS)

*Normal*
Normal ultrasound appearance of liver is homogeneous.

*Abnormal*
- Biliary obstruction
- Stones
- Cystic lesions within the liver and hepatic abscesses
- Tumors
- Detection of fatty liver as well as textural changes of cirrhosis
- Heterogeneity of the parenchyma

## COMPUTED TOMOGRAPHY
*Advantages/Disadvantages*
Advantages:
- Most liver pathology can be visualized by ultrasound but CT improves accuracy and reveals smaller lesions
- Entire liver can be imaged by CT in a single breath-hold in <30s
- This rapid scanning allows optimal utilization of contrast material. The entire liver can be imaged during the arterial phase after injection of a contrast bolus to detect hypervascular lesions, such as hepatomas, that typically enhance more than normal hepatic parenchyma during the arterial phase
- The technique is not operator-dependent; therefore, errors in acquisition of pertinent information are reduced
- CT is an essential tool for evaluating and staging mass lesions, e.g. for diagnosis of hepatic abscesses and metastases
- In biliary obstruction, CT is very useful in determining the cause of obstruction, including carcinoma of the pancreatic head or the ampulla, especially when ultrasound is inconclusive
- Can assess hepatic fat content
- Identifies idiopathic hemochromatosis in moderately advanced stages
- Early diagnosis of Budd–Chiari syndrome
- Detection of varices and splenomegaly

*Normal*
Normal, homogeneous liver architecture.

*Abnormal*
- Changes in liver size or architecture: e.g. an enlarged, fatty liver or a small, nodular liver
- Hepatic masses: primary or metastatic neoplasia
- Vascular abnormality, such as a hemangioma
- Dilated hepatic ducts
- Masses in the pancreas or surrounding region

# TREATMENT

## CONSIDER CONSULT
- Refractory ascites may respond to large-volume paracentesis
- Management of refractory ascites, encephalopathy, variceal bleeding, and uncommon etiologies of cirrhosis (e.g. primary biliary cirrhosis, Wilson's disease, hemochromatosis) should be in consultation with a gastroenterologist or hepatologist
- Depending upon the circumstances, referral to a hepatologist involved with a liver transplant program may be indicated
- Patient showing the first sign of decompression should be referred to a gastroenterologist or hepatologist
- If urine output falls in the absence of a clear-cut explanation, a nephrologic consultation may be of considerable help, especially because creatinine level may not adequately reflect renal function

## IMMEDIATE ACTION
Prompt hospitalization is required for patients with:
- Gastrointestinal bleeding
- Worsening encephalopathy
- Increasing azotemia
- Signs of peritoneal irritation
- Unexplained fever

## PATIENT AND CAREGIVER ISSUES
### Impact on career, dependants, family, friends
Alcoholic cirrhosis results from long-standing substance abuse that may have resulted in alienation of family. Active participation on the part of members of the family in the patient's care and lifestyle changes may be difficult.

### Patient or caregiver request
- Patient may already think of cirrhosis as a terminal illness with no hope
- Alternatively, the patient may have an unrealistic hope of cure from a liver transplant and that they should and will receive one

## MANAGEMENT ISSUES
### Goals
- Remove or alleviate the underlying cause of cirrhosis
- Prevent further liver damage
- Prevent complications

### Management in special circumstances
COEXISTING MEDICATION
Patients should avoid all medications and substances that may be toxic to the liver, further worsening the underlying cirrhosis.

SPECIAL PATIENT GROUPS
- Cirrhosis may worsen during pregnancy, and higher rates of spontaneous abortion, premature birth, and perinatal death are seen in pregnant cirrhotic patients
- Pregnancy in a cirrhotic patient has additional implications. Pregnant women with cirrhosis have an approximately 25% chance of experiencing variceal bleeding, especially in the latter half of gestation. In addition, as the gravid uterus enlarges, there may be an obstruction of the inferior vena cava with peripheral venous return forced through collateral systems. Despite the risk of variceal bleeding and associated maternal and fetal mortality, no clear guidelines are available regarding therapy

PATIENT SATISFACTION/LIFESTYLE PRIORITIES
Many patients are chronic alcoholics with low self-esteem. A nonjudgmental, sympathetic approach can provide support, raise self-esteem, and improve compliance.

## SUMMARY OF THERAPEUTIC OPTIONS
### Choices
Lifestyle:
- A proper diet and activity are crucial to a favorable outcome, irrespective of etiology

Drugs:
- Large esophageal varices seen at endoscopy prior to clinical bleeding – nonselective beta-blocker, e.g. propranolol, at a dose to decrease the resting pulse by 25% or to a baseline heart rate of 60 beats/min
- Ascites: spironolactone may be given; it takes 3 days before onset of action. Add furosemide if needed
- Encephalopathy (under care of specialist): lactulose can be given to produce two or three soft stools per day
- Spontaneous bacterial peritonitis (under care of specialist): cefotaxime alone as initial treatment; norfloxacin, ciprofloxacin, and trimethoprim-sulfamethoxazole can decrease the risk of subsequent development of spontaneous bacterial peritonitis after treatment

Specific treatment based on etiology (under care of specialist):
- Wilson's disease: penicillamine, 125–250mg four times daily (give on empty stomach to avoid inactivation by metal binding). In patients intolerant to penicillamine, trientine may be used
- Hemochromatosis: remove excess body iron with phlebotomy and/or desferrioxamine
- Autoimmune chronic hepatitis: corticosteroids with or without azathioprine
- Therapy for chronic hepatitis B and chronic hepatitis C would be instigated and followed by a specialist
- Primary biliary cirrhosis: ursodiol (ursodeoxycholic acid), 12–15mg/kg/day in a twice-daily dose
- Cholestatic disease: ursodiol (ursodeoxycholic acid)

Surgical therapy:
- Possible procedures for portal hypertension include splenorenal or portacaval anastomosis and transjugular intrahepatic portal-systemic shunt
- Liver transplantation in suitable candidate (substance-free, motivated, and adherent to all advice). Liver transplant is the ultimate therapy but the efficacy of this treatment depends on the etiology of the cirrhosis and the overall general health of the patient prior to transplantation

### Clinical pearls
- All patients with a history of spontaneous bacterial peritonitis should be placed on secondary prophylaxis with norfloxacin, ciprofloxacin, or trimethoprim-sulfamethoxazole DS
- Diuretic treatment of patients with ascites usually follows the ratio of 100mg aldactone to 40mg furosemide
- Protein restriction should only be used if there is a documented susceptibility to encephalopathy from protein
- All patients with decompensated liver disease should be considered for referral for evaluation for liver transplantation

### Never
Never forget to emphasize at each visit the importance of remaining abstinent from alcohol.

## FOLLOW UP
- In a stable patient – yearly review and repeat liver tests
- Consider alpha fetoprotein and imaging to screen for hepatocellular carcinoma

- In an unstable patient – tests may be repeated at weekly intervals
- Patient should monitor weight and maintain a daily diary of fluid intake
- Screen for esophageal varices with upper endoscopy and if present can give beta-blocker for primary prophylaxis for hemorrhage
- Vaccinate for hepatitis A and B if not immune

## Plan for review
- Maintain a caloric intake of at least 2000–3000kcal/day
- Monitor prothrombin time, serum albumin, and bilirubin to assess the severity and progression of hepatocellular dysfunction
- Check stools at each visit for evidence of occult bleeding
- Check abdomen for evidence of ascites (shifting dullness, fluid wave, bulging flanks). Ultrasound examination is useful to confirm presence of ascites and rule out veno-occlusive disease

## Information for patient or caregiver
- Prognosis can often be greatly improved and symptoms lessened by careful adherence to the prescribed medical program
- Dietary discipline and omission of alcohol are central to a successful outcome and should be stressed

## DRUGS AND OTHER THERAPIES: DETAILS
### Drugs
PROPRANOLOL
- Nonselective beta-adrenergic blocker
- This is an off-label indication

*Dose*
120–240mg/day in three divided doses.

*Efficacy*
Effective in preventing bleeding in cirrhosis.

*Risks/benefits*
Risks:
- May further elevate liver function tests – false increase in bilirubin
- May worsen hepatic encephalopathy
- Use caution in diabetes mellitus, thyroid disease, renal disease
- Use caution in peripheral vascular disease, Raynaud's syndrome
- Use caution prior to surgery or anesthesia
- Use caution in pregnancy and breast-feeding
- Do not withdraw abruptly

*Side effects and adverse reactions*
- Cardiovascular system: bradycardia, congestive heart failure, heart block, peripheral vascular disease
- Central nervous system: lethargy, depression, dizziness, vivid dreams
- Eyes, ears, nose, and throat: dry eyes, sore throat
- Gastrointestinal: nausea, vomiting, diarrhea, dry mouth, ischemic colitis
- Hematologic: agranulocytosis, thrombocytopenia
- Metabolism: hyperglycemia, hyperlipidemia, masked hypoglycemia
- Respiratory: bronchospasm, dyspnea, wheezing
- Skin: alopecia, bruising, rash

*Interactions (other drugs)*
- Adenosine
- Alpha-adrenergic blockers
- Amiodarone
- Amoxicillin, ampicillin
- Antacids
- Antidiabetics
- Beta agonists
- Calcium channel blockers
- Clonidine
- Cocaine
- Digoxin
- Dipyridamole
- Lidocaine
- Neostigmine
- Neuroleptics
- Nonsteroidal anti-inflammatory drugs (NSAIDs)
- Physostigmine
- Prazosin
- Tacrine
- Theophylline
- Verapamil

*Contraindications*
- Severe chronic obstructive pulmonary disease
- In treatment of myocardial infarction, patients with hypotension
- Bronchospastic diseases, asthma
- Cardiogenic shock
- Congestive heart failure
- Advanced atrioventricular heart block
- Severe bradycardia
- Hepatic disease
- Pregnancy category C
- Breast-feeding
- High serum propranolol levels have been noted in patients with Down syndrome, suggesting that the bioavailability of propranolol may be increased in patients with this condition

*Acceptability to patient*
Well tolerated apart from drowsiness, fatigue.

*Follow up plan*
Monitor blood pressure and pulse as well as other management for varices.

*Patient and caregiver information*
Take pulse at home and notify physician if it falls below 50 beats/min.

SPIRONOLACTONE
Aldosterone antagonist.

*Dose*
- 100mg/day initially, either in a single daily dose or in divided doses
- Range: 25–250mg/day
- Takes 3 days for beneficial effect to be realized

*Efficacy*
- Effective in the treatment of ascites
- Can be given with furosemide for increased effectiveness

*Risks/benefits*
Risks:
- Spironolactone is a potassium-sparing diuretic therefore use caution with potassium supplements and hyponatremia
- Use caution in renal and hepatic impairment; diabetes, acidosis, and dehydration; menstrual problems and gynecomastia; in pregnancy and in the elderly

*Side effects and adverse reactions*
- Cardiovascular system: hypotension, bradycardia
- Central nervous system: headache, drowsiness
- Gastrointestinal: nausea, vomiting, diarrhea, bleeding, abdominal pain
- Genitourinary: menstrual irregularities, gynecomastia, hirsuitism, impotence
- Metabolic: hyperkalemia, hyponatremia, acidosis
- Skin: rashes, pruritus

*Interactions (other drugs)*
- Angiotensin-converting enzyme (ACE) inhibitors
- Ammonium chloride
- Anticoagulants

- Angiotensin II receptor antagonists ■ Cardiac glycosides ■ Carbenoxolone ■ Cyclosporine, tacrolimus ■ Disopyramide ■ Lithium ■ Mitotane ■ Potassium ■ Salicylates

*Contraindications*
■ Severe renal disease ■ Anuria ■ ACE inhibitors and angiotensin receptor antagonists in antikaliuretic therapy ■ Hyperkalemia

*Acceptability to patient*
Well tolerated apart from potential gastrointestinal side effects and pruritus.

FUROSEMIDE
Loop diuretic.

*Dose*
- Adult: initiate with 20–80mg as a single oral dose; may increase by 20 or 40mg no sooner than 6–8h after previous dose until desired diuretic effect is obtained
- Child: 2mg/kg bodyweight as a single oral dose; may be increased by 1 or 2mg/kg no sooner than 6–8h after previous dose. Not to exceed 6mg/kg

*Efficacy*
Can be given with spironolactone for increased effectiveness.

*Risks/benefits*
Risks
- Excessive diuresis may cause dehydration and blood volume reduction with circulatory collapse and possibly vascular thrombosis and embolism, particularly in elderly patients
- Use caution in diabetes mellitus, systemic lupus erythematosus; renal and liver disease; pregnancy and nursing mothers; hypertension, gout, porphyria

Benefit: reduces fluid congestion.

*Side effects and adverse reactions*
- Cardiovascular system: chest pain, circulatory collapse, orthostatic hypotension
- Central nervous system: dizziness, headache, paresthesia, fever
- Eyes, ears, nose, and throat: visual disturbances, ototoxicity, tinnitus, hearing impairment, thirst
- Gastrointestinal: ischemic hepatitis, vomiting, pancreatitis, nausea, diarrhea, anorexia
- Genitourinary: glycosuria, hyperuricemia, bladder spasm, polyuria
- Hematologic: blood disorders, agranulocytosis
- Metabolic: hyperglycemia, hyponatremia, hypokalemia, hypomagnesemia, hypovolemia, hypochloremia, hypercholesterolemia, hypertriglyceridemia
- Skin: erythema multiforme, exfoliative dermatitis, urticaria

*Interactions (other drugs)*
■ ACE inhibitors ■ Alpha-adrenergic antagonists ■ Amphotericin ■ Antibiotics (aminoglycosides, polymixins, vancomycin, cephalosporins) ■ Antidiabetics
■ Antidysrhythmics (amiodarone, cardiac glycosides, disopyramide, flecainide, mexelitine, quinidine, sotalol) ■ Beta-2 adrenergic agonists ■ Carbenoxolone ■ Cholestyramine, colestipol ■ Cisplatin ■ Clofibrate ■ Corticosteroids ■ Digitalis – increased risk of digitalis toxicity ■ Diuretics (thiazides, metolazone, acetazolamide) ■ Lidocaine ■ Lithium ■ NSAIDs
■ Phenobarbital ■ Phenytoin ■ Pimozide ■ Reboxetine ■ Selective serotonin reuptake inhibitors ■ Terbutaline ■ Tubocurarine

*Contraindications*
- Renal failure with anuria
- Hepatic coma

*Acceptability to patient*
Diuresis may interfere with normal daily activity.

*Follow up plan*
Monitor serum electrolytes, calcium, glucose, uric acid, creatinine, and blood urea nitrogen in first months of therapy.

*Patient and caregiver information*
- Should be taken with food or drink – may cause gastrointestinal upset
- Should be taken early in the day
- Prolonged exposure to sunlight should be avoided

LACTULOSE
Synthetic disaccharide analog of lactose.

*Dose*
30–45mL three or four times daily, adjusted to produce two or three soft stools per day.

*Risks/benefits*
Risks:
- A theoretical hazard may exist for patients being treated with lactulose solution who may be required to undergo electrocautery procedures during proctoscopy or colonoscopy
- Preparations will contain galactose (<2.2g/15mL) and lactose (<1.2g/15mL); should be used with caution in diabetics
- In the overall management of portal-systemic encephalopathy, it should be recognized that there is serious underlying liver disease with complications such as electrolyte disturbance (e.g. hypokalemia) for which other specific therapy may be required
- Use with caution in breast-feeding women

Benefits:
- Has cathartic effect
- Decreases serum ammonia level
- Improves hepatic encephalopathy
- Minimal systemic absorption
- May be used concomitantly with antibiotic therapy
- May be used for long-term therapy

*Side effects and adverse reactions*
- Gastrointestinal: abdominal discomfort, nausea, gaseous distension with flatulence
- Excessive dosage can lead to diarrhea with potential complications such as loss of fluids, hypokalemia, and hypernatremia

*Interactions (other drugs)*
- Benzodiazepine receptor ligand (reduces the efficacy of these drugs, and contributes to its positive effect on encephalopathy)
- Neomycin (may interfere with the degradation of lactulose)
- Other laxatives (may interfere with lactulose dosing)
- Nonabsorbable antacids (may inhibit the lactulose-induced drop in colonic pH)

*Contraindications*
- Patients requiring low galactose diet
- Safety and efficacy in children have not been

established ■ Pregnancy category B ■ Other laxatives should not be used, especially during the initial phase of therapy for portal-systemic encephalopathy, because the loose stools resulting from their use may falsely suggest that adequate lactulose dosage has been achieved

*Patient and caregiver information*
Can be mixed with fruit juice, water, or milk to improve palatability.

## Surgical therapy
LIVER TRANSPLANTATION
- Liver transplantation is definitive treatment for patients with decompensated liver disease
- Under the auspices of the United Network of Organ Sharing, patients are ranked according to their Mathematical Endstage Liver Disease Score (MELD), which predicts 90-day survival. Values used to generate a MELD score include creatinine, total bilirubin, and international normalized ratio (INR)
- Most patients receive cadaveric grafts. Because of organ shortage, there has been increasing interest using grafts from living donors and split livers

*Efficacy*
- In properly selected patients, 5-year survival may be as high as 85%
- Patients with acute liver failure who are treated in a transplant center can do very well
- Best candidates are those who are highly motivated, emotionally stable, and willing to comply with a medical program
- Primary indications for which clear benefit has been established: postnecrotic cirrhosis, primary biliary cirrhosis, viral hepatitis, primary sclerosing cholangitis, and alcoholic liver disease (but only if sobriety has been sustained for at least 6 months and adequate social support is available)
- Relative contraindications: hepatocellular carcinoma (depending on size and number of lesions) and renal failure
- AIDS, extrahepatic sepsis, metastatic cancer, active alcohol or drug abuse, and severe cardiopulmonary disease are absolute contraindications

*Risks/benefits*
Risks:
- Morbidity or mortality from surgery or the medications used to prevent rejection
- Increased risk of infection and some forms of neoplasia following transplantation
- Certain complications occur following transplantation, such as biliary stenosis and leaks
- Certain forms of liver disease, especially hepatitis C, tend to recur. The benefits of active therapy to prevent recurrences is being evaluated
- Return to alcohol consumption only occurs in about 10% of patients transplanted for alcoholic cirrhosis but has a bad prognostic impact

Benefit: Improved survival and return to a normal quality of life for the majority of patients who do well after transplantation

*Acceptability to patient*
Transplantation is arduous for patients and their families, but most patients do well and accept the transplant.

*Follow up plan*
Patients need to be closely monitored by a liver transplant specialist for appropriate drug levels and periodic monitoring.

*Patient and caregiver information*
- Patients with advanced liver disease should be instructed to seek consultation and follow the often challenging regimens offered
- Compliance with the regimen and avoidance of alcohol are essential for survival

## LIFESTYLE

Diet:
- Adequate protein (1g/kg) and generous calories to help regenerate the liver
- In the presence of hepatic encephalopathy, protein restriction may be necessary
- In the presence of ascites, salt restriction is necessary (2g or less/day)
- In the presence of hyponatremia (sodium <130mEq (<130mmol)), fluid restriction may be necessary (<1L)
- Avoid alcohol
- A trained nutritionist is required to give advice on appropriate and acceptable nutrition plan

Activity:
- Keep as active as possible
- With peripheral edema, leg elevation is necessary

RISKS/BENEFITS
Benefit: a proper diet and activity are crucial to a favorable outcome, irrespective of etiology.

FOLLOW UP PLAN
Periodic review, reinforcement, and encouragement.

PATIENT AND CAREGIVER INFORMATION
Thorough explanation of dietary advice and reasons why compliance is so important.

# OUTCOMES

## EFFICACY OF THERAPIES
- Main goal is to slow progression of disease. End-stage liver disease cannot be treated, except by transplantation. However, the following actions can reduce the risk of developing or worsening cirrhosis: abstinence for alcohol abuse, specific therapy for hepatitis B and C (e.g. interferon and ribavirin), phlebotomy for primary and chelation for secondary hemochromatosis, and chelation for Wilson's disease
- Efficacy of any treatment requires patient's understanding and compliance
- Efficacy depends on stage of liver disease and etiology

### Review period
Depends on severity of liver dysfunction, precise etiology, and presence of complications.

## PROGNOSIS
- Depends on nature, severity, and activity of the underlying illness
- For alcoholic cirrhosis, survival is affected by alcohol ingestion. Five-year survival is 60–85% in those who abstain, compared with 40–60% for those who continue to drink
- Onset of jaundice or ascites further decreases 5-year survival (to 30% in drinkers)
- Irrespective of etiology, development of ascites, encephalopathy, hyperbilirubinemia, hypergammaglobulinemia (from bypass of the hepatic reticuloendothelial system), and hypoalbuminemia are poor prognostic signs, as is decreased liver size
- Mortality rate exceeds 80% in patients with hepatorenal syndrome

### Clinical pearls
- Patients waiting for liver transplantation will need regular tests for creatinine, total bilirubin, and international normalized ratio (INR)
- Active correspondence is essential between the primary provider and the transplant center
- There are no pharmacologic treatments for cirrhosis; liver transplantation is the only definitive treatment of patients with decompensated liver disease
- Patients should be encouraged to follow a low-salt diet and eat at least three meals a day and a bedtime snack
- Patients with hepatic cirrhosis should be asked during clinic visits about the interval development of jaundice, ascites, encephalopathy, or gastrointestinal bleeding
- Patients with hepatic cirrhosis should be screened on a regular basis for hepatocellular carcinoma
- Hepatorenal syndrome is suggested by a rising creatinine and decreasing urine output
- In ascites, a ratio of spironolactone 100mg:furosemide 40mg will usually maintain normokalemia

### Therapeutic failure
- Any patient deteriorating despite their management regimen will need to be referred for specialist review
- Liver transplantation – last resort for a selected group of patients

### Terminal illness
Liver failure, with or without renal failure, will lead to difficulties in management of the terminally ill patient. These include:
- Nausea and vomiting
- Anorexia and cachexia
- Anemia from hematemesis and malabsorption
- Severe pruritus
- Coagulopathy

## COMPLICATIONS
- Portal hypertension
- Hepatic encephalopathy
- Coagulopathy
- Ascites
- Bleeding esophageal varices
- Liver failure
- Hepatocellular carcinoma
- Susceptibility to infections
- Spontaneous bacterial peritonitis
- Hepatorenal syndrome

## CONSIDER CONSULT
Any patient deteriorating despite their management regimen will need to be referred for specialist review immediately.

## PREVENTION

### RISK FACTORS
Hepatotoxic medications, hepatitis C, hereditary liver disease such as hemochromatosis, alcohol.

### MODIFY RISK FACTORS
**Lifestyle and wellness**
ALCOHOL AND DRUGS
- Limit use of alcohol and other liver toxins, especially if the patient has hepatitis C
- No sharing of syringes for intravenous drug abusers
- Liver test surveillance while on hepatotoxic drugs

SEXUAL BEHAVIOR
Safer sex – condoms, monogamy.

FAMILY HISTORY
Screening of family members when a genetic disease is recognized.

DRUG HISTORY
Awareness of potential mortality from acetaminophen.

IMMUNIZATION
Hepatitis A and B vaccines for at-risk groups.

*Cost/efficacy*
Both vaccines are inexpensive and widely available.

### PREVENT RECURRENCE
Avoid liver toxins, especially alcohol.

# RESOURCES

## ASSOCIATIONS
American Liver Foundation
75 Maiden Lane, Suite 603
New York, NY 10038
Tel: (800) GO-LIVER (465-4837)
E-mail: info@liverfoundation.org
http://www.liverfoundation.org

National Digestive Diseases Information Clearinghouse
Box NDDIC
Bethesda, MD 20892
Tel: (301) 468-6344
http://www.niddk.nih.gov

## KEY REFERENCES
- Caldwell SH, Oelsner DH, Iezzoni JC, et al. Cryptogenic cirrhosis: clinical characterization and risk factors for underlying disease. Hepatology 1999;29:664–9
- Poynard T, Bedossa P, Opolon P. Natural history of liver fibrosis progression in patients with chronic hepatitis C. Lancet 1997;349:825–32
- McCullough AJ, O'Connor JF. Alcoholic liver disease: proposed recommendations for the American College of Gastroenterology. Am J Gastroenterol 1998;93:2022–36
- Borowsky SA, Strome S, Lott E. Continued heavy drinking and survival in alcoholic cirrhotics. Gastroenterology 1981;80:1405
- Campra JL, Reynolds TB. Effectiveness of high-dose spironolactone therapy in patients with chronic liver disease and relatively refractory ascites. Dig Dis Sci 1978;23:1025
- Conn HO, Leevy CM, Vlahcevic ZR, et al. Comparison of lactulose and neomycin in the treatment of chronic portal-systemic encephalopathy; a double-blind controlled trial. Gastroenterology 1977;72:573
- Pagliaro L, D'Amico G, Sorensen TIA, et al. Prevention of first bleeding in cirrhosis: a meta-analysis of randomized trials of nonsurgical treatment. Ann Intern Med 1992;117:59–70
- Poynard T, Cales P, Pasta L, et al. Beta-adrenergic antagonist drugs in the prevention of gastrointestinal bleeding in patients with cirrhosis and esophageal varices. N Engl J Med 1991;324:1532–8
- Starzl TE, Demetris AJ, Van Thiel D. Liver transplantation. N Engl J Med 1989;321:1014-22, 1092–9
- Sleisenger & Fordtran's gastrointestinal and liver disease, 6th edn. Philadelphia, PA: W.B. Saunders, 1998

## FAQS
### Question 1
When should a patient with cirrhosis and ascites be evaluated for liver transplantation?

### ANSWER 1
Because the one-year survival rate after liver transplantation is >75% patients with cirrhosis and ascites or any other complications should be evaluated for transplantation. The one-year survival without transplantation in this setting is 50%, and 20% at 5 years.

### Question 2
Who is at risk of developing spontaneous bacterial peritonitis?

### ANSWER 2
Patients with fulminant hepatic failure, cirrhotics with ascites and low ascitic fluid total protein, and cirrhotics with gastrointestinal hemorrhage.

### Question 3
What clinical events precipitate hepatic encephalopathy in cirrhotic patients?

ANSWER 3
Infection, gastrointestinal hemorrhage, dehydration, renal failure, drugs, toxins, medications, and dietary indiscretion (excessive protein intake).

## CONTRIBUTORS
Russell C Jones, MD, MPH
Andrew H Soll, MD
Rudolph A Bedford, MD
Hetal A Karsan, MD
J Adrian Lunn, MD

# CROHN'S DISEASE

- Summary Information — 132
- Background — 133
- Diagnosis — 135
- Treatment — 148
- Outcomes — 161
- Prevention — 163
- Resources — 164

## SUMMARY INFORMATION

### DESCRIPTION
- Characterized by inflammation of the gastrointestinal tract; usually inflammation of the full thickness of the bowel but in a patchy, noncontinuous distribution
- Any portion of the gastrointestinal tract from mouth to anus may be involved; the terminal ileum and colon are most commonly affected
- Chronic, recurrent condition, marked by remissions and exacerbations
- Complications include fistulas, abscesses, perianal disease, and strictures
- Mainstays of therapy include 5-aminosalicylic acid derivatives, corticosteroids, and other immunosuppressive therapies

### URGENT ACTION
Crohn's disease patients are immunosuppressed and may not have overt symptoms; therefore, the threshold for office or emergency room visit should be low.

### KEY! DON'T MISS!
Symptoms should not be ascribed to irritable bowel syndrome if there is evidence of loss of mucosal integrity (rectal bleeding) or of an inflammatory disorder (fever, weight loss).

# BACKGROUND

## ICD9 CODE
555.9 Crohn's disease

## SYNONYMS
Chronic idiopathic inflammatory bowel disease.

## CARDINAL FEATURES
- Insidious onset of symptoms
- Weight loss, lethargy, fever, and general malaise
- Diarrhea, which may be bloody and can be intermittent
- Often vague abdominal pain, typically right lower quadrant or central, cramping or constant ache in nature
- Severe acute pain mimicking acute appendicitis
- Palpable, tender mass may be present in the lower abdomen, which represents thickened or matted loops of inflamed intestine or an abscess
- Frequently perianal disease with abscess and fistulas
- Radiographic evidence of ulceration, stricturing, or fistulas of small intestine or colon
- Any part of the gastrointestinal tract may be involved, and involvement is not continuous
- Extraintestinal manifestations are common (15%) and include stomatitis, oral aphthous ulceration, ocular disease (iritis, conjunctivitis, episcleritis), skin lesions (erythema nodosum and pyoderma gangrenosum), arthritis, clubbing, venous thrombosis, gallstones due to the malabsorption of bile salts from the terminal ileum and nephrolithiasis with urate or calcium oxalate stones, liver disease

## CAUSES
### Common causes
- Substantial alteration in diet in last half-century; incidence of Crohn's disease is increasing
- Possible breakdown in the tolerance of the intestinal mucosa to many bacterial and food antigens, leading to an unrestrained inflammatory process
- Improved sanitary and hygiene conditions during childhood reduces antigen exposure and, therefore, weakens immune tolerance in adults
- Possible involvement of a chronic, persistent gastrointestinal infection
- Stress can exacerbate symptoms and may be involved in pathogenesis
- Obvious link with cigarette smoking, Crohn's disease being more common in incidence and relapse in smokers
- 20% of patients with Crohn's disease have an affected relative, suggesting a genetic predisposition in some individuals

### Contributory or predisposing factors
- Genetic predisposition
- Cigarette smoking

## EPIDEMIOLOGY
### Incidence and prevalence
INCIDENCE
Crohn's disease: 2–6/100,000 population.

PREVALENCE
Crohn's disease: 30–50/100,000 population.

## Demographics

### AGE
- Occurs among all age groups but peak incidence at 15–35 years and a smaller second peak at 55–75 years
- 25–30% of patients first manifest the disease when younger than 20 years
- Rare before 10 years of age, whereas ulcerative colitis may be seen as early as infancy

### GENDER
Females may be slightly more disposed to develop Crohn's disease.

### RACE
- Seen in all ethnic groups
- Higher prevalence in Jews who have immigrated from northern Europe (less common in Sephardic Jews of Mediterranean or Middle Eastern origin)
- Less common in African races

### GENETICS
Inflammatory bowel disease has a strong genetic component:
- If a family member is affected, the chance of developing Crohn's disease is 10–15%
- If one of identical twins is affected, the risk to the other is 50%
- If a young adult has inflammatory bowel disease, the likelihood of a sibling or parent being affected by Crohn's disease is 3–8%
- The risk to a child of a parent with inflammatory bowel disease is 2%

### GEOGRAPHY
- More common in urban areas
- More common in northern Europe and North America

### SOCIOECONOMIC STATUS
- May be linked to a high standard of living – incidence in Japan and southern Europe has risen in line with increasing standards of living
- Within a specific region, incidence does not vary between socioeconomic groups

# DIAGNOSIS

## DIFFERENTIAL DIAGNOSIS
Crohn's disease can mimic almost any gastrointestinal condition.

### Ulcerative colitis
Ulcerative colitis is a chronic, recurrent condition marked by remissions and exacerbations.

FEATURES
- Diarrhea with bloody stools containing mucus and pus
- Proctitis with tenesmus may be present
- Confined to the colon
- A 10-year history of ulcerative colitis increases risk of cancer of the colon
- 10–20% of patients with inflammatory bowel disease have an indistinguishable form of colitis termed 'colitis intermediate'
- About three times as common as Crohn's disease

### Irritable bowel syndrome
Irritable bowel syndrome is a chronic, relapsing functional bowel disorder.

FEATURES
- Commonly there is a long duration of symptoms, usually not severe, with chronic, cramping abdominal pain, bloating, and intermittent loose stool
- Typically, variable bowel habit with some normal days, possibly with some fluctuation between constipation and diarrhea
- No rectal bleeding, weight loss, or systemic features
- X-rays and endoscopic studies (both macroscopically and histologically) are normal
- Normal inflammatory markers

### Celiac disease
Celiac disease is an inflammatory condition of the small intestine.

FEATURES
- Malabsorption syndrome; gluten intolerance produces villous atrophy in the small intestine
- Characterized by weight loss, diarrhea, abdominal bloating, and steatorrhea
- Aphthous ulcers may occur

### Appendicitis
Appendicitis is the acute inflammation of the appendix.

FEATURES
- Acute onset and rapid progression if untreated
- Fever
- Right lower quadrant pain

### Yersinia enterocolitica enteritis
FEATURES
- Acute onset with symptoms persisting beyond one week
- Fever
- Right lower quadrant pain
- Rare and tends to occur in epidemics
- Typically, systemic features such as polyarthritis, sacroiliitis, Reiter's syndrome, osteomyelitis
- Diagnosed by positive stool culture or serology
- Typically involves ileum

## Intestinal lymphoma

FEATURES
- Weight loss and malaise
- Diarrhea
- Pain not always a feature
- May have protein-losing enteropathy (low albumin)
- Fever
- Abnormal small bowel X-rays may mimic Crohn's disease
- Can present with intussusception

## Diverticulitis with abscess formation

Diverticulitis implies microperforation of a diverticulum with ensuing localized inflammation contained by pericolonic fat and mesentery.

FEATURES
- Fever and systemic malaise
- Abdominal pain and mass (most often left lower quadrant)
- Nausea, vomiting
- Elevated white blood cell count
- Acute abdomen

## Acute ischemic colitis

Acute vascular insufficiency of the colon usually involving the portion supplied by the inferior mesenteric artery.

FEATURES
- Often associated with risk factors for cardiovascular disease, most commonly diabetes and smoking
- Usually precipitated by a systemic low blood flow state; less frequently occurs secondary to embolic disease
- May present with symptoms identical to ulcerative colitis: fever, abdominal pain, and bloody diarrhea; abdominal pain generally more severe than in ulcerative colitis
- Generally older age at presentation (>50 years)
- Colonoscopy usually shows ulceration in transverse, descending, and sigmoid colon, with most intense involvement around splenic flexure
- Rectum is usually spared; usually affected in ulcerative colitis
- Self-limiting in 90% of cases and resolves without specific therapy
- May be recurrent or lead to chronic stricture in <10% of cases

## Radiation colitis

Colitis resulting from radiation therapy to the abdominal region.

FEATURES
- Nausea and vomiting
- Diarrhea
- Cramping pain
- Obstruction secondary to stricture formation may occur
- Perforation and fistula formation may rarely occur

## Viral gastroenteritis

Gastroenteritis is the acute inflammation of the lining of the stomach and intestines caused by a virus.

### FEATURES
- Typically lasts only 1–4 days and is self-limiting
- No rectal bleeding
- Negative stool culture

### Bacterial/amebal gastroenteritis
Bacterial/amebal gastroenteritis is the acute inflammation of the lining of the stomach and intestines caused by bacterial pathogens.

### FEATURES
- Most bacterial pathogens produce self-limiting disease lasting 7–14 days or less
- Rectal bleeding, fever, fecal leukocytes, and mucosal appearance may be indistinguishable from ulcerative colitis or Crohn's disease in acute phase
- Positive cultures obtained in 40% of cases
- *Shigella, Salmonella, Escherichia coli, Campylobacter,* and *Entamoeba histolytica* are the main causative organisms; herpes simplex virus (HSV), chlamydial and gonorrheal proctitis should be considered in patients who have had recent unprotected anal intercourse

### Clostridium difficile infection
FEATURES
- Symptoms and endoscopic appearance can mimic those of Crohn's disease or ulcerative colitis
- Often occurs in hospitalized patients, the immunocompromised, and the elderly
- History of taking antibiotics in past 2 months

## SIGNS & SYMPTOMS
### Signs
- Insidious onset with weight loss and fever (and associated diarrhea)
- Overt lower gastrointestinal bleeding is less typical
- Signs of anemia may be present
- Tender, right lower quadrant mass representing thickened or matted loops of inflamed intestine
- Perianal disease, frequently with abscess or fistulas
- Signs of intestinal obstruction, e.g. distension, dehydration, abdominal tenderness, hyperactive bowel sounds
- Extraintestinal manifestations occur less frequently than in ulcerative colitis: oral aphthous lesions, erythema nodosum, pyoderma gangrenosum, episcleritis, oligoarticular nondeforming arthritis, iritis, uveitis

### Symptoms
- Frequently nonspecific and vary according to the affected site in the gastrointestinal tract, severity of inflammation, and presence of complications
- Intermittent bouts of low-grade fever, diarrhea, and right lower quadrant and/or periumbilical pain
- General malaise, frequently associated with weight loss and loss of energy
- Diarrhea, not necessarily bloody and often intermittent
- Proctitis usually characterized by small-volume diarrhea with urgency and tenesmus
- Upper gastrointestinal involvement typically manifests with nausea, vomiting, epigastric pain, or obstruction
- Obstruction often causes postprandial cramping abdominal pain; this is seen most often in patients with active disease or late in the course of the disease from chronic fibrosis

## ASSOCIATED DISORDERS
The inflammatory bowel diseases (IBD) are associated with a number of extraintestinal manifestations, which can serve as markers for disease. 10% of patients present with extraintestinal manifestations.

Arthritis (ankylosing spondylitis and seronegative arthritis):
- Migratory, often involving the hip, ankle, wrist, or elbow
- Usually monoarticular and asymmetric, with no synovial destruction
- Course of the arthritis parallels that of the colitis

Nutritional and metabolic abnormalities:
- Hypoalbuminemia, as a result of nutritional, protein-losing enteropathy
- Deficiency of minerals such as iron, calcium, magnesium and zinc, as a result of decreased absorption in the gastrointestinal tract

Hepatic and biliary manifestations:
- Sclerosing cholangitis – chronic inflammation of the bile ducts with associated biliary obstruction
- Gallstones

Renal manifestations:
- Kidney stones
- Obstructive uropathy and fistulas to the urinary tract
- Amyloidosis

Eye manifestations:
- Conjunctivitis
- Iritis, which tends to follow a course independent of the course of the bowel disease
- Episcleritis, which often parallels the activity of the bowel disease
- Uveitis (when patients are HLA-B27 positive)

Hematologic abnormalities:
- Anemia
- Leukocytosis
- Thrombocytosis
- Megaloblastic anemia secondary to B12 deficiency if chronic terminal ileal disease or ileal resection

Skin manifestations:
- Pyoderma gangrenosum is an ulcerating lesion, which often leads to secondary infection and may be difficult to heal
- Erythema nodosum is an inflammation of the subcutaneous tissues (panniculitis) and is most commonly seen on the anterior shins
- Stomatitis with multiple aphthous ulcers

## KEY! DON'T MISS!

Symptoms should not be ascribed to irritable bowel syndrome if there is evidence of loss of mucosal integrity (rectal bleeding) or of an inflammatory disorder (fever, weight loss).

## CONSIDER CONSULT

All patients should be referred to a gastroenterologist initially for confirmation of diagnosis and ruling out of other conditions.

Urgent and emergent referral:
- Abscess – suggested by a tender abdominal mass with diarrhea, fever, and leukocytosis. Abdominal mass not always palpable, but abscess should still be considered in a toxic-appearing patient with history of Crohn's disease and abdominal pain
- Fistula formation, which may occur between affected intestine and urinary bladder, vagina, or skin. This may result in chronic cystitis, hematuria, and pneumaturia in vesicular fistulas;

leakage of fecal contents per vagina in vaginal fistulas; and skin drainage in cutaneous fistulas
- Small bowel obstruction in Crohn's disease, suggested by postprandial pain with distension, nausea, and vomiting
- Perforation – toxic-appearing patient with severe constant abdominal pain, rebound tenderness, guarding, and absent bowel sounds
- Anemia from chronic blood loss, dehydration, or hypovolemia from acute bleeding (suggested on clinical examination by tachycardia and orthostatic hypotension)
- Severe gastrointestinal bleeding is a medical emergency for which surgery is the definitive treatment
- Patients with pyoderma gangrenosum should be referred urgently to a specialist
- Patients with ophthalmologic symptoms should be promptly referred to an ophthalmologist

## INVESTIGATION OF THE PATIENT
### Direct questions to patient

**Q** Do you have abdominal pain? Where is it located and what is its quality? Location and quality of pain may help in differential diagnosis

**Q** How many bowel movements are you having each day? Are they loose and watery? Frequency of bowel movements can help determine severity of disease. However, loose bowel movements are characteristic of many gastrointestinal disorders

**Q** Have you had any rectal bleeding? Has there been blood in your bowel movements? Is it mixed in with the stool or streaking the outside of a hard stool? Bloody bowel movements are characteristic of inflammatory bowel disease but sometimes patients can mistake bleeding from hemorrhoids, especially when constipated, i.e. blood mixed in with stool is more likely to be an indicator of inflammatory bowel disease

**Q** Have you recently had any fever? Are the episodes of increasing abdominal pain associated with fever or myalgia? Frequently flares of Crohn's disease will be associated with constitutional symptoms such as fever and myalgia

**Q** Does the abdominal pain or diarrhea wake you from sleep? Symptoms of irritable bowel syndrome seldom wake patients from sleep

**Q** Does anything relieve your abdominal pain? Is your pain relieved by defecation? Symptoms of irritable bowel syndrome are more likely to be relieved by defecation whereas the abdominal pain characteristic of Crohn's disease is often unremitting during a flare-up

**Q** Do you have pain on defecation and tenesmus? Rectal symptoms are characteristic of anal Crohn's disease

**Q** Do you frequently get aphthous ulcers or other mouth lesions? Do you get red nodules on the skin that sometimes come and go? These extraintestinal manifestations are characteristic of Crohn's disease

**Q** Have you been lethargic or noticed recent weight loss? These symptoms usually accompany bowel symptoms, but may be the only presenting features

### Contributory or predisposing factors

**Q** Do you smoke? Cigarette smoking is associated with Crohn's disease

**Q** Have you participated in any unprotected anal intercourse? This may predispose patients to proctitis secondary to HSV, gonorrhea, or chlamydia, which can present with symptoms similar to Crohn's disease

**Q** Have you recently been to any underdeveloped countries or drunk potentially unclean water? Drinking unpurified water may lead to infection with *Entamoeba histolytica*, which can result in a dysenteric syndrome similar to Crohn's disease

**Q** Have you been on antibiotics in the last 2 months? This may be a risk factor for development of pseudomembranous colitis secondary to *Clostridium difficile* infection

**Q** Have you ever been treated with radiation therapy, particularly for uterine or prostatic malignancy? Radiation proctitis/colitis may occur during therapy, immediately following therapy, or months to years following completion of radiation

**Q** Do you have HIV or risk factors for HIV? Are you immunosuppressed due to another condition, such as organ or bone marrow transplantation? Immunosuppressed patients are at risk for diarrhea secondary to cytomegalovirus, which can present with similar symptoms to Crohn's disease. *Mycobacterium avium* complex can also affect the terminal ileum, leading to diarrhea and malabsorption

Q  Do you have tuberculosis, a history of tuberculosis, or previous exposure to tuberculosis? *Mycobacterium tuberculosis* often affects the terminal ileum, which can lead to fever, diarrhea, malabsorption, and occasionally perforation

Q  Are you taking nonsteroidal anti-inflammatory drugs (NSAIDs)? NSAIDs are associated with ulcers and rarely strictures throughout the gastrointestinal tract, and can flare Crohn's disease

### Family history

Q  Is there a family history of Crohn's disease or ulcerative colitis? Patients with a family history of inflammatory bowel disease have a predisposition to developing the disease themselves

Q  Does anyone in your family have problems with an 'irritable bowel' or other chronic and nonspecific gastrointestinal complaints that have never been firmly diagnosed? Patients may have a family member with inflammatory bowel disease that has never been diagnosed

### Examination

- **Record vital signs.** Tachycardia, hypotension, fever, reduced capillary refill, pallor, or dry mucous membranes are suggestive of dehydration, sepsis, or shock
- **Perform general inspection.** Patients with Crohn's disease are usually thin and look unwell prior to treatment
- **Look for clinical evidence of anemia.** Anemia is a common feature of Crohn's disease and is secondary to malabsorption and blood loss from the gastrointestinal tract
- **Check for signs of peritoneal inflammation**, including rebound tenderness and involuntary guarding. This could indicate an acute abdomen associated with bowel perforation
- **Examine for an inflammatory mass.** Usually seen in the right lower quadrant, which is tender to palpation
- **Check for blood in the stool and tenderness on rectal examination.** These findings may indicate rectal involvement
- **Check for the presence of perianal disease.** Fistulas, fissures, and anorectal abscesses are markers for Crohn's disease
- **Examine for any sign of extraintestinal disease.** Check for arthritis, skin lesions, clubbing of the fingers, uveitis, and episcleritis, which are all associated with Crohn's disease

### Summary of investigative tests

All investigative tests should be performed in conjunction with a gastrointestinal specialist.

Diagnostic:
- Colonoscopy with ileoscopy is the diagnostic test of choice for patients with colonic involvement and will usually confirm or exclude the diagnosis of inflammatory bowel disease. Pattern of affected bowel may indicate whether the disease is Crohn's or ulcerative colitis. Abnormal mucosa should be biopsied at colonoscopy to confirm diagnosis histologically
- Sigmoidoscopy has an important role in diagnosis of inflammatory bowel disease. It is perhaps best used to screen patients with colonic symptoms such as bleeding and urgency. It will accurately diagnose ulcerative colitis and Crohn's disease involving the left colon. Sigmoidoscopy plus small bowel X-ray will identify most patients with untreated inflammatory bowel disease
- Esophagogastroduodenoscopy and biopsy may be more appropriate for patients with upper abdominal symptoms. Typical mucosal changes of Crohn's disease can sometimes be found in this area and histologic identification can be helpful
- Upper gastrointestinal series with a small bowel follow-through can be used to diagnose Crohn's disease and demonstrate the extent of small bowel involvement. Can also be used to

determine whether the patient has associated complications such as fistulas, strictures, or abscess
- Abdominal computed tomography (CT) with oral contrast. Most often indicated for a suspected abscess but can also identify fistulas and strictures. Bowel wall thickening seen on CT may also represent areas of affected intestine

Exclusion of infection:
- Laboratory stool examination for culture, sensitivity, parasite ova and *C. difficile* toxin, and cytomegalovirus

Assessment of complications:
- Abdominal plain films (obstructive series). Used to evaluate an acute abdomen. Will demonstrate perforation (air under the diaphragm in an upright patient)

Assessment of associated disorders and complications:
- Serum laboratory tests, including electrolytes, complete blood count, albumin, and ESR, are useful in determining if there is active inflammatory disease with diarrhea. Liver enzymes may indicate if there is complicating liver disease. Vitamin B12 may be low in cases of Crohn's disease affecting terminal ileum or Crohn's disease leading to malabsorption

## DIAGNOSTIC DECISION
Definitive diagnosis can be made with biopsy of the abnormal mucosa to confirm pattern of histologic inflammation is consistent with the clinical suspicion of Crohn's disease.

## CLINICAL PEARLS
- Sigmoidoscopy with biopsy and small bowel series will identify all patients with ulcerative colitis and virtually all patients with Crohn's disease. These should be regarded as the sine qua non to rule out IBD
- Crohn's disease should be considered in the evaluation of any patient with anemia or with weight loss even in the absence of overt gastrointestinal symptoms, especially in relatively young individuals
- Nonbloody diarrhea is a sign of Crohn's disease and not ulcerative colitis
- Severe abdominal pain is more common in Crohn's disease than ulcerative colitis either due to obstruction or to abscess

## THE TESTS
### Body fluids
SERUM ELECTROLYTES AND BLOOD UREA NITROGEN (BUN)
*Description*
Venous blood sample.

*Advantages/Disadvantages*
Advantages:
- Inexpensive
- Easy to perform

Disadvantage: nonspecific.

*Normal*
Normal values depend on the accepted standards of a particular laboratory or institution.
- Sodium: 135–147mEq/L (135–147mmol/L)
- Potassium: 3.5–5mEq/L (3.5–5mmol/L)
- Urea: 10–20mg/dL (2.5–6.7mmol/L)

*Abnormal*
- Results outside the normal reference range
- Keep in mind the possibility of a false-positive result

*Cause of abnormal result*
- Dehydration secondary to diarrhea may cause electrolyte and BUN disturbance
- Hypokalemia may be caused by chronic diarrhea
- Multiple medical conditions may cause electrolyte disturbance; this is not specific to Crohn's disease

## LIVER FUNCTION TESTS
*Description*
Venous blood sample.

*Advantages/Disadvantages*
- Advantage: simple, inexpensive test
- Disadvantage: nonspecific

*Normal*
- Bilirubin (direct): 0–0.2mg/dL (0–2.0mg/L)
- Bilirubin (indirect): 0–1.0mg/dL (0–10.0mg/L)
- Alanine aminotransferase (ALT): 0–35U/L
- Aspartate aminotransferase (AST): 0–35U/L
- Alkaline phosphatase: 30–120U/L
- Serum albumin: 4–6g/dL (40–60g/L)
- Prothrombin time (PT): 10–12s

*Abnormal*
- Results outside the normal reference range
- Keep in mind the possibility of a false-positive result

*Cause of abnormal result*
- Increased alkaline phosphatase or transaminase levels may indicate hepatobiliary involvement
- Hypoalbuminemia indicates active inflammatory bowel disease
- Malabsorption or protein-losing enteropathy may contribute

*Drugs, disorders and other factors that may alter results*
- Low albumin is also caused by cirrhosis, nephrotic syndrome, chronic illness, or malignancy
- Many other medical conditions may cause abnormal liver function tests

## COMPLETE BLOOD COUNT
*Description*
Venous blood sample.

*Advantages/Disadvantages*
- Advantage: simple blood test
- Disadvantage: nonspecific

*Normal*
- Hemoglobin: men 13.6–17.7g/dL (8.4–11.0mmol/L); women 12.0–15.0g/dL (7.4–9.3mmol/L)
- White cell count: 3200–9800/mm$^3$
- Platelet count: 130,000–300,000/mm$^3$

*Abnormal*
- Results outside the normal reference range
- Keep in mind the possibility of a false-positive result

*Cause of abnormal result*
- Leukocytosis may indicate active inflammation
- Anemia can result from malabsorption and occult blood loss
- Thrombocytosis favors the diagnosis of IBD over infectious diarrhea

*Drugs, disorders and other factors that may alter results*
- Anemia can be caused by many conditions and chronic illness
- Infection or inflammatory conditions cause leukocytosis

## ESR
*Description*
Venous blood sample.

*Advantages/Disadvantages*
- Advantage: simple, inexpensive test
- Disadvantage: nonspecific

*Normal*
- Men: 0–15mm/h
- Women: 0–20mm/h

*Abnormal*
- Results outside the normal reference range
- Keep in mind the possibility of a false-positive result

*Cause of abnormal result*
Raised ESR is secondary to active inflammation.

*Drugs, disorders and other factors that may alter results*
- Any inflammatory, infectious, or malignant condition may cause a raised ESR
- Anemia will give a falsely high ESR

## VITAMIN B12 LEVEL
*Description*
Venous blood sample.

*Advantages/Disadvantages*
- Advantage: simple, inexpensive test
- Disadvantage: nonspecific

*Normal*
>120pg/dL (1200pg/L).

*Abnormal*
- Results below the normal range
- Keep in mind the possibility of a false-positive result

*Cause of abnormal result*
Levels may be low due to B12 malabsorption with terminal ileal disease.

*Drugs, disorders and other factors that may alter results*
Many factors alter B12 levels, namely normal intake (abnormal in strict vegetarians), binding and subsequent removal of protein factors in gastric and small bowel lumen (abnormal in pernicious anemia), and an intact distal terminal ileum where B12 is absorbed (abnormal in tuberculosis, Crohn's disease, or after small bowel surgery). Patients with Crohn's disease not affecting the terminal ileum may have normal levels.

## LABORATORY STOOL EXAMINATION
*Description*
Fresh stool sample to identify presence of infection, cysts, or ova.

*Advantages/Disadvantages*
Advantages:
- Very nonspecific investigation but does help rule out bacterial or parasitic infections
- Cheap and easy to perform

*Abnormal*
Presence of noncommensal gut organisms such as *Salmonella, Shigella, Campylobacter*, cysts, and ova.

*Cause of abnormal result*
Infection.

*Drugs, disorders and other factors that may alter results*
Antibiotic use.

## STOOL FOR CLOSTRIDIUM DIFFICILE TOXIN
*Description*
Assay of stool to assess for toxins produced by *C. difficile*. May check for toxin A and/or toxin B, depending on the laboratory.

*Advantages/Disadvantages*
Advantages:
- Useful if positive; a negative result does not rule out infection
- Cheap and easy to perform

*Abnormal*
Presence of toxin.

*Cause of abnormal result*
Presence of toxin-producing strain of *C. difficile*.

## Biopsy
*Description*
Biopsy may be obtained using biopsy forceps at time of endoscopy. Generally required to confirm diagnosis and to rule out other causes.

*Advantages/Disadvantages*
Disadvantage: invasive procedure.

*Abnormal*
- Inflammatory infiltrate generally seen in the mucosa and submucosa; may also be seen into the muscularis propria if deep biopsies obtained

- Findings may otherwise be similar to ulcerative colitis, with distortion of the normal crypt architecture and loss of crypt density
- Noncaseating granulomas are relatively specific for Crohn's disease, but are only seen in 20% of patients
- Patchy distribution of inflammation favors Crohn's disease over ulcerative colitis

*Cause of abnormal result*
Inflammatory lesions are seen in Crohn's disease, ulcerative colitis, and inflammation associated with NSAID use and infection.

## Imaging
### UPPER GASTROINTESTINAL SERIES WITH SMALL BOWEL FOLLOW-THROUGH
*Advantages/Disadvantages*
- Advantage: useful in Crohn's disease because of the frequent involvement of the small intestine
- Disadvantage: small intestine is generally inaccessible to endoscopy, thus contrast X-rays are required if this area is to be investigated

*Abnormal*
- Loss of normal architecture of the mucosal contour. Mucosa loses its normal feather-like appearance. Extent of involvement can be determined by the radiologist
- String sign – thin column of barium produced as a result of luminal narrowing (stricture) or fistula formation associated with ileal Crohn's disease

*Cause of abnormal result*
- Inflammatory changes (including ulceration and edema) and strictures will distort the outline of the small bowel
- Ileal narrowing can be seen with other causes of ileitis, including infections (notably tuberculosis) or NSAID-induced ulcers

### ABDOMINAL PLAIN FILM (OBSTRUCTIVE SERIES)
*Description*
- An obstructive series includes a supine and erect abdominal film. It can evaluate for free air under the diaphragm, a marker for bowel perforation, as well as air-fluid levels
- A series of films taken on consecutive days can be used for comparison to identify response to therapy or continued deterioration

*Advantages/Disadvantages*
Advantages:
- Simple and quick
- Safe investigation, although it involves a modest dose of radiation

*Abnormal*
- Air-fluid levels
- Dilated loops of bowel
- Air under the diaphragm

*Cause of abnormal result*
Obstruction or perforation secondary to stricture or edema and inflammation.

### ABDOMINAL CT SCAN
*Advantages/Disadvantages*
Advantage: may be useful to evaluate for intra-abdominal abscess and to gauge extent of disease.

Disadvantages:
- Relatively insensitive for mild disease; findings also not specific for colitis
- Moderate radiation exposure; avoid in women of childbearing age

*Abnormal*
- Abscess may be seen as an intra-abdominal fluid collection, occasionally with air-fluid levels
- Bowel wall thickening and fat stranding can be appreciated in small or large intestinal inflammation
- Fistulas can sometimes be identified if oral contrast is seen in nongastrointestinal organs (i.e. bladder in enterovesicular fistula)

*Cause of abnormal result*
Any cause of inflammation may cause thickening and fat stranding.

## Special tests
SIGMOIDOSCOPY
*Description*
- Involvement in Crohn's disease tends to be patchy, therefore a negative sigmoidoscopy does not rule out Crohn's disease. Also, if pathology seen on sigmoidoscopy is suspicious for Crohn's disease, a colonoscopy is indicated to gauge extent of disease
- Test of choice only when attempting to make the initial diagnosis in a patient with colonic symptoms
- Perform with caution in patients with severe, active disease because of risk of bowel perforation
- Biopsy may be performed

*Advantages/Disadvantages*
- Advantage: an advantage of sigmoidoscopy is in the regular follow up of patients with inflammation or stricture within the reach of the sigmoidoscope
- Disadvantage: the main disadvantage is the inability to identify lesions in the right or transverse colon

*Abnormal*
- Crohn's disease is suggested by focal inflammation with aphthous ulcers, linear or stellate ulcers with normal intervening mucosa, or inflammatory changes beginning above the rectum, referred to as rectal-sparing
- A cobblestone appearance is characteristic (course irregularity of the mucosa secondary to inflammation)
- Transmural inflammation with skip areas of intervening normal bowel on histologic examination, although superficial inflammation alone does not rule out Crohn's disease
- Noncaseating granulomas are characteristic but not found universally

*Cause of abnormal result*
Inflammation of the colon.

*Drugs, disorders and other factors that may alter results*
Some laxatives used to prepare the bowel for colonoscopy can also lead to minute bowel erosions that might be mistaken for colitis.

COLONOSCOPY WITH ILEOSCOPY
*Description*
Endoscopic examination of the entire colon to the terminal ileum is possible. Experienced endoscopists can cannulate the terminal ileum 80–90% of the time, although this may be more difficult if scarring and structuring are present.

*Advantages/Disadvantages*
- Advantage: may be used to determine extent of colonic involvement in either ulcerative colitis or Crohn's disease, and screen for cancer in long-standing ulcerative colitis
- Disadvantage: uncomfortable for patient with acute inflammation and carries a risk of perforation

*Abnormal*
- Crohn's disease is suggested by focal inflammation with aphthous ulcers, linear or stellate ulcers with normal intervening mucosa, or inflammatory changes beginning above the rectum, referred to as rectal-sparing
- A cobblestone appearance is characteristic (course irregularity of the mucosa secondary to inflammation)
- Transmural inflammation with skip areas of intervening normal bowel on histologic examination, although superficial inflammation alone does not rule out Crohn's disease
- Noncaseating granulomas are characteristic but not found universally

*Cause of abnormal result*
Inflammation of the mucosa of the large intestine.

*Drugs, disorders and other factors that may alter results*
- Some laxatives used to prepare the bowel for colonoscopy can lead to minute bowel erosions that might be mistaken for colitis. However, biopsy of these lesions will be essentially normal
- Ischemic colitis, Crohn's disease, *C. difficile* colitis, and other infectious colitides can present with similar or identical endoscopic findings

## ESOPHAGOGASTRODUODENOSCOPY
*Description*
Endoscopic examination of the upper gastrointestinal tract. Often accompanied by biopsy.

*Advantages/Disadvantages*
- Advantage: may demonstrate the presence of Crohn's disease
- Disadvantage: negative examination does not exclude Crohn's disease

*Abnormal*
Crohn's disease is suggested by focal inflammation with aphthous ulcers, linear or stellate ulcers with normal intervening mucosa.

*Cause of abnormal result*
- Inflammation
- Gastric ulceration and duodenal ulceration may be independent of Crohn's disease

*Drugs, disorders and other factors that may alter results*
NSAIDs are a common cause of gastric erosions, which may resemble those seen in upper gastrointestinal Crohn's involvement.

# TREATMENT

## PATIENT AND CAREGIVER ISSUES
### Patient or caregiver request
Is there an association between Crohn's disease and measles or the measles vaccine, or with cows' milk contaminated with a specific bacterium? There have been television and press reports of an association between Crohn's disease and these entities, but patients need to be made aware that there is no convincing proof that vaccines or bacteria cause the disease.

## MANAGEMENT ISSUES
### Goals
- To achieve remission, defined by the FDA Gastrointestinal Advisory Panel as the absence of inflammatory symptoms (rectal bleeding or diarrhea) in conjunction with evidence of mucosal healing (absence of ulceration, significant granularity or friability). In Crohn's disease, remission is difficult to define because the correlation between clinical activity and endoscopic/radiologic findings is poor
- To adopt a regimen of maintenance therapy to prevent a recurrence of clinical or endoscopic signs of active disease. Patients requiring continuous steroid therapy are not in remission
- To treat, or refer for treatment, extraintestinal manifestations and complications

### Management in special circumstances
SPECIAL PATIENT GROUPS
Pregnancy:
- Pregnant patients with active disease are at greater risk of miscarriage, premature delivery, or a low-birthweight baby
- Investigation with X-rays and lower endoscopy should be avoided
- Medical management of Crohn's disease is usually effective during pregnancy and is less harmful than untreated disease. Sulfasalazine and corticosteroids are safe. Immunosuppressants should be avoided where possible, as should metronidazole

## SUMMARY OF THERAPEUTIC OPTIONS
### Choices
Diet:
- Elemental diets are almost as effective as oral corticosteroid treatment in acute attacks of Crohn's disease; however, relapse is more likely than in patients on corticosteroid treatment
- Elemental diets may be useful for patients with acute disease to promote bowel rest; such diets should be prescribed in conjunction with a gastroenterologist
- Elemental diets are rarely prescribed because they are not very palatable
- Patients with active disease often gain symptomatic relief from a low-roughage diet, especially if there is lumenal narrowing from severe inflammation or stricture
- Patients with malabsorption may require supplemental folate, iron, vitamin D, and monthly B12 injections

Acute attacks:
- Resuscitation if patient is hypovolemic or septic
- Severe disease should be referred to a specialist for intravenous administration of corticosteroid and consideration of total parenteral nutrition and antibiotic therapy
- Mild-to-moderate disease requires oral corticosteroid (prednisone) treatment with or without an oral 5-ASA (olsalazine, sulfasalazine, and mesalamine) – consider urgent referral depending on the patient's condition and response to treatment
- Mild disease - an oral 5-ASA (olsalazine and mesalamine) is the treatment of choice. Metronidazole is an appropriate alternative. Consider addition of an oral corticosteroid if the patient fails to make a rapid improvement (resolution within 2 weeks) or if deterioration occurs

- For perianal disease, metronidazole is recommended for mild disease. Ciprofloxacin, 6-mercaptopurine, and infliximab are alternatives

Maintenance therapy:
- Mesalamine is generally the preferred maintenance therapy because it is associated with fewer side effects than corticosteroids
- Corticosteroids (prednisone) should not be considered maintenance drugs because their long-term side effects are so devastating
- Mesalamine enema may be used in Crohn's disease limited to the rectosigmoid region
- Corticosteroid enema may be used in Crohn's disease limited to the rectosigmoid region; systemic absorption may be significant and mesalamine enema is generally preferred
- Metronidazole is generally not recommended as maintenance therapy because long-term use is associated with irreversible peripheral neuropathy
- Azathioprine and mercaptopurine are excellent alternatives where mesalamine has failed. Risk of pancreatitis is significant
- Methotrexate intramuscularly may be used in selected patients with refractory, steroid-dependent Crohn's disease
- Infliximab has been used for moderate-to-severe Crohn's disease unresponsive to steroid management, and to aid healing of perianal fistulas. Use is limited to specialist supervision as this is a new drug whose role is being defined

Symptomatic treatment:
- Loperamide may be used to treat chronic diarrhea without active disease
- Cholestyramine may be helpful in patients who suffer from diarrhea after ileal resection
- Endoscopic stricturoplasty – colonic strictures secondary to chronic scarring from Crohn's disease can occasionally be dilated with symptomatic relief

Surgery:
- Surgery should only be considered after aggressive medical management with high-dose intravenous steroids and/or infliximab has failed
- Crohn's disease tends to recur at sites of surgical anastomoses
- Emergency surgical intervention for complications of an acute attack
- Failed medical therapy
- Surgery for complications of chronic disease – small bowel strictures may be treated with resection; total colectomy may be performed when the large intestine is involved

## Clinical pearls
- The first step in managing a flare is to maximize the current mesalamine therapy
- Combination of oral and topical treatments is very useful in left colon disease
- Initial use of corticosteroids on an alternate day basis is generally not beneficial; also, rapidly tapering dosages (such as methylprednisolone dose pack) do not work in Crohn's disease
- Although uncommon, mesalamine may cause diarrhea particularly at higher doses
- Azathioprine or 6-mercaptopurine are widely used maintenance drugs in Crohn's disease of all types, whereas mesalamine is best for ileocolonic disease

## Never
- Never prescribe immunosuppressive agents in inflammatory bowel disease without advice from a gastroenterologist as to their indications and safety concerns
- Never delay referring early in acute and chronic disease as both can be more effectively treated at an early stage
- In the presence of fulminant disease and/or toxic megacolon, never prescribe anticholinergic or antidiarrhea drugs as these can precipitate or aggravate toxic megacolon
- Never perform colonoscopy during an acute episode as the risk of perforation is high

## FOLLOW UP
### Plan for review
- As Crohn's disease is a relapsing and remitting illness, it is accepted that patients with quiescent disease or maintained remission do not need to be followed up regularly but do need periodic visits to monitor drug safety
- Review relapses at the first opportunity
- Regularly review, as part of the treatment plan, patients with active, complex, or refractory disease
- Review to check response and any side effects when new medications such as steroids or immunosuppressants are started (some of these drugs require monitoring)
- Review of most patients will be combined with specialist input

### Information for patient or caregiver
- This is an illness which may affect you throughout your life and which, as yet, has no known cause or cure
- There will be times when the activity of the disease settles down and you will be free of symptoms. This is called remission and the aim of treatment is to keep you at this stage
- You may need to take medication periodically or for longer periods of time in order to control symptoms and inflammation. This will help get you into remission as well as prevent relapses
- It is difficult to predict the course of your illness. You may get better and stay that way for years, but you could also rapidly get worse and need to be admitted to hospital – most people fall somewhere in between

## DRUGS AND OTHER THERAPIES: DETAILS
### Drugs
SULFASALAZINE
First-line treatment in the US for colonic disease. Not an expensive medication.

*Dose*
- Recommended starting dosage is 0.5g orally twice daily, slowly increased as tolerated to 0.5–1.0g orally four times daily
- Once in remission, dose range between 2.0g and 3.0g/day
- Should be continued when further medication or treatment is given

*Efficacy*
- Effective in the treatment of mild-to-moderate acute exacerbations of colonic or ileocolic disease, and in maintaining remission
- Not as effective as corticosteroids for inducing remission in patients with moderate or severe disease
- Thought to be less effective for small bowel disease because it disassociates into its active moiety in the colon

*Risks/benefits*
Benefits:
- Only after critical appraisal should sulfasalazine tablets be given to patients with hepatic or renal damage or blood dyscrasias
- Concomitant relief of symptoms of coexisting gastrointestinal inflammatory disease

*Side effects and adverse reactions*
- Cardiovascular system: pericarditis, allergic myocarditis
- Central nervous system: dizziness, drowsiness, headache, seizures
- Eyes, ears, nose, and throat: blurred vision, tinnitus
- Gastrointestinal: abdominal pain, diarrhoea, hepatotoxicity, melena, vomiting

- Genitourinary: renal failure, urinary retention
- Hematologic: blood cell disorders
- Musculoskeletal: arthralgia, myalgia, osteoporosis
- Skin: Stevens–Johnson syndrome

*Interactions (other drugs)*
- Digoxin ■ Methenamine ■ Phenytoin ■ Tolbutamide ■ Warfarin

*Contraindications*
- Contraindicated in porphyria and gastrointestinal or urinary tract obstruction ■ Cross-hypersensitivy with salicylates ■ Caution required in patients with renal or hepatic impairment, glucose-6-phosphate deficiency

*Acceptability to patient*
Well tolerated by patients.

*Follow up plan*
- Patients remaining in remission should be continued on this drug at maintenance dose; stopping the drug increases the risk of relapse
- Some gastroenterologists advocate stopping the drug after 4 years without any evidence of relapse; obviously, if the patient subsequently relapses, the drug needs to be restarted
- Note that follow-up plan should include history of symptoms specific to individual patients, weight during remission, complete blood count (CBC), and albumin

*Patient and caregiver information*
Oral medications should be taken with food if there are significant gastrointestinal side effects.

MESALAMINE
A 5-ASA preparation that can be given orally, as a suppository or as an enema.

*Dose*
- In active disease, the recommended oral dose is 2.4–4.8g/day
- Once the disease is in remission (usually after an 8-week course), these oral dosages can be tapered to 400mg three times a day (or occasionally 800mg three times a day). The higher dosage can be reinstituted if patients have recurrences at these levels
- Micronized preparations of mesalamine are dosed at 2g twice a day for induction therapy and 1g twice a day for maintenance; preferentially deliver drug to the terminal ileum and may be preferred for ileal disease

*Efficacy*
- Effective for treating active disease and maintaining remission
- Patients usually have a gradual response to this medication
- The higher 4.8g dose of oral mesalamine produces significantly better results than the 2.4g dose
- The enema or suppository mesalamine is best for proctosigmoiditis, but has little efficacy in anorectal Crohn's disease

*Risks/benefits*
Risks:
- Use caution when administering to patients with impaired hepatic function
- Mesalamine has been associated with an acute intolerance syndrome that may be difficult to distinguish from inflammatory bowel disease
- Patients with pyloric stenosis may have prolonged gastric retention of mesalamine which could delay release of mesalamine in the colon

- May exacerbate the symptoms of colitis
- Mesalamine suppositories may cause tubular damage and pancolitis
- Mesalamine suspension enema contains potassium metabisulfite, a sulfite that may cause allergic-type reactions including anaphylactic symptoms and life-threatening or less severe asthmatic episodes in certain susceptible people

*Side effects and adverse reactions*
Common side effects include headache, abdominal pain, nausea, fever, rash, dyspepsia, diarrhea, hepatitis, and occasionally bone marrow suppression. Interstitial nephritis occurs in up to one in 300 patients. These can occur with both oral and topical therapies.

*Interactions (other drugs)*
**Absorption of digoxin possibly reduced.**

*Contraindications*
**History of allergy or intolerance to aspirin.**

*Acceptability to patient*
- Patients may be resistant initially to using enemas or suppositories
- Enemas are expensive

*Follow up plan*
Patients need to be followed closely by a specialist. If this first-line agent does not quell disease activity, a more robust drug regimen may be indicated.

*Patient and caregiver information*
- Oral medication should be swallowed whole
- Patients should be advised to lie on their left side during enema administration

### OLSALAZINE
ASA preparation primarily used in patients who are intolerant to sulfasalazine.

*Dose*
1.0g/day in two divided doses.

*Efficacy*
Not enough data available in Crohn's disease.

*Risks/benefits*
Risks: use caution in renal disease, in children, and in breast-feeding and pregnancy.

*Side effects and adverse reactions*
- Central nervous system: fever, depression, dizziness, headache
- Gastrointestinal: nausea, vomiting, diarrhea, abdominal pain, anorexia, bloating, raised liver enzymes, hepatitis
- Hematologic: blood cell dyscrasias
- Musculoskeletal: arthralgia
- Skin: rash, pruritus

*Interactions (other drugs)*
**Digoxin.**

*Contraindications*
- Hypersenstivity to salicylates
- Severe renal impairment

PREDNISONE
An oral corticosteroid useful in patients with acute episodes of mild and moderate Crohn's disease.

*Dose*
- Active Crohn's disease: dose 10–40mg orally for several weeks, then tapering over 2–3 months, and then discontinuing
- Important to start at recommended dosage; a common mistake is to give suboptimal dose in the hope of avoiding side effects
- Intravenous therapy for hospitalized patients with severe fulminant disease: 75–100mg daily; switch to oral prednisone regimen once symptoms improve
- Foam or liquid enema preparations for rectal disease may be used once daily (100mg daily)
- Dosage requirements are variable and must be individualized on the basis of the response of the patient

*Efficacy*
- Indicated only for the treatment of acute exacerbations and should not be used for long-term maintenance
- Response to intravenous therapy usually seen in 3–5 days
- Corticosteroid enemas are generally less effective than 5-ASA enemas

*Risks/benefits*
Risks:
- Use caution when administering to patients with congestive heart failure, diabetes mellitus, glaucoma, renal disease, ulcerative colitis, and peptic ulcer
- Use caution when administering to the elderly
- Prednisone taken in doses higher than 7.5mg for 3 weeks or longer may lead to clinically relevant suppression of the pituitary-adrenal axis

*Side effects and adverse reactions*
- Side effects are minimized by short duration of therapy
- Cardiovascular system: hypertension, thromboembolism
- Central nervous system: insomnia, euphoria, depression, psychosis, seizures
- Endocrine: adrenal suppression, impaired glucose tolerance, growth suppression in children
- Eyes, ears, nose, and throat: cataract, glaucoma, blurred vision
- Gastrointestinal: dyspepsia, peptic ulceration, oesophagitis, oral candidiasis
- Musculoskeletal: proximal myopathy, osteoporosis
- Skin: delayed healing, acne, striae, fragile skin

*Interactions (other drugs)*
- Aminoglutethimide (increased clearance of prednisone) - Antidiabetics (hypoglycemic effect inhibited) - Antihypertensives (effects inhibited) - Barbiturates (increased clearance of prednisone) - Cardiac glycosides (toxicity increased) - Cholestyramine, colestipol (may reduce absorption of corticosteroids) - Clarithromycin, erythromycin, troleandomycin (may enhance steroid effect) - Cyclosporine (may increase levels of both drugs; may cause seizures) - Diuretics (effects inhibited) - Isoniazid (reduced plasma levels of isoniazid) - Ketoconazole - Nonsteroidal anti-inflammatory drugs (NSAIDs) (increased risks of bleeding) - Oral contraceptives (enhanced effects of corticosteroids) - Rifampin (may inhibit hepatic clearance of prednisone) - Salicylates (increased clearance of salicylates) - Warfarin (alters clotting time)

*Contraindications*
- Systemic infection ■ Avoid live virus vaccines in those receiving immunosuppressive doses
- History of tuberculosis ■ Cushing's syndrome ■ Recent myocardial infarction

*Acceptability to patient*
Systemic corticosteroids have an extensive side effect profile, which can be troubling to patients.

*Follow up plan*
- Patients on steroids need to be closely monitored and have their steroid doses carefully tapered
- Patients given long-term (>3 months) steroids should be placed on calcium and vitamin D replacement for osteoporosis prophylaxis. Annual bone mineral densitometry should be considered. Patients who fall >2 standard deviations below the mean should be considered for bisphosphonate therapy

AZATHIOPRINE AND 6-MERCAPTOPURINE
Immunomodulatory drugs.

*Dose*
- Dosing requirements vary. These medications should be administered only by physicians with experience of complicated cases of ulcerative colitis and Crohn's disease
- Azathioprine: usual oral dose 2.0–2.5mg/kg/day
- 6-Mercaptopurine: usual dose 1.0–1.5mg/kg/day

*Efficacy*
- These agents are most commonly used in patients who are unresponsive to first- and second-line medical management
- Onset of action may take 2–6 months, so use of other agents is necessary in the interim. Thus, may not be appropriate for acute disease but should be considered for long-term therapy
- May be effective for perianal disease

*Risks/benefits*
Risks (azathioprine):
- Use caution when administering to patients with bone marrow depression and infection
- Use caution when administering to patients with renal or hepatic impairment
- Severe blood cell disorders may occur
- May increase risk of neoplasia

Risk (6-mercaptopurine): major risks include bone marrow suppression, hepatotoxicity, and pancreatitis.

*Side effects and adverse reactions*
Azathioprine:
- Gastrointestinal: nausea, vomiting, diarrhea, abdominal pain, hepatic failure, jaundice
- Genitourinary: depression of spermatogenensis
- Hematologic: anemia, leukopenia, pancytopenia, thrombocytopenia
- Musculoskeletal: arthralgia, myalgia, malaise
- Skin: rash, alopecia
- Other: fungal, bacterial, protozoal and viral infections, may increase risk of neoplasm (skin cancer, reticulocyte or lymphomatous tumors), teratogenicity

6-Mercaptopurine:
- Major side effects include bone marrow suppression and pancreatitis
- Other side effects include diarrhea, fever, weakness, oral lesions, nausea, vomiting, abdominal

pain, and anorexia. Bone marrow suppression, particularly neutropenia, is dose-dependent
- Pancreatitis develops in 3–15% of patients. It typically develops after several weeks of therapy and resolves spontaneously after the drug has been discontinued. It rapidly recurs if the drug is given again
- Recent studies demonstrate that concern that these drugs may increase the risk of cancer in patients is minimal

*Interactions (other drugs)*
Azathioprine:
- Angiotensin-converting enzyme (ACE) inhibitors ■ Allopurinol ■ Anticoagulants
- Carbamazepine ■ Clozapine ■ Co-trimoxazole (TMP-SMX) ■ Cyclosporine ■ Methotrexate
- Nondepolarizing muscle blockers ■ Vaccines ■ Warfarin

6-Mercaptopurine:
- Bactrim (increases risk of bone marrow suppression with mercaptopurine) ■ Cyclosporine (azathioprine decreases concentration of cyclosporine)

*Contraindications*
Azathioprine:
- Hypersenstitivity to the drug ■ Intramuscular injections ■ Pregnancy or breast-feeding
- Vaccines

6-Mercaptopurine:
- Safety and efficacy not established in children under 12 years

*Acceptability to patient*
- Both drugs are tolerated surprisingly well by patients if they manage to continue past the initial few weeks of treatment
- With encouragement, most patients manage to continue therapy for the required duration to achieve a response

*Follow up plan*
- After therapy is started, complete blood counts should be monitored
- Careful monitoring for toxicity is mandatory
- Drugs should be administered only by physicians with experience of patients with complicated cases of inflammatory bowel disease

## METRONIDAZOLE
*Dose*
- Maximum dose: 2g/day
- In chronic metronidazole therapy, dosages >1g/day can be associated with irreversible peripheral neuropathy

*Efficacy*
- Effective in patients with active Crohn's disease and has a potency similar to that of sulfasalazine
- Metronidazole is particularly effective in patients who have perianal Crohn's disease, with the benefits improving as the dosage is increased, up to a maximum of 2g/day
- Not generally suitable as maintenance therapy because of risk of irreversible peripheral neuropathy

*Risks/benefits*
Risks:
- Nausea and vomiting likely if alcohol is taken

- Caution in hepatic and renal impairment
- Caution in central nervous system disease or history of seizures

*Side effects and adverse reactions*
- Central nervous system: dizziness, headache, seizures, ataxia, peripheral neuropathy
- Gastrointestinal: nausea, vomiting, taste disturbance, diarrhea, abdominal pain, dry mouth, anorexia, constipation
- Genitourinary: urination difficulties, cystitis, vaginal dryness
- Hematologic: blood cell disorders
- Skin: rashes, itching, flushing

*Interactions (other drugs)*
- **Alcohol** ■ **Antiepileptics** ■ **Anticoagulants** ■ **Barbiturates** ■ **Carbamazepine** ■ **Cholestyramine** ■ **Cimetidine** ■ **Colestipol** ■ **Disulfiram** ■ **Fluorouracil** ■ **Lithium**

*Contraindications*
- **Pregnancy and breast-feeding** ■ **Blood dyscrasias**

*Acceptability to patient*
Generally well tolerated.

*Patient and caregiver information*
- Take with food to avoid gastrointestinal upset
- Avoid alcohol because of disulfiram-like action (severe vomiting)
- Drug may cause metallic taste
- Do not use during pregnancy because leads to birth defects

## CIPROFLOXACIN
*Dose*
- 500mg twice daily
- Not recommended in children under 12 years of age

*Efficacy*
- Effective in active Crohn's disease
- May be used in patients intolerant of metronidazole or as an addition to metronidazole

*Risks/benefits*
Risks:
- Not suitable for children or growing adolescents
- Caution in adolescents, pregnancy, epilepsy, glucose-6-phosphate dehydrogenase deficiency
- Use caution in renal disease

*Side effects and adverse reactions*
- Central nervous system: anxiety, depression, dizziness, headache, seizures
- Eyes, ears, nose, and throat: visual disturbances
- Gastrointestinal: abdominal pain, altered liver function, anorexia, diarrhoea, vomiting
- Skin: photosensitivity, pruritus, rash

*Interactions (other drugs)*
- **Antacids** ■ **Beta-blockers** ■ **Cyclosporine** ■ **Caffeine** ■ **Didanosine** ■ **Diazepam** ■ **Mineral supplements (zinc, magnesium, calcium, aluminium, iron)** ■ **NSAIDs** ■ **Opiates** ■ **Oral anticoagulants** ■ **Phenytoin** ■ **Theophylline**

*Contraindications*
- Use is not recommended in children because arthropathy has developed in weightbearing joints in young animals ■ Pregnancy category B

*Acceptability to patient*
Ciprofloxacin is generally well tolerated.

## LOPERAMIDE
Anticholinergic agent that increases colonic water absorption and internal sphincter function.

*Dose*
4mg orally initially, then 2mg after each unformed stool to a maximum of 16mg/day.

*Efficacy*
Affords symptomatic relief for patients who do not have systemic symptoms but who continue to have diarrhea despite adequate primary therapy for Crohn's disease.

*Risks/benefits*
Risks:
- Use caution in liver disease, dehydration, severe ulcerative colitis
- Not recommmended in children

*Side effects and adverse reactions*
- Central nervous system: fatigue, dizziness, drowsiness
- Gastrointestinal: nausea, constipation, toxic megacolon, abdominal cramps and bloating, paralytic ileus, vomiting
- Genitourinary: nephrotoxicity
- Respiratory: respiratory depression
- Skin: rash

*Interactions (other drugs)*
- Bethanechol ■ Cholestyramine ■ Cisapride ■ Metoclopramide ■ Erythromycin

*Contraindications*
- Development of abdominal distension or inhibition of peristalsis ■ Acute diarrhea due to infectious organisms such as *Escherichia coli, Salmonella, Shigella* ■ Pseudomembranous colitis associated with broad-spectrum antibiotics ■ Acute dysentery

*Acceptability to patient*
Generally acceptable as it provides symptomatic benefit.

*Patient and caregiver information*
Patients should be instructed not to take this medication when they experience more severe symptoms, and to consult their physician.

## CHOLESTYRAMINE
*Dose*
4g anhydrous cholestyramine resin once or twice per day, and maintenance on 8–16g/day, with maximum 24g/day – increase dose gradually with periodic assessment of lipid/lipoprotein levels.

*Efficacy*
- Gives symptomatic relief only

- Useful in management of patients with bile salt-induced diarrhea after ileal resection and may be effective in patients with bile acid malabsorption due to severe terminal ileal disease

*Risks/benefits*
Risks:
- Use caution in pregnancy and breast-feeding
- Use caution in children
- Use caution if patient is constipated

*Side effects and adverse reactions*
- Cardiovascular system: cardiac arrest, cardiovascular collapse, phlebitis
- Eyes, ears, nose, and throat: hearing disturbances, ototoxicity
- Gastrointestinal: nausea
- Genitourinary: renal damage
- Hematologic: neutropenia, eosinophilia, leukopenia
- Skin: rashes, chills, fever, 'red man's syndrome'

*Interactions (other drugs)*
- Acarbose ■ Acetaminophen ■ Cardiac glycosides ■ Corticosteroids ■ Diuretics
- Levothyroxine ■ Methotrexate ■ Oral anticoagulants ■ Phenylbutazone ■ Raloxifene
- Valproic acid ■ Vancomycin

*Contraindications*
**Biliary obstruction.**

*Acceptability to patient*
- Many patients find cholestyramine powder unpalatable. Mixing it with orange juice may improve palatability
- Acceptable if there is symptomatic improvement and limited side effects

*Patient and caregiver information*
Do not take at the same time as other medications as their absorption may be affected.

## Surgical therapy
### SURGICAL MANAGEMENT OF CROHN'S DISEASE
- 75% of patients with Crohn's disease will eventually require surgery
- Most commonly required for disease refractory to medical management; it may also be indicated for abscess not responsive to percutaneous management, strictures causing bowel obstruction, bleeding, perforation, or intolerable side effects from medication
- Total colectomy with ileostomy may be required for patients with extensive inflammation of the large intestine, and may be curative
- Segmental resection with reanastomosis or ileohemicolectomy with reanastomosis may be done, but there may be recurrence at the anastomotic site
- Stricturoplasty without resection may be done for localized stricture
- Anorectal disease unresponsive to medical management is often managed surgically
- Surgical management with incision is necessary for acute suppurative anorectal disease

*Efficacy*
- Very efficacious for immediate relief of symptoms; however, recurrence over the following months to years at the site of surgery is common
- Patients with large bowel involvement who undergo colectomy usually experience significant improvement in symptoms
- Removal of an affected part of bowel may relieve symptoms, but will not cure the disease

- 50% of patients will relapse after surgery, though risk of anastomotic relapse can be lowered with 6-mercaptopurine or mesalamine

*Risks/benefits*
Risks:
- Risks of anesthesia, infection, and complications associated with any major surgery
- Possibility that anastomosis might fail and precipitate additional surgeries for revision of the initial procedure
- Adhesions secondary to surgery, causing obstruction that may be difficult to differentiate from recurrent stricture
- Bile-salt malabsorption occurs in patients who undergo removal of the terminal ileum; they may require treatment with cholestyramine
- May relieve obstructive symptoms

*Acceptability to patient*
Surgery is often acceptable if medical therapy has failed to treat symptoms.

*Follow up plan*
Patients are routinely followed up postoperatively at 4–8 weeks.

*Patient and caregiver information*
- Patients should be aware that surgery is not curative for Crohn's disease
- Patients requiring a total colectomy should receive pre- and postoperative education and counseling

### Endoscopic therapy
ENDOSCOPIC STRICTUROPLASTY
- Colonic strictures secondary to chronic scarring for Crohn's disease can occasionally be dilated with symptomatic relief
- Performed by passing a balloon dilator across the stricture and inflating it or by passing a bougie
- Can be performed in the outpatient setting
- Used mainly in anastomotic strictures following ileocolic resection, but has also been used in other colonic strictures

*Efficacy*
- Generally effective for benign colonic strictures
- Strictures around flexures cannot be endoscopically dilated

*Risks/benefits*
Risk: risks include perforation, bleeding, and conscious sedation associated with colonoscopy.

*Acceptability to patient*
Generally acceptable, as may allow patient to avoid surgery.

*Follow up plan*
- Patient should be followed for evidence of recurrent stricture that presents with signs and symptoms of large bowel obstruction
- Biopsies should be taken when stricture is seen as it may represent colonic malignancy

## LIFESTYLE
- Elemental diets are almost as effective as oral corticosteroid treatment in acute attacks of Crohn's disease; however, relapse is more likely than in those patients on corticosteroid treatment

- Elemental diets may be useful for patients with acute disease to promote bowel rest; such diets should be prescribed in conjunction with a gastroenterologist
- Patients with active disease often gain symptomatic relief from a low-roughage diet
- Foods that may need to be avoided due to worsening of symptoms include dairy products and spicy foods
- Patients with malabsorption may require supplemental folate, iron, and vitamin D
- B12 injections may be necessary for patients with terminal ileal disease or resection

RISKS/BENEFITS
- Risk: relapses may occur if not used in combination with other therapy
- Benefit: may improve pain and diarrhea in an acute exacerbation

ACCEPTABILITY TO PATIENT
- Generally acceptable if there is an obvious improvement in symptoms
- Enteral diets are often unpalatable and expensive

PATIENT AND CAREGIVER INFORMATION
Information on diet and advice from a dietitian are important.

# OUTCOMES

## EFFICACY OF THERAPIES

- Generally, physicians will escalate therapy with multiple, or increasingly immunosuppressive, agents until remission is induced or chronic, active disease is brought under control
- Sulfasalazine and other 5-ASA medications may be effective for inducing and maintaining remission in Crohn's disease
- Prednisone is used for acute exacerbations of Crohn's disease; it should not be used long-term
- Systemic corticosteroids (conventional) have not been proven to be effective in reducing relapse from remission
- Azathioprine is effective in maintaining remission in Crohn's disease. Response is improved with increased dose and it has a steroid-sparing effect
- Azathioprine and 6-mercaptopurine induce remission in active Crohn's disease. The length of time on therapy should be at least 17 weeks. Some adverse effects are noted with this medication
- Metronidazole is effective in the treatment of mild disease and may be especially useful in the treatment of perianal disease
- Surgery is often used to treat complications and disease which is refractory to medical therapy. It is not curative and patients frequently have recurrence

### Review period

- Patients need to be followed life-long due to the nature of the disease
- Patients on complex drug regimens involving immunosuppressants should be reviewed regularly (in the region of four times a year) and when there are problems with further disease or therapy
- Early assessment is indicated during periods of active disease
- Follow up should be shared between the primary care physician and gastroenterologist
- Patients on long-term corticosteroids should be maintained on calcium and vitamin D supplementation. Annual bone mineral densitometry and bisphosphonate therapy for patients with confirmed osteoporosis should also be considered

## PROGNOSIS

- Response to treatment is highly variable
- Most patients have chronic intermittent disease
- 75% of patients require surgery at some point in the course of their disease for the treatment of complications

### Clinical pearls

- Relapse after surgery is so common that all patients should be on azathioprine/6-mercaptopurine immediately after surgery
- Patients with stenosis or stricture may respond acutely to bowel rest with a liquid diet
- Patients on long-term mesalamine, steroids, or immunomodulators should have a full understanding of the potential risks, even those that are relatively rare, such as aseptic necrosis with steroids or interstitial nephritis with mesalamine
- The natural history of Crohn's disease suggests that it can become dormant and the associated gastrointestinal cancer risk is low

### Therapeutic failure

- Generally, physicians escalate therapy with multiple, or increasingly immunosuppressive, agents until remission is induced or chronic, active disease is brought under control
- Surgery should be considered when medical management has failed

### Deterioration
- High-dose oral or intravenous steroids may be required for acute deterioration
- Surgery may be required for patients who do not respond to high-dose steroids

## COMPLICATIONS
- Perforation or megacolon from long-standing disease requires surgical management. The surgery indicated for perforation will depend on its site and the extent of active disease
- Small bowel obstruction, seen in moderate-to-severe Crohn's disease, requires inpatient management
- Fistulating disease in Crohn's with diarrhea and malabsorption needs to be evaluated for medical or surgical treatment. Symptomatic fistulas (e.g. to bladder, vagina, skin) require surgical treatment
- Abscess formation usually requires percutaneous drainage; if this fails or is not possible, surgery is required
- Severe bleeding needs urgent referral
- Anemia may be secondary to blood loss, malabsorption, or chronic disease
- Malnutrition may be seen in chronic or severe disease
- Lactose intolerance develops in 35% of patients with Crohn's disease
- Patients are at increased risk of small bowel cancer, although this is rare. Screening for small bowel cancer is not routinely recommended; colonic dysplasia screening is recommended for patients with pancolitis with colonoscopy and random biopsy after 8 years of disease

## CONSIDER CONSULT
In addition:
- Refer if there are signs of systemic infection
- Difficulty in maintaining remission is the most common reason for further specialist referral
- Disease refractory to first-line management should be referred at the earliest opportunity to a specialist center for medical and surgical management and follow up

# PREVENTION

## RISK FACTORS
Some studies suggest that certain foods, notably milk or lactose, may act as secondary triggers for Crohn's disease and ulcerative colitis. These findings are not widely accepted.

## MODIFY RISK FACTORS
### Lifestyle and wellness
TOBACCO
Tobacco use is associated with an increased risk of Crohn's disease.

## SCREENING
In the absence of characteristic symptoms, screening is not efficacious.

## PREVENT RECURRENCE
- Treatment aims to maximize duration of remissions; depending on the severity of the disease, different drugs may be taken for extended periods of time to induce and extend remissions
- As the drugs are toxic and regimens have to be tailored, it is generally recommended that a gastroenterologist is consulted
- Smoking may be associated with an increased risk of postsurgical recurrence and should be discouraged

# RESOURCES

## ASSOCIATIONS

**American College of Gastroenterology**
4900 B South 31st Street
Arlington, VA 22206
Tel: (703) 820-7400
Fax: (703) 931-4520
http://www.acg.gi.org

**Crohn's and Colitis Foundation of America**
386 Park Avenue South
17th Floor
New York, NY 10016
Tel: (800) 932-2423
Fax: (212) 779-4098
E-mail: info@ccfa.org
http://www.ccfa.org

## KEY REFERENCES

- Connell WR. Safety of drug therapy for inflammatory bowel disease in pregnant and nursing women. Inflammatory Bowel Dis 1996;2:33–47
- Allan RN, et al, eds. Inflammatory bowel disease. New York: Churchill Livingstone, 1997
- Sandborn WJ. A review of immune modifier therapy for inflammatory bowel disease: azathioprine, 6-mercaptopurine, cyclosporine, and methotrexate. Am J Gastroenterol 1996;91:423–33
- Stenson WF. Inflammatory bowel disease. In: Yamada T, ed. Textbook of gastroenterology, 2nd edn, Vol. 2. Philadelphia: Lippincott, 1995, p1748–805
- Sandborn W, Sutherland L, Pearson D, et al. Azathioprine or 6-mercaptopurine for induction of remission in Crohn's disease (Cochrane Review). In: The Cochrane Library, 1, 2002. Oxford: Update Software
- Steinhart AH, Ewe K, Griffiths AM, et al. Corticosteroids for maintenance of remission in Crohn's disease (Cochrane Review). In: The Cochrane Library, 1, 2002. Oxford: Update Software

## FAQS

### Question 1
What is a screening work-up for inflammatory bowel disease?

### ANSWER 1
Flexible sigmoidoscopy and biopsy plus small bowel series.

### Question 2
How does one distinguish Crohn's disease from ulcerative colitis?

### ANSWER 2
In Crohn's disease, the colon involvement is generally patchy and the rectum is spared. Noncaseating granulomas on biopsy indicate Crohn's disease.

### Question 3
When are steroids indicated?

### ANSWER 3
In the initial management of patients with systemic symptoms such as fever or weight loss, in those with vomiting or severe bleeding, and in those refractory to 5-ASA.

## Question 4
When are immunomodulators indicated?

ANSWER 4
They are really the drug of choice for maintenance in patients with flares requiring steroid therapy and in any patient after surgery.

## Question 5
Is cancer surveillance necessary?

ANSWER 5
Only in patients with extensive colon involvement starting after 8 years of symptoms.

## CONTRIBUTORS
Dennis F Saver, MD
Andrew F Ippoliti, MD
Vijay Yajnik, MD
Laura Targownik, MD, FRCP(C)

# DIVERTICULAR DISEASE

| | | |
|---|---|---|
| ■ | Summary Information | 168 |
| ■ | Background | 169 |
| ■ | Diagnosis | 171 |
| ■ | Treatment | 179 |
| ■ | Outcomes | 186 |
| ■ | Prevention | 188 |
| ■ | Resources | 189 |

## SUMMARY INFORMATION

### DESCRIPTION

- Diverticulosis is a disorder of the digestive tract consisting of sac-like outpouchings of mucosa and submucosa through the muscular layer
- They are generally found along the colon's mesenteric border at the site where the vasa recta penetrate the muscle wall (anatomic weak point)
- Sigmoid colon by far the commonest site in westernized countries, but may occur anywhere in the digestive tract. Certain populations, including nations in Asia and Africa, often have predominantly right-sided disease
- 'Diverticular disease' encompasses all aspects and effects of the condition

### KEY! DON'T MISS!

Younger patients (<40) and immunocompromised patients often present in an atypical way and the condition is more serious in these groups.

# BACKGROUND

## ICD9 CODE
562.10 Diverticulosis of colon
562.11 Diverticulitis of colon

## CARDINAL FEATURES
- Diverticulosis is common and in 70%, asymptomatic
- Bleeding may occur in up to 15% of patients, due to abrasion or erosion of adjacent artery by inspissated feces
- Diverticulosis progresses to diverticulitis in about 20% of those affected
- Diverticulitis implies microperforation of a diverticulum with ensuing localized inflammation contained by pericolonic fat and mesentery
- Complicated diverticulitis implies the added complications of abscess formation, free perforation, or fistula formation

## CAUSES
### Common causes
- The term diverticular disease refers generally to outpouchings in the distal and sigmoid colon. These are actually 'false diverticula', as only the mucosa and submucosa herniate through the colonic wall. True diverticula rarely occur in the colon and classically involve all layers of the enteric wall
- Segmental spasm of the muscular coat of the bowel causes mucosal extrusion at its weakest points – adjacent to the penetrating nutrient artery
- Highly refined Western low-fiber diet is thought to be a major contributing factor

### Rare causes
- Rarely, diverticula formation may occur in the stomach, duodenum, jejunum, or ileum
- Very occasionally a single giant diverticulum is found; treatment is excision
- Less commonly may result from connective-tissue disorders such as Marfan's syndrome

## EPIDEMIOLOGY
### Incidence and prevalence
The incidence and prevalence of colonic diverticular disease is remarkably dependent upon the age and nationality of the patient. In particular, it is much more common in 'westernized' nations that traditionally support low-fiber diets, and is increasingly more common with age.

PREVALENCE
- Less than 10% in those under 40
- Up to 65% of those over the age of 85 in 'westernized nations'

### Demographics
AGE
- Diverticulosis rare below 40 years
- Almost universal over the age of 90 years

GENDER
Male=female

RACE
- Rare in Africans
- Sigmoid colon most commonly affected but people of Japanese, Chinese or Hawaiian ancestry are prone to diverticula in the cecum and ascending colon

### GENETICS
There is no evidence of any genetic predisposition to the disorder.

### GEOGRAPHY
Most common in industrialized western societies.

### SOCIOECONOMIC STATUS
Currently no evidence that socioeconomic status has a bearing on the epidemiology.

# DIAGNOSIS

## DIFFERENTIAL DIAGNOSIS
Of prime importance to exclude malignancy.

### Irritable bowel syndrome
Irritable bowel syndrome is common and shares many of the clinical features of diverticulosis.

FEATURES
- Physical examination normal
- Nonspecific abdominal tenderness, often in left lower quadrant
- Loose stools, often in the morning and after meals, alternating with constipation

### Appendicitis
Right-sided diverticulosis is uncommon, but not rare. If complicated by diverticulitis it may mimic acute appendicitis. Of note, while patients with diverticulitis may suffer for several days prior to presentation, those with acute appendicitis tend to have a more abbreviated and punctuated course.

Age of patient is helpful in differential since diverticulosis is rare before age 40 whereas appendicitis is most frequent before age 20.

FEATURES
- Periumbilical pain migrating to right lower quadrant
- Pyrexia and leukocytosis
- Nausea, vomiting
- Tachycardia
- Psoas sign (pain aggravated by right thigh extension)
- Maximal tenderness at McBurney's point

### Pyelonephritis
Pyelonephritis is an infection, usually bacterial in origin, of the upper urinary tract.

FEATURES
- Flank pain
- Dysuria
- Polyuria
- Costovertebral tenderness

### Inflammatory bowel disease
Inflammatory bowel disease includes Crohn's disease and ulcerative colitis.

FEATURES
- Typically a chronic disorder marked by intermittent flares and relapses
- Abdominal distension and tenderness
- Bloody diarrhea
- Fever, dehydration
- May be associated arthritis, liver disease, etc.
- Suspect Crohn's disease if aphthous ulcers, perianal involvement

### Colorectal cancer
- The early detection of colorectal cancer is of prime importance in the management of older patients with lower-bowel related symptoms

- 10–20% of patients diagnosed with diverticulosis on clinical grounds subsequently found to have carcinoma of the colon

FEATURES
- Rectal bleeding
- Change in bowel habit
- Palpable rectal or abdominal mass
- Abdominal tenderness and distension

## Ovarian cancer

Colorectal cancer and ovarian cancer are the most important conditions to eliminate when considering the diagnosis of diverticular disease.

FEATURES
- Abdominal fullness
- Early satiety
- Pelvic and back pain
- Constipation
- Pelvic mass

## Pelvic inflammatory disease

Pelvic inflammatory disease (PID) is a range of inflammatory disorders of the upper genital tract.

FEATURES
- Lower abdominal pain
- Vaginal discharge
- Abnormal uterine bleeding
- Dysuria
- Dyspareunia
- Pain on manipulation of the cervix
- Adnexal tenderness
- Adnexal mass

## Endometriosis

Endometriosis is the presence of functioning endometrial tissue outside the uterine cavity.

FEATURES
- Dysmenorrhea, dyspareunia, and infertility
- Tender uterosacral ligaments
- Cul-de-sac nodularity
- Induration of rectovaginal septum
- Fixed retroversion
- Adnexal mass

## Pseudomembranous colitis

Pseudomembranous colitis is a disorder characterized by diarrhea and bowel inflammation associated with antibiotic use and due to overgrowth of *Clostridium difficile*.

FEATURES
- History of antibiotic use, especially amoxicillin or clindamycin. May occur with most every antibiotic class
- Abdominal tenderness

- Fever
- Diarrhea

## Ischemic colitis

Ischemic colitis is inflammation of the colon due to interruption of the colonic blood supply.

### FEATURES
- Associated vascular or cardiovascular disease. In particular, is often associated with atrial fibrillation
- Diarrhea with dark clots
- Pyrexia and tachycardia, often in association with progressive hypotension and impending sepsis
- Diffuse and poorly defined colonic tenderness with 'pain out of proportion to palpation'
- 'Thumbprinting' on barium enema

## SIGNS & SYMPTOMS
### Signs
#### Diverticulosis
- Physical examination in patients with uncomplicated diverticulosis generally normal
- Left lower quadrant tenderness may be present
- Only signs are those of complications, e.g. rectal bleeding

#### Diverticulitis
- Left lower quadrant tenderness with or without guarding (but right-sided signs do not preclude the diagnosis)
- Low-grade fever
- Leukocytosis

#### Complicated diverticulitis
More rarely a patient may present with the signs of complicated diverticulitis (abscess, fistula, free perforation, obstruction).

### Symptoms
#### Diverticulosis
- Usually asymptomatic
- Often discovered incidentally on barium enema or during lower endoscopy for colon cancer screening
- Some patients may report constipation, constipation alternating with diarrhea, left lower quadrant discomfort and bloating
- May present as rectal bleeding due to erosion of an artery by inspissated feces; typically described as 'painless hematochezia'

**Diverticulitis** usually presents as:
- Left lower quadrant pain
- Fever
- Malaise
- Change in bowel habit, usually constipation
- Occasionally anorexia, nausea and vomiting
- Very rarely is there concurrent bleeding during a bout of diverticulitis

**Complicated diverticulitis** will present with the typical features of the underlying pathology, i.e. abscess, fistula, obstruction, free perforation.

## KEY! DON'T MISS!
Younger patients (<40) and immunocompromised patients often present in an atypical way and the condition is more serious in these groups.

## CONSIDER CONSULT
Refer:
- When the possibility of colorectal or ovarian malignancy cannot be ruled out
- When significant peritoneal signs present; i.e. signs suggesting free perforation
- If the patient has any fever in association with persistent or progressive abdominal pain
- If significant or increasing rectal bleeding
- If patient on steroid treatment
- If patient immunosuppressed
- When there are signs of obstruction
- If abscess or fistula formation suspected

## INVESTIGATION OF THE PATIENT
### Direct questions to patient
- **Q** Any change in bowel habit? Diarrhea or constipation of recent onset may occur in diverticular disease or colonic cancer. May also be present in the setting of underlying irritable bowel syndrome, which can both mimic diverticular disease and contribute to its formation. Of particular note is the development of 'pencil thin' stools, which may indicate the presence of a left-sided intraluminal lesion.
- **Q** Previous episodes of abdominal pain? How longstanding is the condition? Diverticulitis that is recurrent will be managed more aggressively
- **Q** Have you had any rectal bleeding? The most common cause of painless rectal bleeding is diverticular disease, but always suspect malignancy
- **Q** Any weight loss? No significant weight loss in diverticulosis or mild uncomplicated diverticulitis
- **Q** Have you had a course of antibiotics recently? Exclude pseudomembranous colitis if the patient's major complaint is diarrhea
- **Q** Any urinary problems? Exclude pyelonephritis, urolithiasis, colovesical fistula
- **Q** Any gynecologic problems? Exclude gynecologic causes of pelvic symptoms (e.g. ovarian cysts, neoplasms, endometriosis), colovaginal fistula

### Examination
- **Age?** Commonest in the older patient but more severe in the unusual cases under 40s
- **Is the patient well/unwell?** Uncomplicated diverticulosis will not cause constitutional upset. Diverticulitis causes moderate illness. Complicated diverticulitis may be catastrophic
- **Signs of weight loss?** Remember the possibility of malignancy
- **Clinically anemic?** Possibility of chronic blood loss, must exclude colorectal carcinoma
- **Check for pyrexia.** Moderate pyrexia is usual in diverticulitis, but may be absent in the elderly who are most at risk for diverticular formation. Additionally, immunocompromised patients may not present with fever
- **Check pulse, BP.** General cardiovascular condition satisfactory?
- **Dipstick urine**, useful to rule out urinary tract infection (UTI), kidney stone, possibility of rectovesical fistula
- **Palpate abdomen generally.** Check for masses, hepatosplenomegaly, ascites
- **Palpate the site of maximum pain.** Any guarding? Any rebound tenderness? Any left lower quadrant mass?
- **Auscultation.** Bowel sounds present? Normal? Remember obstruction, perforation in complicated diverticulitis
- **Rectal examination.** Any mass? Any tenderness? Any blood? If so, what color? Usually fresh red arterial blood

- **Pelvic examination.** Any adnexal mass? Any tenderness on manipulation of the cervix? Any discharge?

## Summary of investigative tests
- Complete blood test should be routine and will detect anemia and leukocytosis
- Urinalysis for infection, hematuria
- X-rays may be useful in initial evaluation of suspected perforation, obstruction, urolithiasis
- Abdominal ultrasound useful in suspected gynecologic pathology, hydronephrosis
- Computed tomography (CT) scan helpful in diagnosis of diverticulitis and diverticular abscess
- Endoscopy. Colonoscopy and flexible sigmoidoscopy are gold standards for documenting diverticula. However, endoscopy should be avoided during acute bouts of diverticulitis as colonic insufflation may exacerbate the risk of perforation

## DIAGNOSTIC DECISION
### Diverticulosis
Clinically mild disorder, with:
- Constipation, or
- Constipation alternating with diarrhea
- Left lower quadrant discomfort or bloating

### Diverticulitis
The majority of patients will have:
- Left lower quadrant pain (93–100%)
- Fever (57–100%)
- Leukocytosis (69–83%)

In addition the patient may have some of the common associated features of diverticulitis:
- Nausea
- Vomiting
- Constipation
- Diarrhea

### Guidelines
- The American College of Gastroenterology has published practice guidelines. Stollman NH, Raskin JB for and on behalf of the Ad Hoc Practice Parameters Committee of the American College of Gastroenterology. Diagnosis and management of diverticular disease of the colon in adults [1]
- Practice parameters for the treatment of sigmoid diverticulitis. Standards Task Force, The American Society of Colon and Rectal Surgeons [2]

## THE TESTS
### Body fluids
COMPLETE BLOOD COUNT
*Description*
Venous blood sample.

*Normal*
**White blood cells**
3200–9800/mm$^3$

**Red blood cells**
Male: 4.3–5.9x10$^6$/mm$^3$
Female: 3.5–5x10$^6$/mm$^3$

**Hemoglobin**
Male: 13.6–17.7g/dL
Female: 12–15g/dL

**Hematocrit**
Male: 39–49%
Female: 33–43%

**Mean corpuscular volume**
76–100fL

*Abnormal*
Values outside the normal range.

*Cause of abnormal result*
- Iron-deficiency anemia should suggest a diagnosis of colonic cancer rather than diverticular disease, until proved otherwise
- Raised white cell count usually present in diverticulitis with predominance of polymorphonuclear leukocytes
- Other infectious, inflammatory, or neoplastic disorder

*Drugs, disorders and other factors that may alter results*
Other infectious, inflammatory, or neoplastic disorder.

URINALYSIS
*Description*
Tests on mid-stream urine.

*Advantages/Disadvantages*
Routine test.

*Normal*
- Normal appearance, pH, specific gravity
- No blood, cells, glucose, protein

*Abnormal*
- Altered appearance, pH, specific gravity
- Presence of blood, cells, glucose, or protein

*Cause of abnormal result*
- Presence of white blood cells if inflammatory process is adjacent to ureter or bladder
- Frank infection may signify colovesicular fistula. In extreme instances the patients may pass frank feces in the urine, which is pathognomonic for a colovesicular fistula
- Hematuria may indicate infection or neoplasm of genitourinary tract or urolithiasis

**Imaging**
X-RAYS
*Advantages/Disadvantages*
- Plain film supine and upright may be useful where perforation is suspected. In particular, an upright chest film is most sensitive for detecting free intraperitoneal air
- Barium enema the best method of diagnosis of diverticulosis, but avoid in diverticulitis – risk of extravasation from a perforation

- Barium enema may convert a contained microperforation to generalized peritonitis
- Water-soluble contrast enema is safer but still carries some risk
- Gentle, single-contrast study is preferred

*Abnormal*
Contrast studies will demonstrate:
- Colonic wall thickening
- Diverticula
- Fistula formation
- Displacement of the colon by abscess

## CT SCAN
*Advantages/Disadvantages*
### Diverticulosis
- Not very useful in differentiating cancer from diverticulosis and should be supplemented by contrast enema or endoscopy

### Diverticulitis
- Useful, noninvasive investigation in the diagnosis of diverticulitis
- The procedure of choice in cases of moderate severity or where the diagnosis is in doubt
- Expensive, but not generally necessary in mild cases

Should be considered if:
- Diverticulitis is of moderate severity
- The condition occurs in an immunocompromised patient
- The diagnosis is unclear

## ABDOMINAL ULTRASOUND
*Advantages/Disadvantages*
Abdominal ultrasound is usually readily available and is:
- Noninvasive
- May demonstrate colonic wall thickness
- Very sensitive for detecting fluid collections such as an abscess
- May be helpful in women to exclude gynecologic pathology
- Useful to rule out hydronephrosis as a cause of abdominal pain

*Drugs, disorders and other factors that may alter results*
Accuracy and usefulness very dependent on the examiner's skill.

## Other tests
### ENDOSCOPY
*Description*
- Colonoscopy
- Flexible sigmoidoscopy

### Diverticulosis
- Gold standard for demonstrating presence of diverticula
- Extremely valuable in excluding colorectal cancer
- Useful for treatment of bleeding, in expert hands

### Diverticulitis
- Usually avoided during an attack of acute diverticulitis – risk of perforation by the instrument or by insufflation of excessive air

- However, limited proctoscopy with minimal insufflation may help to exclude other diagnoses, e.g. inflammatory bowel disease

*Abnormal*
Visualization of diverticula.

*Cause of abnormal result*
Presence of diverticula.

# TREATMENT

## CONSIDER CONSULT
**Refer if, despite treatment:**
- Pain persists for >3 days
- Increasing pain or increasing fever
- White cell count continues to rise
- Inability to tolerate oral fluids

## IMMEDIATE ACTION
- Free perforation with purulent peritonitis will require urgent surgery
- This is a surgical emergency with a mortality rate approaching 35%
- Primary resection of the diseased segment and anastomosis is the procedure of choice
- Hartmann's resection appropriate if substantial contamination
- Significant and persistent bleeding requires blood replacement, identification of bleeding site, and surgical resection if it persists

## PATIENT AND CAREGIVER ISSUES
### Health-seeking behavior
Ask about the patient's intake of dietary fiber since low fiber intake is a risk factor for diverticulosis.

## MANAGEMENT ISSUES
### Goals
The aim of management is:
- Diverticulosis: control of symptoms and prevention of complications
- Diverticulitis: bed rest, control of infection, bowel rest (low residue, fluid only diet, or nil per mouth in severe cases) and maintenance of hydration
- Severe or complicated diverticulitis: early detection and hospitalization

### Management in special circumstances
**Bleeding in diverticulosis:**
- May be severe and is usually painless
- Presents as large volume maroon or red stool
- Emergency management similar to that for any gastrointestinal bleeding, i.e. appropriate volume replacement and supportive care
- Surgical consultation is required
- Early colonic purge with urgent colonoscopy has been shown, in limited series, to improve outcomes by ensuring rapid hemostasis

### COEXISTING MEDICATION
- **Nonsteroidal anti-inflammatory drugs (NSAIDs):** concurrent use of NSAIDs should probably be stopped because of the risk of both upper and lower intestinal bleeding with this class of drugs
- **Steroids:** refer early as the risk of complications is high

### SPECIAL PATIENT GROUPS
#### Immunocompromised patients
- Includes transplant patients, patients with renal failure, AIDS, chronic steroid use and those receiving chemotherapy
- Diverticulitis may present in an atypical way, with few of the classical signs and symptoms being present
- These patients should be referred for specialist management. Postoperative mortality is reported to be as high as 40% in this group

### Younger age groups
- Diverticular disease uncommon in patients under 40 (2–5% of the total)
- Often not considered in this age group and may be misdiagnosed as appendicitis
- Obesity is a comorbid factor
- Young patients present with a higher incidence of complicated diverticulitis
- A much higher proportion of these patients require emergency surgery on presentation (50–75%)
- Elective surgery should be considered after a single episode of acute diverticulitis because of high-risk recurrence

### Recurrent diverticulitis after resection
- Only 4–7% of patients have recurrence of diverticulitis after resection
- Referral usually indicated

## SUMMARY OF THERAPEUTIC OPTIONS
### Choices
For pain control:
- Simple analgesics may be adequate
- Meperidine may be used for severe pain. However, its short duration of action predisposes to a 'rebound' pain effect. Moreover, it has a potentially toxic metabolite – normeperidine – which may induce seizures, myoclonus, and tremors. Therefore, use this preparation with caution
- Morphine and other opioids may increase intracolonic pressure. However, it is unclear if this theoretic disadvantage translates into clinically meaningful ill effects

Diverticulosis:
- High-fiber diet
- Dietary fiber supplementation with bran (15g daily is recommended), or fecal bulking agents (psyllium or methylcellulose preparations)
- Antispasmodic (anticholinergic) drugs

Diverticulitis:
- Bowel rest
- Broad-spectrum oral or intravenous antibiotics effective against anaerobes and Gram-negative rods are generally prescribed for 7–10 days
- Maintenance of hydration

Patients who do not respond to medical therapy of acute diverticulitis may require surgical intervention:
- Laparoscopic surgery is useful in the management of diverticular disease
- Initial treatment of abscess by CT-guided percutaneous drainage
- If not amenable to this, or if symptoms persist, laparotomy with the aim of primary resection of the diseased segment and anastomosis
- If much inflammation or contamination, Hartmann's resection is performed (a two-stage procedure usually revised in 3–6 months)
- Other indications for surgery include: perforation, persistent tender mass, narrowing or deformity of sigmoid on X-ray (possibility of cancer), dysuria associated with diverticulitis in men and hysterectomized women – may presage fistula formation; clinical, endoscopic or X-ray signs that do not rule out cancer
- Early colonic purge with urgent colonoscopy has been shown, in limited series, to improve outcomes by ensuring rapid hemostasis. When this is inadequate or unsuccessful, surgical evaluation should be obtained

## Guidelines
- The American College of Gastroenterology has produced practice guidelines. Stollman NH, Raskin JB for and on behalf of the Ad Hoc Practice Parameters Committee of the American College of Gastroenterology. Diagnosis and management of diverticular disease of the colon in adults [1]
- Practice parameters for the treatment of sigmoid diverticulitis. Standards Task Force, The American Society of Colon and Rectal Surgeons [2]

## FOLLOW UP
Follow up 4–6 weeks after resolution of symptoms of an attack of diverticulitis.

### Plan for review
After recovery from an initial episode of diverticulitis patients should be re-evaluated. This will include:
- Flexible sigmoidoscopy and
- Barium enema or colonoscopy

### Information for patient or caregiver
- High-fiber diet advised – for life
- Control of obesity should be recommended.
- Report any significant recurrence of symptoms of diverticulitis

## DRUGS AND OTHER THERAPIES: DETAILS
### Drugs
PSYLLIUM PREPARATIONS
- Absorb water in intestine
- Promote peristalsis
- Reduce gastrointestinal (GI) transit time

*Dose*
Oral: 1–2 rounded teaspoonfuls or 1–2 packets in 8oz glass of liquid one to four times per day; 1–2 wafers with 8oz glass of liquid one to four times per day

*Efficacy*
While psyllium preparations may help guard against future diverticular formation by minimizing intraluminal pressures, they may also exacerbate the condition if taken incorrectly. In particular, the patient must be reminded to drink up to 8 glasses of water a day. If not, the psyllium forms a sort of 'cement' rather than a 'slurry,' and may promote rather than relieve constipation.

*Risks/benefits*
- Dietary modification and bran is cheaper
- Use caution in phenylketonuria

*Side effects and adverse reactions*
- Gastrointestinal: anorexia, nausea, vomiting, abdominal pains, diarrhea, constipation, bloating, bowel obstruction

*Interactions (other drugs)*
- No significant interactions noted

*Contraindications*
- Intestinal obstruction
- Fecal impaction

*Acceptability to patient*
*Patient and caregiver information*
- Maintain adequate fluid intake – up to 8 glasses of water per day
- Avoid inhalation

## METHYLCELLULOSE PREPARATIONS
- Attract water
- Expand in intestine to increase peristalsis
- Absorb excess water in stool
- Decrease diarrhea

*Dose*
Oral: 1 heaped tablespoon in 8oz cold water, one to three times a day.

*Risks/benefits*
- Dietary modification and bran is cheaper
- Use caution in phenylketonuria
- Do not use other laxatives
- Able to use in pregnancy
- Use caution in rectal, esophageal or intestinal ulcerations, bleeding or stenosis

*Side effects and adverse reactions*
- Gastrointestinal: anorexia, nausea, vomiting, abdominal pains, diarrhea, constipation, bloating, bowel obstruction

*Interactions (other drugs)*
- Surfactants

*Contraindications*
- Patients who require a low galactose diet ■ Acute surgical abdomen ■ Nausea, vomiting or other symptom of appendicitis ■ Fecal impaction ■ Undiagnosed abdominal pain
- Intestinal obstruction

*Evidence*
A small, double-blind crossover trial examined the efficacy of methylcellulose versus placebo in the management of symptomatic diverticular disease. Methylcellulose was not shown to have a significant effect on a symptom score [3] *Level P*

*Patient and caregiver information*
- Notify clinician of unrelieved constipation, rectal bleeding
- Ensure adequate fluid intake

## ANTISPASMODIC (ANTICHOLINERGIC) DRUGS
*Dose*
**Hyoscyamine preparations:**
- Oral/sublingual: 0.125–0.25mg three to four times a day as required before food
- Time release capsules 0.375mg 12-hourly
- Subcutaneous/intravenous: 0.25–0.5mg 6-hourly as required

**Dicyclomine preparations:**
- Oral: 10–40mg three to four times a day as required
- Intramuscular: 20mg 4–6 hourly as required
- Available as capsules, uncoated tablets, syrup, and injection solution

*Efficacy*
- Antispasmodics may be tried in cases where spasm is a prominent feature
- They are of unproven efficacy and probably of limited value

*Risks/benefits*
- Use caution in the elderly and children
- Use caution in hepatic and renal disease

*Side effects and adverse reactions*
- Cardiovascular system: palpitations, tachycardia
- Central nervous system: confusion, stimulation, dizziness, drowsiness
- Eye, ears, nose, and throat: increased intraocular pressure, blurred vision, mydriasis
- Gastrointestinal: dry mouth, constipation, nausea and vomiting
- Skin: rash, urticaria

*Interactions (other drugs)*
- Amantadine
- Tricyclic antidepressants
- Monoamine oxidase inhibitors (MAOIs)
- Antihistamines
- Phenothiazines
- Levodopa
- Ketoconazole

*Contraindications*
- Narrow-angle glaucoma
- GI atony and obstruction
- Prostatic hypertrophy

## MEPERIDINE

*Dose*
Oral/intramuscular/intravenous/subcutaneous: 50–150mg every 3–4h.

*Efficacy*
Provides effective pain relief where there is pain of moderate severity.

*Risks/benefits*
- Use caution in head injury, respiratory conditions including asthma, renal and hepatic impairment, hypothyroidism and Addison's disease
- Use caution in the elderly
- Use caution in patients with supraventricular tachycardias

*Side effects and adverse reactions*
- Cardiovascular system: tachycardia, bradycardia, palpitations, postural hypotension
- Central nervous system: drowsiness, sedation, seizures, dizziness, tremors
- Gastrointestinal: nausea, vomiting, constipation, anorexia
- Respiratory: respiratory depression
- Skin: rash

*Interactions (other drugs)*
- Antihistamines
- Anxiolytics/hypnotics (chloral hydrate, glutethimide)
- Barbiturates
- Cimetidine
- Ciprofloxacin
- Ethanol
- MAOIs
- Methocarbamol
- Metoclopramide
- Mexiletine
- Neuroleptics
- Phenytoin
- Ritonavir
- Selegiline
- Tricyclic antidepressants

*Contraindications*
- Existing CNS depression
- Alcohol abuse
- MAOI therapy (within 14 days)
- Severe renal impairment
- Severe or acute bronchial asthma
- Respiratory depression

## ANTIBIOTICS

Effective regimen should cover typical enteric Gram-negative organisms along with anaerobic flora, especially if there is a concurrent abscess. If no evidence of peritonitis or perforation, may start with ciprofloxacin or ampicillin along with metronidazole orally or intravenously, depending upon the patients' ability to take orals. Clindamycin may be substituted for ampicillin in penicillin-allergic patients. In the setting of peritonitis consider a second or third generation cephalosporin combined with gentamicin or a combination of ampicillin, gentamicin, and metronidazole.

### Dose
- **Ampicillin:** 500mg orally every 6h
- **Amoxicillin clavulanate:** 500mg orally every 8h
- **Ciprofloxacin:** 500–750mg orally every 12h
- **Metronidazole:** 250–500mg orally four times a day
- **Clindamycin:** 400–900mg every 8h
- **Cefotetan:** 1g intravenously every 12h
- **Gentamicin:** 3–5mg/kg/day in patients with normal renal function

### Efficacy
The inflammatory process in mild to moderate diverticulitis generally settles after 6–7 days of antibiotic treatment combined with rest and liquid diet.

### Risks/benefits
- Bear in mind the potential side effects of antibiotic therapy particularly in the elderly
- Renal insufficiency
- Thrush
- Pseudomembranous colitis
- Abdominal discomfort, bloating, and diarrhea
- Do not administer for prolonged or repeated treatment

### Side effects and adverse reactions
- Cardiovascular system: palpitations
- Central nervous system: seizures, hallucinations, coma, anxiety, convulsions
- Gastrointestinal: nausea, diarrhea, vomiting, altered liver function tests, pseudomembraneous colitis, abdominal pain
- Genitourinary: urinary problems, renal damage, moniliasis, vaginitis, nephrotoxicity
- Hematologic: bleeding disorders, bone marrow depression, agranulocytosis
- Respiratory: anaphylaxis
- Skin: erythema multiforme, rash, urticaria

### Interactions (other drugs)
- Alcohol
- Aminoglycosides
- Amphotericin B
- Antacids
- Anticholinesterases (neostigmine, pyridostigmine)
- Antibiotics (penicillins, cephalosporins, polymixins, vancomycin)
- Anticholinesterases (neostigmine, pyridostigmine)
- Anticoagulants
- Atenolol
- Barbiturates
- Caffeine
- Cyclosporine
- Diazepam
- Loop diuretics
- Methotrexate
- Mineral supplements (zinc, magnesium, calcium, aluminium, iron)
- Neuromuscular blocking agents (atracurium, vecuronium)
- NSAIDs
- Opiates
- Oral contraceptives
- Phenytoin
- Platinum compounds (carboplatin, cisplatin)
- Probenecid
- Succinylcholine
- Theophylline

### Contraindications
- Hypersensitivity to antibiotic

*Evidence*
Inpatient management of diverticulitis with a cephalosporin (cefoxitin) was compared with a combination of gentamicin and clindamycin in a small randomized controlled trial. Patients requiring surgery were excluded. The two treatments had similar efficacy [4] *Level P*

## LIFESTYLE

All patients with diverticular disease should be encouraged:
- To adopt a high-fiber diet
- To reduce obesity

### ACCEPTABILITY TO PATIENT
- High-fiber diet and bran may both cause flatulence
- Bloating and flatulence generally resolve after a few weeks

### FOLLOW UP PLAN
Colonic evaluation is indicated after resolution of clinically diagnosed diverticulitis to exclude neoplasm.

## OUTCOMES

### EFFICACY OF THERAPIES
#### Uncomplicated diverticulitis
- Conservative management results in resolution in 70–100% of patients

#### Complicated diverticulitis
- Abscess formation: if amenable to CT-guided percutaneous drainage 70–90% may be successfully treated
- Free perforation: outcome depends on degree of fecal contamination, magnitude of sepsis and timeliness of intervention. Mortality approaches 35%

#### Evidence
- There is some evidence that medical management of acute, uncomplicated diverticulitis confers high clinical cure rates and low mortality, however there is a chance of recurrent acute diverticulitis [5]
- PDxMD are unable to cite evidence which meets our criteria for evidence for other therapies used in the management of diverticular disease

### PROGNOSIS
#### Diverticulosis
- 70% are asymptomatic
- 5–10% experience diverticular bleeding
- 10–15% proceed to diverticulitis

#### Diverticulitis
- 75% remain as simple diverticulitis. Of these, 15% require surgical intervention
- Of those treated conservatively, 30–40% continue to have symptoms (cramps, etc.). 30–40% are asymptomatic. Out of this group, 20–30% will have a further attack. After a second attack the chance of a third episode is more than 50%
- 25% proceed to complicated diverticulitis

#### Complicated diverticulitis
25% of patients with diverticulitis proceed to complicated diverticulitis, and of these, 90–95% require surgery.

#### Recurrence after surgery
Of all patients treated surgically, 4–10% experience recurrence.

#### Recurrence
Following repeated attacks of diverticulitis, surgical resection may be required:
- Decision individualized to minimize morbidity and mortality, taking into account age of the patient; number, severity and frequency of attacks; speed and degree of response to medical treatment; persistence of symptoms following an acute attack
- Generally, surgery is recommended after resolution of a second attack of acute diverticulitis (except in under 40s where it should be considered after the first episode)
- When resection is required for recurrent uncomplicated diverticulitis a one-stage procedure is standard; the affected segment is removed and end-to-end anastomosis performed
- Follow up in 4–6 weeks after surgery. Following surgery, only 4–7% of patients may have further attacks of diverticulitis

### COMPLICATIONS
Complications which require surgery include fistula and obstruction.

### Surgical treatment of fistula
- Other causes of fistula formation should be excluded, e.g. colorectal cancer and inflammatory bowel disease
- The commonest types of fistula are colovesicular (65% of all fistulas), colovaginal, colocutaneous, coloenteric and colouterine
- Treatment involves resection of the diseased section of colon and repair of the contiguous organ

### Surgical treatment of obstruction
- Expeditious surgery is the aim
- Hartmann's resection is the usual approach

## CONSIDER CONSULT
### Refer for surgery if:
- There are repeated attacks of diverticulitis
- Complications of diverticulitis are suspected
- Patient presents with gastrointestinal hemorrhage

# PREVENTION

## RISK FACTORS
The only known risk factor is the low-residue western diet.

## MODIFY RISK FACTORS
- Adoption of a high-fiber diet should be recommended in all cases
- No evidence to exclude whole pieces of fiber (nuts, corn, seeds)

### Lifestyle and wellness
TOBACCO
There is no proven effect on diverticular disease.

ALCOHOL AND DRUGS
No proven effect on diverticular disease.

DIET
This should contain significant quantities of fruit, vegetables and grains.

PHYSICAL ACTIVITY
- Adequate exercise should be advised, appropriate to age
- Evidence indicates protective effect of physical activity

# RESOURCES

## ASSOCIATIONS
**NIDDK**
National Institutes of Health
31 Center Drive, MSC 2560
Bethesda, MD 20892-2560
http://www.niddk.nih.gov

**American Society of Colon and Rectal Surgeons**
85 W. Algonquin Rd., Suite 550
Arlington Heights, IL 60005
Tel: (847) 290-9184
Fax: (847) 290-9203
http://www.fascrs.org

## KEY REFERENCES
- The Standards Task Force American Society of Colon and Rectal Surgeons. Practice parameters for sigmoid diverticulitis. Dis Colon Rectum 1995;38(2):125–32
- Stollman NH, Raskin JB. Diagnosis and management of diverticular disease of the colon in adults. Am J Gastroenterol 1999;94(11):3110–21 (available from the American College of Gastroenterology and at http://www-east.elsevier.com/ajg/issues/9411/ajg1501fla.htm)
- Kohler L, et al. Diagnosis and treatment of diverticular disease. Surg Endosc 1999;4:430–6
- Stollman NH, et al. Diverticular disease of the colon. J Clin Gastroenterol 1999;29(3):241–52
- Conti A, et al. Complications of colonic diverticulosis. Ann Ital Chir 1995;66(1):53–60
- Ozick LA, et al. Pathogenesis, diagnosis and treatment of diverticular disease of the colon. Gastroenterologist 1994;4:299–310
- Glauser R, et al. Diverticular disease of the colon. Dtch Med Wochenschr 1997;102(200):755–9
- Cheskin LJ, et al. Diverticular disease. Drugs Aging 1995;6(1):55–63
- Stollman NH, et al. Diagnosis and management of diverticular disease of the colon. Am J Gastroenterol 1999;94(11):3110–21
- Halphen M, et al. Natural history of colonic diverticulosis. Rev Prat 1995;45(8):952–8
- Wilcox CM, et al. Nonsteroidal antiinflammatory drugs are associated with both upper and lower gastrointestinal bleeding. Dig Dis Sci 1997;92(3):419–24
- Longstreth GF. Epidemiology and outcome of patients hospitalized with acute lower gastrointestinal hemorrhage. Am J Gastroenterol 1997;92(3);419–24
- Moreaux J, et al. Diagnostic pitfalls of complicated diverticulitis. Rev Prat 1995;45(8):990–3
- Vernava AM, et al. Lower gastrointestinal bleeding. Dis Colon Rectum 1997;40(7):846–58
- Sadousky R. Causes of occult and obscure gastrointestinal bleeding. Gastroenterology 2000;118:202–21
- McCarthy DW, et al. Etiology of diverticular disease. J Natl Med Assoc 1996;88(6):389–90
- Padidar AM, et al. Differentiating sigmoid diverticulitis from carcinoma. Am J Roentgenol 1994;163(1):81–3
- Farthmann EH, et al. Evidence-based surgery: diverticulitis – a surgical disease? Langenbecks Arch Surg 2000;385(2):143–51
- Jensen DM, et al. Urgent colonoscopy for the diagnosis and treatment of severe diverticular hemorrhage. N Engl J Med 2000;342(2):125–7
- Foutch PG, et al. Diverticular bleeding. Am J Gastroenterol 1996;91(12):2589–93
- Gostout CJ. The role of endoscopy in managing acute lower gastrointestinal bleeding. N Engl J Med 2000;342(2):125–7
- Boulez J, et al. Colonic diverticulosis and laparoscopy. Ann Chir 1999;53(10):1033–8
- Wong SK, et al. Clinical behavior of complicated right-sided and left-sided diverticulosis. Dis Colon Rectum 1997;40(3):344–8
- Chow DC, et al. Jejunoileal diverticula. Gastroenterologist 1997;5(1):78–84
- Krishnamurthy S, et al. Jejunal diverticulosis. Gastroenterology 1983;85(3):538–47
- Akhrass R, et al. Small bowel diverticulosis. Journal of the American College of Surgeons 1997;184(4):383–8
- Chia EJ, et al. Diverticular disease of the small bowel. Hepatogastroenterology 2000;47(31):181–4
- Giuffrida MC, et al. Diverticula of the right colon. Minerva Chir 1997;52(12):1503–12

- Carus T, et al. Surgical therapy of right-sided colonic diverticulitis. Langenbecks Arch Chir 1995;380(5):288–91
- Custer TJ, et al. Giant colonic diverticulum. J Gastrointest Surg 1999;3(5):543–8
- Aldoori WH, et al. A prospective study of dietary fibre types and symptomatic diverticular disease. J Nutrit 1998;128(4):714–9
- Setti Carraro PG, et al. Predictive value of a pathophysiological score in the surgical treatment of perforated diverticular disease. Chir Ital 1999;51(1):31–6
- D'Abbicco D, et al. The indications and surgical treatment in the complications of colonic diverticular disease. Chir Ital 1999;51(4):277–82
- Ferzoco LB, et al. Current concepts: acute diverticulitis. N Engl J Med 1998;338(21):1521–6
- Formento E, et al. Diverticular disease and its treatment. Minerva Chir 1997;52(3):261–70
- Rao PM. Helical CT of appendicitis and diverticulitis. Radiol Clin North Am 1999;37(5):895–910
- Ambrosetti P, et al. Computed tomography in acute left colonic diverticulitis. Br J Surg 1997;84(4):532–4
- Iber FL. Dambro: Griffith's 5-minute clinical consult. Philadelphia: Lippincott Williams & Wilkins, 1999, 328
- Goroll AH, et al. Primary care medicine. Philadelphia: Lippincott-Raven, 1995
- Feldman M, et al. Sleisenger and Fordtran's gastrointestinal and liver disease. Philadelphia: WB Saunders, 1998
- Rosen P. Emergency medicine: concepts and clinical practice. St Louis: Mosby-Year Book, 1998, 2022–7
- Smith JW. Rakel: Conn's Current Therapy 2000. Philadelphia: WB Saunders, 2000, 478–82
- Ferri FF. Ferri's Clinical Advisor. St Louis: Mosby, 2000, 185
- Jaret P. The case for high-fiber diets. Hippocrates 2000;14(5). http://www.hippocrates.com/archive/May2000/05features/05featfiber.html
- Gostout C. The role of endoscopy in managing acute lower gastrointestinal bleeding. N Engl J of Med Created January 13 2000 http://content.nejm.org/cgi/content/short/342/2/125
- Mishra G. Diverticulitis: is there any science to the pain? University of Florida College of Medicine. Created: September 17, 1999 Modified: June 8, 2000 http://www.medinfo.ufl.edu/cme/grounds/mishra/index.html

### Evidence references and guidelines

1 Stollman NH, Raskin JB for and on behalf of the Ad Hoc Practice Parameters Committee of the American College of Gastroenterology. Diagnosis and management of diverticular disease of the colon in adults. Am J Gastroenterol 1999;94:3110–21
2 Practice parameters for the treatment of sigmoid diverticulitis. Standards Task Force, The American Society of Colon and Rectal Surgeons. Dis Colon Rectum 2000;43:2890–97. Available online at the National Guideline Clearinghouse
3 Hodgson WJ. The placebo effect. Is it important in diverticular disease? Am J Gastroenterol 1977;67:157–62. Reviewed in Clinical Evidence 2001;5:296–302
4 Kellum JM, Sugerman HJ, Coppa GF, et al. Randomized, prospective comparison of cefoxitin and gentamicin-clindamycin in the treatment of acute colonic diverticulitis. Clin Ther 14;376–84. Reviewed in Clinical Evidence 2001;5:296–302
5 Simpson J, Spiller R. Clonoic diverticular disease: Digestive system disorders. Clinical Evidence 2001;5:296–302. London: BMJ Publishing Group

# FAQS
## Question 1
Do all patients with active diverticular bleeding require immediate surgical evaluation upon admission to hospital?

ANSWER 1
It depends on the severity of bleeding. Patients with massive bleeding should be evaluated by a surgeon on admission to the hospital. However, it is important to remember that while early surgical evaluation may expedite care later on, the first priority is to ensure that a trained gastroenterologist has considered the case. In particular, administration of a rapid colonic purge in association with urgent colonoscopy (within 12h of presentation) has been associated with rapid hemostasis and improved outcomes and may successfully divert patients away from surgery. Clearly, if bleeding persists despite initial attempts at endoscopic therapy, then surgical evaluation must be rightfully pursued.

## Question 2
All things being equal, which lesion is more likely to bleed: a sigmoid or a cecal diverticulum?

### ANSWER 2
Actually, while left-sided diverticula are more common, right-sided diverticula are more apt to bleed. The thin walls and wide lumen of the cecum potentiate Laplacian forces and subject the penetrating arteries to relatively higher pressures than the sigmoid colon. The end result is a higher propensity for cecal lesions to bleed.

## Question 3
Do diverticula mimic irritable bowel syndrome, or does irritable bowel syndrome promote diverticula?

### ANSWER 3
Most likely both. Constipation-predominant irritable bowel syndrome may exacerbate and potentially help generate sigmoid diverticula, though the association has not been definitively proven. Likewise, sigmoid diverticula may cause bloating and left lower quadrant discomfort, which are also hallmarks of irritable bowel syndrome.

## CONTRIBUTORS
Fred F Ferri, MD, FACP
Andrew H Soll, MD
Brennan Spiegel, MD

# GASTROESOPHAGEAL REFLUX DISEASE IN ADULTS

| | | |
|---|---|---|
| ■ | Summary Information | 194 |
| ■ | Background | 195 |
| ■ | Diagnosis | 198 |
| ■ | Treatment | 208 |
| ■ | Outcomes | 221 |
| ■ | Prevention | 223 |
| ■ | Resources | 224 |

## SUMMARY INFORMATION

### DESCRIPTION
- Passive reflux of gastric contents into the esophagus that causes symptoms or histopathologic changes in the esophageal epithelium (or both)
- Typical symptoms are heartburn, acid regurgitation, and dysphagia
- Atypical symptoms reflect upper airway consequences of reflux and noncardiac chest pain
- Typical histopathologic changes are epithelial erosion, ulceration, and inflammation; severe disease can cause severe epithelial injury; mild disease can cause thickening of the basal zone and lengthening of the papillae
- Typical symptoms frequently occur in the absence of endoscopic change (nonerosive reflux disease) or histologic change
- Repair of esophageal ulceration may result in strictures, scars, pseudodiverticula, or Barrett's esophagus
- Barrett's esophagus is the most severe histologic consequence of chronic gastroesophageal reflux disease (GERD) in which the normal esophageal epithelium is replaced by columnar epithelium; intestine goblet cells are the marker of an increased risk of adenocarcinoma

### KEY! DON'T MISS!
- Symptoms of ischemic heart disease are not infrequently confused with GERD
- Acute inferior myocardial infarction in particular may present with upper abdominal complaints

## BACKGROUND

### ICD9 CODE
- 530.81 Gastroesophageal reflux
- 530.11 Reflux with esophagitis
- 530.1 Esophagitis
- 530.2 Barrett's syndrome or ulcer (chronic peptic ulcer of esophagus)
- 787.1 Heartburn

### SYNONYMS
- Peptic esophagitis
- Reflux esophagitis
- GERD
- GORD (gastro-oesophageal reflux disease)
- Hiatus hernia is incorrectly used as a synonym; hiatal hernia is an independent structural abnormality that is an important risk factor for severe acid reflux. However, hiatal hernias often occur without acid reflux and gastroesophageal reflux disease (GERD) occurs in the absence of hiatal hernias

### CARDINAL FEATURES
- Reflux of gastric contents into the esophagus causing symptoms and/or inflammatory change in the esophageal epithelium
- Reflux occurs from: transient relaxation of the lower esophageal sphincter (LES) or reduced LES pressure allowing spontaneous reflux (free reflux); or reflux induced by increased abdominal pressure (stress reflux)
- There are two predominant forms of reflux that differ with respect to pathophysiology, clinical presentation, natural history, and response to therapy: a severe form due to impaired resting LES and gastroesophageal barrier function; and a mild form due to transient, inappropriate relaxation of the LES
- Gastroesophageal reflux episodes of short duration commonly occur several times a day in normal subjects but do not constitute GERD
- GERD with esophageal changes demonstrated on endoscopy is known as endoscopy-positive (or erosive) GERD; disease with no demonstrable esophageal changes is known as endoscopy-negative (or nonerosive) GERD
- Typical symptoms are heartburn, acid regurgitation, and dysphagia
- Important atypical features are upper airway-induced symptoms and noncardiac chest pain
- Typical histopathologic changes of endoscopy-positive GERD are epithelial erosion, ulceration, and inflammation; severe disease can cause severe epithelial injury or even mucosal destruction (erosive esophagitis); mild disease can cause thickening of the basal zone and lengthening of the papillae
- Esophageal pathology and severity of symptoms do not always correlate well: many patients with symptoms of GERD have either no or only very minor histopathologic changes, and not all patients with histopathologic changes of GERD have symptoms
- Healing of esophageal ulceration may result in strictures, scars, pseudodiverticula, or Barrett's esophagus
- Barrett's esophagus is the most severe histologic consequence of chronic GERD in which the normal esophageal epithelium is replaced by columnar epithelium; the presence of intestinal goblet cells imparts an increased risk of adenocarcinoma

### CAUSES
#### Common causes
GERD results from a combination of factors. However, there are two predominant forms of reflux:
- Impaired resting LES and gastroesophageal barrier function resulting in the more severe or

'classic' form of gastroesophageal reflux
- Transient, inappropriate relaxation of the LES resulting in the milder and more common form

Other factors:
- Decreased clearance of acid from the esophagus due to decreased peristalsis or salivary secretion
- Reduced resistance of esophageal mucosa to gastric contents (increased 'sensitivity' of the esophagus to reflux)
- Delayed gastric emptying
- Although there is some controversy regarding whether increased acid secretion is an important predictor of severe acid reflux, it is clear that gastric acid and peptic activity are critical factors for reflux disease. Profound inhibition of acid secretion heals almost all cases of acid hypersecretion. Furthermore, there is no controversy that in defined hypersecretory states, such as gastrinoma, acid reflux is a common problem until acid secretion is adequately inhibited

### Contributory or predisposing factors
- Hiatal hernia is an important risk factor for severe reflux. Displacement of the LES from the diaphragm removes the diaphragmatic support for the gastroesophageal barrier and intra-abdominal segment of the esophagus. If the LES is already weak, the result is severe reflux. A hiatal hernia can also pool gastric acid, which can then be easily refluxed into the esophagus
- Pregnancy: GERD results from the effects of progesterone, which tends to reduce LES pressure; increased abdominal pressure probably also plays a role
- Diabetes mellitus type 1 or type 2: diabetic gastroparesis can predispose to GERD because of retarded emptying of gastric contents
- Connective tissue disorders (especially scleroderma, but also rheumatic disorders, Sjögren's syndrome, and mixed connective tissue disease). Sicca syndrome, with reduced salivary secretion, is also associated with acid reflux
- Obesity (often observed clinically, although systematic data are lacking)
- Foods and drinks that lower LES or have an irritant effect on the esophagus (chocolate, caffeine, alcohol, peppermint; exact list differs for each patient)
- Drugs, including nonsteroidal anti-inflammatory drugs, opioids, anticholinergic agents, and drugs with anticholinergic activity, e.g. tricyclic antidepressants

## EPIDEMIOLOGY
### Incidence and prevalence
- Epidemiologic data vary according to definitions and diagnostic methods used for GERD; most epidemiologic figures are based on estimates
- Very common and many people with symptoms do not bring themselves to medical attention

FREQUENCY
- Up to 60% of adults report having heartburn at some time, with perhaps 7% having it daily and 20% weekly; about 10% of those with frequent heartburn would probably be found to have endoscopy-positive GERD if they were tested
- Up to 80% of pregnant women report having heartburn
- Up to 20% of adults use antacids or over-the-counter histamine $H_2$ receptor antagonists at least once a week

### Demographics
AGE
All ages are affected, but older people are probably more likely to consult a primary care physician about symptoms.

## GENDER

- Men and women are equally commonly affected
- Men are two to three times more commonly affected by esophagitis and 10 times more commonly affected by Barrett's esophagus

# DIAGNOSIS

## DIFFERENTIAL DIAGNOSIS
Because gastroesophageal reflux disease (GERD) is common, as are many of its differential diagnoses, acid reflux frequently accompanies other disorders.

### Infectious esophagitis
- Usually associated with immunosuppression due to disease or steroid medication
- Common infecting agents are cytomegalovirus, herpes virus, *Candida albicans*, and HIV
- HIV, diabetes mellitus, and transplantation can predispose to infectious esophagitis

FEATURES
- Odynophagia is usually a prominent symptom (mild odynophagia occurs with an irritable esophagus sometimes associated with GERD; sudden, severe odynophagia is rare in GERD)
- Endoscopic appearance is of a diffuse esophagitis, with the proximal esophagus involved more often than in GERD
- Candidal esophagitis usually causes a white, cheesy exudate visible on endoscopy

### Pill-induced esophagitis
May be associated with: nonsteroidal anti-inflammatory drugs (NSAIDs), tetracyclines, potassium supplements, quinidine, corticosteroids, and alendronate.

FEATURES
- History includes use of a medication that can cause esophagitis, and patients often report swallowing pills with little water or while recumbent
- Odynophagia is prominent
- Endoscopic appearance is of deep, isolated ulcerations, typically at points of stasis, especially near the arch of the aorta. Distal esophagus is less involved

### Peptic ulcer disease
Includes gastric and duodenal ulcers. GERD often accompanies peptic ulcer disease, especially if there is hypersecretion of gastric acid.

FEATURES
- Abdominal pain, often described as 'gnawing' and usually midepigastric, is typically the main feature
- Classically, food relieves pain of a duodenal ulcer but may aggravate symptoms of gastric ulcer, although neither pattern is specific or sensitive
- Epigastric tenderness is sometimes present, but is a nonspecific finding
- Symptoms are not usually aggravated by lying down or bending over (unlike symptoms of GERD)

### Esophageal carcinoma
FEATURES
- Progressive dysphagia (starting with solid foods and progressing to soft foods and then liquids), often of relatively recent onset
- Weight loss, usually rapid
- Cervical lymphadenopathy may be present
- Gastrointestinal bleeding, which may be massive
- Secondary spread in advanced disease

### Biliary tract disease
Biliary tract disease is commonly due to calculi impacted in the cystic duct or biliary tree.

FEATURES
- Right upper quadrant pain
- Nausea and vomiting often present
- Jaundice, if common bile duct is blocked
- Abnormal liver function tests, especially if common bile duct is blocked, or transiently with biliary colic from a stone impacted in the cystic duct

### Ischemic heart disease
- Chest pain caused by ischemic heart disease can be easily confused with GERD, especially if patient has a history of heartburn. Generally, a change in features provides a clue as to the etiology
- Inferior myocardial infarction in particular may present with pain centered in the upper abdomen

FEATURES
- History and physical examination may suggest that ischemic heart disease is present (e.g. risk factors, chest pain induced by exercise, other features such as dyspnea, tachycardia), although none of these features rules out GERD
- Reflux is usually a problem that people have intermittently over decades, whereas cardiac disease has a time-limited presentation. New or changing symptoms deserve attention
- ECG and exercise stress test likely to show signs of cardiac ischemia

### Noncardiac chest pain
- Substernal discomfort or pain in the absence of demonstrated cardiac disease
- Diagnosis cannot be made until a cardiac etiology has been ruled out
- Increasing evidence points to a functional disorder with an irritable or sensitive esophagus as an underlying factor

FEATURES
- Angina-like, substernal chest pain
- Odynophagia is common
- Esophageal spasm can be associated, but manometry and barium studies show unco-ordinated, diffuse esophageal spasm to be inconsistently present and causality remains controversial
- Often associated with acid reflux, but lower esophageal sphincter (LES) pressure and endoscopy are often normal

## SIGNS & SYMPTOMS
### Signs
- Physical examination is usually normal
- Signs of anemia may be present if patient has an iron-deficiency anemia caused by blood loss as a result of esophageal ulcerations or erosions
- Pharyngitis and dental decay
- Halitosis

### Symptoms
Common:
- Heartburn (pyrosis) is reported by most patients; it often (but not always) occurs after meals, may be aggravated by bending over or lying down, and is often relieved by antacids. Importantly, heartburn may occur only after meals and not at night (upright reflux due to transient relaxation of the LES)
- Acid regurgitation (regurgitation of gastric contents into mouth)

Other gastrointestinal symptoms:
- Indigestion and dyspepsia
- Sour taste in mouth
- Epigastric pain
- Early satiety, abdominal fullness, and bloating
- Belching
- Globus (lump in throat)
- Hypersalivation ('water brash')
- Odynophagia (pain on swallowing food)
- Nausea
- Bad breath (halitosis)
- Gastrointestinal bleeding

Other symptoms:
- Wheezing
- Nocturnal cough
- Nocturnal choking or aspiration of gastroesophageal contents
- Hoarseness
- Noncardiac chest pain
- Enamel erosion

## KEY! DON'T MISS!
- Symptoms of ischemic heart disease are not infrequently confused with GERD
- Acute inferior myocardial infarction in particular may present with upper abdominal complaints

## CONSIDER CONSULT
- Refer patients who have gastrointestinal bleeding, dysphagia, or odynophagia
- Refer patients with chest pain of uncertain etiology who need to have cardiac disease firmly excluded

## INVESTIGATION OF THE PATIENT
### Direct questions to patient

Q Do you have heartburn, acid regurgitation, or difficulty in swallowing (either when eating or not)? These are the most common symptoms of GERD. Investigative tests may be warranted in patients with difficulty in swallowing

Q Do you have any other symptoms related to eating or swallowing? Patients with GERD may complain of indigestion, dyspepsia, a sour taste in the mouth or frank regurgitation of gastric contents into the mouth, a globus sensation, painful swallowing of food, nausea, epigastric pain, early satiety, abdominal fullness or bloating, and belching. Investigative tests are indicated in patients with persistent swallowing symptoms

Q When do your symptoms occur? Are they made worse by bending over or lying down? Are they worse at night? Symptoms are often aggravated by bending over or lying down

Q Are your symptoms related to meals or eating in any way? Symptoms are often worst after meals. Importantly, symptoms may occur only after meals (upright reflux)

Q Does anything relieve your symptoms? Do you take antacids or other medications for the symptoms? Most patients with symptoms of GERD use over-the-counter (OTC) antacids or histamine $H_2$ receptor antagonists, either regularly or from time to time

Q How long have you had your symptoms? Have they become worse recently? Have you been treated for these sorts of symptoms before and, if so, when? New onset of symptoms (especially in someone over the age of 45–50 years), worsening of symptoms, frequent recurrence of symptoms, or lack of response to treatment may warrant investigative tests

Q Have you lost weight recently? Weight loss related to GERD may warrant investigative tests

Q Have you been vomiting recently? Recurrent, unexplained vomiting warrants investigative tests

- **Q** What medications do you take? Pill-induced esophagitis may be due to the use of NSAIDs, tetracycline, potassium supplements, quinidine, corticosteroids, and alendronate
- **Q** Do you wheeze or have asthma, especially at night? Do you have a cough, especially at night? Do you ever wake up at night with a feeling of choking? Asthma, nocturnal cough, and nocturnal choking sometimes occur in patients with GERD
- **Q** Do you ever get chest pain? GERD can cause noncardiac chest pain, but chest pain of cardiac origin needs to be excluded
- **Q** Are you ever hoarse? Hoarseness and laryngitis may occur
- **Q** How are your teeth? Have you or your dentist noticed problems? Chronic GERD can cause erosion of tooth enamel

## Contributory or predisposing factors
- **Q** Are you pregnant? Pregnancy is the most common predisposing factor; up to 80% of pregnant women report having heartburn
- **Q** Do you have diabetes? Gastroparesis resulting from diabetes mellitus type 1 or type 2 can predispose to GERD because of retarded emptying of gastric contents
- **Q** Do you find that your hands are sensitive to cold? Do you have joint pains or arthritis? Connective tissue disorders (especially scleroderma, but also rheumatic disorders, Sjögren's syndrome, and mixed connective tissue disease) are often associated with GERD
- **Q** Do you find that alcohol or some foods cause your symptoms? Alcohol and some foods lower the LES pressure or have an irritant effect on the esophagus; chocolate, caffeine, alcohol, peppermint, and spicy foods very commonly exacerbate symptoms, although list differs for each patient
- **Q** Have you gained weight recently? Patients who are clinically obese are more likely to suffer from reflux

## Examination
In most cases, GERD causes no abnormalities that can be detected on routine physical examination. Signs that should be looked for include:
- Iron-deficiency anemia, e.g. pallor of skin or conjunctivae. These may be present if patient has significant, long-term blood loss as a result of esophageal ulcerations or erosions; if confirmed by a blood count, anemia related to GERD warrants investigative tests
- Pharyngitis
- Halitosis

## Summary of investigative tests
- For patients with typical symptoms, simple treatment measures can often be instituted without the need for investigative tests
- Patients in whom testing is warranted include those: over the age of 45–50 years with new onset of symptoms; with long-term (>5 years) or frequently recurring symptoms; with symptoms unresponsive to treatment; with 'alarm' symptoms – weight loss, recurrent vomiting, evidence of gastrointestinal bleeding or anemia, dysphagia, or odynophagia
- Most investigative tests for GERD require referral

Specific tests:
- Upper gastrointestinal endoscopy (or esophagoscopy) is a standard test to evaluate chest and abdominal symptoms of presumed gastrointestinal etiology. Although it can diagnose esophagitis and peptic ulcer disease, it cannot exclude acid reflux, since majority of cases are 'endoscopy-negative'
- Endoscopic biopsies can be taken if indicated for suspected Barrett's esophagus and gastric lesions
- Esophageal barium radiography studies may be better than endoscopy at showing an esophageal ring or stricture; otherwise endoscopy is the preferred investigation

- Esophageal manometry and ambulatory 24h pH monitoring is indicated for persistent atypical symptoms. These investigations are required prior to antireflux surgery
- All these tests are either invasive or relatively difficult to perform, and a proton pump inhibitor (PPI; omeprazole, lansoprazole, rabeprazole, pantoprazole, or esomeprazole) can be given as an empirical acid-suppression test; often useful in symptomatic patients with normal endoscopy findings

Other tests:
- All patients undergoing investigative tests for GERD should have a blood count to look for iron-deficiency anemia, which may result from esophageal bleeding
- Patients over the age of 45–50 years and any patients with features suggestive of ischemic heart disease should have an ECG and other cardiac tests, as appropriate; acute inferior myocardial infarction sometimes presents with only upper abdominal complaints

## DIAGNOSTIC DECISION
- Most cases of GERD in primary care can be diagnosed on the basis of clinical history. Diagnosis can generally be made with reasonable certainty if patient complains of heartburn and regurgitation of gastric contents. Relief of symptoms with acid inhibition provides strong supporting evidence for the diagnosis of GERD
- Diagnosis is more difficult when symptoms are less clear-cut, especially when patient complains of chest pain that is not typical heartburn. After cardiac disease has been excluded, relief by acid inhibitors supports the diagnosis of reflux
- It is important to distinguish the two predominant patterns of reflux as this has important implications for management
- Severe reflux due to impaired resting LES pressure and gastroesophageal barrier function: reflux occurs spontaneously when lying down (free reflux), bending over or otherwise increasing abdominal pressure (stress reflux), as well as after meals. Night-time reflux is often predominant, relentless and longstanding, and particularly concerning because episodes are usually prolonged due to the absence of gravity and peristalsis
- Mild reflux due to transient, inappropriate relaxation of the LES: relaxation of the LES is a vagal nerve reflex that occurs with a full stomach and in an upright posture, but is suppressed at night and with an empty stomach. This is 'reflex-reflux'. Often the resting LES is normal so that night-time reflux is not a problem. Symptoms of this form of reflux often occur after meals and not at night; in its relatively pure form, this can be referred to as 'upright' reflux
- If upright reflux is the predominant pattern and night-time reflux is minimal, erosive esophagitis is unlikely and there is a low risk of Barrett's esophagus. Endoscopy is generally not warranted. In contrast, if the patient has chronic night-time reflux symptoms, there is a higher risk of underlying esophagitis
- A proton pump inhibitor trial is appropriate in patients with upper airway symptoms that may be due to acid reflux or noncardiac chest pain
- Patients with symptoms suggestive of more severe disease or a more serious disorder ('alarm' features: weight loss, recurrent vomiting, evidence of gastrointestinal bleeding or anemia, dysphagia, or odynophagia) should be investigated further

### Guidelines
- The American College of Gastroenterology. ACG treatment guideline: Updated guidelines for the diagnosis and treatment of gastroesophageal reflux disease [1]

## CLINICAL PEARLS
- Esophageal disorders present across the full spectrum of visceral sensation. At the hypersensitive end are disabling symptoms in the absence of esophagitis or even an abnormal degree of acid reflux, and at the low sensitivity end is complicated esophagitis in the absence of typical heartburn. Although the symptom pattern can be useful in determining how to

approach GERD, even with nonerosive GERD, the severity of symptoms is highly variable among individuals
- Majority of patients with typical symptoms of GERD do not have macroscopic or microscopic esophagitis. In nonerosive GERD, the level of acid reflux that provokes symptoms is often in the normal range and symptomatic improvement with acid inhibition provides the evidence, albeit indirect, that reflux is the cause. The most plausible explanation for this is that patients with reflux symptoms have become sensitized to perceived acid present in their esophagus

## THE TESTS
### Body fluids
BLOOD COUNT
*Description*
Venous blood sample.

*Advantages/Disadvantages*
Advantages:
- Simple, readily available test
- Diagnoses anemia
- Provides baseline measurement

Disadvantage: nonspecific.

*Normal*
- Hemoglobin: men 13.6–17.7g/dL (136–177g/L); women 12.0–15.0g/dL (120–150g/L)
- Hematocrit: men 39–49%; women 33–43%
- Mean corpuscular volume (MCV): 76–100mcm$^3$ (76–100fL)

*Abnormal*
- Values outside the normal ranges
- Hemoglobin reduced in iron-deficiency anemia; hematocrit and MCV may also be reduced
- Keep in mind the possibility of a false-positive result

*Cause of abnormal result*
Iron-deficiency anemia caused by esophageal bleeding in GERD.

### Biopsy
ESOPHAGEAL BIOPSY TAKEN DURING ENDOSCOPY
*Description*
- Biopsies of the lesions and mucosa are taken for pathology analysis during endoscopy
- Main value is to exclude Barrett's esophagus. Sensitivity for detecting acid reflux in absence of erosive esophagitis is sufficiently low as to not justify biopsy as a diagnostic tool for routine reflux

*Advantages/Disadvantages*
Advantages:
- Easy to perform in context of an endoscopy
- Provides definitive histologic diagnosis of abnormalities of the esophageal mucosa
- Can confirm presence of metaplasia (as in Barrett's esophagus), dysplasia, or frank neoplasia
- Can diagnose infective esophagitis

Disadvantages:
- Invasive procedure
- Biopsy specimen may miss abnormalities, especially if disease is discrete and widely spaced
- Costs are considerable and add to costs of endoscopy alone

*Abnormal*
Histopathologic changes in esophageal mucosa:
- In mild disease, thickening of basal zone and lengthening of papillae
- In moderate disease, epithelial erosion, ulceration, and inflammation
- In severe disease, epithelial injury or destruction

In Barrett's esophagus:
- Normal esophageal epithelium is replaced by metaplastic, columnar, intestine-like epithelium
- Cytology most commonly shows villi of columnar epithelium with goblet cells that stain positive with period acid-Schiff stain and Alcian blue stain. Goblet cells, which impart risk of adenocarcinoma, must be present for diagnosis of Barrett's
- Cytology features may be redolent of gastric, small intestinal, large intestinal, or colonic epithelium; a mixture of these may occur
- Barrett's epithelium may be contiguous or separated by areas of other epithelium

## Imaging
ESOPHAGEAL BARIUM RADIOGRAPHY STUDIES
*Description*
X-rays of esophagus with barium as a contrast medium.

*Advantages/Disadvantages*
Advantages:
- Sensitive test for detection of esophageal rings and strictures
- Relatively noninvasive compared with endoscopy
- When used with a bolus, such as a barium-soaked marshmallow, test can be quite helpful for evaluating dysphagia, even when endoscopy is negative

Disadvantages:
- Uses ionizing radiation
- Cannot usually detect esophagitis or Barrett's esophagus
- Does not enable biopsies to be taken
- Normal study does not usually rule out need for endoscopy, whereas a normal endoscopy result usually means that barium studies are not required (except possibly for unexplained dysphagia)
- Physiologic reflux is often demonstrated, which does not always correlate with symptoms

*Abnormal*
- Esophageal stricture
- Grossly abnormal esophageal mucosa

## Special tests
ESOPHAGEAL MANOMETRY STUDIES
*Description*
Indicated for:
- Persistence of symptoms while on antireflux therapy
- Investigation of atypical symptoms
- Prior to antireflux surgery

*Advantages/Disadvantages*
Advantages:
- Allows assessment of lower esophageal sphincter function
- Defines function of lower esophageal body (peristalsis)
- Diagnoses peristalsis abnormalities

Disadvantages:
- Invasive
- Specialized test
- Expensive
- Sometimes hard to interpret

*Abnormal*
Peristalsis wave formation abnormal.

## AMBULATORY 24H PH MONITORING
*Description*
Indicated for:
- Persistence of symptoms while on antireflux therapy
- Investigation of atypical symptoms
- Prior to antireflux surgery

*Advantages/Disadvantages*
Advantages:
- Criterion standard for diagnosis of GERD
- Quantifies GERD
- Correlates GERD clinical features and episodes of reflux

Disadvantages:
- Invasive
- Specialized test
- Expensive
- Requires correct positioning of probe for 24h pH monitoring and instructing patient about continuing normal activities. Variability can be quite high when repeat tests are done
- Not needed if clinical history or endoscopy confirms GERD
- Frequently overlaps with normal, especially in nonerosive disease. This is not a test to exclude acid reflux

*Abnormal*
Excessive reflux with low pH recording.

## Other tests
ECG
*Advantages/Disadvantages*
Advantages:
- Simple test that can easily be performed in the office
- Results available immediately
- May establish presence of ischemic heart disease
- ECG taken during a symptomatic episode may show transient ischemic changes if ischemic heart disease is the cause

Disadvantage: normal or abnormal result does not rule out GERD or ischemic disease as a cause for symptoms.

*Abnormal*
- Signs of ischemia
- ECG taken during a symptomatic episode may show transient ischemic changes such as T-wave inversion or ST-segment depression
- Keep in mind the possibility of a falsely abnormal result

*Cause of abnormal result*
Ischemic heart disease.

## UPPER GASTROINTESTINAL ENDOSCOPY
*Description*
Indications:
- Patients with symptoms that suggest severe GERD or a more serious disorder (weight loss, recurrent vomiting, evidence of gastrointestinal bleeding or anemia, dysphagia, or odynophagia)
- Screen for Barrett's esophagus

*Advantages/Disadvantages*
Advantages:
- Best test to establish details of esophageal mucosa; can establish presence or absence of esophagitis, Barrett's esophagus, and cancer
- Can diagnose some of the most common and significant complications of GERD, including Barrett's esophagus and esophageal stricture
- Enables biopsies to be taken

Disadvantages:
- Invasive procedure
- Presence of a normal esophageal mucosa does not rule out GERD, since reflux can cause symptoms in patients whose esophagus is 'sensitive' to acid in the absence of mucosal changes

*Normal*
Light, flesh-colored mucosa without ulceration, with transition point from squamous esophageal to gastric mucosa (squamocolumnar junction or z-line) at the gastroesophageal junction, marked by the upper extent of the gastric folds.

*Abnormal*
- Esophagitis: erosions and ulceration with or without hemorrhage in distal esophagus
- Barrett's esophagus: proximal displacement of squamocolumnar junction above the gastroesophageal junction
- Neoplasia: friable mass, nodule, or stricture arising from esophageal mucosa
- Bacterial or fungal esophagitis: diffuse exudative lesions throughout esophagus

*Cause of abnormal result*
Damage to esophageal epithelium by refluxed, acidic gastric content.

## ACID-SUPPRESSION TEST
*Description*
Empirical trial of a PPI (omeprazole, lansoprazole, rabeprazole, pantoprazole, or esomeprazole) given at a therapeutic dose for 1–2 weeks.

*Advantages/Disadvantages*
Advantages:
- Noninvasive assessment that is simple to perform and very acceptable to patients
- A randomized trial has shown that symptomatic relief from omeprazole has a sensitivity similar to that of esophageal pH monitoring in diagnosing GERD
- Positive result also provides symptomatic relief
- Predicts therapeutic response to PPIs
- Useful in patients with symptoms of GERD in whom endoscopy has not revealed esophageal abnormalities

Disadvantages:
- Symptomatic relief does not preclude presence of Barrett's esophagus, erosive esophagitis, or esophageal or other gastrointestinal malignancy
- May also treat pain secondary to gastric ulcer
- May also represent placebo effect

# TREATMENT

## CONSIDER CONSULT
- Refer patients with long-standing reflux symptoms (>5 years) in whom it is appropriate to exclude Barrett's esophagus
- Refer patients whose symptoms and signs suggest gastric malignancy, stricture, or erosive esophagitis
- Refer patients whose symptoms are unexplained

## PATIENT AND CAREGIVER ISSUES
### Patient or caregiver request
**Q Is it possible that my symptoms are due to cancer or heart disease?** Patients may need to be reassured that the diagnosis of gastroesophageal reflux disease (GERD) does not indicate that they have cancer, heart disease, or another feared condition

**Q Will I have to take medication or modify my lifestyle forever?** Some patients may want to know whether the condition can be 'cured' or whether recurrence is likely

**Q Should I make any changes to my diet?** Foods such as chocolate, peppermints, tomatoes, onions, and others decrease lower esophageal sphincter (LES) pressure, and may lead to more reflux. Avoiding trigger foods may decrease frequency and/or severity of reflux episodes. However, no foods are absolutely contraindicated in reflux patients. There is also no need to exclude foods that do not cause symptoms, except if part of a weight-loss diet

### Health-seeking behavior
**Q Have you been using any over-the-counter (OTC) treatments? If so, how often and for how long?** Many patients with GERD who present to their primary care physician have tried OTC antacids or histamine $H_2$ receptor antagonists; if they have not, these may be worth trying if symptoms are mild; if they have, it is important to know if these treatments have become less effective

**Q Have you tried doing anything else to relieve your symptoms?** Some patients may have tried lifestyle modifications that they have read or heard about or that they have discovered for themselves; if so, it is worth knowing if these have had any benefit; if not, it is worth discussing them with the patient

## MANAGEMENT ISSUES
### Goals
- To provide symptomatic relief
- To prevent complications

### Management in special circumstances
SPECIAL PATIENT GROUPS
Pregnancy: use of pharmacologic treatment should generally be kept to a minimum; $H_2$ receptor antagonists are the medication of choice.

## SUMMARY OF THERAPEUTIC OPTIONS
### Choices
- Simple OTC antacids are often adequate for patients with occasional, mild symptoms; however, most patients will have tried these and more aggressive therapy is often required
- Lifestyle modifications (including raising the head of the bed, avoiding foods that can aggravate GERD, large meals or eating just before lying down, stopping smoking, avoiding tight clothing, and losing weight) are helpful for many patients and should always be recommended if appropriate
- $H_2$ receptor antagonists (cimetidine, ranitidine, nizatidine, and famotidine) bring symptomatic relief to most patients (up to 85%) by reducing gastric acid secretion

- Proton pump inhibitors (PPIs; omeprazole, lansoprazole, rabeprazole, pantoprazole, or esomeprazole) also act by reducing gastric acid secretion; they are more effective than $H_2$ receptor antagonists, and are particularly valuable for severe disease
- Occasional patients with demonstrated night-time gastroesophageal acid reflux may benefit from an $H_2$ receptor antagonist at bedtime in addition to a PPI in the morning
- Surgery to correct gastroesophageal reflux is usually reserved for patients with severe symptoms, symptoms that are refractory to treatment or complications such as Barrett's esophagus, esophageal bleeding, or aspiration
- Although there is some debate in the literature, there is no proof that either surgical or medical therapy prevents the development of Barrett's esophagus or reduces the low, but finite, risk of developing high-grade dysplasia or adenocarcinoma. Therefore, the only guideline that is universally accepted for treating Barrett's esophagus is to control symptoms with appropriate medical therapy or surgery

### Guidelines
- The American College of Gastroenterology. ACG treatment guideline: updated guidelines for the diagnosis and treatment of gastroesophageal reflux disease [1]
- Society of American Gastrointestinal Endoscopic Surgeons. Guideline for surgical treatment of gastroesophageal reflux disease (GERD) [2]

## Clinical pearls
- If a PPI is taken while $H_2$ receptor antagonists are active (a period lasting 6-8h), this will, by inhibiting the acid-secreting parietal cells, attenuate the effects of the PPI. However, some evidence indicates that in patients who have failed to respond fully to a standard, once-daily dose of PPI, adding a night-time $H_2$ receptor antagonist can help control night-time secretion and effectively complement a PPI taken in the morning at a lower cost than taking a second PPI. The key point is to avoid simultaneously taking a PPI and an $H_2$ receptor antagonist
- Tolerance can develop to $H_2$ receptor antagonist inhibition in as short as 7 days of therapy. This may explain the poor clinical response to them in some patients. Tolerance does not appear to develop with PPIs, which is probably one reason for their added effectiveness
- Rebound acid hypersecretion has been observed following cessation of one or more months of $H_2$ receptor antagonist or PPI therapy. This may underlie exacerbation of acid peptic diseases and prompts caution regarding the abrupt discontinuation of long-term antisecretory therapy in patients at risk for complications or recurrence. After prolonged therapy with the most potent agents, therapy should be tapered down slowly

## FOLLOW UP
- Patients with typical symptoms of GERD in whom there is no reason for investigative tests do not usually need to be followed up unless symptoms persist on therapy or change in nature. Generally, they will be seen once if their symptoms respond to a PPI and an endoscopy is not indicated
- When erosive esophagitis is found at endoscopy, Barrett's is hard to evaluate and biopsies difficult to interpret for dysplasia. Therefore, patients with moderate or severe erosive change should be re-endoscoped when healed after taking a PPI for 8 weeks. Barrett's esophagus without dysplasia should be followed up with endoscopy in 2–3 years, although optimal management for Barrett's is highly controversial

## Plan for review
- Patients with mild and occasional symptoms can usually be reviewed only if treatment fails to relieve symptoms
- Patients with more significant symptoms should be reviewed at the end of their course of treatment

- Erosive esophagitis should be re-endoscoped after 8 weeks of PPI therapy to exclude Barrett's esophagus
- Barrett's esophagus should be followed up with periodic endoscopy; the optimal interval remains to be established

## DRUGS AND OTHER THERAPIES: DETAILS
### Drugs
OTC ANTACIDS
- Numerous OTC antacid preparations are available, in tablet and liquid form; liquid preparations tend to be the more effective
- Most antacids contain aluminum and/or magnesium compounds as their active ingredient; calcium and bismuth compounds are found in some
- Sodium bicarbonate dissolved in water (up to one teaspoon in a glass of water) is also often effective

*Dose*
- Aluminum hydroxide suspension: two teaspoonfuls followed by a sip of water if desired, five or six times daily, between meals and on retiring
- Aluminum hydroxide tablets: two tablets of the 0.3g strength, or one tablet of the 0.6g strength, five or six times daily between meals and on retiring
- Aluminum hydroxide with magnesium hydroxide preparations available as oral suspension: two to four teaspoonfuls, four times per day, or as directed by physician
- Calcium carbonate chewable tablets: regular strength, chew two to four tablets as symptoms occur; maximum strength, chew one to two tablets as symptoms occur

*Efficacy*
- Provide effective relief from symptoms of GERD
- Less effective than either $H_2$ receptor antagonists or PPIs
- Not effective for healing esophagitis

*Risks/benefits*
Risks:
- Long-term or frequent use may mask symptoms of GERD that would benefit from more appropriate treatment
- May mask symptoms of a complication (e.g. Barrett's esophagus) or a more serious disorder (e.g. peptic ulcer or esophageal carcinoma). However, long-term, sustained use of antacids in itself is indicative of more severe reflux disease and warrants endoscopy to detect Barrett's esophagus in appropriate patients
- Overdosing of these products may produce milk-alkali syndrome. Treatment of symptoms is not treatment of condition; these drugs do not treat the underlying disorder. Symptomatic relief does not preclude malignancy
- Prolonged use of aluminum-containing antacids in patients with renal failure may worsen dialysis osteomalacia

Benefits:
- Available OTC and so useful for patients with only occasional, mild symptoms
- Relatively inexpensive

*Side effects and adverse reactions*
- Aluminum can cause constipation
- Magnesium can have a laxative effect
- Sodium bicarbonate can interfere with acid-base balance if used in excess or in patients at risk for salt retention

- Bismuth can be neurotoxic if absorbed; it can also cause constipation
- Calcium can cause rebound acid secretion, and prolonged use can induce hypercalcemia and alkalosis

*Interactions (other drugs)*
- **Prescription drugs (may react with prescription drugs)** - Magnesium-containing antacids may reduce effects of $H_2$ receptor antagonists

*Contraindications*
**None listed.**

*Acceptability to patient*
Generally high.

*Follow up plan*
Patients should be told to return if they need to use antacids frequently or for long periods.

*Patient and caregiver information*
Avoid taking antacids at the same time as other medications, especially enteric-coated tablets.

CIMETIDINE
$H_2$ receptor antagonist that inhibits action of histamine on the parietal cells of the stomach and so reduces gastric acid secretion.

*Dose*
1600mg/day in two or four divided doses for 12 weeks.

*Efficacy*
- Effective at inhibiting gastric acid secretion, but much less effective than PPIs
- Occasional patients with demonstrated GERD at night-time may benefit from taking an $H_2$ receptor antagonist at bedtime, in addition to a PPI in the morning

*Risks/benefits*
Risks:
- Drug interactions are greater with $H_2$ receptor antagonists than with other forms of treatment for peptic ulcer disease. Patients may have limited choices due to concomitant drug issues
- Symptomatic response does not preclude possible gastric malignancy
- Rare instances of cardiac arrhythmias and hypotension have been reported following the rapid administration of cimetidine HCl injection by intravenous bolus

Benefits:
- Inhibits gastric acid production and provides relief for many patients
- Generally less expensive than PPIs and available OTC
- Can be used in GERD in pregnancy

*Side effects and adverse reactions*
- Central nervous system: headache, mental state abnormalities (lethargy, confusion, depression, hallucinations)
- Genitourinary: antiandrogenic properties may be possible with cimetidine use, causing reversible impotence and gynecomastia
- Hematologic: rare hematologic toxicity (thrombocytopenia, leukopenia)
- Other: hepatitis

*Interactions (other drugs)*
- Cimetidine interacts with theophylline, warfarin, phenytoin, lidocaine via inhibition of cytochrome P450 isozymes, leading to reduced drug clearance. Avoid use of cimetidine with interacting drugs
- Ranitidine and famotidine have rarely been associated with increased theophylline levels
- Avoid magnesium-containing antacids while taking $H_2$ receptor antagonists

*Contraindications*
- If patients have known renal insufficiency (glomerular filtration rate <30mL/min), $H_2$ receptor antagonist use should be discouraged
- Therapy cannot be recommended for pediatric patients under 16
- Pregnancy category B
- Breast-feeding

*Evidence*
- A systematic review found that $H_2$ antagonists are more likely to relieve heartburn than placebo in patients with endoscopy-negative reflux disease [3] *Level M*
- The systematic review also compared PPIs with $H_2$ antagonists. PPIs are more effective than $H_2$ antagonists in the empirical treatment of typical GERD symptoms, but the difference was not significant for heartburn remission [3] *Level M*
- A systematic review found that $H_2$ antagonists achieved faster healing rates than placebo in patients with erosive esophagitis, however they were not as effective as PPIs (Note: results were pooled across treatment arms, so that the benefits of randomization were lost) [4] *Level M*

*Acceptability to patient*
Generally good.

*Follow up plan*
Review in 6–8 weeks to gauge effectiveness of treatment.

*Patient and caregiver information*
Smoking reduces the effectiveness of cimetidine.

## RANITIDINE, NIZATIDINE, FAMOTIDINE
$H_2$ receptor antagonists that inhibit the action of histamine in the parietal cells of the stomach and so reduce secretion of gastric acid.

*Dose*
- Rantidine: 150mg or 10mL (two teaspoonfuls equivalent to 150mg of ranitidine) twice daily
- Nizatidine: 150mg twice daily
- Famotidine: 20mg twice daily for up to 6 weeks. The recommended oral dosage for the treatment of adult patients with esophagitis including erosions and ulcerations and accompanying symptoms due to GERD is 20 or 40mg twice daily for up to 12 weeks

*Efficacy*
- Effective at inhibiting both nocturnal and daytime gastric acid secretion, but much less effective than PPIs
- Occasional patients with demonstrated gastroesophageal acid reflux at night-time may benefit from a $H_2$ receptor antagonist at bedtime in addition a PPI in the morning

*Risks/benefits*
Risks:
Ranitadine
- Use caution with renal and hepatic disease, gastric malignancy and immunocompromised patients

- Use caution in pregnancy and nursing mothers, and the elderly

Nizatidine
- Drug interactions are greater with $H_2$ receptor antagonists than with other forms of treatment for peptic ulcer disease. Patients may have limited choices due to concomitant drug issues
- Symptomatic response does not preclude possible gastric malignancy

Famotidine
- Drug interactions are greater with $H_2$ receptor antagonists than with other forms of treatment for peptic ulcer disease. Patients may have limited choices due to concomitant drug issues
- Symptomatic response does not preclude possible gastric malignancy

Benefits:
- Inhibit gastric acid production and provide relief for many patients
- Generally less expensive than PPIs and some preparations are available OTC
- Can be used in GERD in pregnancy

*Side effects and adverse reactions*
Generally safe; rarely cause thrombocytopenia (1:1000).

Ranitidine:
- Cardiovascular system: atrioventricular block, palpitations
- Central nervous system: dizziness, vertigo
- Gastrointestinal: abdominal pain, constipation, diarrhea, hepatitis, pancreatitis
- Hematologic: granulocytopenia, leukopenia, thrombocytopenia
- Musculoskeletal: arthralgia, myalgia
- Skin: alopecia, erythema multiforme, rash

Nizatidine:
- Central nervous system: headache, mental state abnormalities (lethargy, confusion, depression, hallucinations)
- Genitourinary: antiandrogenic properties may be possible with cimetidine use, causing reversible impotence and gynecomastia
- Hematologic: thrombocytopenia, leukopenia
- Other: hepatitis

Famotidine:
- Central nervous system: headache, dizziness, fever, asthenia
- Gastrointestinal: constipation, diarrhea
- Genitourinary: antiandrogenic properties may be possible with cimetidine use, causing reversible impotence and gynecomastia
- Hematologic: rare hematologic toxicity (thrombocytopenia, leukopenia)
- Other: hepatitis

*Interactions (other drugs)*
Avoid magnesium-containing antacids while taking $H_2$ receptor antagonists.

Ranitidine:
- Cephalosporins
- Calcium channel blockers
- Enoxacin
- Glipizide
- Ketoconazole

Nizatidine:
- No other interactions listed

Famotidine:
- Famotidine has rarely been associated with increased theophylline levels

*Contraindications*
Ranitidine:
- Known to have hypersensitivity to the drug ■ Pregnancy and breast-feeding

Nizatidine:
- If patients have known renal insufficiency (glomerular filtration rate <30mL/min), $H_2$ receptor antagonist use should be discouraged ■ Pregnancy and breast-feeding ■ Safety and eficacy in pediatric patients have not been established

Famotidine:
- If patients have known renal insufficiency (glomerular filtration rate <30mL/min), $H_2$ receptor antagonist use should be discouraged ■ Pregnancy category B ■ Breast-feeding ■ Safety and efficacy in children under one year have not been established

*Evidence*
- A systematic review found that $H_2$ antagonists are more likely to relieve heartburn than placebo in patients with endoscopy negative reflux disease [3] *Level M*
- The systematic review also compared PPIs with $H_2$ antagonists. PPIs are more effective than $H_2$ antagonists in the empirical treatment of typical GERD symptoms, but the difference was not significant for heartburn remission [3] *Level M*
- A randomized controlled trial (RCT) compared lansoprazole with ranitidine in patients with endoscopy negative reflux disease. Significantly lower heartburn scores were seen in patients treated with lansoprazole after 8 weeks of treatment [5] *Level P*
- A systematic review found that $H_2$ antagonists achieved faster healing rates than placebo in patients with erosive esophagitis, however they were not as effective as PPIs (Note: results were pooled across treatment arms, so that the benefits of randomization were lost) [4] *Level M*

*Acceptability to patient*
Generally good.

*Follow up plan*
Review in 6–8 weeks to gauge effectiveness of treatment.

## OMEPRAZOLE, LANSOPRAZOLE, PANTOPRAZOLE, RABEPRAZOLE, ESOMEPRAZOLE
PPIs act by irreversibly blocking the hydrogen-potassium adenosine triphosphatase enzyme system (proton pump) in the gastric parietal cells, thereby blocking the final step in the production of gastric acid; gastric acid secretion is therefore inhibited until additional enzyme can be synthesized.

*Dose*
PPIs need to be in the bloodstream at the time when the acid-secreting parietal cells are activated; therefore, best taken 30–60min before meals. Taking a PPI in a fasting state or at bedtime renders them less effective.

Acute dose:
- Omeprazole: 20mg once daily for 4–12 weeks
- Lansoprazole: 30mg once daily for 4–12 weeks
- Pantoprazole: 40mg once daily for 4–12 weeks
- Rabeprazole: 20mg once daily for 4–12 weeks
- Esomeprazole magenesium: 20mg once daily for 4–12 weeks

Maintenance dose:
- Omeprazole: 20mg once daily
- Lansoprazole: 15–30mg once daily
- Pantoprazole: 20–40mg once daily
- Rabeprazole: 20mg once daily
- Esomeprazole magnesium: 20mg once daily

*Efficacy*
- Most effective medical therapy available
- PPIs relieve symptoms, promote healing of esophagitis, and prevent recurrence
- Particularly useful in patients with severe disease
- PPIs fail in about 10% of patients; in some cases improvements simply require adjusting the time when PPIs are taken

*Risks/benefits*
Risks:
Omeprazole
- Use caution in the elderly and children
- Gastric malignancy may still be present even if symptoms lessen with treatment

Lansoprazole
- Symptomatic response to therapy with lansoprazole does not preclude the presence of gastric malignancy

Pantoprazole
- Symptomatic response to therapy with pantoprazole does not preclude the presence of gastric malignancy

Rabeprazole
- Symptomatic response to therapy with rabeprazole does not preclude the presence of gastric malignancy
- Use caution when administering to patients with hepatic impairment

Esomeprazole magnesium
- Symptomatic response to therapy with esomeprazole magnesium does not preclude the presence of gastric malignancy
- Atrophic gastritis has been noted occasionally in gastric corpus biopsies from patients treated long-term with omeprazole, of which esomeprazole magnesium is an enantiomer

Benefits:
- Provide rapid relief of symptoms
- Promote healing in esophagitis
- Prevent recurrence
- Can prevent recurrence of peptic strictures and reduce overall costs

*Side effects and adverse reactions*
Omeprazole:
- Central nervous system: headache, dizziness
- Gastrointestinal: nausea, vomiting, diarrhea, constipation, flatulence, abdominal pain, hepatitis, pancreatitis
- Genitourinary: interstitial nephritis, gynecomastia, urinary problems, urinary infections
- Hematologic: agranulocytosis, thrombocytopenia, anemia, neutropenia, and other blood cell disorders

- Hypersensitivity: angioedema, rashes, anaphylactoid reactions
- Skin: purpura, Stevens–Johnson syndrome, alopecia, erythema multiforme

Lansoprazole:
- Gastrointestinal: diarrhea due to antibiotics (may resolve by changing amoxicillin to tetracycline), nausea, vomiting
- Genitourinary: urinary retention
- Hematologic: agranulocytosis, aplastic anemia, hemolytic anemia, leukopenia, neutropenia, pancytopenia, thrombocytopenia, and thrombotic thrombocytopenic purpura
- Skin: Stevens–Johnson syndrome (rare)
- Other: pseudomembranous colitis (treat with vancomycin), anaphylaxis

Pantoprazole:
- Central nervous system: headache, asthenia, back pain, chest pain, neck pain, influenza syndrome, infection, pain, migraine, insomnia, anxiety, dizziness, hypertonia
- Gastrointestinal: diarrhea, flatulence, abdominal pain, eructation, constipation, dyspepsia, gastroenteritis, gastrointestinal disorder, nausea, rectal disorder, vomiting
- Metabolic: hyperglycemia, hyperlipemia
- Musculoskeletal: arthralgia
- Respiratory: bronchitis, cough increased, dyspnea, pharyngitis, rhinitis, sinusitis, upper respiratory tract infection
- Skin: rash

Rabeprazole:
- Cardiovascular system: hypertension, myocardial infarction, ECG abnormal, migraine, syncope, angina pectoris, bundle branch block, palpitation, sinus bradycardia, tachycardia
- Central nervous system: insomnia, anxiety, dizziness, depression, nervousness, somnolence, hypertonia, neuralgia, vertigo, convulsion, abnormal dreams, libido decreased, neuropathy, paresthesia, tremor, asthenia, fever, allergic reaction, chills, malaise, chest pain substernal, neck rigidity, photosensitivity reaction
- Eyes, ears, nose, and throat: cataract, amblyopia, glaucoma, dry eyes, abnormal vision, tinnitus, otitis media
- Gastrointestinal: diarrhea, nausea, abdominal pain, vomiting, dyspepsia, flatulence, constipation, dry mouth, eructation, gastroenteritis, rectal hemorrhage, melena, anorexia, cholelithiasis, mouth ulceration, stomatitis, dysphagia, gingivitis, cholecystitis, increased appetite, abnormal stools, colitis, esophagitis, glossitis, pancreatitis, proctitis
- Genitourinary: cystitis, urinary frequency, dysmenorrhea, dysuria, kidney calculus, metrorrhagia, polyuria
- Hematologic: anemia, ecchymosis, lymphadenopathy, hypochromic anemia
- Musculoskeletal: myalgia, arthritis, leg cramps, bone pain, arthrosis, bursitis
- Respiratory: dyspnea, asthma, epistaxis, laryngitis, hiccup, hyperventilation
- Skin: rash, pruritus, sweating, urticaria, alopecia

Esomeprazole magnesium:
- Central nervous system: headache
- Gastrointestinal: diarrhea, nausea, flatulence, abdominal pain, constipation, dry mouth

*Interactions (other drugs)*
Omeprazole:
- Calcium channel antagonists (nifedipine, nimodipine, nisoldipine, nitrendipine)
- Carbamazepine ■ Cefpodoxime, cefuroxime ■ Clarithromycin ■ Diazepam ■ Digoxin
- Enoxacin ■ Glipizide, glyburide ■ Itraconazole, ketoconazole ■ Methotrexate ■ Phenytoin
- Sucralfate ■ Tacrolimus ■ Tolbutamide ■ Warfarin

Lansoprazole:
- Sulcralfate
- Lansoprazole may interfere with the absorption of drugs where gastric pH is an important determinant of bioavailability (e.g. ketoconazole, ampicillin esters, iron salts, digoxin)

Pantoprazole:
- Digoxin
- Itraconzaole
- Ketoconazole

Rabeprazole:
- Digoxin
- Itraconzaole
- Ketoconazole

Esomeprazole magnesium:
- Diazepam
- Drugs where gastric pH is an important determinant of bioavailability (e.g. ketoconazole, iron salts, and digoxin)

*Contraindications*
Omeprazole:
- Pregnancy and breast-feeding
- Gastric carcinoma
- Hepatic impairment

Lansoprazole:
- Pregnancy and breast-feeding
- Gastric carcinoma
- Hepatic impairment
- Safety and efficacy in pediatric patients have not been established

Pantoprazole:
- Pregnancy and breast-feeding
- Gastric carcinoma
- Hepatic impairment
- Safety and efficacy in pediatric patients have not been established

Rabeprazole:
- Pregnancy and breast-feeding
- Rabeprazole is contraindicated in patients with known hypersensitivity to rabeprazole, substituted benzimidazoles, or to any component of the formulation
- Safety and efficacy in pediatric patients have not been established

Esomeprazole magnesium:
- Known hypersensitivity to any component of the formulation or to substituted benzimidazoles
- Pregnancy category B
- Breast-feeding
- Safety and efficacy in pediatric patients have not been established

*Evidence*
There is evidence that PPIs are effective in the treatment of nonerosive esophagitis (endoscopy negative reflux disease).
- A systematic review found that PPIs were significantly more effective than placebo for the treatment of heartburn in patients with endoscopy-negative reflux disease [3] *Level M*
- The systematic review also compared PPIs with $H_2$ antagonists. PPIs are more effective than $H_2$ antagonists in the empirical treatment of typical GERD symptoms, but the difference was not significant for heartburn remission [3] *Level M*
- A RCT compared lansoprazole with ranitidine in patients with endoscopy-negative reflux disease. Significantly lower heartburn scores were seen in patients treated with lansoprazole after 8 weeks of treatment [5] *Level P*
- Omeprazole was found to be significantly more effective than ranitidine for the maintenance of remission after one year in a RCT [6] *Level P*

There is evidence that PPIs are effective for the treatment of erosive esophagitis.
- A systematic review found that treatment of erosive esophagitis with PPIs produced a faster

healing rate than placebo. PPIs were also superior to $H_2$ antagonists after 12 weeks of treatment (Note: results were pooled across treatment arms, so that the benefits of randomization were lost) [4] *Level M*
- A RCT compared omeprazole with placebo for the prevention of relapse in patients with erosive esophagitis. Omeprazole achieved significantly higher remission rates at one year [7] *Level P*
- Lansoprazole has also been shown to be more effective than placebo for the prevention of relapse in a RCT [8] *Level P*
- Two RCTs compared omeprazole with ranitidine in the management of people with endoscopically confirmed esophagitis, who had already received omeprazole for 4 weeks. Relapses were significantly less likely in patients taking daily omeprazole at one year [9,10] *Level P*
- A RCT compared intermittent, symptomatic treatment with ranitidine or omeprazole over one year. Moderate control of symptoms was achieved with both medications, and no significant difference was found between the groups in terms of long-term relapse rates. Symptom control was achieved more rapidly with omeprazole [11] *Level P*

*Acceptability to patient*
Generally very good.

*Follow up plan*
- At 6–8 weeks to ensure response to therapy
- Consider increasing dose to twice a day and performing endoscopy if reflux symptoms persist
- May also consider switching from one PPI to another. Metabolism differs among the drugs, so some variation in response does occur

*Patient and caregiver information*
- Medication should be taken 30–60min before meals; treatment at bedtime is less effective
- Capsule should be swallowed whole
- Medication can be given long-term

### Surgical therapy
SURGERY TO CORRECT GASTROESOPHAGEAL REFLUX
Surgical procedures include:
- Fundoplication: indicated for patients with: symptoms refractory to PPI treatment that has been confirmed by 24h pH testing and esophageal manometry; and possibly for complicated GERD, including Barrett's esophagus or nonhealing erosive esophagitis. The valve created by the stomach's fundus is folded around the esophagus at the LES; operation reduces risk of a hiatal hernia by narrowing the esophageal hiatus. Laparoscopic fundoplication is superceding the open procedure. It is performed under general endotracheal anesthesia and takes around 3h; there is an inpatient stay of 2 days
- All patients require preoperative 24h pH monitoring and esophageal manometry to confirm moderate-to-severe reflux and exclude achalasia and severely impaired peristalsis
- Return of the esophagogastric junction to below the diaphragm
- Crural tightening

*Efficacy*
- Often provides symptomatic relief in patients with complicated GERD (e.g. Barrett's esophagus, erosive esophagitis, esophageal stricture, esophageal ulceration) or with extraesophageal manifestations (e.g. hoarseness, aspiration)
- Fundoplication is not curative for all GERD. Many patients will have GERD symptoms requiring PPI therapy even after fundoplication. Patients who failed to respond to PPI therapy before surgery are probably the ones most at risk for failure with surgery
- >90% of patients have complete resolution of symptoms within 6 weeks. However, long-term

benefits remain controversial; number who remain symptom-free and off other therapy over time has not been firmly established
- The success of antireflux surgery depends upon the expertise of the operator, especially with laparoscopic fundoplication
- Patients with poor esophageal motility prior to surgery are at increased risk for dysphagia after surgery. Experienced surgeons claim that this problem can be reduced by adjusting the pressure of the wrap

*Risks/benefits*
Risks:
- Usual risks of anesthesia and surgery
- Less likely to be effective and more likely to be complicated in older patients
- May cause problems with belching and gastric emptying, which can produce a persistent feeling of bloating
- Repairs may break down after 5 years or so; benefits of reoperation are controversial and reoperation should be done only by the most experienced surgeons
- Impact on progression of GERD to Barrett's esophagus is controversial

Benefits:
- Useful in patients who fail to respond to medical therapy and lifestyle changes
- Reduces risk of aspiration of gastric acid
- Can be used for patients with complications of GERD (e.g. Barrett's esophagus, esophageal stricture or bleeding, aspiration), though it has not been definitively proven to heal Barrett's esophagus
- Can be used for patients with extraesophageal symptoms of GERD (e.g. hoarseness, asthma, aspiration)
- Laparoscopic fundoplication has more rapid recovery than conventional surgery; overall risks may be less, but only in the hands of the most experienced laproscopic surgeons

*Evidence*
- A RCT compared medical and surgical management in patients with complicated GERD (erosive esophagitis, Barrett's esophagus, stricture, esophageal ulcer). Continuous medical treatment (with antacids, ranitidine, metoclopramide, or sucralfate), symptomatic treatment, and open fundoplication were compared. Significantly improved symptom scores and degree of esophagitis were achieved in patients treated with fundoplication [12] *Level P*
- Preliminary data from a RCT suggest that omeprazole may have similar efficacy to fundoplication for patients with erosive esophagitis at 3-year follow-up [13] *Level P*

*Acceptability to patient*
Generally good given that patients who come to surgery usually have severe disease or disease that is refractory or recurrent.

*Follow up plan*
Usual postoperative follow up, and check for:
- 'Gas-bloat' syndrome: 10–15% develop bloating after meals due to their inability to belch. Advice concerning eating small meals and avoiding sodas will help. Fundal wrap at the LES may need loosening if problem persists
- Refractory reflux symptoms may require further investigations including esophageal manometry to check function of the fundoplication. A PPI can be prescribed to reduce these symptoms. A revision fundoplication is rarely required, but needs to be approached with caution since results of reoperation are generally not as good as the first operation
- Regular endoscopic follow up as fundoplication has not been proven to prevent progression of Barrett's esophagus, or development of dysplasia or carcinoma

## LIFESTYLE

Lifestyle modifications should always be tried and are potentially helpful for mild and severe GERD if adapted to the specific patient:
- Raising the head of the bed: can be helpful for patients with night-time symptoms or erosive or complicated esophagitis but not daytime upright reflux
- Avoiding foods that may precipitate attacks (e.g. chocolate, caffeine, peppermint, spices, onions); list needs to be individualized for each patient
- Avoiding or reducing alcohol intake
- Losing weight if obese
- Stopping smoking (or cutting down)
- Avoiding large meals or lying down within 3h or so of a meal
- Avoiding clothing that is tight or constrictive around the abdomen or lower chest

RISKS/BENEFITS
Benefits:
- May lessen or stop symptoms
- Several of these lifestyle modifications promote healthier living in their own right

ACCEPTABILITY TO PATIENT
Patients may be resistant to some of these lifestyle modifications (especially weight loss and smoking reduction).

# OUTCOMES

## EFFICACY OF THERAPIES
- Most patients respond well to lifestyle modifications and pharmacologic therapy
- Proton pump inhibitors (PPIs) are generally more effective than $H_2$ receptor antagonists at relieving symptoms, preventing recurrence, and promoting healing in endoscopy-positive gastroesophageal reflux disease (GERD), and both are more effective than placebo
- Surgery (fundoplication) often provides symptomatic relief in patients with complicated GERD (e.g. Barrett's esophagus, erosive esophagitis, esophageal stricture, esophageal ulceration) or with extraesophageal manifestations (e.g. hoarseness, aspiration)

### Evidence
#### Nonerosive esophagitis (endoscopy negative reflux disease)
- A systematic review found that $H_2$ antagonists and PPIs are more likely to relieve heartburn than placebo in patients with endoscopy-negative reflux disease [3] *Level M*
- PPIs are more effective than $H_2$ antagonists in the empirical treatment of typical GERD symptoms [3] *Level M*
- Omeprazole was found to be significantly more effective than ranitidine for the maintenance of remission after one year in a RCT [6] *Level P*

#### Erosive esophagitis
- A systematic review of indirect comparisons found that $H_2$ antagonists and PPIs achieved faster healing rates than placebo in patients with erosive esophagitis. PPIs were superior to $H_2$ antagonists after 12 weeks of treatment [4] *Level M*
- Omeprazole and lansoprazole have been shown to be more effective than placebo for the prevention of relapse [7,8] *Level P*
- Omeprazole (daily treatment) was found to be more effective than ranitidine for the prevention of relapses in people with endoscopically confirmed esophagitis [9,10] *Level P*
- Relapse rates were similar for omeprazole and ranitidine when used as intermittent, symptomatic treatment [11] *Level P*
- Fundoplication has been found to be more effective than antacids, ranitidine, metoclopramide, or sucralfate for the management of patients with complicated GERD (erosive esophagitis, Barrett's esophagus, stricture, esophageal ulcer). Significantly improved symptom scores and degree of esophagitis were achieved in patients treated with fundoplication [12] *Level P*
- Preliminary data from a randomized controlled trial suggests that omeprazole may have similar efficacy to fundoplication for patients with erosive esophagitis at 3-year follow-up [13] *Level P*

### Review period
6 months.

## PROGNOSIS
- GERD is generally a benign condition with little mortality, although moderate-to-severe disease can have a markedly deleterious effect on quality of life
- Prognosis depends on whether mild, largely nonerosive disease or severe, erosive disease is being treated. Symptoms in mild disease are frequently intermittent and respond well to on-demand therapy. In contrast, patients with severe erosive disease who require PPI therapy to heal will generally require this therapy indefinitely to prevent recurrences
- Reflux is generally not a progressive disease. Patients with an initial normal endoscopy usually have a normal follow up and patients with mild disease generally remain with mild symptoms

### Clinical pearls
- Term 'maintenance' therapy is often a misnomer for severe, erosive esophagitis. Patients who require aggressive therapy to heal often require full-dose therapy to maintain remission

- Severe, erosive esophagitis is difficult to heal and to keep healed. PPIs are generally indicated for both healing and maintenance therapy. In contrast, mild reflux without esophagitis improves or is nonprogressive in 95% of cases and can be treated symptomatically
- Psychosocial stressors are not commonly mentioned for reflux disease. However, reflux symptoms are often exacerbated by stressful life situations and get better when the situations resolve. Refractory symptoms are also commonly associated with psychosocial issues; when a patient fails to respond to therapy, a psychosocial evaluation should be considered
- In refractory patients where symptoms are not obviously explained by persisting acid reflux, other diagnoses should be explored
- In general, patients who are being considered for surgery should have an attempt to control their symptoms with aggressive medical therapy (twice or three times daily PPI); in patients who respond there is little question about the diagnosis. However, if patients refractory to high-dose PPI (taken appropriately twice daily 30min before breakfast and dinner), there is a lingering question regarding the diagnosis and it is critical to confirm that symptoms while on therapy are associated with persisting, uncontrolled acid reflux. Often, symptoms persist with acid reflux that is very well controlled. This is not the place to do surgery for acid reflux

### Therapeutic failure

Patients in whom lifestyle modifications and pharmacologic treatments fail require referral to a specialist for assessment, investigation of complications of GERD, and treatment as required, including surgery.

### Recurrence

- Suggest reinstatement of lifestyle modifications if these were effective and have been stopped. If these were not effective, analyze whether they were properly used
- Restart pharmacologic treatment if this has been stopped; some patients may respond better to a different treatment regimen
- Consider referral if recurrence is frequent, if it occurs rapidly after cessation of therapy, or if it occurs despite apparently adequate therapy

### Deterioration

Consider referral for evaluation and endoscopy, especially if deterioration has been preceded by a quiescent period or a period in which symptoms have been adequately controlled on pharmacologic treatment.

## COMPLICATIONS

- Barrett's esophagus (up to 20% of patients)
- Esophageal stricture (1–20%, depending on the series)
- Esophageal ulceration (about 5%)
- Esophageal bleeding (about 2%)
- Pulmonary and upper airway disorders, e.g. asthma, aspiration, chronic laryngitis, and chronic cough. A single exposure to acid is enough to cause marked irritation of the upper airway mucosa, which is much more sensitive to acid that the esophagus or stomach

## CONSIDER CONSULT

- Refer patients whose symptoms are unresponsive to treatment
- Refer patients whose symptoms are only partially responsive and require a PPI more than once daily for control
- Refer patients whose symptoms recur quickly when treatment is stopped
- Refer patients with complications

## PREVENTION

Not specifically preventable in the general population.

### SCREENING
Screening of the general population for gastroesophageal reflux disease (GERD) or Barrett's esophagus is not warranted.

#### UPPER GASTROINTESTINAL SURVEILLANCE ENDOSCOPY AND BIOPSY
- Patients who have had GERD for 5 years or more should probably be offered endoscopic screening for Barrett's esophagus with mucosal biopsy if they are willing and able to submit to surgery if severe dysplasia is found
- An initially normal endoscopy result remains normal in most patients, so repeat screening of these patients is not warranted, unless pattern of symptoms changes
- Patients who have an endoscopic diagnosis of Barrett's esophagus without dysplasia should have a surveillance endoscopy with mucosal biopsy every 2–3 years, although optimal interval remains to be established. Barrett's esophagus has columnar epithelium with intestinal metaplasia (goblet cells), which increases the risk of adenocarcinoma
- Patients with low-grade dysplastic changes in the esophageal mucosa require more frequent surveillance
- Patients with high-grade dysplastic changes in the esophageal mucosa should be closely followed up. Risk of development of adenocarcinoma is 15–60% in one year. These patients should be considered for surgery after the diagnosis has been confirmed by repeat endoscopy and review by an expert pathologist

*Cost/efficacy*
Screening patients with endoscopically proven Barrett's esophagus every 3 years was cost effective in retrospective clinical studies, although this conclusion is controversial.

### PREVENT RECURRENCE
- Lifestyle modifications need to be continued indefinitely in most patients
- Appropriate pharmacologic therapy can be used on-demand in patients with mild disease, whereas continual therapy is indicated for patients with severe, protracted symptoms, or a history of severe erosive or complicated disease

# RESOURCES

## ASSOCIATIONS

**American Gastroenterological Association**
7910 Woodmont Avenue, 7th Floor
Bethesda, MD 20814-3015
Tel: (301) 654-2055
Fax: (301) 652-3890
http://www.gastro.org

**Society of American Gastrointestinal Endoscopic Surgeons**
2716 Ocean Park Boulevard, Suite 3000
Santa Monica, CA 90405
Tel: (310) 314-2404
Fax: (310) 314-2585
http://www.sages.org

**American Society for Gastrointestinal Endoscopy**
13 Elm Street
Manchester, MA 01944-1314
Tel: (978) 526-8330
Fax: (978) 526-4018
http://www.asge.org

## KEY REFERENCES

- American Society for Gastrointestinal Endoscopy. The role of endoscopy in the management of GERD. Guidelines for clinical application. Gastrointest Endosc 1999;49:834–5
- Anonymous. Barrett's esophagus: an overrated cancer risk factor [editorial]. Gastroenterology 2000;119:587-9
- Anonymous. Evaluation of dyspepsia. Gastroenterology 1998;114:579–81 (Guidelines produced by the American Gastroenterological Assocation, available online at the National Guideline Clearinghouse)
- Anonymous. Guideline for surgical treatment of gastroesophageal reflux disease (GERD). Surg Endosc 1998;12:186–8 (Guidelines produced by the Society of American Gastrointestinal Endoscopic Surgeons, available online at the National Guideline Clearinghouse)
- Bardhan KD, Muller Lissner S, Bigard MA, et al. Symptomatic gastro-oesophageal reflux disease: double-blind controlled study of intermittent treatment with omeprazole or ranitidine. Br Med J 1999;318:502–7
- Bate CM, Green JR, Axon AT, et al. Omeprazole is more effective than cimetidine for the relief of all grades of gastro-oesophageal reflux disease-associated heartburn, irrespective of the presence or absence of endoscopic oesophagitis. Aliment Pharmacol Ther 1997;11:755–63
- Chiba N, Hunt RH. Gastroesophageal reflux disease. In: McDonald JWD, Burroughs AK, Feagen BG, eds. Evidence based gastroenterology and hepatology. London: BMJ Books, 1999, p16–65
- Fass R, Ofman JJ, Sampliner RE, et al. The omeprazole test is as sensitive as 24-h oesophageal pH monitoring in diagnosing gastro-oesophageal reflux disease in symptomatic patients with erosive oesophagitis. Aliment Pharmacol Ther 2000;14:389–96
- Jones R. Management of gastroesophageal reflux disease: the primary care stragegy. Yale J Biol Med 1999;72:203–9
- Kahrilas PJ. Gastroesophageal reflux disease and its complications. In: Feldman M, Scharschmidt BF, Sleisenger MH, eds. Sleisenger and Fortran's gastrointestinal and liver disease, 6th edn. Philadelphia, PA: WB Saunders, 1998, p498–517
- Maton PN, Orland R, Joelsson B. Efficacy of omeprazole versus ranitidine for symptomatic treatment of poorly responsive acid reflux disease: a prospective, controlled trial. Aliment Pharmacol Ther 1999;13:819–26
- Moayyedi P, Delaney B, Katzka D, Forman D. Gastroesophageal reflux disease. In: Barton S, ed. Clinical evidence. London: BMJ Publishing Group; 2001, p311–23
- Revicki DA, Sorenson S, Maton PN, Orland RC. Health-related quality of life outcomes of omeprazole versus ranitidine in poorly responsive symptomatic gastroesophageal reflux disease. Digest Dis 1998;16:284–91

- Richter JE. Extraesophageal manifestations of gastroesophageal reflux disease. Clin Perspect 1998;1:28–39
- Richter JE, Peura D, Benjamin SB, et al. Efficacy of omeprazole for the treatment of symptomatic acid reflux disease without esophagitis. Arch Intern Med 2000;160:1810–16. Reviewed in: Clinical Evidence 2001;6:351–63
- Richter JM. Approach to the patient with heartburn and reflux (gastroesophageal reflux disease). In: Gorroll AH, Mulley AG Jr, eds. Primary care medicine: office evaluation and management of the adult patient, 4th edn. Philadelphia, PA: Lippincott Williams and Wilkins; 2000, p395–9
- Rusch VWS, Levine DS, Haggitt R, Reid BJ. The management of high grade dysplasia and early cancer in Barrett's esophagus. Cancer 1994;74:1225–9
- Sampliner RE. Heartburn. In: Greene HL, Johnson WP, Maricic MJ, eds. Decision making in medicine, 2nd edn. St Louis, MO: Mosby, 1998
- Soll AH, Fass R. Gastroesophageal reflux: practical management of a common, challenging disorder. Clin Cornerstone 1999;1:1–17
- Sonnenberg A, El-Serag HB. Clinical epidemiology and natural history of gastroesophageal reflux disease. Yale J Biol Med 1999;72:81–92
- van Pinxteren B, Numans ME, Bonis PA, Lau J. Short-term treatment with proton pump inhibitors, H2-receptor antagonists and prokinetics for gastro-oesophageal reflux disease-like symptoms and endoscopy negative reflux disease (Cochrane Review). In: The Cochrane Library, 3, 2001. Oxford: Update Software
- Schenk BE, Kuipers EJ, Klinkenberg-Knol EC, et al. Omeprazole as a diagnostic tool in gastroesophageal reflux disease. Am J Gastroenterol 1997;92:1959–60

### Evidence references and guidelines

1. The American College of Gastroenterology. ACG treatment guideline: updated guidelines for the diagnosis and treatment of gastroesophageal reflux disease. Am J Gastroenterol 1999;94:1434–42
2. Society of American Gastrointestinal Endoscopic Surgeons. Guideline for surgical treatment of gastroesophageal reflux disease (GERD). Surg Endosc 1998;12:186–8. Available at the National Guideline Clearinghouse
3. van Pinxteren B, Numans ME, Bonis PA, Lau J. Short-term treatment with proton pump inhibitors, H2-receptor antagonists and prokinetics for gastro-oesophageal reflux disease-like symptoms and endoscopy negative reflux disease (Cochrane Review). In: The Cochrane Library, 1, 2002. Oxford: Update Software
4. Chiba N, DeGara CJ, Wilkinson JM, Hunt RH. Speed of healing and symptom relief in grade II to IV gastroesophageal reflux disease: a meta-analysis. Gastroenterology 1997;112:1798–1810. Reviewed in: Clinical Evidence 2001;6:351–63
5. Richter JE, Campbell DR, Kahrilas PJ, et al. Lansoprazole compared with ranitidine for the treatment of nonerosive gastroesophageal reflux disease. Arch Intern Med 2000;160:1803–9. Reviewed in: Clinical Evidence 2001;6:351–63
6. Festen HPM, Shenk E, Tan G, et al. Omeprazole versus high-dose ranitidine in mild gastroesophageal reflux disease: short and long-term treatment. Am J Gastroenterol 1999;94:931–6. Reviewed in: Clinical Evidence 2001;6:351–63
7. Bate CM, Booth SN, Crowe JP, et al. Omeprazole 10mg or 20mg once daily in the prevention of recurrence of reflux esophagitis. Gut 1995;36:492–8. Reviewed in: Clinical Evidence 2001;6:351–63
8. Robinson M, Lanza F, Avner D, Haber M. Effective maintenance treatment of reflux esophagitis with low-dose lansoprazole: a randomized double blind placebo-controlled trial. Ann Intern Med 1996;124:859–67. Reviewed in: Clinical Evidence 2001;6:351–63
9. Dent J, Yeomans ND, Mackinnon M, et al. Omeprazole v ranitidine for prevention of relapse in reflux esophagitis: a controlled double blind trial of their efficacy and safety. Gut 1994;35:590–8. Reviewed in: Clinical Evidence 2001;6:351–63
10. Vigneri S, Termini R, Leandro G, et al. A comparison of five maintenance therapies for reflux esophagitis. N Engl J Med 1995;333:1106–10. Reviewed in: Clinical Evidence 2001;6:351–63
11. Bardhan KD, Muller-Lissner S, Bigard MA, et al. Symptomatic gastro-oesophageal reflux disease: double-blind controlled study of intermittent treatment with omeprazole or ranitidine. BMJ 1999;318:502–7. Reviewed in: Clinical Evidence 2001;6:351–63
12. Spechler SJ. Comparison of medical and surgical therapy for complicated gastroesophageal reflux disease in veterans. N Engl J Med 1992;326:786–92. Reviewed in: Clinical Evidence 2001;6:351–63
13. Lundell L, Dalenback J, Hattlebakk J, et al. Omeprazole or antireflux surgery in the long term management of gastroesophageal reflux disease: results of a multicenter, randomized clinical trial. Gastroenterology 1998;114:A207. Reviewed in: Clinical Evidence 2001;6:351–63

# FAQS

## Question 1
When should endoscopy be done early in the course of evaluating a patient with presumed reflux?

### ANSWER 1
To evaluate alarm features (e.g. dysphagia, anemia, blood in the stool, or weight loss) or to establish the diagnosis. If the diagnosis is clear, then treatment should be started without awaiting endoscopy. Often the response to treatment becomes an important piece of evidence confirming the diagnosis. If the patient has had long-standing, frequent reflux, especially with a prominent night-time pattern, and is a candidate for surgery, endoscopy is appropriate to exclude Barrett's. However, it is better to delay endoscopy until the patient has been on proton pump inhibitor (PPI) treatment for about 8 weeks so that any erosive changes can heal. At this point it will be possible to more confidently detect Barrett's endoscopically and, if present, to evaluate dysplasia in any regions of Barrett's mucosa.

## Question 2
When do you need to do endoscopy to assess the severity of cases or monitor therapy?

### ANSWER 2
A few years ago, experts advised doing endoscopy to identify patients with severe erosive disease because these patients would need more aggressive management. However, it is now clear that symptomatic responses usually are adequate to monitor therapy. If symptoms resolve, the esophagitis usually has also responded. If symptoms have not resolved, then therapy probably needs to be stepped up to see if control can be achieved. For patients who are refractory to treatment, endoscopy is necessary to exclude other diagnoses and determine if esophageal erosions are present. With the exception of an occasional complicated case, symptomatic responses (resolution of heartburn or acid regurgitation) are adequate endpoints to monitor therapy. If a patient responds well to $H_2$ receptor antagonists, then this is probably adequate therapy. If he/she does not respond, then patient should have an acid-suppression test with a PPI.

## Question 3
Should I start therapy with lifestyle measures and antacids or over-the-counter or prescription-dose $H_2$ receptor antagonists, or a PPI?

### ANSWER 3
It is always worth advising lifestyle measures; they never hurt and they can help some patients quite a bit. For other than mild cases, however, they are rarely sufficient. Regarding pharmacotherapy, there is heated debate as to which of two approaches to use: step-down (start with a PPI, and then reduce therapy to a $H_2$ receptor antagonist ) or step-up (start with a $H_2$ receptor antagonist and step up to PPI in patients who fail to respond). Rather than a firm rule, it makes sense to base this decision on the patient's presentation. With severe symptoms or evidence of severe underlying gastroesophageal reflux disease (GERD), or with known erosive esophagitis or a history of complications, start with a PPI. In fact, with very severe disease where a rapid response is desired, it is reasonable to start with a twice-daily PPI to rapidly control the symptoms, and then reduce to a single dose. This aggressive approach is only needed in about 10% of patients. Intermittent therapy works well in the majority of patients with milder disease and in this setting $H_2$ receptor antagonists perform quite well against PPIs. If such a patient fails to respond adequately, then switch to a PPI.

## Question 4
Is there still a role for a barium esophogram?

ANSWER 4
The esophogram is very useful when dealing with dysphagia as it can define the anatomy and show peristalsis. However, the test is not useful for the large majority of other cases with GERD.

## Question 5
Is there an association between GERD and *Helicobacter pylori*?

ANSWER 5
Current dogma is that there is no direct association, and there is no accepted role of testing or treating for *H. pylori* in GERD patients. However, there are several puzzling aspects. If patients with *H. pylori* are put on long-term antisecretory therapy, atrophic gastritis can progress and over several decades there is a theoretical risk of gastric cancer, although this is controversial. Another controversial aspect is the possibility that reflux may worsen after *H. pylori* is cured. This effect is explained by the reversal of *H. pylori*-induced atrophic gastritis, which can theoretically lower acid secretion. With the rebound in acid secretion, patients are at higher risk for GERD. An epidemiologic association is evident in developed countries: incidence of GERD and esophageal adenocarcinoma in particular have been rising in parallel with a fall in *H. pylori*. There are occasional patients with *H. pylori* who report GERD plus other dyspeptic symptoms (e.g. belching, bloating, upper abdominal pain). Appropriate management has not been established by controlled studies, but many gastrointestinal specialists will cure the *H. pylori*, especially if the patient fails to respond to PPI alone.

## CONTRIBUTORS
Kathleen M O'Hanlon, MD
Andrew H Soll, MD
Laura Targownik, MD, FRCP(C)

# HEMORRHOIDS

| | | |
|---|---|---|
| ■ | Summary Information | 230 |
| ■ | Background | 231 |
| ■ | Diagnosis | 233 |
| ■ | Treatment | 238 |
| ■ | Outcomes | 253 |
| ■ | Prevention | 255 |
| ■ | Resources | 256 |

## SUMMARY INFORMATION

### DESCRIPTION

- Hemorrhoids are responsible for most anorectal complaints
- Masses of dilated vascular tissue occur in and around the anus and rectum
- Internal hemorrhoids are located above the dentate line, are covered by mucosa, and do not have sensory innervations; external hemorrhoids are located below the dentate line, are covered by squamous epithelium, and are extremely sensitive
- Course may be acute, chronic, or relapsing
- Hemorrhoids are normal features of anatomy; the presence of hemorrhoids without accompanying symptoms (pain, pruritus, bleeding) does not necessitate treatment

### URGENT ACTION

- Internal hemorrhoids, usually Grade IV, can strangulate, leading to gangrene and creating a surgical emergency. Although much less common than external hemorrhoids, internal hemorrhoids also can develop thrombosis
- Hemorrhoids that prolapse out of anus and are irreducible (strangulated) also can constitute a surgical emergency

# BACKGROUND

## ICD9 CODE
455 Hemorrhoids

## SYNONYMS
Piles

## CARDINAL FEATURES
- Bright red bleeding/staining of toilet paper
- Perianal irritation
- Pain, itching, swelling, thrombosis
- Mucofecal staining of underclothes
- Prolapse
- Constipation (particularly hard stools and straining) is frequently present

## CAUSES
### Common causes
Hemorrhoidal bulging and distension into the lumen of the anal canal results from deterioration of connective tissue that supports hemorrhoids and occurs as a normal part of aging. Veins become distended as they lose support. Conditions that increase intra-abdominal pressure may accelerate deterioration of supporting connective tissue.

### Serious causes
Any cause of portal hypertension (i.e. cirrhosis) can worsen hemorrhoidal veins pressure.

### Contributory or predisposing factors
- Low fiber, high fat diets
- Constipation
- Diarrhea
- Straining during defecation – passing hard stools
- Pregnancy
- Childbirth – associated with thrombosed hemorrhoids
- Heavy lifting – associated with thrombosed hemorrhoids
- Prolonged sitting
- Malignancy of gastrointestinal tract
- Rectal surgery/episiotomy
- Chronic cough
- Anal intercourse

## EPIDEMIOLOGY
### Incidence and prevalence
INCIDENCE
Due to the chronic relapsing nature of hemorrhoids, data are usually expressed as prevalence rather than incidence

PREVALENCE
Estimated at 50% of adults

### Demographics
AGE
- More common with advancing age: peaks between 45–65 years of age
- Uncommon in infants: if present, look for underlying cause (venacaval or mesenteric obstruction, cirrhosis, portal hypertension)

## GENDER
Equal incidence between males and females.

## RACE
Increased frequency among Caucasians.

## GENETICS
May have a familial predisposition.

## GEOGRAPHY
Absent in African populations presumably because of high-residue diets.

## SOCIOECONOMIC STATUS
- Unclear
- Hemorrhoidal prevalence may be related to occupation rather than to social class
- Frequency of hemorrhoids is higher among rural dwellers than urban dwellers in the United States

# DIAGNOSIS

## DIFFERENTIAL DIAGNOSIS
### Anal fissure
FEATURES
- Linear tear in anal canal
- Extends from dentate line to anal verge
- Most common cause of painful defecation

### Skin tag
FEATURES
- Stretched, enlarged perianal skin, painless and does not itself bleed
- Occurs secondarily to a previous thrombosed external hemorrhoid
- May interfere with anal hygiene

### Anorectal abscess/fistula
FEATURES
- Anorectal abscess and fistula represent acute and chronic phases, respectively, of the same disease process
- Obstruction of anal gland, which discharges into anal crypt at dentate line, produces an infection
- Throbbing perianal pain: perianal drainage may be present

### Carcinoma
FEATURES
- Painless nodules or plaques
- Change in bowel habits
- Pruritus
- Mucoid drainage
- Pain – late in disease

### Proctalgia fugax
FEATURES
- Transient, severe rectal pain related to spasm of levator ani and coccygeal muscles
- Symptoms may last for 30min

### Proctitis
FEATURES
- Inflammatory disease of rectum
- Mucopurulent discharge
- Rectal bleeding
- Rectal pain and tenesmus
- May be ulcerative or infectious
- Infectious proctitis occurs primarily in homosexual males who engage in frequent anal intercourse with multiple partners

### Condyloma acuminata
FEATURES
- Sexually transmitted viral disease caused by human papillomavirus
- Lesions (anogenital warts) usually asymptomatic, but if infected may cause pain, odor, or bleeding

### Pruritus ani
**FEATURES**
- Intense anal itching
- Many causes: anorectal disease, fecal contamination, parasitic, bacterial, or venereal infections, dermatologic diseases, local irritants

### Rectal prolapse
**FEATURES**
- Protrusion of either mucosa or entire thickness of rectum; may protrude from anus by as much as 12cm
- Most common in women over the age of 40 years: laxity of pelvic musculature is typical cause

## SIGNS & SYMPTOMS
### Signs
- One or more tender, bluish, spherical masses present at anal verge; may range from a few millimeters to several centimeters in size
- Overlying skin is tense and edematous; sometimes skin is thin, ulcerated, and partially extruded
- Painless, perianal skin tags, secondary to previous thrombosed external hemorrhoids
- Incomplete defecation
- Internal hemorrhoids (examined via anoscopy) appear as pinkish-blue swellings of mucosa – may bleed when touched

### Symptoms
- Bright red bleeding onto toilet tissue – more common with internal hemorrhoids
- Anorectal pain – external hemorrhoids
- Painful lump at anus – external hemorrhoids
- Anorectal itching

## CONSIDER CONSULT
Prolapsed hemorrhoids that are irreducible should be referred to a colorectal surgeon.

## INVESTIGATION OF THE PATIENT
### Direct questions to patient
**Q** What symptoms are you experiencing? Pain and itching localized to anal area are indicative of acute external hemorrhoids. Painless bleeding associated with defecation may indicate internal hemorrhoids

**Q** When did you begin having anorectal symptoms? Hemorrhoidal symptoms may be acute, chronic, or relapsing. If patient presents within 72h of onset of acute symptoms, thrombosed hemorrhoids may be surgically excised

**Q** Are there any abdominal symptoms, weight loss, or accompanying change in bowel habits? If present, a colonoscopy may be necessary to rule out malignancy/inflammatory bowel diseases

**Q** Have you noticed any masses/nodules near the anus? Swellings may indicate prolapsed internal hemorrhoids; painless nodules or plaques may indicate neoplasms of perianal skin or anorectal tract

**Q** How is your diet? Low fiber, high fat diets are associated with a higher incidence of hemorrhoids

**Q** Do you frequently experience difficulty passing stools? Straining during defecation may contribute to hemorrhoidal development

**Q** Have you recently experienced constipation or diarrhea? Both constipation and diarrhea contribute to development of hemorrhoids

**Q** What is your occupation? Prolonged periods of sitting or standing contribute to development of hemorrhoids

- **Q** Women: Are you pregnant or have you had any children? Provides insight into recent trauma (episiotomy); pregnancy and childbirth contribute to development of hemorrhoids
- **Q** What medications have you tried? Assists in determining the severity of pain and evaluates previous treatment failures

### Contributory or predisposing factors
- **Q** Are you pregnant? Pregnancy predisposes to hemorrhoidal development
- **Q** Women: Have you had any children? Childbirth predisposes to hemorrhoidal development particularly if trauma (episiotomy) occurred

### Family history
Given a 50% population incidence, family history is not helpful.

### Examination
- Are tender bluish masses present upon visual inspection of peritoneal area? Hemorrhoids may prolapse or thrombose
- Are masses, tenderness, mucoid discharge, or blood noted on digital rectal examination? Internal hemorrhoids are often not palpable unless thrombosed
- Are internal hemorrhoids visible with anoscope? If not, consider fissures, abscesses, and obtain cultures
- Is malignancy or inflammatory bowel disease suspected? Consider performing sigmoidoscopy or referral for colonoscopy; sigmoidoscopy should be performed for all patients over 40 years presenting with new perianal bleeding

### Summary of investigative tests
- Complete blood count, specifically check hematocrit and rule out infection
- Internal hemorrhoids may be visualized via anoscopy

## DIAGNOSTIC DECISION
External hemorrhoids may be assessed via direct visual examination. Pain, incomplete defecation, constipation, excessive moisture, bleeding, and prolapsed masses are commonly found. Internal hemorrhoids frequently bleed but are not palpable unless thrombosed. Internal hemorrhoids may be visualized via anoscopy. Hemorrhoids are classified as first degree if they merely bleed (small in size); second degree if they prolapse under pressure but return spontaneously (medium in size); third degree when anal suspensory ligament has stretched such that permanent prolapse is present, but can be reduced manually (large in size); and fourth degree when prolapse is irreducible (large in size).

### Guidelines
The Society for Surgery of the Alimentary Tract has produced guidelines with diagnostic information. Surgical management of hemorrhoids. Patient Care Committee, 2000 [1]

## CLINICAL PEARLS
- Both hemorrhoids and lower gastrointestinal (GI) bleeding are very common. Because there are other causes of bleeding, especially neoplasia, it is essential to appropriately evaluate patients with bleeding hemorrhoids. Hemorrhoidal bleeding should be a diagnosis of exclusion arrived at after endoscopy to rule out neoplasia and other causes of bleeding. Flexible sigmoidoscopy and anoscopy in low-risk, young patients or colonoscopy in most other patients is the indicated strategy
- Hemorrhoidal bleeding is usually painless and associated with a bowel movement. Blood usually coats the stool at the end of defecation, drips into the bowl, or is found on the toilet paper. Bleeding associated with painful defecation is often due to an anorectal fissure
- Long-standing blood loss from hemorrhoids can lead to iron-deficiency anemia, but before this conclusion is reached other causes must be excluded

# THE TESTS
## Body fluids
### COMPLETE BLOOD COUNT
*Description*
Venous blood.

*Advantages/Disadvantages*
Advantages:
- Identify anemia, secondary to blood loss
- Assist in identifying infection, if present

Disadvantages: needle stick.

*Normal*
Hematocrit: male: 40.7–50.3% (SI: 0.407–0.503)
Hematocrit: female: 36.1–44.3% (SI: 0.361–0.443)
White blood cell count: 3800–9800/mcL (SI: 3.8–9.8x$10^9$/L)
Neutrophils: 1800–7500/mcL (SI: 1.8–7.5x$10^9$/L)
Lymphocytes: 900-4500/mcL (SI: 0.9–4.5x$10^9$/L)

*Abnormal*
- Low hematocrits may indicate significant blood loss
- Elevated white blood cell count may indicate presence of infection
- Neutrophils may be elevated in response to bacterial infections; lymphocytes are often elevated in viral infections
- Keep in mind the possibility of a false-positive result

*Cause of abnormal result*
- Blood loss (low hematocrit)
- Infection (elevated white blood cell counts)

*Drugs, disorders and other factors that may alter results*
- Low hematocrit: anemia, genitourinary bleeding, peptic ulcer disease
- Elevated hematocrit: dehydration, chronic obstructive pulmonary disease, smoking
- Decreased lymphocytes: steroids, AIDS, chemotherapy, aplastic anemia, adrenocortical hyperfunction, multiple sclerosis, myasthenia gravis
- Elevated lymphocytes: chronic lymphocytic leukemia, Hodgkin's disease, ulcerative colitis, hypoadrenalism
- Neutropenia: vitamin B12 deficiency, folic acid deficiency
- Neutrophilia: pregnancy, smoking, stress, exercise, inflammation, malignancy

## Imaging
### ANOSCOPY
*Advantages/Disadvantages*
Advantages:
- Convenient – no bowel preparation required
- Sedatives/analgesics rarely required
- Direct examination of lower rectal mucosa and anal canal
- Collection of microbiological specimens/cultures
- Biopsy of suspicious masses (caution and experience are necessary because of highly vascular structures in perianal region)
- Allows for hemorrhoidal treatment by coagulation, injection, or banding

Disadvantages:
- Procedure may cause pain, bleeding, bowel perforation
- Embarrassment/anxiety for patient
- Depth of visualization is approximately 10cm

*Normal*
Mucosa is pink with visible submucosal vessels

*Abnormal*
- Presence of blood, pus, masses, vesicles, inflammation
- Pinkish-blue swellings of mucosa; may bleed when touched
- Keep in mind the possibility of a false-positive result

*Cause of abnormal result*
Hematoma, carcinoma, polyps, fissures, infection, thrombosed hemorrhoids.

*Drugs, disorders and other factors that may alter results*
- Inflammatory bowel diseases
- Other anorectal diseases (polyps, fissures, infection, carcinoma)

# TREATMENT

## CONSIDER CONSULT
If pain/bleeding are present and hemorrhoids are absent, refer to gastroenterologist for colonoscopy. Even if hemorrhoids are present, they are common and bleeding could be coming from another source. Bleeding hemorrhoids are an excellent indication for 'screening' colonoscopy or at least a flexible sigmoidoscopy.

## IMMEDIATE ACTION
If presenting within 72h of onset, thrombosed external hemorrhoids can be excised.

## PATIENT AND CAREGIVER ISSUES
### Patient or caregiver request
- Q **Do hemorrhoids cause cancer?** Hemorrhoids do not cause cancer; however, both hemorrhoids and cancer can cause rectal bleeding
- Q **How can I get relief from the anorectal pain and irritation?** Hot sitz baths are recommended two to three times daily for one week. Ice packs may also provide some symptomatic relief
- Q **What treatments are available?** Topical anesthetic and steroid preparations may provide relief from pain and inflammation
- Q **Can hemorrhoids be removed?** External hemorrhoids may be excised within 72h of flare-up; symptomatic care is typically provided following 72h. Internal hemorrhoids are usually treated by various endoscopic procedures
- Q **What should I do to prevent hemorrhoids?** Good bowel habits, a high fiber diet with supplements of psyllium products (Konsyl, Metamucil, etc.), and possibly stool softeners

### Health-seeking behavior
- Q **When did symptoms begin?** Hemorrhoids may be excised within 72h of symptom onset; otherwise, treatment is typically symptomatic
- Q **What therapies have you tried?** Provides insight into severity of pain and previous treatment failures

## MANAGEMENT ISSUES
### Goals
- To provide symptomatic relief of pain, swelling, itching
- To prevent complications such as infection, chronic fissures, anemia
- To prevent further attacks

### Management in special circumstances
Endoscopic hemorrhoidal treatments should be considered for hemorrhoids that have failed to respond to bulk agents, suppositories, topical preparations, and sitz baths. However, endoscopic therapies are contraindicated in a variety of concomitant diseases.

### COEXISTING DISEASE
- Endoscopic hemorrhoidal treatment is contraindicated if the following are present: bleeding diathesis, inflammatory bowel disease, anorectal fissures/infections, AIDS or other immunodeficiency states, portal hypertension, rectal wall prolapse, anorectal tumors
- Avoid electrical endoscopic stimulation procedures in patients with pacemakers or defibrillators
- Extreme caution should be used when treating patients at high risk for bacterial endocarditis (previous history of bacterial endocarditis, rheumatic fever, or murmurs); antibiotic prophylaxis may be impractical since treated areas remain open and irritated for 2–3 weeks after endoscopic treatments

COEXISTING MEDICATION
Warfarin, heparin, aspirin, nonsteroidal anti-inflammatory drugs – some endoscopic hemorrhoidal therapies may increase the risk of bleeding.

SPECIAL PATIENT GROUPS
Endoscopic hemorrhoidal management is contraindicated in pregnancy and in the immediate postpartum period (8 weeks).

PATIENT SATISFACTION/LIFESTYLE PRIORITIES
Patients that must sit (e.g. truck drivers) or stand (e.g. pharmacists) for extended periods of time require prompt relief from pain to fulfill occupational responsibilities; sitz baths three times daily may not be feasible.

## SUMMARY OF THERAPEUTIC OPTIONS
### Choices
- Bulk forming agents – retain water, create softer stools for easier passage
- Docusate – stool softener for easier passage of stool
- Lidocaine ointment – local anesthetic
- Dibucaine – local anesthetic
- Benzocaine – local anesthetic
- Dyclonine – local anesthetic
- Pramoxine – local anesthetic
- Hydrocortisone – topical steroid to reduce inflammation
- Hydrocortisone/pramoxine – alleviates pain, itch, inflammation
- Witch hazel – astringent
- External hemorrhoid excision – for thrombosed external hemorrhoids
- Rubber band ligation – therapy of choice for internal hemorrhoids when pharmacologic methods fail, office procedure
- Infrared coagulation – painless office procedure, equipment needed
- Sclerotherapy – associated with more complications than other endoscopic therapies
- DC current – treatment for advanced grades of hemorrhoids
- Bipolar electrocoagulation – painless office procedure, equipment required
- Sitz baths
- High fiber diet

### Guidelines
- Guidelines are available from the Society for Surgery of the Alimentary Tract. Surgical management of hemorrhoids. Patient Care Committee, 2000 [1]
- The American Society of Colon and Rectal Surgeons has prepared treatment guidelines. Practice parameters for the treatment of hemorrhoids. Standards Task Force of the American Society of Colon and Rectal Surgeons; 1998–1999 [2]

## Clinical pearls
- A tender purple, elliptical mass extending from the anal verge is the presentation of thrombosed external hemorrhoid. Conservative therapy is acceptable for mild cases, but when the pain is severe or excruciating surgical excision is indicated
- Bowel habits and diet constitute the main predisposing factors for hemorrhoids. Changing the diet, adding psyllium or similar products and possibly stool softeners are often all that is needed
- The pruritus and irritation that occur with hemorrhoids usually respond well to analgesic creams, hydrocortisone, or warm sitz baths. Therapy should be limited to one week because of adverse effects, such as mucosal atrophy with topical steroids and contact dermatitis with analgesic creams

## FOLLOW UP
Depending upon the treatment utilized, the patient should be seen for a follow up in 1–4 weeks

### Plan for review
Evaluate healing of previously treated hemorrhoids and treat new groups of hemorrhoids if required.

### Information for patient or caregiver
- Keep the anal area clean, using water and gentle dabbing after bowel movements
- Keep the hemorrhoids and anus as dry as possible
- Eat a diet high in fiber to produce soft stools that are easy to pass
- Avoid straining during bowel movements. Use bulk-forming agents (Metamucil, Konsyl, etc.) and stool softeners to assure that stools are soft and straining is avoided. Shake these powders hard in cold juice and drink quickly to make them palatable
- Drink plenty of water to help stools stay soft; fiber alone will not do the job
- When thrombosis pain and tenderness occur, sit in hot bath for 10–20min, four times daily

## DRUGS AND OTHER THERAPIES: DETAILS
### Drugs
BULK-FORMING AGENTS
Psyllium (powder, wafer)
Polycarbophil (tablets)
Methylcellulose (powder)
Cellulose (powder)
Malt soup extract (tablets, powder, liquid)
(This is an off-label indication)

*Dose*
- Psyllium powder – 1–3 tbsp (approximately 3.4–10.0g) administered in 8–12oz of liquid up to four times daily
- Psyllium wafer – 1–2 wafers with 8oz of liquid up to three times daily
- Polycarbophil – 1g one to four times daily or as needed; not to exceed 4g/24h
- Methylcellulose – 1 heaping tbsp administered in 8oz of liquid one to three times daily
- Cellulose – 1 tbsp into 3–4oz of liquid or apple sauce up to three times daily
- Malt soup extract tablets – 12–36g/day, in four divided doses
- Malt soup extract powder – 32g twice daily for 3–4 days, then 16–32g at bedtime
- Malt soup extract liquid – 2 tbsp twice daily for 3–4 days, then 1–2 tbsp at bedtime

*Efficacy*
Retain water in stools, producing soft, bulky stools that are easier to pass with reduced need to strain. Provides some benefit if constipation contributes to hemorrhoids.

*Risks/benefits*
Risks:
- Obstruction has occurred in patients when administered without adequate fluid
- Psyllium – IgE-mediated allergies

Benefits:
- Soft stools facilitate easier passage with less need to strain
- Generally not absorbed; suitable for pregnant women
- Methylcellulose is generally the best tolerated with regard to flatulence

*Side effects and adverse reactions*
- Bloating and flatulence

- Abdominal cramping
- Diarrhea
- Esophageal/bowel obstruction

*Interactions (other drugs)*
No significant interactions recorded.

*Contraindications*
- Intestinal obstruction
- Fecal impaction

*Acceptability to patient*
Generally well tolerated, may cause increased flatus

*Follow up plan*
Re-examine hemorrhoids in 1–2 weeks if symptoms persist.

*Patient and caregiver information*
- Take with full glass of water
- Do not use in presence of abdominal pain, nausea, vomiting
- Avoid inhaling dust from powders
- Phenylketonuronics: sugar-free preparations may contain aspartame

METHYLCELLULOSE (POWDER)
This is an off-label indication.

*Dose*
2g (1 heaping tbsp) in 8oz of water one to three times daily.

*Efficacy*
Retains water in stool, producing soft, bulky stools, which are easier to pass and reduces the need to strain. Beneficial if constipation contributes to hemorrhoids.

*Risks/benefits*
Risks: obstruction has occurred when administered without adequate fluids.

Benefits:
- Soft stools facilitate easier passage with less need to strain
- Generally not absorbed; suitable for pregnant women

*Side effects and adverse reactions*
- Bloating and flatulence
- Abdominal cramping
- Diarrhea
- Esophageal/bowel obstruction

*Interactions (other drugs)*
No significant interactions recorded.

*Contraindications*
- Intestinal obstruction
- Fecal impaction

*Acceptability to patient*
Generally well tolerated.

*Follow up plan*
Re-examine hemorrhoids in 1–2 weeks if symptoms persist.

*Patient and caregiver information*
- Take with a full glass of water
- Do not use in presence of abdominal pain, nausea, vomiting
- Avoid inhaling dust from powders
- Phenylketouronics: sugar-free preparations contain aspartame

## DOCUSATE
Docusate sodium (dioctyl sodium sulfosuccinate)
Docusate calcium (dioctyl calcium sulfosuccinate)
(This is an off-label indication)

*Dose*
Docusate sodium – 50–300mg/day
Docusate calcium 240mg/day

*Efficacy*
Facilitates mixture of fats and water to soften stool. This allows for easier passage and minimizes straining. May be beneficial if constipation is present.

*Risks/benefits*
Risks:
- May cause throat irritation
- Prolonged use to be avoided – may cause elecrolyte disturbances

Benefit: facilitates easier stool passage, minimizes straining.

*Side effects and adverse reactions*
- Throat irritation
- Rash
- Diarrhea
- Electrolyte disturbances in prolonged use

*Interactions (other drugs)*
No signficant interactions reported.

*Contraindications*
- Obstruction
- Fecal impaction
- Nausea or vomiting
- Concomitant use of mineral oil

*Acceptability to patient*
Generally well tolerated.

*Follow up plan*
Re-examine hemorrhoids in 1–2 weeks if symptoms persist.

*Patient and caregiver information*
- Drink plenty of water while using this medication
- Do not use if vomiting, nausea, or abdominal pain is present

## LIDOCAINE OINTMENT
*Dose*
5% ointment applied to affected area as needed.

*Efficacy*
Local anesthetic that reduces hemorrhoidal pain and itching by preventing transmission of nerve impulses.

*Risks/benefits*
Risks:
- Accumulation with repeated administration may lead to significant systemic absorption through mucous membranes, increasing risk of systemic side effects
- Local irritation – burning, stinging
- Cardiovascular depression

Benefit: transient alleviation of hemorrhoidal pain.

*Side effects and adverse reactions*
- Hypersensitivity reactions
- Local irritation
- Central nervous system depression or excitation
- Cardiovascular depression

*Interactions (other drugs)*
**No signficant interactions reported.**

*Contraindications*
**Hypersensitivity to amide local anesthetics.**

*Acceptability to patient*
Generally well tolerated.

*Follow up plan*
Re-examine hemorrhoids in 1–2 weeks if symptoms persist.

*Patient and caregiver information*
- Apply topically to affected area
- Avoid contact with eyes
- Dermal analgesia may be accompanied by loss of all skin sensation in the treated area. Avoid inadvertent trauma by scratching, rubbing, or exposing to extreme hot or cold until complete sensation has returned

DIBUCAINE
Dibucaine ointment, cream (0.5–1.0%).

*Dose*
Apply topically four times daily as needed.

*Efficacy*
Topical anesthetic that alleviates itching and pain associated with hemorrhoids by preventing transmission of nerve impulses from sensory nerves.

*Risks/benefits*
Risk: may cause local irritation.

Benefits:
- Temporary alleviation of hemorrhoidal irritation
- Not as likely as lidocaine to accumulate and cause systemic effects

*Side effects and adverse reactions*
- Hypersensitivity reactions
- Local irritation

*Interactions (other drugs)*
**No significant interactions reported.**

*Contraindications*
**Hypersensitivity to amide anesthetics.**

*Acceptability to patient*
Generally well tolerated.

*Follow up plan*
Re-evaluate hemorrhoids in 1–2 weeks if symptoms persist.

*Patient and caregiver information*
- Apply topically to affected area
- Avoid contact with eyes

BENZOCAINE
Lotion – 6%
Cream – 6%
Aerosol/spray – 5–20%
Liquid – 20%
Gel – 15–20%
Ointment – 20%

*Dose*
Apply topically to affected area as needed.

*Efficacy*
Topical anesthetic that prevents initiation and transmission of nerve impulses to alleviate pain and itching associated with hemorrhoids.

*Risks/benefits*
- Risk: sensitization more common than with other topical anesthetics
- Benefit: rapid onset of anesthetic action – occurs within one minute

*Side effects and adverse reactions*
Local irritation – rash, erythema, edema, stinging, tenderness, urticaria.

*Interactions (other drugs)*
**No significant interactions reported.**

*Contraindications*
**Known hypersensivity.**

*Acceptability to patient*
Generally well tolerated.

*Follow up plan*
Re-evaluate hemorrhoids in 1–2 weeks if symptoms persist.

*Patient and caregiver information*
- Apply topically to affected area
- Avoid use in eyes
- Protect solution from heat and light; discard if brown in color or if precipitate is present

## DYCLONINE
Dyclonine solution (0.5–1.0%)

*Dose*
Apply topically to affected area as needed.

*Efficacy*
Local anesthetic that anesthetizes mucous membranes to relieve pain associated with anogenital lesions – blocks nerve endings in the skin and mucous membranes.

*Risks/benefits*
Benefit: alleviates pain quickly, in 2–10min.

*Side effects and adverse reactions*
- Cardiovascular depression
- Central nervous system excitation or depression
- Respiratory arrest in overdose

*Interactions (other drugs)*
**No significant interactions reported.**

*Acceptability to patient*
Generally well tolerated.

*Follow up plan*
Re-evaluate hemorrhoids in 1–2 weeks if symptoms persist

*Patient and caregiver information*
- Avoid too frequent application to prevent drug accumulation and systemic toxicities
- Drowsiness may be the first indication of toxicity

## PRAMOXINE
Pramoxine (gel, cream, lotion, spray – 1%)

*Dose*
Apply topically three to four times daily; some preparations may be used rectally following bowel movements.

*Efficacy*
Local anesthetic that blocks initiation and nerve impulse conduction to alleviate pain and itching associated with hemorrhoids.

*Risks/benefits*
- Risk: may cause local irritation
- Benefit: alleviates discomfort quickly within 2–5min with an extended duration of action

*Side effects and adverse reactions*
Local irritation – burning, rash, stinging.

*Interactions (other drugs)*
**No significant interactions reported.**

*Acceptability to patient*
Generally well tolerated.

*Follow up plan*
Re-evaluate hemorrhoids in 1–2 weeks if symptoms persist.

*Patient and caregiver information*
- Do not apply to unaffected areas
- Avoid contact with eyes
- Notify physician if condition worsens or fails to improve within 3–4 days

HYDROCORTISONE
Hydrocortisone (suppositories, cream, ointment)

*Dose*
25mg suppositories or 1–2.5% creams/ointments used rectally two to four times daily after bowel movements.

*Efficacy*
Provides symptomatic relief of itching and inflammation associated with anorectal dermatitis, which may accompany hemorrhoids.

*Risks/benefits*
Risks:
- May cause local irritation
- Therapy should be limited to one week

*Side effects and adverse reactions*
- Thin fragile skin, dermatitis, burning, dryness, secondary infections
- Therapy should be limited to one week.

*Interactions (other drugs)*
**No signficant interactions reported.**

*Contraindications*
**Systemic fungal infections.**

*Acceptability to patient*
Generally well tolerated.

*Follow up plan*
Re-evaluate hemorrhoids after one week if symptoms persist.

*Patient and caregiver information*
- Use following bowel movements, after washing and drying affected area
- If symptoms have not improved after 7 days or if bleeding, protrusion, or seepage occurs, notify your physician

HYDROCORTISONE/PRAMOXINE
Hydrocortisone/pramoxine (cream, ointment, lotion, foam) – 1%/1%
Hydrocortisone/pramoxine (cream, ointment, lotion) – 2.5%/1%

*Dose*
Apply topically or rectally as needed.

*Efficacy*
Anesthetic actions of pramoxine combined with anti-inflammatory actions of hydrocortisone alleviate pain, itch, and inflammation associated with hemorrhoids.

*Risks/benefits*
Risks:
- May cause local irritation
- May cause secondary infection

*Side effects and adverse reactions*
- Thin fragile skin
- Dermatitis
- Local irritation
- Skin dryness
- Secondary infection

*Interactions (other drugs)*
No significant interactions reported.

*Contraindications*
Systemic fungal infections.

*Acceptability to patient*
Generally well tolerated.

*Follow up plan*
Re-evaluate hemorrhoids in 1–2 weeks if symptoms persist.

*Patient and caregiver information*
- Use following bowel movements, after washing and drying affected area
- Avoid contact with eyes
- Notify physician if condition worsens or fails to improve after 3–4 days or if bleeding, protrusion, or seepage occur

WITCH HAZEL
Witch hazel or hamamelis water (liquid or 50% pads).

*Dose*
Apply locally up to six times daily or use as a wipe after bowel movements.

*Efficacy*
Provides temporary relief of hemorrhoidal irritation and itching.

*Risks/benefits*
Risk: may cause local irritation.

*Side effects and adverse reactions*
No significant adverse reactions reported.

*Interactions (other drugs)*
No significant interactions reported.

*Acceptability to patient*
Generally well tolerated.

*Follow up plan*
Re-evaluate hemorrhoids in 1–2 weeks if symptoms persist.

*Patient and caregiver information*
- For external use only
- If condition worsens or does not improve within 7 days, notify physician

### Surgical therapy
EXTERNAL HEMORRHOIDAL EXCISION
Hemorrhoidal excision.

*Efficacy*
Removal of thrombosis may alleviate some pain associated with thrombosed external hemorrhoids. The involved external hemorrhoid can be incised and expressed only, or excised.

*Risks/benefits*
Risks:
- Bleeding
- Pain
- Recurrence
- Chronic fissure

Benefits: may alleviate some pain and speed the healing process.

*Evidence*
Surgery should be reserved for symptomatic patients with third or fourth degree hemorrhoids. 95% of patients with fourth degree hemorrhoids can achieve long-term symptom reduction with surgical therapy [1] *Level C*

*Acceptability to patient*
Painful procedure, requires local anesthetic, and usually an assistant to help with positioning the patient. Patient may require oral analgesics to control pain following procedure.

*Follow up plan*
Re-evaluate hemorrhoids for wound check in 48–72h; follow up in 3–4 weeks.

*Patient and caregiver information*
- Perianal area will be painful for 1–2 days
- Sitz baths should be utilized three times daily for one week
- Avoid straining and prolonged sitting on toilet to prevent recurrent thrombosis
- High bulk, high fluid diet is essential

### Endoscopic therapy
RUBBER BAND LIGATION
*Efficacy*
- Endoscopic treatment suited to office use
- Useful for second or third degree hemorrhoidal bleeding or prolapsing internal hemorrhoids
- Hemorrhoidal tissue, ensnared by rubber band placed under direct vision with special instrument, undergoes necrosis and sloughs
- Removes internal hemorrhoids by tissue necrosis and sloughing

- There is a 15–20% recurrence rate of internal hemorrhoids within 5 years but this is the lowest rate of recurrence with any endoscopic procedure

*Risks/benefits*
Risks:
- Bleeding
- Pain
- Thrombosis (rare)
- Sepsis with pelvic cellulitis (rare)
- Avoid in patients with AIDS or other immunodeficiency state

Benefits:
- Removal of internal hemorrhoid
- Relatively inexpensive
- Quick procedure

*Evidence*
- Rubber banding is an appropriate treatment for first, second or third degree hemorrhoids. Resolution of symptoms is seen in at least 90% of patients with first or second degree disease, and 70% of patients with third degree hemorrhoids [1] *Level C*
- The first choice treatment for symptomatic first and second degree hemorrhoids not responsive to medical therapy is rubber band ligation [2] *Level C*

*Acceptability to patient*
Typically well tolerated, with minor discomfort for 2 days following procedure; best tolerance is achieved if only one hemorrhoid is ligated at a time.

*Follow up plan*
- Re-evaluate in 2–4 weeks
- Perform further banding of other hemorrhoidal groups if required

*Patient and caregiver information*
- Mild aching may be present for 2 days following procedure, including a sensation of needing to pass a stool
- Bleeding may occur in 7–10 days when hemorrhoid sloughs; aspirin and nonsteroidal anti-inflammatory drugs should be avoided 2 weeks postprocedure
- Notify physician of severe bleeding, fever, dysuria, urinary retention, or severe pain

## INFRARED COAGULATION
*Efficacy*
Painless procedure that uses infrared light to induce photocoagulation of first, second, and small third degree internal hemorrhoids. Office procedure, requires infrared unit. Painless procedure with long-term results equal to other endoscopic therapies.

*Risks/benefits*
Risks:
- Dull, aching postprocedural pain subsiding within 2 days
- Minor bleeding

Benefits:
- Procedure is painless – only a warm sensation is felt
- No reported perineal sepsis

*Evidence*
- Infrared coagulation is an appropriate treatment for first, second or third degree hemorrhoids. Resolution of symptoms is seen in at least 90% of patients with first or second degree disease [1] *Level C*
- Repetitive treatment may be required for first and second degree hemorrhoids [2] *Level C*

*Acceptability to patient*
Well tolerated; better tolerated if one hemorrhoidal group is treated per session.

*Follow up plan*
- Re-evaluate hemorrhoids in 3–4 weeks
- Treat residual disease or another hemorrhoidal group

*Patient and caregiver information*
Notify physician of pain, fever, or inability to urinate.

## SCLEROTHERAPY
*Efficacy*
Effective procedure to treat first and second degree internal bleeding hemorrhoids. Scarring that occurs as a result of the sclerosant stops internal bleeding.

*Risks/benefits*
Risks:
- Painful thrombosis of hemorrhoids may occur
- Anaphylaxis from sclerosant
- Abscesses
- Bleeding
- Necrosis of anal canal if injection is too superficial

Benefits:
- Eliminates internal bleeding of hemorrhoids
- May treat all hemorrhoidal groups simultaneously
- Inexpensive procedure

*Acceptability to patient*
- Has been associated with significant complications
- It is possible for all three hemorrhoidal sites to be treated at one session

*Follow up plan*
- Re-evaluate hemorrhoids in 3 weeks
- Treat other hemorrhoidal groups if necessary

*Patient and caregiver information*
- Mild rectal discomfort may occur after treatment
- Notify physician of severe symptoms
- Healing will take 3–6 weeks

## DC CURRENT (ULTROID)
*Efficacy*
Effective treatment for all internal hemorrhoidal grades by coagulant effects. Especially effective for more advanced grades of hemorrhoids.

*Risks/benefits*
Risks:
- Deep burns if probe penetrates tissue too deeply
- Bleeding
- Time inefficient – requires 8–14min

Benefits:
- Nearly painless procedure for internal hemorrhoidal treatment
- More than one hemorrhoid may be treated per session

*Acceptability to patient*
Generally well tolerated, although this procedure takes longer than other endoscopic methods at each visit.

*Follow up plan*
Re-evaluate hemorrhoids after anatomic resolution of treated hemorrhoids (3–10 days).

*Patient and caregiver information*
Minor perianal discomfort or bleeding may occur.

### BIPOLAR ELECTROCOAGULATION (BICAP)
*Efficacy*
Effectively treats hemorrhoids by coagulation. Best for higher grades of hemorrhoids.

*Risks/benefits*
Risks:
- Painful ulcer or fissure if probe is placed too closely to anoderm line
- Burns
- Prolonged rectal spasm
- Minor bleeding

Benefits:
- Quick and simple procedure
- Complications are rare
- Higher grades and multiple groups of hemorrhoids can be treated simultaneously

*Acceptability to patient*
Generally well tolerated.

*Follow up plan*
- Re-evaluate hemorrhoids in 3–4 weeks
- Treat until all hemorrhoids have been reduced to zero or first degree

*Patient and caregiver information*
Minor bleeding may occur immediately after procedure or 10–14 days following procedure.

## Other therapies
### SITZ BATHS
*Efficacy*
Sitting in warm-to-hot water for 10–20min three or four times daily may help alleviate pain associated with hemorrhoids. Sitz baths should be initiated at the first sign of a flare-up.

*Risks/benefits*
- Risks: none
- Benefits: transient relief of hemorrhoidal pain and irritation

*Acceptability to patient*
Well tolerated.

*Follow up plan*
Physician should be contacted if rectal bleeding is present or if hemorrhoids fail to spontaneously resolve within one week.

*Patient and caregiver information*
- Water should be as hot as tolerable (careful not to burn)
- If topical anesthetics are used concurrently, use caution to prevent burning or scalding of anesthetized tissue

## LIFESTYLE
High fiber diet and drink six to eight glasses of liquids daily.

### RISKS/BENEFITS
Risks: None

Benefits:
- Provides bulk to stool
- Decreases constipation/straining while stooling
- Fiber may also prevent colon cancer

### ACCEPTABILITY TO PATIENT
Well tolerated.

### FOLLOW UP PLAN
None required.

### PATIENT AND CAREGIVER INFORMATION
- Eat bran, fiber, or roughage
- Many breakfast cereals are high in bran
- Fresh fruits, leafy vegetables, whole grain breads are rich in fiber
- Avoid alcohol – dehydrating and may contribute to constipation

# OUTCOMES

## EFFICACY OF THERAPIES
When bleeding hemorrhoids do not resolve with appropriate pharmacologic therapies, endoscopic therapies are well tolerated by patients with resolution of symptoms typically occurring within 4 weeks.

### Evidence
PDxMD are unable to cite evidence which meets our criteria for evidence.

### Review period
Resolution of hemorrhoids may be re-evaluated in 1–2 weeks following pharmacologic therapy or in 3–4 weeks following endoscopic treatments.

## PROGNOSIS
Hemorrhoidal discomfort may be experienced acutely or chronically and relapses may occur. The recurrence rate is 10–50% over 5 years. Usually, hemorrhoids resolve spontaneously. Rarely is the disease fatal.

### Therapeutic failure
Hemorrhoidectomy – surgical removal of hemorrhoids is performed in patients failing nonsurgical treatments, those with strangulated internal hemorrhoids, and those suffering from both symptomatic internal and external hemorrhoids. Hemorrhoidectomy is reserved for third and fourth grade hemorrhoids accompanied by severe symptoms. Hospitalization may be required and the recovery period may last for weeks. Possible complications include urinary retention, hemorrhage, anal sepsis, and anal stenosis. A risk of compromising anal sphincter competence also exists.

### Recurrence
The following endoscopic therapies may be used to treat hemorrhoids when they recur:
- Rubber band ligation
- Bipolar coagulation
- Infrared coagulation
- DC current
- Sclerotherapy

### Deterioration
Endoscopic therapies may be used if pharmacologic therapies/dietary modifications do not resolve hemorrhoidal symptoms:
- Rubber band ligation
- Bipolar coagulation
- Infrared coagulation
- DC current
- Sclerotherapy

Hemorrhoidectomy is reserved for third and fourth grade hemorrhoids that fail to resolve by nonsurgical methods.

## COMPLICATIONS
- Thrombosis may occur in both internal and external hemorrhoids
- Rare cases of strangulation due to Grade IV internal hemorrhoids
- Secondary infections
- Ulceration
- Anemia (rare) secondary to blood loss
- Incontinence

## CONSIDER CONSULT
Third and fourth grade hemorrhoids accompanied by severe symptoms that have failed nonsurgical treatment options should be referred to anorectal surgeon for hemorrhoidectomy.

# PREVENTION

## RISK FACTORS
**Diet**: high fat, low fiber diets are associated with hemorrhoids
**Sexual behavior**: anal intercourse is associated with increased risk of anorectal complications, such as secondary infections
**Family history**: frequently a familial predisposition is present

## MODIFY RISK FACTORS
Dietary modifications, high fiber and high fluid diets, are the best measures for hemorrhoid prevention.

### Lifestyle and wellness
DIET
Eat a diet high in fiber, low in fat; drink fluids liberally.

SEXUAL BEHAVIOR
Avoid anal intercourse or limit partners to minimize anorectal complications.

## PREVENT RECURRENCE
- Avoid prolonged sitting
- Avoid constipation. Constipation may be a side effect of some drugs including anticholinergics and opioids. Use stool softeners if medications known to cause constipation are necessary to manage concomitant diseases
- Eating a diet high in fiber, low in fat and drinking fluids liberally reduces the risk of constipation
- Pass bowel movements as soon as urge occurs. Avoid lingering on the toilet because time spent sitting puts pressure on the hemorrhoids. Avoid straining while stooling. Avoid vigorous wiping; pat rather than rub. At first sign of recurrent symptoms, initiate frequent sitz baths
- Walk or exercise to help move stools through body more quickly

### Reassess coexisting disease
Prolonged pushing during childbirth and episiotomies may worsen hemorrhoids.

INTERACTION ALERT
Opioids, anticholinergics – may cause constipation, worsening hemorrhoids.

# RESOURCES

## ASSOCIATIONS

**American Gastroenterological Association**
7910 Woodmont Ave., Seventh Floor,
Bethesda, MD 20814
Tel: (301) 654-2055
Fax: (301) 652-3890
Email: ctheokas@gastro.org

**American Society of Gastrointestinal Endoscopy**
Thirteen Elm Street
Manchester, MA 01944-1314
Tel: (978) 526-8330
Fax: (978) 526-4018

**Society of Gastroenterology Nurses and Associates**
401 North Michigan Avenue
Chicago, IL 60611-4267
Tel: (800) 245-7462, in Illinois - (312) 321-5165
Fax: (312) 527-6658
http://www.sgna.org

## KEY REFERENCES

- Linehan IP. The patients with anal problems. Practitioner 2000; 244:329–34
- Johanson JF, Sonnenberg A. The prevalence of hemorrhoids and chronic constipation: an epidemiologic study. Gastroenterology 1990; 98:380–6
- Haas PA, Fox TA Jr, Haas GP. The pathogenesis of hemorrhoids. Dis Colon Rectum 1984; 27: 442–50

### Guidelines

1. Society for Surgery of the Alimentary Tract. Surgical management of hemorrhoids. Patient Care Committee, 2000. Also available at the National Guideline Clearinghouse
2. Practice parameters for the treatment of hemorrhoids. Standards Task Force of the American Society of Colon and Rectal Surgeons; 1998–1999. Available at the National Guideline Clearinghouse

## CONTRIBUTORS

Dennis F Saver, MD
Andrew H Soll, MD

# ALCOHOLIC HEPATITIS

| | | |
|---|---|---|
| ■ | Summary Information | 258 |
| ■ | Background | 259 |
| ■ | Diagnosis | 261 |
| ■ | Treatment | 276 |
| ■ | Outcomes | 288 |
| ■ | Prevention | 290 |
| ■ | Resources | 292 |

# SUMMARY INFORMATION

## DESCRIPTION
- One manifestation of alcoholic liver disease, alcoholic hepatitis is characterized by an acute inflammatory process in the liver
- Occurs in 10–35% of long-term heavy abusers of ethanol
- Probable multifactorial etiology related to multiple toxic, metabolic, and immunologic effects of ethanol on the liver
- Often occurs following an episode of ethanol intake greater than usual for the patient
- Most often presents clinically with acute jaundice, malaise, fever, and abdominal pain
- Can be accompanied by signs of hepatic decompensation, including ascites, hepatic encephalopathy, variceal bleeding, and coagulopathy. It can also be accompanied by any of the severe sequelae of alcoholism, including withdrawal, seizures, and delirium tremens
- Can be the first presentation of alcoholic liver disease in the relatively young alcoholic
- Even with adequate intervention, those patients presenting with severe acute alcoholic hepatitis and a biochemical discriminant function score >32 or spontaneous hepatic encephalopathy can have a 50% mortality rate at one month

## URGENT ACTION
- Alcoholic hepatitis is a potentially fatal condition, even with appropriate treatment
- Patients should be referred to the emergency room for admission to hospital
- Broad-spectrum antibiotics should be instituted if sepsis is suspected
- The use of acetaminophen should be stopped
- If the patient has presented with seizures (which are commonly related to alcohol withdrawal), benzodiazepines should be commenced
- If the patient is bleeding and a coagulopathy is documented by prolonged prothrombin time and the international normalized ratio (INR), treat with 10mg vitamin K by subcutaneous injection daily for 3 days and immediate transfusion of fresh frozen plasma

## KEY! DON'T MISS!
- Physical signs and symptoms of advanced chronic liver disease, which may point toward underlying alcoholism
- History suggestive or overtly confirmatory of chronic alcohol abuse
- Signs and symptoms of encephalopathy may be difficult to distinguish from alcohol intoxication or withdrawal
- Evidence of Wernicke's encephalopathy, which if not treated, can have devastating consequences, including progression to Korsakoff's psychosis
- Sepsis

## BACKGROUND

### ICD9 CODE
- 303. Alcohol dependence syndrome
- 571.1 Acute alcoholic hepatitis

### CARDINAL FEATURES
- One manifestation of alcoholic liver disease, alcoholic hepatitis is characterized by an acute inflammatory process in the liver
- Occurs in 10–35% of long-term heavy abusers of ethanol
- History of chronic alcohol intake continuing to current presentation
- Often occurs following an episode of ethanol intake greater than usual for the patient
- Can be the first presentation of alcoholic liver disease in the relatively young alcoholic
- Most often presents clinically with acute jaundice, malaise, fever, and right upper quadrant abdominal pain
- Hepatomegaly and anorexia are often present
- Can be accompanied by signs of hepatic decompensation, including ascites, hepatic encephalopathy, variceal bleeding, and coagulopathy
- Can also be accompanied by any of the severe sequelae of alcoholism, including withdrawal, seizures, and delirium tremens
- Liver function tests are abnormal: elevated aminotranferases (aspartate aminotranferases (AST) two to five times normal; alanine aminotranferases (ALT), two to three times normal; AST:ALT ratio <2), elevated gamma-glutamyl transpeptidase, elevated bilirubin
- Elevated prothrombin time and international normalized ratio (INR)
- Positive blood alcohol level
- Often elevated serum ferritin level
- Macrocytosis
- Typical histopathologic features on liver biopsy
- Even with adequate intervention, those patients presenting with severe acute alcoholic hepatitis and a biochemical discriminant function score >32 or spontaneous hepatic encephalopathy can have a 50% mortality rate at one month

## CAUSES
### Common causes
- Ongoing alcohol abuse
- Binge drinking or increased alcohol intake preceding presentation, in the context of chronic alcohol abuse

### Contributory or predisposing factors
- Heavy alcohol intake over a period of many years (average: >80g/day of ethanol with mean duration of 25 years)
- Binge drinking
- Specific polymorphisms of the alcohol dehydrogenase (ADH), cytochrome P450 2E1 (CYP2E1), and acetaldehyde dehydrogenase (ALDH) genes
- Female sex (women have a higher risk of developing alcoholic liver disease of all types than men do; thus, women require less ingestion of alcohol to develop complications of alcoholic liver disease)
- Poor diet and nutrition
- Concurrent hepatitis C virus or hepatitis B virus infection

## EPIDEMIOLOGY
### Incidence and prevalence
The actual incidence of acute alcoholic hepatitis is difficult to determine. What is known is that

approx. 90% of heavy drinkers develop fatty liver and that only about 10–35% of these go on to develop alcoholic hepatitis, with 10–20% eventually developing cirrhosis. The following numbers are calculated based on these statistics.

## INCIDENCE
Incidence of alcohol abuse or dependence in the US is approx. 7%, or 70/1000 among people aged over 18 years.

## PREVALENCE
- Prevalence of alcoholic liver disease: 70/1000 of the population
- Prevalence of alcoholic hepatitis: 9–25/1000 of the population (extrapolated)

## FREQUENCY
10–35% (100–350/1000) of heavy drinkers develop alcoholic hepatitis.

## Demographics

### AGE
There is no one age group in which acute alcoholic hepatitis is more prevalent. The predominant age group for alcoholism as a whole is between 20 and 40 years of age.

### GENDER
- Lifetime risk of alcoholism for males is 8–10%
- Lifetime risk of alcoholism for females is 3–5%
- Women are more susceptible to alcoholic liver damage than men, with a lower threshold of alcohol intake before serious liver disease occurs (7 units/week for women; 21 units/week for males; one unit is 7g ethanol)

### RACE
- There is a wide range of alcohol clearance rates among various ethnic groups
- People of Asian descent tend to not drink to excess or at all. But if they do drink, they tend to suffer a higher incidence of alcoholic liver disease than those of northern European descent, owing to genetic differences in metabolic enzymes

### GENETICS
- Susceptibility to alcoholic liver disease has a genetic component
- The genes coding for the enzymes ADH, ALDH, and the CYP2E1 system may all contribute to susceptibility to alcoholic liver disease

### SOCIOECONOMIC STATUS
Alcoholic hepatitis affects all socioeconomic groups.

# DIAGNOSIS

## DIFFERENTIAL DIAGNOSIS
### Viral hepatitis
- Viral hepatitis is a common accompaniment to alcoholic liver disease
- Up to 40% of patients with alcoholic liver disease are also seropositive for hepatitis C virus
- A smaller percentage show evidence of hepatitis B virus infection or other viral hepatitides. Because the current treatment of hepatitis C virus infection often involves the use of interferon, distinction from alcoholic hepatitis is essential, since immune stimulation can cause increased hepatocellular damage in patients receiving interferon
- Thus, active alcohol use is a contraindication to interferon-based treatment regimens for chronic viral hepatitis

FEATURES
- Fever, jaundice, malaise, abdominal pain, and nausea are clinical features common to both alcoholic and viral hepatitis
- Preferential rise in alanine aminotransferase (ALT) helps distinguish active hepatitis C virus infection from alcoholic hepatitis
- Active viral infection can usually be distinguished from inflammation due to alcoholic hepatitis on liver biopsy, since each entity has specific patterns of inflammation and hepatocellular damage

### Toxic and drug-induced hepatitis
- Hepatitis may result from the ingestion of various medications or chemicals
- Jaundice, abnormal liver function tests, and a history of exposure to, or ingestion of, chemicals should alert the clinician
- Two types of chemical hepatotoxicity are recognized: the direct toxic type (e.g. caused by carbon tetrachloride, acetaminophen) and the idiosyncratic type (e.g. caused by phenytoin, isoniazid)

### Nonalcoholic steatohepatitis
Nonalcoholic steatohepatitis, or NASH, is defined as fatty liver accompanied by inflammation, without a history of ethanol abuse.

FEATURES
- No history of significant alcohol intake elicited by rigorous history taking from patient and/or family, or by CAGE* questionnaire or other similar profiling instrument
- Frequently asymptomatic (>50% of patients). Variable nonspecific symptoms of right upper quadrant or generalized abdominal pain, weakness, and fatigue are present in a small percentage of patients
- Aminotransferases can be normal to moderately elevated (two to three times normal) with alanine aminotransferases (ALT) usually raised more than the aspartate aminotransferases (AST)
- Bilirubin, prothrombin time, and serum albumin are usually normal
- Serum ferritin may be elevated
- Common associations or concurrent disorders include obesity, noninsulin-dependent diabetes mellitus, and hyperlipidemia

(*CAGE: Cutdown, Annoyed by critcism, Guilt about drinking, Eye-opener drinks)

### Hemochromatosis
- Hereditary hemochromatosis is caused by a defect in the regulation of iron absorption, usually secondary to a mutation in the HFE gene, resulting in toxic iron overload in the liver
- Secondary iron overload can result from hemophilia with multiple blood transfusions, from alcoholism, and (rarely) from nonalcoholic steatohepatitis and hepatitis C

FEATURES
- Patients can present with hyperferritinemia and mild liver enzyme elevations as the only initial finding, making distinction from alcoholic liver disease necessary
- Aminotransferase levels usually normal or slightly elevated in hemochromatosis
- Liver biopsy showing markedly increased iron staining and a high calculated hepatic iron index (>1.9)
- Positive for an HFE gene mutation (C282Y/C28Y) in most cases of hereditary hemochromatosis

### Alpha-1-antitrypsin deficiency
- Alpha-1-antitrypsin deficiency is an autosomal recessively inherited disease occurring with great prevalence in Caucasians of northern European descent (1/1700 to 1/2000 people)
- In the homozygous form, 70% of patients have persistent low level elevation of aminotransferases and 10% progress to cirrhosis with liver failure as adults
- The heterozygous adult appears to be predisposed to end-stage liver damage and liver cancer when there are also insults from other sources, such as alcohol or hepatitis B virus or hepatitis C virus infection

FEATURES
- In the homozygous neonatal patient, jaundice appears within the first 4 months of life and lasts for 2–3 months with hepatosplenomegaly and signs of cholestasis and hepatocellular damage
- There may be no symptoms until adulthood, when evidence of chronic or end-stage liver disease appears
- Serum alpha-1-antitrypsin levels <25% lower limit of normal
- Serum protein electrophoresis with decreased alpha-1-globulin
- Immunophenotype demonstrating PiZZ homozygosity or, in occasional cases, PiZ, PiMZ, or PiSZ heterozygosity

## SIGNS & SYMPTOMS
### Signs
Signs of acute alcoholic hepatitis:
- Jaundice
- Fever, up to 103°F (39.4°C) in 50% of cases
- Spontaneous encephalopathy (in severe cases)
- Seizures and tremor if alcohol withdrawal is present
- Tender hepatomegaly
- Splenomegaly is seen in one-third of patients

Signs related to underlying advanced alcoholic liver disease:
- Spider nevi
- Facial telangiectasia
- Collateral veins visible on abdominal wall (caput medusae)
- Portal venous bruit (hum)
- Bleeding esophageal varices
- Ascites
- Gynecomastia
- Testicular atrophy
- Parotid gland enlargement
- Palmar erythema

### Symptoms
- Mildly affected patients may be asymptomatic or complain of recent onset of generalized malaise
- Pruritus
- Nausea

- Vomiting
- Anorexia
- Fever
- Abdominal pain
- Symptoms due to acute alcohol withdrawal (agitation, anxiety)
- Confusion
- Jaundice

## ASSOCIATED DISORDERS
Disorders associated with alcoholic hepatitis are other conditions caused by chronic ethanol abuse:
- Neurologic manifestations
- Gastrointestinal manifestations
- Endocrine manifestations
- Other manifestations

Neurologic manifestations:
- Acute alcohol withdrawal syndrome – the sudden cessation of alcohol intake following a period of prolonged alcohol dependence can precipitate withdrawal symptoms, sometimes within only a few hours. The initial symptom is usually a tremor, often accompanied by nausea, sweating, irritability, and a craving for alcohol for 24–48h. In approx. 25% of such patients, these symptoms are followed by auditory and/or visual hallucinations, which resolve over the next 2–3 days
- Neurologic diseases caused by chronic excessive alcohol abuse include: central pontine myelinolysis, cerebellar atrophy, generalized cortical atrophy, and Wernicke-Korsakoff syndrome (secondary to thiamine deficiency, which is present in many chronic alcoholics and therefore in the setting of alcoholic hepatitis)
- Peripheral neuropathy caused by malnutrition is seen in the setting of chronic excessive alcohol ingestion and thus can be an accompaniment of acute alcoholic hepatitis

Gastrointestinal manifestations:
- Fatty liver is common, and cirrhosis may be present
- Spontaneous bacterial peritonitis often accompanies acutely decompensated alcoholic liver disease and is seen frequently in the setting of acute alcoholic hepatitis. The mechanism is suspected to relate to an impaired mucosal barrier to enteric organisms caused by poor nutrition as well as the direct effects of alcohol on the bowel mucosa. It can lead to generalized sepsis
- Malabsorption (alcohol causes changes in the function of duodenal and jejunal villi, leading to mild malabsorption)
- Gastritis can occur after severe alcohol ingestion
- Acute and chronic pancreatitis, hemorrhagic pancreatitis
- Esophageal varices

Endocrine manifestations:
- Hypogonadism (as a result of direct effect of alcohol on testicular function, as a result of the underlying liver dysfunction, or because of decreased gonadotropic hormones from more central effects of alcohol on the endocrine axes)
- A variety of effects are noted including decreased libido, impotence, and gynecomastia
- Pseudo-Cushing's syndrome, which is biochemically and clinically indistinguishable from its primary adrenocortical counterpart, caused by direct stimulation of adrenocorticotropic hormone secretion by alcohol
- Hypoglycemia, caused by the prolonged fasting that often accompanies alcoholism. It is essential that glucose levels be checked in any patient presenting with stigmata of alcoholic liver disease and encephalopathy, stupor, or coma

Other manifestations:
- Hypertension
- Cardiomyopathy
- Skeletal muscle disease (e.g. rhabdomyolysis, progressive painless muscle wasting primarily of the proximal lower limb groups)
- Hypoproteinemia secondary to poor nutrition
- Macrocytic anemia from nutritional deficiency of vitamin B12 or folate
- Microcytic anemia from chronic occult blood loss
- Hyperammonemia

## KEY! DON'T MISS!
- Physical signs and symptoms of advanced chronic liver disease, which may point toward underlying alcoholism
- History suggestive or overtly confirmatory of chronic alcohol abuse
- Signs and symptoms of encephalopathy may be difficult to distinguish from alcohol intoxication or withdrawal
- Evidence of Wernicke's encephalopathy, which if not treated, can have devastating consequences, including progression to Korsakoff's psychosis
- Sepsis

## CONSIDER CONSULT
Those patients presenting with symptoms and signs of severe hepatic decompensation (seizures, encephalopathy, variceal bleeding, spontaneous bacterial peritonitis, sepsis, hepatorenal syndrome) need immediate hospitalization, stabilization, and, in many cases, consultation with a gastroenterologist.

## INVESTIGATION OF THE PATIENT
### Direct questions to patient
If the patient has full cognitive function, the CAGE questionnaire or the more detailed Michigan Alcoholism Screening Test (MAST) should be administered. If cognitive function is impaired for any reason, family members or friends might offer the only resource.

- **Q** What type of alcohol is consumed? The type of alcohol is important. A patient who consumes two beers or similar beverage a day can be ingesting up to 85g/day of ethanol
- **Q** How often do you drink? How much do you drink? Even though a patient may drink alcohol to excess only sporadically, his or her threshold dose for alcoholic liver disease may nevertheless be reached
- **Q** Where do you drink (e.g. at home, in a bar)? With patients who drink alcohol primarily at home it may be easier to quantify the amount drunk by asking, for example, how often they buy spirits and how many bottles of wine they buy each week. Patients who drink primarily at home can consume large quantities of alcohol a little at a time
- **Q** What is the degree of alcohol dependence? The following questions constitute the CAGE questionnaire, with two or more affirmative answers indicating a high probability of alcohol dependence: have you ever felt you should Cut down on your drinking? Have other people Annoyed you by criticizing your drinking? Have you ever felt Guilty about your drinking?; Have you ever taken a drink first thing in the morning (Eye opener) to steady your nerves or get rid of a hangover?
- **Q** Over what period of time and when did the current symptoms develop? When was the last time you had a drink? Typically, alcoholic hepatitis develops during a bout of drinking with cessation occurring because of the acute appearance of jaundice often with nausea, vomiting, anorexia, abdominal pain, or diarrhea
- **Q** Have you noticed discoloration of the skin, abdominal discomfort, or any bleeding (e.g. nosebleeds)? The presence of clinical features of alcoholic hepatitis, and their severity, should be determined

## Contributory or predisposing factors

- **Q** Have you recently had an episode where you drank more than usual? Binge drinking in a setting of chronic excessive alcohol intake
- **Q** Are you aware of any genetic or enzyme deficiencies you may have? Polymorphisms of the alcohol dehydrogenase (ADH), acetaldehyde dehydrogenase (ALDH), and cytochrome P450 2E1 (CYP2E1) gene systems may lead to increased susceptibility to liver damage
- **Q** Is there any history of intravenous drug use? These questions address the possible contribution of hepatitis C or B virus infection to the current illness
- **Q** Is there any history of a transfusion of blood or blood products? This may cause jaundice through either infected blood products or a transfusion reaction
- **Q** Have you been diagnosed with viral hepatitis? Concurrent hepatitis C or B virus infection may accelerate liver injury
- **Q** What is your usual diet like? Poor nutrition may contribute to the evolution of alcoholic liver disease to alcoholic hepatitis
- **Q** Is there any history of occupational exposures? A wide variety of industrial exposures can cause chemical hepatitis or be directly hepatotoxic. Direct queries as to the nature of a person's occupation are essential
- **Q** Is there any habitual use of large quantities of nonsteroidal anti-inflammatory agents (NSAIDs) or acetaminophen? Acetaminophen is one of the safest drugs to use in the setting of mildly impaired liver function even though it is cleared by the liver. However, in alcohol abusers, even standard doses of acetaminophen may be hepatotoxic. NSAIDs can occasionally be severely hepatotoxic and contribute to decreased renal function in a hepatocompromised patient

## Family history

Do either of your parents or any of your siblings have liver-related disease and, if so, do they drink excessively? There exists an inheritable predisposition to liver injury separate from and in addition to that governing drinking behavior.

## Examination

- Examine the patient's vital signs. Signs of occult blood loss or cardiac disease secondary to alcoholism may be detected. Fever is an important initial indicator of possible early sepsis
- Examine the skin for jaundice and cutaneous stigmata of chronic liver disease
- Perform an abdominal examination. There may be evidence of ascites, abdominal tenderness, or palpable tender hepatomegaly with or without splenomegaly. Of alcoholic patients, 80% present with an enlarged liver caused either by fatty infiltration or by hepatocellular ballooning degeneration. The liver may not be palpable in patients with established cirrhosis, but in that setting there is usually sufficient portal hypertension to produce splenomegaly
- Examine the body habitus and appearance. The cardinal features to look for include evidence of muscle wasting, Dupuytren's contractures, gynecomastia, Cushingoid features, spider angiomas, facial telangiectases, palmar erythema, parotid gland enlargement, cutaneous venous collaterals, and testicular atrophy
- Examine for the presence of neurologic deficits. Because the presence of encephalopathy is one of the poor prognostic indicators for acute alcoholic hepatitis, assessment of the cognitive functions of the presenting patient is essential. Also, the presence or absence of cerebellar disease can yield insight into the degree of liver failure, and therefore testing for asterixis (flapping tremor of the hands), although simple, can be useful in these patients. Finally, peripheral neuropathy is a sign of long-standing excessive alcohol abuse, so a detailed peripheral neurologic examination is important
- Examine for any recent evidence of bleeding. Coagulopathy may be seen in alcoholic hepatitis and is an indicator of more severe disease; examine the nares and oropharynx for epistaxis and gingival hemorrhage

## Summary of investigative tests

- Serum aminotransferases test for hepatocellular damage. Both are usually <300 IU/L with the aspartate (AST) two to three times higher than the alanine aminotransferase (ALT). Very high elevations tend to rule in favor of a nonalcoholic cause for the hepatic dysfunction. Gamma-glutamyl transferase is usually elevated in heavy drinkers irrespective of the presence of liver disease and can therefore be used to suspect alcohol as the etiologic agent
- Serum alkaline phosphatase (ALP) is usually only mildly elevated in alcoholic liver disease of all types, being markedly elevated in biliary obstruction. It can therefore be utilized to identify the suspected cause of jaundice if necessary
- Bilirubin (total, direct, and indirect) is almost always elevated in acute alcoholic hepatitis and reflects significant hepatocellular dysfunction
- Serum albumin is a test of hepatic synthetic function and is frequently low in significant chronic liver injury of any cause. Usually, by the time a chronic alcoholic patient presents with alcoholic hepatitis, serum albumin is depressed
- Prothrombin time (PT) and international normalized ratio (INR) is an important test of hepatic synthetic function and can be used in conjunction with the bilirubin to assess the severity of alcoholic hepatitis in a given patient
- Serum glucose is often low in the alcoholic patient secondary to the attendant malnutrition and cirrhosis. This parameter should be checked in all patients who present with encephalopathic changes
- Serum sodium can provide important information concerning the patient's renal status and may relate to mental status changes as well. Almost all patients with cirrhosis of any cause will have a low serum sodium. Because the blood urea nitrogen may not be elevated in the setting of hepatorenal syndrome, serum creatinine should be measured
- Serum lipid profile may show hypertriglyceridemia and increased high density lipoproteins, both of which should normalize with abstinence
- Serum uric acid may be elevated but will normalize with abstinence if secondary to alcohol intake
- Complete blood count can provide information important in the management of these patients. Chronic alcoholics typically show a macrocytic anemia with depressed platelets. Anemia may also be secondary to bleeding. Patients with acute alcoholic hepatitis frequently display an elevated white cell count in the leukemoid range. Thrombocytopenia may result from alcohol-induced bone marrow suppression or hypersplenism
- Serologies for hepatitis B and C virus infections are an essential part of the assessment of any patient presenting with the constellation of symptoms shared by alcoholic hepatitis, in order to rule out the participation of viral hepatitis in the patient's illness
- Blood culture is indicated in all patients who present with fever and an elevated white cell count. Chronic alcoholics can be immunocompromised secondary to nutritional and protein synthetic factors and are susceptible to a broad spectrum of bacterial, fungal, and viral infections. Cultures should be directed at the bacterial and fungal pathogens
- Serum ammonia levels are increased in hepatic failure and hepatic encephalopathy
- Carbohydrate-deficient transferrin is used by some hepatologists because it is a marker that is related to chronic high-level alcohol ingestion (>10g/day); it may be used to establish the alcoholic etiology of the presenting illness when there is high suspicion and patient denial. The test is not available at all laboratories. There is some recent indication that the ratio of carbohydrate-deficient transferrin to carbohydrate-rich transferrin may be a more accurate reflection of an alcoholic history
- Abdominal ultrasound examination is usually ordered. It has 94% sensitivity for detecting fatty infiltration of the liver, and it can evaluate the bile ducts for obstruction. Doppler ultrasound can assess portal vein blood flow. A small, irregular, nodular liver by ultrasound is virtually diagnostic of cirrhosis
- Abdominal computed tomography scan may also be useful for determining the extent of liver disease secondary to alcohol; it would probably be ordered by a specialist

- Liver biopsy is frequently ordered and performed by a gastroenterologist or radiologist. Alcoholic hepatitis is reflected in a variety of histopathologic features that can usually distinguish it from hepatitis caused by other agents (except nonalcoholic steatohepatitis). In patients presenting with a prolonged prothrombin time and decreased platelets, the percutaneous route is deferred in favor of the transjugular approach

## DIAGNOSTIC DECISION
- A history of alcoholism is the cornerstone of diagnosis to distinguish alcoholic hepatitis from other causes of liver failure
- The diagnosis of alcoholic hepatitis is specifically established by histologic examination of the liver showing the characteristic findings of steatosis, Mallory bodies, neutrophil infiltration, and ballooning degeneration of hepatocytes with the history of alcohol ingestion. Although liver biopsy and histology establish the diagnosis, in the vast majority of cases such an examination is not necessary because the diagnosis can be made with a high degree of confidence using other clinical information
- The clinical diagnosis of acute alcoholic hepatitis rests on the constellation of jaundice, fever, abdominal pain, anorexia, malaise, hepatomegaly, the characteristic elevations in aminotransferases, elevated bilirubin, and coagulopathy with a history of chronic excessive alcohol use
- In the arena of severe alcoholic hepatitis, a discriminant function (DF) can be calculated using biochemical laboratory data (the prothrombin time and bilirubin) to assess the severity of the disease
- DF = 4.6 x [prothrombin time (seconds) – control time (seconds)] + serum bilirubin (mg/dL) after vitamin K replacement has been administered; a result >32 predicts a mortality within one month of approx. 50%

## CLINICAL PEARLS
- Diagnosis of acute alcoholic hepatitis presenting with fever, jaundice, and tender hepatomegaly is obvious. These patients either have never seen a physician or have not seen their primary care provider (PCP) in months, have poor nutrition, and positive blood alcohol levels
- Diagnosis of alcoholic hepatitis presenting with asymptomatic mild aminotransferase elevations is challenging and is always based on history. Most patients in clinic visits will confess to use of alcohol but may underestimate the quantity used. However, quantity is not relevant if liver enzymes are abnormal
- Discriminant function is an index for assessing the severity of liver dysfunction but it is not an indicator for cirrhosis. Liver biopsy, the definitive test for the diagnosis of cirrhosis, is almost always contraindicated because of the risk of life-threatening bleeding. It is only physical examination that helps the clinician in the diagnosis of cirrhosis
- In patients presenting with acute hepatic decompensation secondary to alcohol use, the clinical care provider has to determine whether there is underlying cirrhosis. This is important because in the absence of cirrhosis there is greater chance of hepatic recovery
- An alcoholic patient found to have an enlarged liver on physical examination is less likely to have cirrhosis than a patient with a small, shrunken liver. Similarly, an acutely ill patient with alcoholic hepatitis who presents with spider nevi, caput medusae, testicular atrophy, or other signs of end-stage liver disease most likely has underlying cirrhosis. Since cirrhosis is a progressive disease, the older the patient, the greater the chances of underlying cirrhosis

## THE TESTS
### Body fluids
SERUM AMINOTRANSFERASES
*Description*
Venous blood sample sent to the laboratory in a tube without anticoagulant.

*Advantages/Disadvantages*
Advantages:
- Provides identification and evaluation of hepatic injury
- Simple test with rapid result

Disadvantage: does not correlate with the extent of liver damage.

*Normal*
- ALT: 6–37 IU/L
- AST: 5–30 IU/L
- Gamma-glutamyl transferase (GGT): males 6–45 IU/L; females 5–30 IU/L

*Abnormal*
- Values for AST greater than five to 10 times normal and values for ALT two to three times normal suggest nonalcohol-related liver disease
- An AST:ALT ratio of 2–3 suggests alcoholic hepatitis, but does not correlate to the severity of disease
- Elevations of GGT also suggest alcohol history
- Keep in mind the possibility of a falsely abnormal result

*Cause of abnormal result*
Acute hepatocellular injury.

*Drugs, disorders and other factors that may alter results*
- Probably the most common source of potential error for the AST determination is hemolysis during collection
- Since AST is widely distributed in the body, with the highest concentrations found in cardiac and skeletal muscle, liver, and kidney, any disorder causing cellular injury to these organs can cause elevations. Erythromycin can also cause AST elevation
- Metronidazole and rifampin can decrease the measured activity of AST
- Erythromycin can cause spurious elevations of the ALT
- Warfarin, phenobarbital, and phenytoin can cause spurious elevations in GGT, sometimes to four times normal values

SERUM SODIUM
*Description*
Venous blood sample.

*Advantages/Disadvantages*
Advantages:
- Simple test with fast result
- Hyponatremia can be used to support a diagnosis of decompensated alcoholic cirrhosis in the appropriate setting

*Normal*
135–145mEq/L (135–145mmol/L).

*Abnormal*
- <135mEq/L (135mmol/L)
- Keep in mind the possibility of a false-positive result

*Drugs, disorders and other factors that may alter results*
- Thiazide diuretics

- Prolonged body fluid loss from any origin (vomiting, diarrhea, sweating)
- Adrenocortical dysfunction
- Salt wasting renal disease
- Water or volume overload

## SERUM GLUCOSE
*Description*
Venous blood sample sent to the laboratory in a tube without anticoagulant.

*Advantages/Disadvantages*
Advantages:
- Indicates nutritional status of the patient
- Indicates metabolic capacity of the liver

*Normal*
- Fasting: 70–110mg/dL (3.9–6.0mmol/L)
- Nonfasting: 70–150mg/dL (3.9–8.3mmol/L)

*Abnormal*
- Hypoglycemia: <70mg/dL (3.9mmol/L) fasting or nonfasting
- Hyperglycemia: >110mg/dL (6.0mmol/L) fasting; >150mg/dL (8.3mmol/L) nonfasting
- Keep in mind the possibility of a false-positive result

*Cause of abnormal result*
In alcoholic liver disease, hypoglycemia may be secondary to malnutrition, with a variable component of decreased gluconeogenesis caused by the inhibitory effects of alcohol and hepatocellular injury.

*Drugs, disorders and other factors that may alter results*
Hyperuricemia and hyperbilirubinemia can interfere with some test methodologies.

## SERUM CREATININE
*Description*
Venous blood sample sent to the laboratory in a tube without anticoagulant.

*Advantages/Disadvantages*
- Advantage: enables assessment of renal function independent of diet
- Disadvantage: relatively insensitive and may not be measurably increased until glomerular filtration has deteriorated more than 50%

*Normal*
- Adult male: 0.6–1.2mg/dL (53–106mmol/L)
- Adult female: 0.3–0.7mg/dL (27–62mmol/L)

*Abnormal*
- Results outside normal reference range
- Keep in mind the possibility of a false-positive result

*Cause of abnormal result*
- Renal failure of any cause
- Hepatorenal syndrome

*Drugs, disorders and other factors that may alter results*
- Hemolytic, icteric, and lipemic specimens can give erroneous results

- Spurious elevations can occur in the presence of glucose, uric acid, alpha-ketoacids, and ascorbate when certain methods of measurement are used
- Cephalosporin antibiotics, dopamine, lidocaine, and 5-fluorocytosine can all cause artifactual elevations of the results

## COMPLETE BLOOD COUNT
*Description*
- Test should include red cell count and red cell indices, white cell count with differential, and platelet count
- Venous blood sample sent to the laboratory in a tube without anticoagulant

*Advantages/Disadvantages*
Advantage: simple, inexpensive.

*Normal*
Red blood cells:
- Hemoglobin: 13.6–17.7g/dL (males); 12.0–15.0g/dL (females)
- Mean cell volume: 76–100mcm$^3$ (76–100fL)
- Mean cell hemoglobin: 27–33pg
- Mean cell hemoglobin concentration: 33–37g/dL (330–370g/L)
- Hematocrit: 39–49% (males); 33–43% (females)

White blood cells:
- White cell count: 3200–9800 cells/mm$^3$ (3.2–9.8x10$^9$ cells/L)
- Basophils: 10–1000 cells/mm$^3$ (<0.01–1.0x10$^9$ cells/L)
- Eosinophils: 40–400 cells/mm$^3$ (0.04–0.4 x10$^9$ cells/L)
- Lymphocytes: 1500–4000 cells/mm$^3$ (1.5–4.0x10$^9$ cells/L)
- Monocytes: 200–800 cells/mm$^3$ (0.2–0.8x10$^9$ cells/L)
- Neutrophils: 3500–7500 cells/mm$^3$ (3.5–7.5x10$^9$ cells/L)

Platelets:
- 130–400x10$^3$ cells/mm$^3$ (130–400x10$^9$ cells/L)

*Abnormal*
- Results outside normal reference range
- Keep in mind the possibility of a false-positive result

*Cause of abnormal result*
- Anemia seen in liver disease is usually macrocytic (mean cell volume >100mcm$^3$)
- Megaloblastic changes due to combined vitamin B12, folate, and vitamin B6 deficiencies commonly occur
- Anemia may be due to gastrointestinal blood loss, hypersplenism, or a direct suppressive effect on the bone marrow from alcohol
- Leukocytosis in patients presenting with alcoholic hepatitis may be suggestive of sepsis
- A leukemoid elevation in the range of 20,000 cells/mm$^3$ often signals sepsis, especially in the presence of fever
- Thrombocytopenia may be due to hypersplenism or a direct suppressive effect of alcohol on the bone marrow

## SERUM ALBUMIN
*Description*
Venous blood sample sent to the laboratory in a tube without anticoagulant.

*Advantages/Disadvantages*
Advantages:
- Measures protein synthetic activity of the liver
- Level correlates well with the severity of the liver disease

*Normal*
3.5–5.5g/dL (35–55g/L).

*Abnormal*
- <3.5g/dL (<35g/L)
- >5.5g/dL (>55g/L)
- Keep in mind the possibility of a false-positive result

*Cause of abnormal result*
Decreased serum albumin can be caused by:
- Inadequate nutrition
- Decreased hepatic synthetic activity
- Gastrointestinal loss due to inflammatory conditions such as inflammatory bowel disease
- Kidney diseases causing loss of albumin in urine

Increased serum albumin is artifactually caused by volume contraction.

*Drugs, disorders and other factors that may alter results*
Genetic abnormalities leading to absence of albumin or abnormal molecular forms.

## SERUM BILIRUBIN
*Description*
Venous blood sample.

*Advantages/Disadvantages*
Advantage: serves as a general assessment of hepatic cellular uptake, synthetic and secretory functions.

*Normal*
- Total: 0.2–1.0mg/dL (3–17mcmol/L)
- Conjugated: 0–0.2mg/dL (0–3mcmol/L)

*Abnormal*
- Any value above the upper limit of the normal range
- Keep in mind the possibility of a false-positive result

*Cause of abnormal result*
- Hepatocellular injury
- Biliary obstruction

*Drugs, disorders and other factors that may alter results*
- Hemolysis
- Lipemia
- Exposure of the specimen to light, especially ultraviolet light or sunlight, causes rapid loss of bilirubin from specimen

## PROTHROMBIN TIME AND INTERNATIONAL NORMALIZED RATIO
*Description*
- The PT is a measure of the activity of the extrinsic and common coagulation pathways
- The INR is a standardized calculation of the PT that measures all commercial assays against a World Health Organization reference thromboplastin
- Venous blood sample must be collected in a vessel that contains an anticoagulant that does not contain calcium

*Advantages/Disadvantages*
Advantage: can evaluate the competency of the extrinsic and common coagulation pathways, in which factors synthesized in the liver are involved.

*Normal*
- PT: 10–14s
- INR: 1.0

*Abnormal*
- Any value outside the control range
- In the arena of acute alcoholic hepatitis, a discriminant function (DF) can be calculated using the PT and bilirubin to assess the severity
- DF = 4.6 x [prothrombin time (seconds) – control time (seconds)] + bilirubin (mg/dL) calculated after vitamin K replacement is given
- A result >32 predicts a mortality from liver failure within one month of approx. 50%
- Keep in mind the possibility of a false-positive result

*Cause of abnormal result*
Liver disease.

*Drugs, disorders and other factors that may alter results*
- Vitamin K deficiency, often seen as part of the poor nutrition of patients with chronic alcoholism, can cause prolongation of the PT in spite of adequate synthetic ability
- Genetic abnormalities of the coagulation factors (congenital factor VII deficiency)
- Warfarin therapy

## SERUM AMMONIA
*Description*
Venous blood.

*Advantages/Disadvantages*
Advantage: Relatively simple test that correlates with degree of hepatic failure.

*Normal*
10–80mcg/dL (5–50mcmol/L).

*Abnormal*
- Values outside the normal range
- Keep in mind the possibility of a false-positive result

*Cause of abnormal result*
Hepatic failure.

*Drugs, disorders and other factors that may alter results*
- Portacaval shunt
- Drugs (including diuretics, methicillin, polymyxin B)

## Biopsy
### LIVER BIOPSY
*Description*
Can be performed by a certified gastroenterologist or radiologist. Most common approach is percutaneous liver biopsy; a transjugular approach is used in selected circumstances.

*Advantages/Disadvantages*
- Advantage: liver parenchyma obtained is suitable for histology and iron studies, giving specific diagnosis for therapeutic decisions
- Disadvantage: invasive procedure, with approx. 1–5% risk of serious bleeding. Patients experience pain, can develop secondary infections, pneumothorax, and perforation of the luminal gastrointestinal tract or gallbladder

*Normal*
Normal liver parenchyma and architecture.

*Abnormal*
- Steatosis, Mallory's hyaline, inflammatory infiltrate with neutrophils being the predominant cells
- Fibrosis is always abnormal and is an indicator of cirrhosis risk

*Cause of abnormal result*
The results of a liver biopsy in alcoholic hepatitis are believed to be due to direct toxic effects of alcohol on the liver. The longer the duration of inflammation is, the greater are the chances that fibrosis will be seen.

*Drugs, disorders and other factors that may alter results*
Nonalcoholic steatohepatitis is indistinguishable from early alcoholic hepatitis.

## Imaging
### ABDOMINAL ULTRASOUND
*Advantages/Disadvantages*
Advantages:
- Can detect parenchymal changes typical of fatty liver
- Can detect changes typical of advanced cirrhosis
- Can evaluate portal venous blood flow when coupled with Doppler examination
- Can detect masses and cysts
- Can detect secondary splenomegaly

Disadvantage: imaging abnormalities observed are common to all progressive diseases of the liver and are not specific to alcoholic liver disease.

*Normal*
Smooth liver of normal size.

*Abnormal*
- Enlarged liver of decreased density indicative of fatty change
- Small liver with irregular contours indicative of cirrhosis

- Decreased portal venous flow
- Keep in mind the possibility of a falsely abnormal result

*Cause of abnormal result*
- Parenchymal liver disease
- Portal venous compression due to cirrhosis
- Congestive splenomegaly
- Masses and cysts of abdominal organs

*Drugs, disorders and other factors that may alter results*
Other progressive diseases of the liver will show the same changes on ultrasound; they are not specific to alcoholic liver disease.

## Special tests
VIRAL HEPATITIS SEROLOGIES
*Description*
Serum is the preferred sample, collected via routine venepuncture into nonanticoagulated tubes or syringes.

*Advantages/Disadvantages*
Advantage: allows evaluation of the possible role of viral hepatitis in the genesis of the current illness.

*Normal*
Hepatitis B markers:
- Hepatitis B surface antigen: negative
- Hepatitis B e-antigen: negative
- Hepatitis B anticore antibody: negative or positive (positivity indicates past exposure if other two markers are negative)

Hepatitis C markers:
- Hepatitis C virus RNA (by polymerase chain reaction): negative
- Antihepatitis C virus antibody (by enzyme-linked immunoassay): negative
- Hepatitis C virus antibody (by recombinant immunoblot assay): negative

*Abnormal*
Hepatitis B markers (acute infection):
- Hepatitis B surface antigen: positive
- Hepatitis B e-antigen: positive (indicates active viral replication)
- Hepatitis B DNA: positive
- Hepatitis B anticore antibody: positive (IgM)

Hepatitis B markers (chronic infection):
- Hepatitis B surface antigen: positive
- Hepatitis B e-antigen: positive or negative
- Hepatitis B DNA: positive
- Hepatitis B anticore antibody: positive (IgG)

Hepatitis C markers:
- Hepatitis C virus RNA: positive
- Antihepatitis C virus antibody: positive

Keep in mind the possibility of a falsely abnormal result.

*Cause of abnormal result*
Active or chronic hepatitis B or C virus infection.

*Drugs, disorders and other factors that may alter results*
- Immunocompromised status can result in false-negative antibody results, especially in detection of hepatitis C virus infection
- Viral parameters below limits of detection

## Other tests
BLOOD CULTURE
*Description*
- Venous blood is obtained from at least two sterile sites according to the procedures established by the laboratory providing the cultures
- The cultures should be directed at detecting aerobic, anaerobic, and fungal micro-organisms

*Advantages/Disadvantages*
- Advantage: can detect infecting micro-organism and antibiotic sensitivities
- Disadvantage: time delay before results are available

*Normal*
No growth.

*Abnormal*
- Growth of micro-organisms
- Keep in mind the possibility of a falsely abnormal result, especially as a result of contamination

*Cause of abnormal result*
Sepsis.

*Drugs, disorders and other factors that may alter results*
- Prior antibiotic therapy may cause a false-negative result
- Contamination of the specimen with normal skin flora may cause a false-positive result

# TREATMENT

## CONSIDER CONSULT
Although the clinical severity varies widely, from a mild illness to fatal hepatic insufficiency, the initial and immediate stabilization should be performed by the primary care physician (PCP). The specialist (gastroenterologist or hepatologist) may then be consulted for further evaluation and management; however, even in the best care of specialists, this illness can have a 50% hospital mortality in its most severe form.

## IMMEDIATE ACTION
- Control any seizure activity with benzodiazepine
- Institute broad-spectrum antibiotic treatment after appropriate work-up if signs or symptoms of sepsis are present
- Administer vitamin K for coagulopathy
- Treat severe ascites with paracentesis and colloid replacement; paracentesis can also rule out spontaneous bacterial peritonitis
- Institute measures to correct encephalopathy (lactulose)
- Stop diuretics and hydrate to preserve renal function
- Control any gastrointestinal bleeding (volume resuscitation, correct coagulopathy and/or thrombocytopenia, then endoscopic sclerotherapy or endoscopic variceal ligation, if indicated)

## PATIENT AND CAREGIVER ISSUES
### Health-seeking behavior
Abstinence and nutrition are the cornerstones of therapy for alcoholic liver disease and alcoholic hepatitis. Inquire from the patient or family and friends about:
- Attempts to participate or participation in counseling and support groups that could ensure long-term abstinence from alcohol
- Socioeconomic and environmental issues affecting the possibility of adequate nutrition

## MANAGEMENT ISSUES
### Goals
- Attend to immediately life-threatening presentations (e.g. bleeding esophageal varices, sepsis, hepatorenal syndrome, encephalopathy, withdrawal seizures)
- Admit to hospital or care facility
- Consult gastroenterologist for management after calculating the discriminant function
- Determine whether presentation is alcohol-related
- Encourage the patient to abstain from alcohol in the future

### Management in special circumstances
COEXISTING DISEASE
- Viral hepatitis can confound the diagnosis and accelerate hepatic injury
- Underlying advanced cirrhosis decreases functional hepatic reserve, thereby creating urgency to the restoration of liver function

COEXISTING MEDICATION
- Acetaminophen, nonsteroidal anti-inflammatory drugs (NSAIDs), and salicylates should be discontinued immediately because of their potentiating effect on liver injury
- Warfarin derivatives can exacerbate bleeding and should be discontinued upon presentation
- Many popular herbal preparations, most notably those containing *Ginkgo biloba*, can have potent anticoagulant effects, and therefore should be discontinued immediately

SPECIAL PATIENT GROUPS
Women have a lower threshold for developing alcoholic liver disease than men do, and women

progress more rapidly once it has developed. For this reason the index of suspicion for alcohol-related illness should be higher in the right setting for women, even though the alcohol intake might not appear adequate to warrant this diagnosis.

### PATIENT SATISFACTION/LIFESTYLE PRIORITIES
- Because abstinence and nutrition play key roles in the long-term survival of patients with alcoholic hepatitis and alcoholic liver disease in general, lifestyle changes are often essential in realizing this goal. This sometimes means avoiding social circles and situations that encourage alcohol ingestion, and this may be objected to by the patient
- Because nutrition plays a major role in the survival of these patients, changes in dietary habits are usually in order, emphasizing more feeding in the day, especially before retiring at night and after waking in the morning
- The patient may need to be placed in an environment in which adequate nutrition is assured, and this may mean loss of some independence. This may be unacceptable to the patient, and hinder attempts to salvage the patient in the long-term

## SUMMARY OF THERAPEUTIC OPTIONS
### Choices
Treatment in the acute phase:
- Control of esophageal variceal bleeding via balloon tamponade or transjugular intrahepatic portosystemic shunt may be necessary if endoscopic band ligation or sclerotherapy is initially not successful in controlling the bleeding
- Lactulose is required for encephalopathy. If encephalopathy is present, patient would most likely be managed in hospital
- Antibiotic therapy is instituted to treat sepsis, if present
- Prednisolone treatment has been shown to reduce short-term mortality in severe acute alcoholic hepatitis. This treatment would be instituted by a subspecialist in an intensive care setting, since the patients who benefit from this treatment are those with a discriminant function >32 or those with spontaneous hepatic encephalopathy. Exclusion criteria for the use of corticosteroids include renal failure, infection, active gastrointestinal hemorrhage, pancreatitis, and severe comorbid illness
- Benzodiazepines are the first-line treatment for seizures and withdrawal symptoms
- Paracentesis with colloid replacement is the standard treatment for severe ascites and is also required to rule out spontaneous bacterial peritonitis. This procedure is performed as an inpatient
- Aggressive nutrition with supplements is a necessary part of treatment for patients who drink excessive alcohol

Long-term treatment:
- Transjugular intrahepatic portosystemic shunt may be inserted by a specialist for refractory ascites or variceal bleeding
- Aggressive nutrition is essential in the promotion of recovery from alcoholic hepatitis. The severe protein and calorie malnutrition that is prevalent in patients who present with acute alcoholic hepatitis has been well documented along with the kind of supplementation and intake required to correct the various deficiencies and promote resumption of hepatic functions. Thiamine supplementation may be required to prevent Korsakoff's psychosis
- Abstinence/rehabilitation/counseling are essential to prolonging survival
- Liver transplantation is a last resort treatment in cases of fulminant hepatic failure. However, transplantation is generally not performed in patients who are actively drinking
- Treatment with pentoxifylline (a tumor necrosis factor-alpha inhibitor) dosed at 400mg orally three times daily for 4 weeks has recently been shown to decrease mortality and the incidence of hepatorenal syndrome in acute alcoholic hepatitis, but confirmatory studies are not available yet; thus, it cannot be recommended for use at this time

### Clinical pearls
Control of volume status, sepsis, coagulopathy, gastrointestinal bleeding, alcohol withdrawal syndrome, encephalopathy, and hypoglycemia is essential to decrease mortality and morbidity.

### FOLLOW UP
- Routine assessment of liver function by measuring serum bilirubin, prothrombin time, and albumin
- Routine assessment of renal function, neurologic state, and nutritional status
- Monitor degree of abstinence

### Plan for review
- Follow-up liver function tests, bilirubin, and prothrombin time
- Follow-up renal function tests, and determine volume status on physical examination
- Routinely assess neurologic state
- Monitor protein and calorie intake and nutritional state
- Review prescription and over-the-counter (OTC) medications

### Information for patient or caregiver
- Alcoholic hepatitis is a serious life-threatening disorder caused by ingestion of alcohol
- Abstinence from alcohol is essential to avoiding progression of liver disease and death
- Good nutrition is also essential to avoiding progression of liver disease and death

### DRUGS AND OTHER THERAPIES: DETAILS
#### Drugs
LACTULOSE
A synthetic disaccharide that acidifies that colon contents, thereby preventing the absorption of ammonia from the bowel lumen and mitigating its participation in producing hepatic encephalopathy.

*Dose*
- 160g/day orally, or 20% solution administered as a retention enema, 1000mL three times daily
- Dose should be titrated to achieve three or four soft bowel movements per day

*Efficacy*
Effective in over 80% of patients in decreasing blood ammonia levels and improving encephalopathy.

*Risks/benefits*
Risks:
- A theoretical hazard may exist for patients being treated with lactulose solution who may be required to undergo electrocautery procedures during proctoscopy or colonoscopy
- Preparations will contains galactose (<2.2g/15mL) and lactose (<1.2g/15mL) and should be used with caution in diabetics
- In the overall management of portal-systemic encephalopathy, it should be recognized that there is serious underlying liver disease with complications such as electrolyte disturbance (e.g. hypokalemia) for which other specific therapy may be required
- Use with caution when administering to breast-feeding women

*Side effects and adverse reactions*
- Gastrointestinal: abdominal discomfort, nausea, gaseous distension with flatulence
- Excessive dosage can lead to diarrhea with potential complications such as loss of fluids, hypokalemia, and hypernatremia

*Interactions (other drugs)*
- Benzodiazepine receptor ligand (reduces the eficacy of these drugs, and contributes to its positive effect on encephalopathy) ■ Neomycin (may interfere with the degradation of lactulose) ■ Other laxatives (may interfere with lactulose dosing) ■ Nonabsorbable antacids (may inhibit the lactulose-induced drop in colonic pH)

*Contraindications*
- Patients requiring low galactose diet ■ Safety and efficacy in children have not been established ■ Pregnancy category B ■ Other laxatives should not be used especially during the initial phase of therapy for portal-systemic encephalopathy, because the loose stools resulting from their use may falsely suggest that adequate lactulose dosage has been achieved

*Acceptability to patient*
- Generally well tolerated by the patient
- Diarrhea may limit compliance in some patients

*Follow up plan*
Titrate the amount of lactulose to produce three or four soft stools per day.

*Patient and caregiver information*
- Inform patients of possible side effects (cramping, diarrhea, flatulence) and warn them about dehydration
- Indicate the therapeutic end-point (three or four soft stools per day)
- Other laxatives should be avoided while on lactulose therapy

## BROAD-SPECTRUM ANTIBIOTIC
- Broad-spectrum antibiotic coverage is often essential in the treatment of infection in alcoholic patients because of their severe immunocompromised state and because of the decreased effectiveness of the mucosal barriers to intraluminal colonic organisms
- Sepsis, when it occurs, is frequently manifested at first as spontaneous bacterial peritonitis
- The most common organisms isolated are *Escherichia coli* and the pneumococcus
- Cefotaxime is the current drug of choice for this complication

*Dose*
Cefotaxime: 2g three times a day intravenously or intramuscularly for at least 5 days for spontaneous bacterial peritonitis.

*Efficacy*
Antibiotics are effective in controlling infections caused by a wide variety of pathogens to which alcoholic patients are susceptible, including spontaneous bacterial peritonitis.

*Risks/benefits*
Risks:
- Use caution with hypersensitivity to penicillins
- Use caution with renal impairment
- Risk of pseudomembranous colitis
- Potentially life-threatening arrhymias following rapid (<60s) bolus administration via central venous catheter have been observed

*Side effects and adverse reactions*
- Central nervous system: headache, sleep disturbance, confusion, dizziness
- Gastrointestinal: anorexia, nausea, diarrhea, abdominal pain, bleeding, raised liver enzymes, colitis, vomiting, pseudomembranous colitis

- Genitourinary: moniliasis, vaginitis
- Hematologic: neutropenia, transient leukopenia, eosinophilia, thrombocytopenia, agranulocytosis
- Hypersensitivity manifestations (pruritus, fever, eosinophilia, urticaria, and (rarely) anaphylaxis: 2.4%)
- Skin: rash, dermatitis, injection site reaction
- Other: interstitial nephritis and transient elevations of blood urea nitrogen and creatinine have been occasionally observed with cefotaxime sodium, transient elevations in aspartate aminotranferase, alanine aminotransferase, serum lactate dehydrogenase, and serum alkaline phosphatase levels have been reported

*Interactions (other drugs)*
- Aminoglycosides
- Chloramphenicol
- Oral anticoagulants
- Probenecid
- Vancomycin
- Polymyxin B

*Contraindications*
- Hypersensitivity to cefotaxime
- Age less than one month

*Acceptability to patient*
- Generally well tolerated by patient
- Can be administered parenterally

*Follow up plan*
- Monitor patient for infectious processes
- Monitor renal function and adjust dose accordingly

## PREDNISOLONE
- A glucocorticoid representing the active form of its sister compound prednisone
- In severe alcoholic hepatitis, in which there is decreased hepatic function, prednisolone (as opposed to prednisone) was considered the preferred drug in the past, but it now seems that the metabolism of prednisone is not affected in severe alcoholic hepatitis and so prednisone may be used
- Patients requiring this treatment should be treated as inpatients, owing to the severity of their disease

*Dose*
Prednisolone or prednisone 40mg/day for 4 weeks followed by doses tapered to zero.

*Efficacy*
- The efficacy of corticosteroids in alcoholic hepatitis is controversial
- Corticosteroid therapy for acute alcoholic hepatitis may reduce short-term mortality in those patients presenting with severe disease (spontaneous encephalopathy or discriminant function >32). However, some studies have found no beneficial effect with corticosteroid therapy
- In all other subgroups there is no solid evidence that corticosteroid therapy improves outcome
- Efficacy of corticosteroid therapy is reduced in patients with acute gastrointestinal bleeding

*Risks/benefits*
Risks:
- Overwhelming septicemia if patient has an infection
- Loss of control of blood glucose in those with diabetes
- Prolonged use causes adrenal suppression
- Use caution in elderly due to risk of diabetes and osteoporosis
- Use caution in patients with psychosis, seizure disorders, or myasthenia gravis

- Use caution in congestive heart failure, hypertension
- Use caution in ulcerative colitis, peptic ulcer, or esophagitis

*Side effects and adverse reactions*
- Side effects are minimized by short duration of therapy
- Cardiovascular system: hypertension, thromboembolism
- Central nervous system: insomnia, euphoria, depression, psychosis
- Endocrine: adrenal suppression, impaired glucose tolerance, growth suppression in children
- Eyes, ears, nose, and throat: cataract, glaucoma, blurred vision
- Gastrointestinal: dyspepsia, peptic ulceration, esophagitis, oral candidiasis
- Musculoskeletal: proximal myopathy, osteoporosis
- Skin: delayed healing, acne, striae

*Interactions (other drugs)*
- Aminoglutethimide ■ Barbiturates ■ Cholestyramine ■ Clarithromycin, erythromycin
- Colestipol ■ Isoniazid ■ Ketoconazole ■ NSAIDs ■ Oral contraceptives ■ Rifampin
- Salicylates ■ Troleandomycin ■ Warfarin

*Contraindications*
- Systemic infection ■ Avoid live virus vaccines in those receiving immunosuppressive doses

*Acceptability to patient*
- Many of the numerous side effects are unacceptable to patients over the long-term
- The prospect of prolonging survival in a potentially life-threatening situation as well as the limited term of treatment might serve to mitigate these apprehensions

*Follow up plan*
The patient should be monitored closely for signs of the development of any infectious process or of the potentially life-threatening effects of corticosteroid therapy.

*Patient and caregiver information*
- The patient should be fully informed as to the possible side effects of corticosteroid treatment
- Aspirin and its derivatives should be avoided

## BENZODIAZEPINE
- The benzodiazepines are a class of agents that have antianxiety and sedative effects, along with appetite stimulating and weak analgesic actions
- Chlordiazepoxide is the original drug in this class and is the most widely used for acute alcohol withdrawal
- Oxazepam is also used commonly because it undergoes little hepatic metabolism

*Dose*
- Chlordiazepoxide hydrochloride: 10–30mg every 6h, tapering over 3–6 days
- Oxazepam: 10–30mg three or four times daily, tapering over 3–6 days

*Efficacy*
Effective in treating symptoms of acute alcohol withdrawal, including seizures.

*Risks/benefits*
Risks:
- Use caution in hepatic and renal disease and in status epilepticus
- Use caution in the elderly and children
- May cause drowsiness (40–75%) or confusion (15%)

- Inadvisable in the elderly and in drivers
- Ineffective in major depression; may worsen depressive symptoms
- Risk of dependency (though risk small with therapeutic use) and withdrawal symptoms

*Side effects and adverse reactions*
- Central nervous system: extrapyramidal neurologic signs
- Gastrointestinal: nausea, constipaton (with long-term use)
- Genitourinary: changes in libido, menstrual irregularities
- Hypersensitivity reactions
- Other: exacerbation of porphyria

*Interactions (other drugs)*
- **Monoamine oxidase (MAO) inhibitors (potentiation of MAO inhibitors)** - Oral anticoagulants (potentiation of anticoagulant effect)

*Contraindications*
- **Known hypersensitivity to benzodiazepines** - **Pregnancy** - **Known porphyria** - **Pregnancy and breast-feeding**

*Acceptability to patient*
The suppression of withdrawal symptoms without the production of sedation makes this drug highly acceptable to patients.

*Follow up plan*
Monitor the patient for appropriate dosage:
- Somnolence indicates overdosage
- Persistence of withdrawal symptoms indicates underdosage

*Patient and caregiver information*
- Information pertaining to side effects is important in longer-term use
- However, in the setting of acute alcohol withdrawal, patients are frequently not of sufficient cognition as to comprehend this information
- Furthermore, duration of treatment is usually sufficiently limited as to avoid serious side effects

## Surgical therapy
- Surgical intervention can benefit the patient with complications of decompensated alcoholic cirrhosis
- Persistent re-bleeding of esophageal varices may require portosystemic shunt surgery if permanent relief of portal venous pressure needs to be accomplished; however, surgery of any kind is contraindicated in the setting of acute alcoholic hepatitis
- Total intractable liver failure may require orthotopic liver allograft, as the only therapeutic option remaining. However, transplantation of an actively drinking patient is controversial and is rarely performed

TRANSJUGULAR INTRAHEPATIC PORTOSYSTEMIC SHUNT INSERTION
Insertion of a transjugular intrahepatic portosystemic shunt (TIPS) consists of the placement of an intrahepatic shunt between a major intrahepatic branch of the portal vein and the vena cava.

Contraindications to TIPS include:
- Known polycystic liver disease
- Cholangitis or any condition causing bile duct dilation
- Portal/hepatic vein occlusion
- Active hepatic encephalopathy

*Efficacy*
- Current experience indicates that, with successful TIPS placement, reduction of portal pressure and elimination of varices can occur in almost all patients
- Although stenosis of the shunt occurs in one-third to one-half of all patients, stent patency and portal decompression can be maintained by repeated radiologic intervention, if needed

*Risks/benefits*
The risks of the procedure itself are small with current techniques and technology.

Risks:
- Inadvertent puncture of the hepatic capsule leading to hemoperitoneum
- Puncture of a dilated biliary radical leading to hemobilia or bile embolism
- Inadvertent puncture of the gallbladder or other adjacent organs such as the kidney or large bowel, leading to complications related to those sites
- Contrast media-induced renal failure
- Cardiac failure or transient arrhythmias
- Infection

Future complications of the TIPS procedure include:
- Encephalopathy (20–30%) caused by hepatofugal flow of the portal circulation
- Accelerated hepatic failure caused by decreased hepatic perfusion (5%); this is partially related to the severity of the underlying liver disease
- Recurrent variceal bleeding caused by shunt dysfunction (<25%)

Benefit: portal venous decompression reducing or eliminating the risk of life-threatening esophageal hemorrhage, and halting the formation of ascites.

*Acceptability to patient*
- TIPS is much less invasive than traditional portosystemic shunt procedures and therefore carries a lower degree of operative mortality or morbidity
- This fact alone makes the procedure more acceptable to the patient

*Follow up plan*
- Doppler ultrasonography of portal venous flow every 3–6 months
- Venography is indicated if shunt insufficiency is suspected (e.g. reversal of intrahepatic flow, maximal peak flow velocity within the shunt is <0.5m/s)
- Percutaneous shunt revision if indicated

*Patient and caregiver information*
- Any signs of encephalopathy or gastroesophageal bleedingshould be reported
- Abstinence from alcohol ingestion is required
- Maintenance of adequate nutrition is important

## PARACENTESIS
- Paracentesis is the evacuation of fluid from the abdominal cavity
- It is usually performed by inserting a soft catheter into the abdominal cavity through a sterile site located in the lower abdomen
- When large volumes (>1L) are to be removed, colloid should be replaced in the form of human albumin at the rate of 10g/L of fluid removed, especially if renal failure is present
- In the setting of hepatic failure of any cause, paracentesis may be used to reduce severe intractable ascites causing volume depletion secondary to 'third spacing' of fluid
- Paracentesis of high volumes may provide only temporary relief in inflammatory states such as alcoholic hepatitis

*Efficacy*
- Paracentesis is an effective way to reduce ascites if salt restriction and diuretics have not been successful
- Effective when there is an acute need to reduce patient pain, discomfort or shortness of breath
- Useful for obtaining ascitic fluid for culture and analysis
- There are no patient-specific parameters during the procedure other than to remain still during the procedure to avoid unnecessary morbidity

*Risks/benefits*
Risks:
- Hypovolemic shock and renal failure may be precipitated by removing too much fluid too quickly without adequate replacement by colloid and appropriate crystalloid
- Perforation of a hollow viscus during insertion of the catheter and a resultant secondary peritonitis

Benefits:
- Relieves patient pain/discomfort
- Allows analysis of ascitic fluid (neutrophils >250/mcL is indicative of peritonitis, and culture and Gram stain of the ascitic fluid will help to determine which organisms are the culprits if peritonitis is present. Albumin concentration can be used to diagnose portal hypertension)

*Acceptability to patient*
The following points must be made to the patient when paracentesis is contemplated in the treatment of complications of alcoholic liver disease:
- The procedure is relatively benign
- Paracentesis will provide relief from the pain and discomfort of ascites
- Paracentesis will provide important diagnostic information

### LIVER TRANSPLANTATION
Liver transplantation is the treatment of last resort for end-stage liver disease, be it from cirrhosis or fulminant failure. It is not indicated in patients who have adequate liver function and who present with acute esophageal bleeding, and is not indicated in patients who currently have alcoholic hepatitis. Furthermore, it is generally not performed in patients who are actively drinking alcohol.

*Efficacy*
- Patients with end-stage cirrhotic alcoholic liver disease have a 5-year survival of 80–90%, equivalent to patients transplanted for other causes of hepatic failure
- Those patients transplanted for fulminant failure secondary to acute alcoholic hepatitis have a lower 5-year survival rate

*Risks/benefits*
Risks:
- Infection from lifelong immunosuppression
- Recurrence of liver disease from continued alcohol abuse

Benefit:
- Cures the systemic manifestations of liver failure

*Acceptability to patient*
The question is not only of acceptability to the patient but also of availability of a donor organ. There are approx. 26,000 cirrhosis-related deaths each year in the US, but only about 3000 livers available for transplantation.

The patient with an impending demise from alcohol-related liver disease must consider the following conditions for this procedure:
- Most centers require at least 6 months of documented abstinence from alcohol before the transplant and complete abstinence after the transplant
- Patient must be able to comply with a regimen of lifelong immunosuppressive therapy and antimicrobial prophylaxis and follow-up appointments
- Patient must recognize the possibility of life-threatening intercurrent infections

*Follow up plan*
- Monitor immunosuppression
- Monitor liver function for signs of rejection
- Monitor for signs of infection

*Patient and caregiver information*
- The patient must be made aware of the risks inherent in organ transplantation and the necessary lifelong commitment to therapy and follow up
- In the alcoholic patient, beneficial lifestyle changes that affect outcome must be stressed

## Complementary therapy
NUTRITIONAL THERAPY
In the presentation of severe alcoholic liver disease, one universal feature is that of severe protein and calorie malnutrition. Such malnutrition is responsible for many of the metabolic and immunologic dysfunctions of these patients. Consequently, a major part of therapy is directed towards putting these patients back into positive nitrogen balance. The components of such therapy are:
- Protein: 1.0g/kg body weight should be consumed, even in patients with encephalopathy (except perhaps initially)
- Total calories: 1.2–1.4 times the resting energy expenditure with a minimum of 30kcal/kg body weight; 50–55% should be consumed as carbohydrate and 30–35% as fat, preferably as unsaturated fat rich in essential fatty acids
- Nutrition should be taken orally or by small bore nasogastric feeding tube
- Salt and water intake should be adjusted to patient's fluid volume
- Liberal multivitamins and minerals are required
- Intramuscular thiamine is advised in encephalopathic patients
- Specialized branched chain amino acids (BCAA) are useful in patients with recurrent encephalopathy (mixed with other sources of amino acids since BCAAs do not promote positive nitrogen balance), but they are expensive
- Essential amino acids (choline, cystine, taurine, and tyrosine)
- S-adenosyl methionine instead of methionine

*Efficacy*
Establishment of a positive nitrogen balance and caloric intake can help to reverse many of the hepatic and systemic effects of acute alcoholic liver disease.

*Risks/benefits*
Benefits:
- Improves immunocompetence
- Encourages hepatic regenerative activity
- Provides substrates for hepatic function

*Acceptability to patient*
- In the acute period, patient acceptability is not an issue
- After the patient is stabilized, compliance with nutritional issues may become a factor in the eventual outcome for the patient

- One must strive to present nutritional goals of therapy within the resources of the patient
- A professional nutritionist or dietitian should be consulted

*Follow up plan*
Formally evaluate nutritional status on a regular basis, every 3–6 months once the patient leaves the hospital.

*Patient and caregiver information*
- Emphasize the importance of multiple daily meals, especially upon waking and before retiring
- Emphasize higher than normal caloric intake

### Endoscopic therapy
Endoscopic therapy is indicated in severe variceal bleeding or in variceal bleeding that persists despite standard medical and endoscopic therapy.

ENDOESOPHAGEAL COMPRESSION (BALLOON TAMPONADE)
- Balloon tamponade is a method of intraluminal compression of varices to control bleeding that is effective in many cases when the other modalities have initially failed at controlling hemorrhage
- It consists of the insertion of an inflatable tube with balloon apparatus, either the Sengstaken-Blakemore tube or the newer Minnesota tube, into the esophagus, inflating the balloon and exerting upward traction

*Efficacy*
When the tube is placed properly without complications, balloon tamponade is very effective in controlling the acute presentation of bleeding.

*Risks/benefits*
Risks:
- High rate of rebleeding upon balloon deflation
- High rate of complications, including asphyxiation, esophageal rupture, and aspiration pneumonia
- Some studies have demonstrated a 25% mortality with the actual placement of the tube

Benefits:
- Can be used quickly
- Can be used in urgent situations
- Good for temporizing until a more definitive procedure can be instituted

*Follow up plan*
Usually transjugular intrahepatic portosystemic shunting or insertion of a surgical shunt follows balloon tamponade since typically the endoscopic sclerotherapy or band ligation, which was initially performed, failed to control the hemorrhage.

### LIFESTYLE
Since chronic alcoholism is a behavioral malady and abstinence is the most important factor in recovery from alcoholic hepatitis, major revisions in lifestyle are essential:
- Abstinence is essential to prolonged survival
- Adequate nutrition is essential to prolonged survival, indicating a probable necessary change in feeding habits
- Intensive counseling, enrollment in a rehabilitative program, and the intercession of support groups are usually necessary to promote lifestyle changes

- Abstinence often requires some change in the social milieu of the patient, a difficult and sometimes impossible task for the patient

## RISKS/BENEFITS
Benefits:
- Abstinence and good nutrition can often mitigate much hepatic damage and prolong survival; failure to abstain from alcohol in a patient presenting with severe acute alcoholic hepatitis results in almost certain mortality within 5 years of initial presentation
- Abstinence is a requirement for consideration for transplantation, should the liver disease progress

## ACCEPTABILITY TO PATIENT
Compliance is the main issue in accomplishing abstinence; it may be extremely difficult for patients to engage in the social changes required to become abstinent.

## FOLLOW UP PLAN
Provide resources for the patient to contact:
- Counseling services
- Twelve-step or other support groups

## PATIENT AND CAREGIVER INFORMATION
The patient needs to be made aware of and understand the consequences of continued drinking.

## OUTCOMES

### EFFICACY OF THERAPIES
- Abstinence is essential for hope of recovery in all patients with alcoholic hepatitis. About 25–30% of abstainees with mild-to-moderate disease and without cirrhosis will show histologic normalization, while 55–60% will show histologic alcoholic hepatitis for up to 14 months. About 15–20% of abstaining patients will progress to cirrhosis despite their abstention
- Establishment of a positive nitrogen balance and caloric intake can reverse many of the hepatic and systemic effects of acute alcoholic hepatic decompensation
- Prednisolone is effective in reducing the short-term mortality in the subgroup of patients with severe alcoholic hepatitis (those with discriminant function >32 and those with spontaneous encephalopathy after specific criteria are met) as concluded by recent meta-analysis of published trials. Long-term prognosis (>1 year) is unaffected by this treatment

### Review period
- Once a patient has been diagnosed with alcoholic hepatitis, continuous surveillance with serum aminotransferase levels, bilirubin levels, and prothrombin times is necessary to detect and prevent early recurrences of alcoholic hepatitis
- There are no standard intervals of testing, and follow up needs to be determined on a case by case basis
- The most rational approach would be slowly increasing intervals as one is convinced that recovery is proceeding as desired

### PROGNOSIS
- Even with adequate intervention, those patients presenting with severe acute alcoholic hepatitis and a discriminant function >32 and those with spontaneous encephalopathy have a mortality rate of approx. 50% at one month
- Patients who present with a very high bilirubin level, a raised creatinine level, an increased international normalized ratio (INR), and ascites or encephalopathy have a very poor short-term prognosis
- In severe alcoholic hepatitis with spontaneous encephalopathy, patients have almost a zero 5-year survival rate and a 20% one-year survival rate without transplantation
- With continued drinking 50% of patients experiencing an episode of mild-to-moderate alcoholic hepatitis will develop cirrhosis, and 40% of these will die within 5 years
- Once cirrhosis has developed, the 5-year survival drops to 16–25% in patients who continue to drink
- Abstinence can reduce mortality by 50% at 5 years, regardless of the degree of liver damage at the time of presentation

### Clinical pearls
- Discriminant function has two components: elevation in prothrombin time and bilirubin. Once appropriate therapy is initiated and gastrointestinal bleeding is under control, the first sign of good prognosis is the correction of prothrombin time. The bilirubin almost always stays elevated and could take weeks to months to come to near normal. Bilirubin may continue to rise even if the patient shows good prognostic signs
- Serum creatinine is elevated and there is intravascular volume depletion in the setting of total sodium overload. Long-acting diuretics should be avoided and serum electrolytes should be measured daily to aid in patient management. If serum creatinine continues to rise on diuretics, stop diuretics and start hydration until the creatinine level drops to a level <1.8mg/dL. These adjustments help to prevent hepatorenal syndrome, which is a negative prognostic marker. Once sepsis and peritonitis are under control, fluid and electrolyte management gets easier
- It is also important to ascertain the contribution of alcohol in patients with chronic hepatitis B or C. Abstinence can delay the time course of progression to cirrhosis

### Therapeutic failure
- Insertion of a transjugular intrahepatic portosystemic shunt (TIPS) is the procedure of choice for persistent esophageal variceal hemorrhage following failed attempts at endoscopic therapy
- Metronidazole or neomycin can be added to the regimen if lactulose alone fails to improve encephalopathy significantly
- Transplantation is the only treatment for fulminant hepatic failure in the face of aggressive medical management

### Recurrence
Since recurrent alcoholic hepatitis often presents with a rapidly downhill course, liver transplantation remains the best option (if criteria are met) for patient salvage in recurrences of alcoholic hepatitis.

### Deterioration
- Deterioration of a patient (determined by the appearance of encephalopathy and/or a discriminant function approaching or >32) who initially presents with mild alcoholic hepatitis requires the institution of appropriate measures. Such treatment would be instituted by a specialist in the hospital setting
- Cefotaxime should be started if there is evidence of bacterial peritonitis
- Deterioration of a patient who initially presented with severe alcoholic hepatitis requires referral to a center for urgent care, including liver transplantation

### Terminal illness
- The patient with alcoholic liver disease whose condition deteriorates to total hepatic failure experiences a secondary multiorgan failure syndrome as a result
- These patients are terminally ill. Such patients will slip into encephalopathic coma, and intractable renal and cardiopulmonary failure. Disseminated intravascular coagulation (DIC) is often part of the terminal presentation. A bleeding diathesis may be part of the picture, secondary to both the DIC and the loss of clotting factors (caused by lack of hepatic synthesis)
- No specific therapies can be recommended, other than those directed at comfort, since even transplantation will not reverse the multisystem deterioration

## COMPLICATIONS
- Alcoholic hepatitis is a major precursor to cirrhosis of the liver
- Spontaneous bacterial peritonitis is a well-described phenomenon in many of these patients
- Coagulopathy
- Hepatic failure may result from acute, severe alcoholic hepatitis
- Hepatic decompensation, including bleeding esophageal varices, ascites, hepatorenal syndrome, and hepatic encephalopathy

## CONSIDER CONSULT
- When there is progression of hepatic failure in a patient originally presenting with mild disease
- When there is accelerated progression in a patient presenting with moderate-to-severe disease
- Any presenting complication not within the treatment repertoire of the physician (e.g. variceal bleeding, encephalopathy)

## PREVENTION

### RISK FACTORS
The only risk factor amenable to change is chronic alcohol abuse.

### MODIFY RISK FACTORS
To avoid the risk of developing alcoholic hepatitis, patients who meet the criteria for alcohol abuse must be counseled to undergo treatment for their addiction. Even though alcoholic hepatitis affects only a small fraction of chronic alcoholics, abstention from excessive alcohol intake is the only sure way of avoiding this complication.

#### Lifestyle and wellness
ALCOHOL AND DRUGS
Patients must abstain from alcohol to avoid this complication of alcoholic liver disease. In addition to finding the motivation to embrace counseling and support programs such Alcoholics Anonymous, the patient often faces giving up the social grouping that has supported their drinking. In some cases this is extremely difficult, especially if the social drinking environment includes the immediate family.

DIET
Patients with chronic alcoholism are usually malnourished or of borderline nutritional status. Emphasis must be placed on a consistent well-balanced diet. Depending on the economic status of the patient, accomplishing adequate nutrition may not be easy, necessitating the intervention of social service agencies.

ENVIRONMENT
Changing social environment may be key in the success of any given patient to abstain from alcohol. On the other hand, a social circle supporting the patient's attempts, including family members, may be enlisted to encourage positive alcohol-free behavior and good nutritional habits.

### PREVENT RECURRENCE
- Abstention from alcohol and improved nutritional habits offer the best hope for preventing a recurrence of alcoholic hepatitis
- Vigorous encouragement to enter a treatment center or a 12-step or other support program should be part of preventive efforts
- Unfortunately, patients must recognize the reality of their alcohol abuse and frequently this realization occurs only with life-threatening end-stage liver disease
- Enlisting family and friends can be helpful, but the social dynamics of alcoholism are often very complicated

#### Reassess coexisting disease
- Hepatitis B or C virus infection is a frequent accompaniment of alcoholic liver disease and can sometimes be mistaken for alcoholic hepatitis
- Similarly, latent alcoholic liver disease can be missed in a patient who is known to have viral hepatitis
- Certain aspects of treatment for viral hepatitis can precipitate acute alcoholic hepatitis

INTERACTION ALERT
Interferon alfa-2b or interferon alfa-2a is part of mainstream therapy for chronic hepatitis B and C infection. It has been shown to precipitate biopsy-proven acute alcoholic hepatitis in patients with only moderate alcohol intake or to increase the severity of alcoholic hepatitis.

PATIENT SATISFACTION/LIFESTYLE PRIORITIES
- The presence of excessive alcohol consumption and coexisting viral hepatitis infection is not infrequently the result of engaging in a high-risk lifestyle
- While social and behavioral alterations can affect the progression of alcoholic liver disease, hepatitis C or chronic hepatitis B will continue to progress regardless of these changes in lifestyle
- However, abatement of the alcoholic disease may allow for more aggressive treatment of the viral hepatitis, a point that should be emphasized to a patient who finds it difficult to embark on a course of alcohol abstention

# RESOURCES

## ASSOCIATIONS

**National Institute on Alcohol Abuse and Alcoholism (NIAAA)**
6000 Executive Boulevard - Willco Building
Bethesda, MD 20892-7003
http://www.niaaa.nih.gov

**Alcoholics Anonymous (International Office)**
Grand Central Station
PO Box 459
New York, NY 10163
Tel: (212) 870-3400
http://www.alcoholics-anonymous.org

**Women for Sobriety, Inc.**
PO Box 618
Quakertown, PA 18951-0618
Tel: (215) 536-8026
Fax: (215) 538-9026
E-mail: NewLife@nni.com
http://www.womenforsobriety.org

## KEY REFERENCES

- Alexander JF, Lischner MW, Galambos JT. Natural history of alcoholic hepatitis. II. The long-term prognosis. Am J Gastroenterol 1971;56:515–25
- Bass NM, Somberg KA. Portal hypertension and gastrointestinal bleeding. In: Feldman M, Scharschmidt BF, Sleisenger MH, eds. Sleisinger and Fordtran's gastrointestinal and liver disease. 6th edn. Philadelphia, PA: WB Saunders, 1998, p1284–309
- Becker U, Sorensen TI, Borch-Johnsen K, et al. Prediction of risk of liver disease by alcohol intake, sex, and age: a prospective population study. Hepatology 1996;23:1025–9
- Bell H, Tallaksen CM, Try K, Haug E. Carbohydrate-deficient transferrin and other markers of high alcohol consumption: a study of 502 patients admitted consecutively to a medical department. Alcohol Clin Exp Res 1994;18:1103–8
- Berlakovich GA, Windhager T, Freundorfer E, et al. Carbohydrate deficient transferrin for detection of alcohol relapse after orthotopic liver transplantation for alcoholic cirrhosis. Transplantation 1999;67:1231–5
- Halm U, Tannapfel A, Mossner J, Berr F. Relative versus absolute carbohydrate-deficient transferrin as a marker of alcohol consumption in patients with acute alcoholic hepatitis. Alcohol Clin Exp Res 1999;23:1614–8
- Cabre E, Rodriguez Iglesias P, Caballeria J, et al. Short- and long-term outcome of severe alcohol-induced hepatitis treated with steroids or enteral nutrition: a multicenter randomized trial. Hepatology 2000;32:36–42
- Carithers RL Jr. Liver transplantation. Liver Transplant 2000;6:122 (Critical review of guidelines for liver transplantation)
- Fitz G. Systemic complications of liver disease. In: Feldman M, Scharschmidt BF, Sleisenger MH, eds. Sleisinger and Fordtran's gastrointestinal and liver disease. 6th edn. Philadelphia, PA: WB Saunders, 1998, p1334–54
- Fujimoto M, Uemura M, Kojima H, et al. Prognostic factors in severe alcoholic liver injury. Nara Liver Study Group. Alcohol Clin Exp Res 1999;23(4 Suppl):338–88
- Ganne-Carrie N, Christidis C, Chastang C, et al. Liver iron is predictive of death in alcoholic cirrhosis: a multivariate study of 229 consecutive patients with alcoholic and/or hepatitis C virus cirrhosis: a prospective follow-up study. Gut 2000;46:277–82
- Gulberg V, Bilzer M, Gerber AL. Long-term therapy and retreatment of hepatorenal syndrome type I with ornipressin and dopamine. Hepatology 1999;30:870–5
- Habeeb KS, Harrera JL. Management of ascites. Paracentesis as a guide. Postgrad Med 1997;101:191–2,195–200
- Imperiale TF, O'Connor JB, McCullough AJ. Corticosteroids are effective in patients with severe alcoholic hepatitis. Am J Gastroenterol 1999;94:3066–8

- Jaffe DL, Chung RT, Friedman LS. Management of portal hypertension and its complications. Med Clin North Am 1996;80:1021–34
- Jalan R, Hayes PC. Sodium handling in patients with well compensated cirrhosis is dependent on the severity of liver disease and portal pressure. Gut 2000;46:527–33
- Lieber CS. Alcoholic liver disease: new insights in pathogenesis lead to new treatments. J Hepatol 2000;32(1 Suppl):113–28
- Maher JJ. Alcoholic liver disease. In: Feldman M, Scharschmidt BF, Sleisenger MH, eds. Sleisinger and Fordtran's gastrointestinal and liver disease. 6th edn. Philadelphia, PA: WB Saunders, 1998, p1199–214
- Mathurin P, Duchatelle V, Ramond MJ, et al. Survival and prognostic factors in patients with severe alcoholic hepatitis treated with prednisolone. Gastroenterology 1996;110:1847–53
- Mendenhall CL, Anderson S, Weesner RE, et al. Protein-calorie malnutrition associated with alcoholic hepatitis. Veterans Administration Cooperative Study Group on Alcoholic Hepatitis. Am J Med 1984;76:211–22
- Mendenhall CL, Anderson S, Garcia-Pont P, et al. Short and long term survival in patients with alcoholic hepatitis treated with oxandrolone and prednisolone. N Engl J Med 1984;311:1464–70
- Mendenhall CL, Moritz TE, Roselle GA, et al. A study of oral nutritional support with oxandrolone in malnourished patients with alcoholic hepatitis: results of a Department of Veterans Affairs Cooperative Study. Hepatology 1993;17:564–76
- McCullough AJ, O'Connor JFB. Alcoholic liver disease: proposed recommendations for the American College of Gastroenterology. Am J Gastroenterol 1998:93:2022–36
- Mezey E, Caballeria J, Mitchell MC, et al. Effect of parenteral amino acid supplementation on short-term and long-term outcomes in severe alcoholic hepatitis: a randomized controlled trial. Hepatology 1991;14:1090–6
- Nanji AA, Zakim D. Alcoholic liver disease. In: Zakim D, Boyer TD, eds. Hepatology: a textbook of liver disease, 3rd edn. Philadelphia, PA: WB Saunders, 1996, p891–961
- Nompleggi DJ, Bonkovsky HL. Nutritional supplementation in chronic liver disease: an analytical review. Hepatology 1994;19:518–33
- O'Beirne J, Patch D, Holt S, et al. Alcoholic hepatitis: the case for intensive management. Postgrad Med J 2000;76:504–7
- Ong JP, Sands M, Younossi ZM. Transjugular intrahepatic portosystemic shunts (TIPS): a decade later. J Clin Gastroenterol 2000; 30:14–28 (Critical review of 10 years of experience with this procedure)
- Orlandi F, Brunelli E, Benedetti A, Macani A. Clinical trials of non-absorbable disaccharide therapy in hepatic encephalopathy. In: Conn HO, Bircher J, eds. Hepatic encephalopathy: syndromes and treatment. Bloomington, IL: Medical Education Press, 1994, p209–12
- Rosa H, Silverio AO, Perini RF, Aruda CB. Bacterial infection in cirrhotic patients and its relationship with alcohol. Am J Gastroenterol 2000;95:1290–3
- Rosen HR, Martin P. Liver transplantation. In: Schiff ER, Sorrell MF, Maddrey WC, eds. Schiff's diseases of the liver, 8th edn. Philadelphia, PA: Lippincott-Raven, 1999, p1589–614
- Runyon BA. Management of adult patients with ascites caused by cirrhosis. Hepatology 1998;27:264–72
- Runyon BA. Ascites and spontaneous bacterial peritonitis. In: Feldman M, Scharschmidt BF, Sleisenger MH, eds. Sleisinger and Fordtran's gastrointestinal and liver disease. 6th edn. Philadelphia, PA: WB Saunders; 1998, p1310–33
- Sheron N. Alcoholic liver disease. In: O'Grady JG, Lake JR, Dowdle PD, eds. Comprehensive clinical hepatology. New York: Mosby, 2000, p19.1–19.18
- Soberon S, Pauley MP, Duplantier R, et al. Metabolic effects of enteral formula feeding in alcoholic hepatitis. Hepatology 1987;7:1204–9
- Sort P, Navasa M, Arroyo V, et al. Effect of intravenous albumin on renal impairment and mortality in patients with cirrhosis and spontaneous bacterial peritonitis. N Engl J Med 1999;341:403–9
- Souba WW. Nutritional support. N Engl J Med 1997;336:41–8
- Such J, Runyon BA. Spontaneous bacterial peritonitis. J Clin Infect Dis 1998;27:669–74
- Addiction Resource Guide. Website devoted to listing resources for various addiction problems, including alcohol. Areas for both patients and healthcare professionals
- The Drug and Alcohol Assessment Screening System, Danya International, Inc.

# FAQS
## Question 1
What is the most important risk factor for progression of alcoholic liver disease?

ANSWER 1
Continued alcohol consumption.

## Question 2
What are some of the contraindications to the use of corticosteroids for the treatment of severe alcoholic hepatitis?

### ANSWER 2
Active gastrointestinal bleeding, renal failure, and infections.

## Question 3
How long after clinical recovery does jaundice resolve?

### ANSWER 3
Several weeks to months.

## Question 4
How does one diagnose cirrhosis in a patient with acute alcoholic hepatitis?

### ANSWER 4
Given circumstances of liver function decompensation, physical examination is the best way; ultrasound also may be suggestive.

## CONTRIBUTORS
Russell C Jones, MD, MPH
Lawrence S Friedman, MD
Vijay Yajnik, MD
Hetal A Karsan, MD
J Adrian Lunn, MD

# VIRAL HEPATITIS

| | | |
|---|---|---|
| ■ | Summary Information | 296 |
| ■ | Background | 297 |
| ■ | Diagnosis | 299 |
| ■ | Treatment | 310 |
| ■ | Outcomes | 314 |
| ■ | Prevention | 316 |
| ■ | Resources | 318 |

## SUMMARY INFORMATION

### DESCRIPTION

- A major public health problem worldwide
- An acute infection of the liver sometimes with chronic sequelae
- Caused by more than five unrelated aetiological agents
- Commonly subclinical but can present with jaundice
- Most cases are self-limiting and do not require active treatment
- Occasional fulminant cases occur

### URGENT ACTION

- Intravenous fluid therapy if severely dehydrated through vomiting
- Urgent referral for bleeding esophageal varices (due to chronic liver disease)
- Urgent referral for fulminant cases with encephalopathy and/or coagulopathy

# BACKGROUND

## ICD9 CODE
070.1 Viral hepatitis A
070.3 Viral hepatitis B
070.51 Viral hepatitis C
070.52 Hepatitis D
070.53 Hepatitis E
070.59 Other specified viral hepatitis

## SYNONYMS
- Hepatitis A: infectious hepatitis, epidemic hepatitis, short incubation hepatitis
- Hepatitis B: serum hepatitis, long incubation hepatitis
- Hepatitis C and E: non-A, non-B hepatitis (NANBH)
- Hepatitis C: intermediate incubation hepatitis

## CARDINAL FEATURES
- Marked elevation of aminotransferase levels
- Presentation in the prodromal period is nonspecific and only detected with a high level of suspicion or fortuitous testing

## CAUSES
### Common causes
- Hepatitis A virus: a single stranded RNA hepatovirus
- Hepatitis B virus: a double stranded DNA hepadnavirus
- Hepatitis C virus: a single stranded RNA virus related to flaviviruses

### Rare causes
- Hepatitis D virus: a single stranded RNA virus that requires a hepadnavirus (hepatitis B) to replicate
- Hepatitis E virus: a single stranded RNA virus related to the caliciviruses
- Hepatitis G virus: a flavivirus closely related to hepatitis C virus and GBV-C
- The GB flaviviruses (GBV-A, GBV-B and GBV-C)

### Serious causes
- With hepatitis A, fulminant hepatic failure occurs more commonly in patients with underlying liver disease, particularly chronic hepatitis C virus infection
- Hepatitis B and D coinfection or superinfection result in more serious disease than hepatitis B infection alone
- Hepatitis E infection has a high mortality (up to 20%) among females in their last trimester of pregnancy

### Contributory or predisposing factors
- Foreign travel to countries with inadequate hygiene or sanitation: hepatitis A and E
- Needlestick injury – occupational, injecting drug use, tattooing, acupuncture or body piercing: hepatitis B, C, and D
- Unprotected heterosexual and homosexual intercourse: hepatitis A, B, C, and probably D
- Individuals with other sexually transmitted infections: probably at a greater risk of exposure to hepatitis B, C, and D
- Recipients of unscreened blood or blood products: hepatitis B, C, D, and rarely A
- Residents and workers in daycare centers and institutions: hepatitis A
- Patients on hemodialysis or recipients of transplanted organs: hepatitis B, C, and D

## EPIDEMIOLOGY
### Incidence and prevalence
Viral hepatitis is estimated to affect more than 500,000 people in the US each year, but the rates are dropping dramatically with the advent of vaccines for hepatitis A and B viruses. However, the incidence of hepatitis C has also dropped dramatically over the past two decades.

#### INCIDENCE
- Hepatitis A: 0.375 to 0.6/1000 (125,000–200,000 infections/year)
- Hepatitis B: 0.42 to 0.96/1000 (140,000–320,000 infections/year)
- Hepatitis C: 0.1 – 0.54/1000 (36,000–180,000 infections/year)

#### PREVALENCE
- Hepatitis B among Caucasians: 30/1000
- Hepatitis B among African-Americans: 140/1000
- Hepatitis C: 18/1000

#### FREQUENCY
- Hepatitis D virus is present in 1% of hepatitis B virus infections
- Hepatitis G virus accounts for 0.3% of acute viral hepatitis (900–2000 infections/year)

### Demographics
#### AGE
- Hepatitis A: 2–5 years old (often asymptomatic) and young adults. Clinical manifestations vary with age. Hepatitis A virus infection is usually subclinical in children, whereas infection in adults varies in severity from a flu-like illness to fulminant hepatitis
- Hepatitis A: more severe in persons over 50 years old
- Hepatitis B: 20–45 years old
- Hepatitis C: 18–39 years old

#### GENDER
- Male homosexual and injecting drug users more commonly infected
- Chronic hepatitis B infection more common in males than females (approx. 2:1)

#### RACE
- Hepatitis A infection rates higher among American Indians and Hispanics
- Hepatitis B and C infection more common among African-Americans than Caucasians

#### GENETICS
Possible genetic susceptibility to progression from acute to chronic hepatitis C infection.

#### GEOGRAPHY
- Hepatitis A infection more prevalent in less developed areas due to inadequate sanitation
- Overall, the western states have the highest rates of hepatitis A infection in the US

#### SOCIOECONOMIC STATUS
Hepatitis A infection more prevalent among lower socioeconomic groups due to inadequate sanitary conditions, poverty and crowding.

# DIAGNOSIS

## DIFFERENTIAL DIAGNOSIS
- Other viral causes of systemic disease
- Nonviral causes of hepatitis, most importantly drugs and other hepatotoxins
- Obstructive causes of jaundice (extrahepatic cholestasis)
- Liver disease in pregnancy
- Reye's syndrome

Differential diagnosis of fulminant failure includes the ABCs (adapted from Goldberg and Sanjit, UpToDate, 2000).
A: Hepatitis A, acetaminophen, autoimmune hepatitis
B: Hepatitis B
C: Hepatitis C
D: Hepatitis D plus B, drugs
E: Esoteric causes: Budd–Chiari, Wilson's disease
F: Fatty liver of pregnancy, Reye's

### Other viral hepatitis
FEATURES
- All presentations of viral hepatitis have a similar clinical picture
- History of risk exposure is useful to differentiate causes
- Serum antibodies provide diagnosis
- Confirmation with advanced techniques, such as polymerase chain reaction (PCR)

### Other viral causes of hepatitis
FEATURES
- Mononucleosis: pharyngitis, lymphadenopathy and splenomegaly
- Cytomegalovirus: cervical adenopathy, hepatosplenomegaly, and jaundice
- Acute human immunodeficiency virus: sore throat, lymphadenopathy, headache, and rash
- Rubella: headache, lymphadenopathy, rash, splenomegaly, and hepatitis
- Measles: maculopapular rash, Koplik spots, lymphadenopathy
- Herpes simplex: myalgia, lymphadenopathy, vesicular rash
- Herpes zoster: localized pain preceding maculopapular rash

### Nonviral causes of hepatitis
FEATURES
- Alcohol: signs of acute intoxication and/or chronic liver disease
- Severe leptospirosis (Weil's disease): a spirochete infection involving the liver, kidneys, and vasculature
- Toxoplasmosis: a protozoal infection with nonspecific features and ocular involvement
- Wilson's disease: a disorder of copper transport that leads to accumulation in the brain, liver, kidneys, and eyes
- Drug induced: estrogens, phenothiazines, captopril, labetalol, isoniazid
- Toxic exposures: carbon tetrachloride and benzene

### Obstructive causes of jaundice
FEATURES
- Cholecystitis: right upper quadrant pain and tenderness (Murphy's sign), guarding, fever, nausea, and vomiting
- Cholangitis: acute onset right upper quadrant pain and tenderness, fever, rigors, and jaundice
- Pancreatic cancer: weight loss, abdominal pain, nausea, and jaundice
- Pancreatitis: epigastric tenderness and guarding, fever, tachycardia, ileus, and jaundice (due to compression of common bile duct)

### Liver disease in pregnancy
FEATURES
- Hyperemesis gravidarum: nausea, vomiting, and mild jaundice in first or second trimester
- Pre-eclampsia and eclampsia: upper abdominal pain, edema, hypertension, mental state change, and jaundice in second or third trimester
- Intrahepatic cholestasis: pruritus followed by jaundice in second or third trimester
- Biliary tract disease: right upper quadrant pain, nausea, vomiting, fever, and jaundice in any trimester
- Acute fatty liver: upper abdominal pain, nausea, vomiting, confusion, and jaundice in third trimester

## SIGNS & SYMPTOMS
### Signs
- Low grade fever may precede the onset of jaundice
- Hepatitis B serum-sickness-like syndrome: early presentation with urticaria, rash and arthralgias
- Hepatitis B surface antigen-antibody complex disease: early presentation with arthritis, arteritis and glomerulonephritis
- Evidence of jaundice: yellow discoloration of skin and sclera, dark colored urine and pale stool
- Injection ('track') marks on the skin might suggest injecting drug use
- Hepatomegaly and right upper quadrant tenderness
- Spider angiomata (rare) in hepatitis B: resolve during recovery
- Splenomegaly (rare)
- Evidence of fulminant hepatic failure: portal hypertension (periumbilical veins), hepatic encephalopathy (flapping tremor) and coagulopathy (bruising), cirrhosis or chronic hepatitis

### Symptoms
- Presentation is often asymptomatic or subclinical especially in children and in hepatitis C infection
- When symptomatic, all types of viral hepatitis have a similar clinical picture
- Coinfection or superinfection of hepatitis B with hepatitis D virus may have a more serious presentation
- Early presentation is usually a flu-like illness **(prodromal phase)**: headache, fever, malaise, lethargy, anorexia, nausea, and vomiting
- Individuals sometimes notice a change in their sense of taste and smell; cigarette smokers may lose their desire for tobacco
- Urticarial eruptions and arthralgias sometimes occur, particularly in hepatitis B infection
- As jaundice develops **(icteric phase)** systemic symptoms often resolve
- Features of cholestasis include pruritus and pain in the right upper quadrant
- Jaundice peaks within 1–2 weeks and resolves in another 2–4 weeks **(recovery phase)**

## ASSOCIATED DISORDERS
- Infection with the human immunodeficiency virus may be associated with hepatitis B, C, and D infection due to their common routes of transmission
- Hepatitis C virus infection is associated with essential mixed cryoglobulinemia, porphyria cutanea tarda, and possibly glomerulonephritis
- A large proportion of patients with decompensated alcoholic liver disease have hepatitis C virus infection

## CONSIDER CONSULT
Refer to gastroenterologist or infectious disease specialist for management of:
- Fulminant hepatitis: rapid clinical deterioration with coma, cerebral edema, and bleeding (due to hepatocellular failure and disseminated intravascular coagulation)

- Persistent (more than 6 months) hepatitis B and/or D infection
- Life-threatening sequelae of chronic hepatitis, e.g. esophageal varices
- Hepatitis of uncertain etiology
- Pregnant patients with liver function abnormalities

## INVESTIGATION OF THE PATIENT
### Direct questions to patient
**Q** When did you first start to feel unwell? To establish approximate time of exposure by incubation period (hepatitis A: 2–6 weeks; hepatitis B: 6–25 weeks; hepatitis C: 3–16 weeks)
**Q** Have you ever had jaundice before? Establish if first acute illness, recurrence or manifestation of chronic disease
**Q** Is anyone else at home or in close contact with you unwell at present? Identify contact with other cases of hepatitis: transmission by feco-oral or parenteral routes
**Q** What kind of work do you do? Find out if individual may have become infected through occupational exposure, or is likely to have transmitted infection on to others, e.g. food handler
**Q** What drugs are you taking? Identify potential hepatotoxins
**Q** Have you been vaccinated for hepatitis? If so, to A or B or both?
**Q** Have you had any blood transfusions? Risk for hepatitis C, B

### Contributory or predisposing factors
**Q** Have you traveled outside the US in the last 3 months? Risk of exposure in endemic areas to hepatitis A or E and possibly B if long-term travel
**Q** Have you had unprotected sexual intercourse with a new partner in the last 6 months? Transmission of hepatitis B, A, D, or C (unusual)
**Q** Any recent tattooing, piercing, acupuncture or injecting drug use? Transmission of hepatitis B, C, or D (rarely A)
**Q** Any history of needlestick injury or other likely exposure to hepatitis at work? Transmission of hepatitis B, C, or D ( rarely A )
**Q** Any history of blood transfusion, organ transplantation or hemodialysis? Transmission of hepatitis B, C, or D (rarely A) infection

### Family history
**Q** Have any other close family members had jaundice recently? (note that infection may be subclinical) – hepatitis A can be transmitted by close contact in families

### Examination
- Is there a fever? Temperature moderately raised in acute infection
- Any evidence of jaundice? Look for yellow skin and sclera, test urine for bile
- Any puncture wounds, piercing, or tattooing? Look for signs of injecting drug use or other needlestick injury
- Is the liver tender or enlarged? Examine the abdomen for right upper quadrant tenderness and hepatic enlargement. Is there splenomegaly?
- Are there any signs of hepatic encephalopathy? Assess for hepatic tremor, fetor hepaticus

### Summary of investigative tests
- Liver function tests for alanine aminotransferase (ALT), aspartate aminotransferase (AST) and alkaline phosphatase to assess degree of hepatocellular inflammation
- Albumin for an indication of liver function (usually normal)
- Prothrombin time (PT) to check for any clotting abnormality that might indicate fulminant hepatic necrosis
- Urine bile to confirm jaundice (if present) is cholestatic
- Serum bilirubin as an indicator of hepatic function – useful to monitor any subsequent deterioration

- Complete blood count (CBC): usually normal
- Erythrocyte sedimentation rate (ESR): usually normal
- Serology for hepatitis A, hepatitis B, hepatitis C, hepatitis D
- Ultrasonography of liver in fulminant hepatitis and to exclude obstruction

## DIAGNOSTIC DECISION
The clinical diagnosis of viral hepatitis is made on the basis of:
- History of likely exposure (although may not always be present)
- Clinical presentation (although may be asymptomatic)
- Results of liver function tests and hepatitis serological markers

The American Academy of Family Physicians has published an article that covers the diagnosis of hepatitis C. Moyer LA, Mast EE, Alter MJ. Hepatitis C: Part I. Routine serologic testing and diagnosis [1]

## CLINICAL PEARL(S)
- Cases with subclinical jaundice may be missed; consider the diagnosis with a typical prodromal illness that persists beyond a couple days
- Consider drug toxicity, which is uncommon, but extremely important to detect at the earliest possible time
- Offer postexposure prophylaxis for hepatitis A and B virus (HAV, HBV) to others who have been exposed. Persons who have been recently exposed to HAV and who have not previously been administered hepatitis A vaccine should be administered a single intramuscular dose of immunoglobulin (Ig) (0.02mL/kg) as soon as possible but not >2 weeks after exposure. Persons who have been administered one dose of hepatitis A vaccine at least 1 month before exposure to HAV do not need Ig. Prophylaxis of an unvaccinated person after exposure to hepatitis B consists of one dose of hepatitis B Ig (0.006 mL/kg intramuscularly) and initiation of hepatitis B vaccination
- Patients with fulminant liver failure (marked by coma, coagulopathy) should be referred early to a transplant center experienced in management of fulminant hepatic failure

## THE TESTS
### Body fluids
ALANINE AMINOTRANSFERASE (ALT)
*Description*
Blood (serum).

*Advantages/Disadvantages*
Accidental needlestick and biohazard risk with hepatitis B, C, and D.

*Normal*
Normal range: 0–35U/L (0–0.58mckat/L)

*Abnormal*
- Can be more than eight times normal range (up to 1000U/L) at onset of jaundice
- Usually higher than aspartate aminotransferase (AST) – reverse is often true in alcoholic hepatitis
- No correlation with clinical severity
- In acute hepatitis B even a minimal rise occasionally followed by chronic hepatitis
- Keep in mind the possibility of a false-positive result

*Cause of abnormal result*
Abnormal liver function.

*Drugs, disorders and other factors that may alter results*
- Alcohol
- Liver disease, e.g. hepatitis, cirrhosis
- Hepatic congestion
- Infectious mononucleosis
- Myocardial infarction
- Myocarditis
- Severe muscle trauma
- Dermatomyositis
- Polymyositis
- Muscular dystrophy
- Drugs, e.g. antibiotics, antihypertensives, heparin, nonsteroidal anti-inflammatories, amiodarone, chlorpromazine, phenytoin
- Malignancy
- Renal and pulmonary infarction
- Convulsions
- Eclampsia

## ASPARTATE AMINOTRANSFERASE (AST)
*Description*
Blood (serum).

*Advantages/Disadvantages*
Accidental needlestick and biohazard risk with hepatitis B, C, and D.

*Normal*
Normal range: 0–35U/L (0–0.58mckat/L).

*Abnormal*
- Can be more than eight times normal range (up to 1000U/L) at onset of jaundice
- Usually lower than alanine aminotransferase (ALT) – reverse is often true in alcoholic hepatitis
- No correlation with clinical severity
- In acute hepatitis B even a minimal rise occasionally followed by chronic hepatitis
- Keep in mind the possibility of a false-positive result

*Cause of abnormal result*
Abnormal liver function.

*Drugs, disorders and other factors that may alter results*
- Alcohol
- Liver disease, e.g. hepatitis, cirrhosis
- Hepatic congestion
- Infectious mononucleosis
- Myocardial infarction
- Myocarditis
- Severe muscle trauma
- Dermatomyositis
- Polymyositis
- Muscular dystrophy
- Drugs, e.g. antibiotics, antihypertensives, heparin, nonsteroidal anti-inflammatories, amiodarone, chlorpromazine, phenytoin
- Malignancy

- Renal and pulmonary infarction
- Convulsions
- Eclampsia

## ALKALINE PHOSPHATASE
*Description*
Blood (serum).

*Advantages/Disadvantages*
Accidental needlestick and biohazard risk with hepatitis B, C, and D.

*Normal*
30–120U/L (0.5–2mckat/L).

*Abnormal*
- From one to three times normal level in acute infection
- Higher if cholestasis is severe
- Keep in mind the possibility of a false-positive result

*Cause of abnormal result*
Abnormal liver function.

*Drugs, disorders and other factors that may alter results*
- Biliary obstruction, cirrhosis, and other liver disease
- Bone disorders, e.g. Paget's disease, rickets, osteomalacia, neoplasms, and metastases
- Hyperthyroidism and hyperparathyroidism
- Ulcerative colitis
- Infectious mononucleosis
- Cytomegalovirus infection
- Sepsis
- Pulmonary infarction
- Congestive heart failure
- Leukemia
- Multiple myeloma
- Pregnancy
- Puberty
- Drugs, e.g. estrogens, albumin, antibiotics

## ALBUMIN
*Description*
Blood (serum).

*Advantages/Disadvantages*
- Risk of accidental needlestick injury and biohazard with hepatitis B, C, and D
- Indicator of hepatic function – use to monitor any deterioration

*Normal*
4–6g/dL (40–60g/L).

*Abnormal*
- Usually normal unless fulminant hepatic necrosis, then lowered
- Keep in mind the possibility of a false-positive result

*Cause of abnormal result*
Abnormal liver function.

*Drugs, disorders and other factors that may alter results*
Decrease due to:
- Liver disease
- Nephrotic syndrome
- Poor nutritional status
- Rapid intravenous hydration
- Inflammatory bowel disease
- Malignancy, e.g. lymphomas
- Chronic inflammatory diseases, e.g. glomerulonephritis
- Pregnancy
- Drugs, e.g. oral contraceptives
- Prolonged immobilization

## PROTHROMBIN TIME (PT)

*Description*
Blood.

*Advantages/Disadvantages*
Indicator of hepatic function – use to monitor any deterioration that might be indicative of fulminant hepatic failure or as an important marker of end-stage chronic liver disease.

*Normal*
10–12s
The international normalized ratio (INR) is a comparative rating of PT ratios. It represents the observed PT ratio adjusted by the international reference thromboplastin. It provides a universal result indicative of what the patient's PT result would have been if measured using the primary World Health Organization international reference reagent.

*Abnormal*
- Increases with progressive liver damage
- If more than 5s above control and does not correct with parenteral vitamin K likely prognosis is poor
- Keep in mind the possibility of a false-positive result

*Cause of abnormal result*
Abnormal liver function.

*Drugs, disorders and other factors that may alter results*
Increase due to:
- Liver disease
- Anticoagulant drugs, e.g. warfarin and heparin
- Clotting factor and vitamin K deficiency
- Afibrinogenemia and dysfibrogenemia
- Other drugs, e.g. salicylate, chloral hydrate, estrogens, antacids, quinidine, antibiotics, allopurinol, anabolic steroids

Decrease due to:
- Thrombophlebitis
- Vitamin K supplements
- Drugs, e.g. glutethimide, estrogens, diphenhydramine, griseofulvin

## URINE BILE

*Description*
Urine.

*Advantages/Disadvantages*
Easy to perform, immediate result.

*Normal*
Absent bilirubin and urobilinogen.

*Abnormal*
- Presence of bilirubin or urobilinogen in urine (bilirubinuria)
- Keep in mind the possibility of a false-positive result

*Cause of abnormal result*
Inability of liver to excrete bilirubin.

*Drugs, disorders and other factors that may alter results*
- Urine bilirubin: viral, toxic, or drug induced hepatitis
- Urine urobilinogen: viral, toxic, or drug induced hepatitis, hemolytic jaundice, cirrhosis, or hepatic metastases

## SERUM BILIRUBIN

*Description*
Blood (serum).

*Advantages/Disadvantages*
- Allows distinction between obstructive and hepatic jaundice
- Use as a marker of deteriorating liver function

*Normal*
- Direct (conjugated) bilirubin: 0–0.2mg/dL (0–4mcmol/L)
- Indirect (unconjugated) bilirubin: 0–1.0mg/dL (2–18mcmol/L)
- Total bilirubin: 0–1.0mg/dL (2–18mcmol/L)

*Abnormal*
- Both indirect (unconjugated) and direct (conjugated) bilirubin may be elevated in viral hepatitis
- Increase can range from moderate to large
- Keep in mind the possibility of a false-positive result

*Cause of abnormal result*
Inability of liver to excrete bilirubin.

*Drugs, disorders and other factors that may alter results*
Indirect (unconjugated) and total bilirubin are increased in:
- Liver disease, e.g. hepatitis, cirrhosis, neoplasm
- Hemolytic anemia (congenital or acquired)
- Hepatic congestion due to congestive heart failure
- Hereditary disorders, e.g. Gilbert's disease
- Resorption from extravascular sources, e.g. hematoma, pulmonary embolism, or infarct
- Drugs including steroids, antibiotics, captopril, labetalol, isoniazid, indometacin, allopurinol, and methyldopa

## HEPATITIS A VIRUS SEROLOGY
*Description*
Blood (serum).

*Advantages/Disadvantages*
- Risk of accidental needlestick injury and biohazard
- Confirms diagnosis of acute hepatitis A infection or past exposure and immunity

*Normal*
Negative.

*Abnormal*
- Hepatitis A virus antibody (HAV IgM) is a marker of acute infection
- HAV IgM appears around time of clinical symptoms or as liver enzymes start to rise
- HAV IgM levels peak 1–2 weeks after onset of symptoms
- HAV IgM becomes undetectable 3–4 months after onset of symptoms (but can persist for up to 12 months)
- Hepatitis A virus antibody (HAV IgG) appears about 3 weeks after HAV IgM becomes detectable
- HAV IgG levels peak 4–6 weeks after onset of symptoms and remain elevated for life (with gradual decline)
- Keep in mind the possibility of a false-positive result

*Cause of abnormal result*
- HAV IgM: acute hepatitis A infection
- HAV IgG: past infection

*Drugs, disorders and other factors that may alter results*
Possibility of false-positive or false-negative test results.

## HEPATITIS B VIRUS SEROLOGY
*Description*
Blood (serum).

*Advantages/Disadvantages*
- Risk of accidental needlestick transmission and biohazard
- Confirms diagnosis of acute or chronic hepatitis B infection

*Normal*
Absent.

*Abnormal*
- Hepatitis B surface antigen (HBsAg) appears 2–6 weeks after exposure
- HBsAg levels peak around time of onset of symptoms
- HBsAg levels decline and become undetectable about 1–3 months after peak
- Persistence of HBsAg beyond 6 months (without appearance of corresponding antibody) indicates chronic infection (asymptomatic or chronic active hepatitis)
- Hepatitis B surface antibody (HBsAb) appears weeks or months after symptoms have cleared
- HBsAb indicates past infection and relative immunity (through infection or immunization)
- Hepatitis B core antibody (HBcAb-IgM) appears around time of clinical symptoms
- HBcAb-IgM levels peak about 1 week after onset of symptoms
- HBcAb-IgM is a good indicator of acute or recent infection (with HBsAg)
- HBcAb-IgM may remain detectable through convalescence (without HBsAg)

- HBcAb-IgM becomes undetectable 3–6 months after its appearance (but can persist for up to 2 years)
- Hepatitis B core antibody (HBcAb-IgG) is a marker of chronic infection
- Hepatitis B envelope antigen (HBeAg) appears about 3–5 days after HBsAg appears
- HBeAg peaks about the same time as HBsAg
- HBeAg becomes undetectable before or after HBsAg disappears in 90% of cases
- HBeAg persists in chronic carriage (with HBsAg)
- HBeAg is indicative of high infectivity (particularly when hepatitis B envelope antibody is absent)
- Hepatitis B envelope antibody (HBeAb-Total) appears at or shortly after the time HBeAg disappears
- HBeAb-Total is indicative of recovery and lowered case infectivity, and can persist for up to 6 years
- Keep in mind the possibility of a false-positive result

*Cause of abnormal result*
Hepatitis B infection.

*Drugs, disorders and other factors that may alter results*
- Possibility of false-positive or false-negative test results
- Isolated hepatitis B core antibody may represent a false positive or low level infection in which hepatitis B surface antigen is undetectable

## HEPATITIS C VIRUS SEROLOGY
*Description*
Blood (serum).

*Advantages/Disadvantages*
- Risk of needlestick and biohazard
- Confirms diagnosis of hepatitis C infection

*Normal*
Negative antigen and antibody.

*Abnormal*
- Hepatitis C virus (HCV) antigen detectable 3–4 weeks after infection
- HCV antibody (HCV IgG) detectable 3–4 months after infection
- HCV IgG undetectable in few (7%) cases at 18 months
- HCV IgG undetectable in about one-third of patients at 4 years
- Anti-HCV is detected by enzyme immunoassay (EIA). The third-generation test (EIA-3) is more sensitive and specific than previous ones
- The best approach to confirm the diagnosis of hepatitis C is to test for HCV RNA using a sensitive polymerase chain reaction (PCR) assay. The presence of HCV RNA in serum indicates an active infection.
- Testing for HCV RNA is also helpful in patients in whom EIA tests for anti-HCV are unreliable. For instance, immunocompromised patients may test negative for anti-HCV despite having HCV infection because they may not produce enough antibody for detection with EIA
- Keep in mind the possibility of a false-positive result

*Cause of abnormal result*
Hepatitis C infection.

*Drugs, disorders and other factors that may alter results*
- Possibility of false-positive or false-negative test results
- False-positive results are common with first-generation enzyme immunosorbent assay tests
- Second- and third-generation enzyme immunosorbent assay tests have fewer false-positive results

## HEPATITIS D VIRUS SEROLOGY
*Description*
Blood (serum).

*Advantages/Disadvantages*
- Risk of needlestick and biohazard
- Enables accurate diagnosis of hepatitis D infection (with hepatitis B)

*Normal*
Negative.

*Abnormal*
- Two case scenarios of hepatitis D infection exist: coinfection with acute hepatitis D and B; superinfection with acute hepatitis D and chronic hepatitis B
- Hepatitis D virus antigen (HDV Ag) appears before symptoms begin (during prodrome)
- HDV Ag peaks about 2–3 days after appearance
- HDV Ag becomes undetectable 1–4 days after peak
- HDV Ag may persist until after symptoms appear
- Hepatitis D virus antibody (HDV IgM) appears about 10 days after symptoms begin
- HDV IgM peaks about 2 weeks after appearance
- HDV IgM becomes undetectable about 35 days after appearance
- HDV IgM is useful to distinguish acute from chronic infection
- Hepatitis D virus total antibody (HDV-Total) appears about 50 days after symptoms begin
- HDV-Total peaks about 2 weeks after appearance
- HDV-Total becomes undetectable about 7 months after appearance
- HDV-Total is best screening test for infection
- Keep in mind the possibility of a false-positive result

*Cause of abnormal result*
Hepatitis D coinfection or superinfection with hepatitis B virus.

*Drugs, disorders and other factors that may alter results*
Possibility of false-positive or false-negative test results.

# TREATMENT

## CONSIDER CONSULT
Refer to gastroenterologist or infectious disease specialist for management of:
- Chronic hepatitis B and D
- Prolonged cholestasis
- Sequelae of chronic infection, e.g. esophageal varices
- Pregnant patients with abnormal liver function
- Acute or chronic hepatitis C infection for consideration of interferon/ribavirin

## IMMEDIATE ACTION
- Intravenous fluid therapy if severely dehydrated through vomiting
- Postexposure prophylaxis following acute exposure to hepatitis A or B virus

## PATIENT AND CAREGIVER ISSUES
### Patient or caregiver request
Q **What is hepatitis?** An inflammation of the liver
Q **How is hepatitis transmitted?** Outline possible contributory or predisposing factors
Q **Am I infectious to others?** Explain risks related to feco-oral, parenteral and sexual transmission
Q **Is it curable?** Explain that most hepatitis is self-limiting, while a small proportion of people become chronic carriers and some of these go on to develop complications
Q **Can I drink alcohol?** Not during acute infection and then only in moderation after 6–12 months (depends if infection becomes chronic). Eliminating alcohol use is probably the most important single step in therapy for chronic hepatitis C
Q **Should I follow a special diet?** A balanced high carbohydrate diet is suggested
Q **Can I exercise?** Moderate activity is acceptable, when recovery permits

### Health-seeking behavior
- Has the patient taken any over-the-counter or alternative medications to treat their illness? These may be hepatotoxic
- Who else may have been at risk of infection before the patient presented? Try to establish whether the patient is likely to have transmitted their infection on to other persons, both at home and in work environment

## MANAGEMENT ISSUES
### Goals
- To achieve a full and uneventful recovery from the current infection
- To reduce or prevent further transmission of the virus to others (vaccination and lifestyle advice regarding prevention of transmission)
- To avoid serious complications and chronic sequelae

### Management in special circumstances
COEXISTING DISEASE
- Response to treatment of chronic disease suboptimal in HIV coinfection
- Injecting drug users: problems related to continued drug injection, sharing injecting equipment with others, unprotected sexual intercourse

COEXISTING MEDICATION
- HIV and other immunocompromised individuals likely to be on other medications that may exacerbate liver disease
- Avoid drugs metabolized by liver and complementary medicines, many of which may be hepatotoxic

- Patients with chronic illness who may be taking other medications will require special consideration and liaison with relevant specialists

### SPECIAL PATIENT GROUPS
- Pregnancy: need to be aware of possible teratogenic effects of any medications prescribed, consider possible risks of immunization during pregnancy
- Elderly patients: likely to be on other medications, some may have effect on, or be affected by, liver function

### PATIENT SATISFACTION/LIFESTYLE PRIORITIES
- Food handlers, institution and care workers must avoid work until infectious period has passed – usually following onset of jaundice (A and E)
- Elderly patients: often more severe and protracted disease, likely to have longer period of convalescence

## SUMMARY OF THERAPEUTIC OPTIONS
### Choices
- Moderate activity recommended
- A balanced high carbohydrate diet
- Lifestyle issues, namely alcohol consumption, should be addressed
- Colestyramine for symptomatic relief of severe pruritus due to cholestasis in hepatitis A
- No suggested therapy for acute hepatitis A, B, D, or E infection, except that exacerbations and selected acute cases may respond to antiviral therapy, but data are limited
- Therapy for treatment of chronic hepatitis B infection with interferon-alpha (2a and 2b), lamivudine, famciclovir, or adefovir is generally undertaken by specialists
- Therapy for chronic (and possibly acute) hepatitis C infection with interferon-alfa, interferon-beta, or ribavirin requires referral to a specialist

Guidelines for the management of hepatitis C have been published by the National Institutes of Health. Management of hepatitis C. NIH Consensus Statement [2]

### Never
- Never prescribe drugs that may exacerbate liver damage, e.g. acetaminophen
- Never prescribe herbal or complementary therapies that may be hepatotoxic

### FOLLOW UP
- See after results of initial blood tests and again in 6 weeks for repeat tests of liver function and appropriate hepatitis serology
- Advise patient to return sooner if symptoms worsen
- Patients with chronic hepatitis B or C have an increased risk of hepatocellular carcinoma. Periodic ultrasonography of liver and serum alpha-fetoprotein testing is recommended

### Plan for review
- Repeat blood tests after 6 weeks with further follow up based on disease progression (resolving or not)
- Refer if clinical condition deteriorates or disease becomes chronic

### Information for patient or caregiver
- Avoid blood donation, unprotected sexual intercourse, sharing any 'sharps', e.g. needles, jewelry, razors (hepatitis B, C, and D)
- Follow good hygiene practices in relation to food handling (hepatitis A and E)

# DRUGS AND OTHER THERAPIES: DETAILS
## Drugs
COLESTYRAMINE
May be useful for symptomatic relief of severe pruritus in hepatitis A virus infection.

*Dose*
- Adult: 4g orally twice daily (can be up to six times daily – not to exceed 32g/day)
- Child: 240mg/kg orally daily in three divided doses

*Efficacy*
Can be effective.

*Risks/benefits*
- Use caution in children
- Use caution if patient constipated

*Side effects and adverse reactions*
- Central nervous system: dizziness, headache, tinnitus, vertigo
- Gastrointestinal: constipation, nausea, vomiting, abdominal pain, peptic ulceration
- Hematologic: bleeding
- Musculoskeletal: myalgia
- Skin: rashes

*Interactions (other drugs)*
- Acetaminophen
- Amiodarone
- Corticosteroids
- Diclofenac
- Digoxin
- Diuretics
- Methotrexate
- Metronidazole
- Thyroid hormone
- Valproic acid
- Warfarin

*Contraindications*
- Biliary obstruction

*Acceptability to patient*
Not to be taken in conjunction with other medications.

*Follow up plan*
Prescribe for 2 weeks and ask patient to return after this time (maximum effect in 2 weeks).

*Patient and caregiver information*
Not to be taken in conjunction with other medications – take other medications one hour before or 4h after colestyramine.

PREDNISOLONE
May shorten prolonged cholestasis in hepatitis A infection.

*Dose*
30mg orally daily tapered over 1–2 weeks.

*Efficacy*
- Uncertain in hepatitis A
- Unhelpful in hepatitis B and C

*Risks/benefits*
- Overwhelming septicemia if patient has an infection
- Loss of control of blood glucose in those with diabetes
- Prolonged use causes adrenal suppression

*Side effects and adverse reactions*
- Side effects are minimized by short duration of therapy
- Cardiovascular system: hypertension, thromboembolism
- Central nervous system: insomnia, euphoria, depression, psychosis
- Endocrine: adrenal suppression, impaired glucose tolerance, growth suppression in children
- Eyes, ears, nose, and throat: cataract, glaucoma, blurred vision
- Gastrointestinal: dyspepsia, peptic ulceration, esophagitis, oral candidiasis
- Musculoskeletal: proximal myopathy, osteoporosis
- Skin: delayed healing, acne, striae

*Interactions (other drugs)*
- Aminoglutethimide
- Barbiturates
- Colestyramine
- Clarithromycin, erythromycin
- Colestipol
- Isoniazid
- Ketoconazole
- Nonsteroidal anti-inflammatory drugs
- Oral contraceptives
- Rifampin
- Salicylates
- Troleandomycin

*Contraindications*
- Systemic infection
- Avoid live virus vaccines in those receiving immunosuppressive doses

*Acceptability to patient*
Caution may be expressed over steroid use: explain in terms of short duration, decreasing dose and type of steroids (not anabolic steroids).

*Follow up plan*
- Review after completion of course
- Advise to return sooner if symptoms become worse

*Patient and caregiver information*
- Take single dose in morning
- May cause gastrointestinal disturbances
- Do not stop taking abruptly (although at small dose for short period is unlikely to be problematic)

## LIFESTYLE
- Avoid alcohol during acute illness and for 6–12 months after
- Avoid future intake of alcohol if chronic hepatitis B or C infection as excessive consumption (more than 50g/day) likely to increase progression to chronic liver disease. The threshold for where injury occurs has not been established, so that abstinence is the best approach
- Avoid hepatically metabolized medicines, e.g. acetaminophen, during acute illness

RISKS/BENEFITS
- Benefit: reduction in liver damage and improved overall outcome
- Risk: acute alcohol withdrawal

ACCEPTABILITY TO PATIENT
- May need support in stopping alcohol: refer to appropriate organizations
- Provide list of medicines that should be avoided

FOLLOW UP PLAN
- Arrange early follow up if likely to have compliancy problems
- Ask about alcohol consumption/compliance with abstention at follow up

PATIENT AND CAREGIVER INFORMATION
Discuss danger of increased severity of liver damage and possible long term sequelae if therapy is not adhered to.

# OUTCOMES

## EFFICACY OF THERAPIES
- Treatment of acute hepatitis A and B infection is mainly supportive and has little effect on outcome; most cases resolve without complications
- Referral and treatment of hepatitis C can help to improve overall outcome

## Evidence
- Treatment of acute hepatitis A virus infection and acute hepatitis B virus (HBV) infection is mainly supportive and has little effect on outcome; most cases resolve without complications; PDxMD is unable to cite evidence for these treatments which meets our criteria for evidence
- For treatment of chronic HBV infection, interferon-alfa is the only cost-effective drug approved by the FDA; a meta-analysis of 15 randomized controlled trials involving a total of 837 adults who were chronic carriers of HBV and who were positive for HBV surface antigen and HBV e antigen found that interferon-alfa effectively ended viral replication and eradicated the carrier state in actively treated patients compared with controls [3] *Level M*
- Referral for treatment of hepatitis C can help to improve overall outcome

## Review period
- Review after 2 weeks; if symptoms are severe, repeat blood tests
- Review after 6 weeks for routine repeat of blood tests
- Further review pending clinical course and results of blood tests

## PROGNOSIS
- Most cases of viral hepatitis are self-limiting: 85–95% of cases of hepatitis B, D, and E recover within 3 months
- 85% of cases of hepatitis C become chronic carriers
- 20% of chronic hepatitis C carriers develop cirrhosis
- Risk of hepatocellular carcinoma is increased in chronic hepatitis B, C

## Therapeutic failure
- Other formulations of interferon, e.g. interferon-beta and interferon-gamma are undergoing clinical trials
- Interferon in combination with other drugs, e.g. thymosin or prednisone, may have an improved effect over interferon alone
- The antiviral drug ribavirin can be given orally and is being assessed in combination with interferon-alpha
- Iron reduction by phlebotomy has been shown to improve aminotransferase levels in chronic hepatitis C infection

## Recurrence
- 5–10% of cases of viral hepatitis relapse during convalescence
- Clinical and biochemical relapses have been documented in cases of hepatitis A and B. (Some relapses of hepatitis B may represent the clinical expression of simultaneous delta hepatitis infection.)
- Fluctuation in aminotransferase levels is common during acute and chronic hepatitis C – sometimes accompanied by a clinical relapse
- Apparent relapse may actually represent instances of second infections with another hepatitis virus

## Deterioration
- Refer the patient for expert management
- Consider other treatment options
- Liver transplantation if all other treatment fails

## Terminal illness

Terminal illness in viral hepatitis can result from fulminant hepatitis or chronic complications

Management includes:
- Urgent referral of fulminant hepatitis to a liver center capable of assessing for liver transplantation and expert at treating liver failure
- Referral to a transplant center of patients with complicated cirrhosis

Management in patient if there is no option of organ transplantation:
- Pain control: analgesia
- Diet: avoidance of high protein intake
- Lifestyle: stop alcohol consumption
- Nursing care as necessary
- Bowel preparation to reduce colonic ammonia production: lactulose and/or neomycin

## COMPLICATIONS

- Fulminant hepatic necrosis and liver failure: can occur with any of the viral hepatitis agents but is more common with acute hepatitis B (particularly if hepatitis D coinfection) and among pregnant women with hepatitis E infection (and some cases of drug/toxin-induced liver disease)
- Chronic asymptomatic carriage or chronic active hepatitis due to hepatitis B (5–10% of cases) or hepatitis C (75–85% of cases)
- Cirrhosis of the liver following chronic infection (chronic active hepatitis) with hepatitis B or C
- Hepatocellular carcinoma (hepatoma): malignant liver disease following (10–20 years) chronic hepatitis B or C infection
- Hepatic encephalopathy with fulminant hepatic necrosis or cirrhosis

## CONSIDER CONSULT

Refer if:
- Hepatitis infection is not resolving (persistently abnormal liver enzymes) or further deterioration of liver function is noted – fulminant hepatitis: monitor prothrombin time, albumin
- Patient develops chronic active hepatitis B: look for persistent (more than 6 months) hepatitis B surface antigen (HBsAg) and hepatitis B envelope antigen (HBeAg) without corresponding antibody
- Patient develops chronic carriage of hepatitis C (more than 50%): monitor serial alanine aminotransferase (ALT) for fluctuation

# PREVENTION

Prevention of hepatitis acquisition and transmission is primarily through lifestyle changes to avoid known risk factors, and immunization where applicable

## RISK FACTORS

- **Foreign travel:** hepatitis A immunization, advise on food and water safety, personal hygiene
- **Injecting drug use:** avoid sharing ANY item of drug injecting equipment with other users
- **Tattooing, piercing, and acupuncture:** observe or inquire about sterilization procedures and appropriate registration of practitioners, avoid 'back street' establishments
- **Unprotected heterosexual and homosexual intercourse:** reduce numbers of sexual contacts, ALWAYS use condoms
- **Healthcare worker:** vaccination for hepatitis A and B; apply universal precautions for handling hazardous material
- **Patients on dialysis or receiving clotting factor:** vaccination for hepatitis A and B

## MODIFY RISK FACTORS
### Lifestyle and wellness

- Occupational exposure: in high-risk settings, e.g. institutions, daycare centers, animal laboratories (primates) be aware of transmission risk, obtain hepatitis A and B immunization and follow universal precautions for handling potentially infected or contaminated material
- Food handlers: persons working in food handling establishments must be aware of risks of fecal-oral spread of viruses and practice appropriate hygiene procedures, e.g. wash hands thoroughly after use of the toilet

### ALCOHOL AND DRUGS

- Moderate alcohol and/or illegal drug consumption: intoxication can lead to high-risk sexual behavior with risk of hepatitis transmission
- Excessive alcohol consumption is a likely cofactor in progression of hepatitis B and C to chronic disease
- Do not inject illegal drugs (including 'body enhancing' products, e.g. steroids)
- If injecting drugs, use sterile needles, water and syringes if possible and dispose of used equipment appropriately
- Do not share any injecting equipment with other users, i.e. needles, syringes, spoons, bowls, or water

### SEXUAL BEHAVIOR

- Limit number of sexual contacts
- Use male/female condoms for all acts of sexual intercourse
- Do not practice high-risk activities such as those involving breaking skin or contact with urine or feces

### ENVIRONMENT

- Ensure careful disposal of excreta without contamination of water supply
- Ensure access to safe water supply
- Practice good food, water, and personal hygiene (hand washing)

### IMMUNIZATION

- Both passive and active immunizations are available for hepatitis A and hepatitis B
- **Hepatitis A immune globulin** is recommended for postexposure (within 2 weeks) prophylaxis of cases and close contacts, e.g. sexual, family, daycare staff. It may also be administered to travelers to high-risk areas who do not present in adequate time for active immunization to take effect (administer vaccine at same time)

- **Hepatitis A vaccination** is recommended for children at high risk of infection in the US, travelers to high risk areas, homosexual males, injecting drug users, persons with occupational risk of exposure, recipients of clotting factors, and cases of chronic liver disease
- **Hepatitis B immune globulin** should be considered for postexposure (within 7–14 days) prophylaxis of an infant born to a hepatitis B surface antigen (HBsAg) positive mother, percutaneous or permucosal exposure to HBsAg-positive blood, sexual exposure to an HBsAg-positive person, and household exposure of an infant 12 months of age to a primary caregiver who has acute hepatitis B. In all cases give hepatitis B vaccination at the same time (at a different site)
- **Hepatitis B vaccination** is recommended for all infants either at birth or within 2 months of delivery (see screening below), children in high-risk populations or areas, adolescents with high-risk behaviors, persons with occupational risk of exposure, hemodialysis patients and those receiving clotting factors, household contacts and sex partners of an HBsAg-positive person, injecting drug users, persons with multiple sexual partners and/or sexually transmitted infections, and inmates of long-term correctional institutions
- **Hepatitis B vaccination** prevents hepatitis D in those susceptible to hepatitis B

*Cost/efficacy*
Hepatitis B vaccination is cheap and use is cost-effective.

## SCREENING

- Screening pregnant women for hepatitis B surface antigen (HBsAg) is recommended at their first prenatal visit to reduce the possibility of perinatal transmission (immunize infant at birth if positive)
- Repeat testing in the third trimester for women who are HBsAg negative but are at high risk of hepatitis B virus infection, or exposure to the virus is suspected during pregnancy
- Screening asymptomatic, high-risk individuals for hepatitis B virus infection to determine eligibility for immunization may be considered
- Screening for hepatitis C virus infection is recommended for blood, plasma, organ, tissue and semen donors
- Routine testing for hepatitis C virus is recommended for certain at-risk individuals including healthcare workers after needlestick or mucosal exposure to hepatitis C virus positive blood, injecting drug users, persons who were ever on chronic dialysis, persons with persistently abnormal alanine aminotransferase (ALT) levels and children born to hepatitis C virus positive women

Appropriate counseling should be provided and consent obtained before testing.

## PREVENT RECURRENCE

- Most individuals who contract viral hepatitis recover fully and develop lifelong immunity
- A small percentage have chronic infection and complications
- Recurrence of one of the other hepatitis agents is a possibility if transmission relates to lifestyle, e.g. injecting drug users are at risk of hepatitis B, C, and D
- To prevent recurrence of a different hepatitis agent advise about lifestyle changes and recommend immunization as appropriate
- Some individuals may experience periodic relapse of disease

### Reassess coexisting disease
INTERACTION ALERT
Use of hepatotoxic drugs, e.g. acetaminophen, for a coexisting disease may worsen the outcome of viral hepatitis (but is not likely to cause recurrence).

# RESOURCES

## ASSOCIATIONS

**Hepatitis Foundation International**
30 Sunrise Terrace
Cedar Grove, NJ 07009-1423
Tel: (800) 891-0707 (Toll-free)
Tel: (973) 239-1035
Fax: (973) 857-5044
http://www.hepfi.org

**National Center for Infectious Diseases**
Mail Stop G-37
Atlanta, GA 30333
Tel: (888) 443-7232 (Toll-free, Hepatitis 24 Hour Hotline)
Tel: (404) 332-4555 (International Health Hotline)
Fax: (404) 371-5488
http://www.cdc.gov

**Communicable Disease Surveillance and Response (CSR)**
For further information contact Health Communications and Public Relations
WHO
Geneva
Tel: (41 22) 791-4458
Fax: (41 22) 791-4858
http://www.who.int

## KEY REFERENCES

- Bannister BA, Begg NT, Gillespie SH. Infectious disease. London: Blackwell Science, 1996
- Feldman M, et al. Sleisenger and Fordtran's gastroenterology and liver disease, 5th edn. Philadelphia: WB Saunders, 1998
- Goroll AH, et al. Primary care medicine, 3rd edn. Philadelphia: Lippincott-Raven, 1995
- Moyer LA, Mast EE, Alter MJ. Hepatitis C: Part I. Routine serologic testing and diagnosis. Am Fam Phys 1999;59:79–88,91–2 (http://www.aafp.org/afp/990101ap/79.html)
- Schinazi RF, Sommadossi J-P, Thomas HC. Therapies for viral hepatitis. London: International Medical Press, 1997
- Shulman ST. Viral hepatitis. In: Shulman ST, Phair JP, Peterson LR, Warren JR (eds). The biologic and clinical basis of infectious diseases, 5th edn. Philadelphia: WB Saunders, 1997
- Terrault NA, Wright TL. Viral hepatitis A through G. In: Beers MH, Berkow R, eds. The Merck manual of diagnosis and therapy, 17th edn. 2000
- Tine F, Magrin S, Craxi S, et al. Interferon for non-A non-B chronic hepatitis: a meta-analysis of randomized clinical trials. J Hepatol 1991;13:192
- Wong D, Cheung A, O'Rourke K, et al. Effect of alpha-interferon treatment in patients with hepatitis B e antigen-positive chronic hepatitis B: a meta-analysis. Ann Intern Med 1993;19:312
- Wong JB, Koff RS, Tine F, et al. Cost-effectiveness of interferon-alpha 2b treatment for hepatitis B e antigen-positive hepatitis B. Ann Intern Med 1995;122:664
- Center for Disease Control National Center for Infectious Diseases. Viral hepatitis (http://www.cdc.gov/ncidod/diseases/hepatitis/index.htm)
- World Health Organization. Health topics – hepatitis B and hepatitis C (http://www.who.int/health-topics/hepatitis.htm)

### Evidence references and guidelines
1. Moyer LA, Mast EE, Alter MJ. Hepatitis C: Part I. Routine serologic testing and diagnosis. Am Fam Physician 1999;59:79–88,91–2
2. Management of hepatitis C. Consensus Statement 1997;15:1–41; also available online through the National Guideline Clearinghouse
3. Wong D, Cheung A, O'Rourke K, et al. Effect of alpha-interferon treatment in patients with hepatitis B e antigen-positive chronic hepatitis B: a meta-analysis. Ann Intern Med 1993;19:312–23

## CONTRIBUTORS
Fred F Ferri, MD, FACP
Andrew H Soll, MD

# FEMORAL AND INGUINAL HERNIA

| | | |
|---|---|---|
| ■ | Summary Information | 322 |
| ■ | Background | 323 |
| ■ | Diagnosis | 325 |
| ■ | Treatment | 329 |
| ■ | Outcomes | 334 |
| ■ | Prevention | 335 |
| ■ | Resources | 337 |

## SUMMARY INFORMATION

### DESCRIPTION

- Protrusion of intra-abdominal contents through an abnormal fascial opening
- Reducible hernia: a hernia that can be manually or spontaneously repositioned into the abdominal cavity
- Incarcerated hernia: a hernia that cannot be reduced. May lead to bowel obstruction but is not associated with vascular compromise
- Strangulated hernia: a nonreducible hernia that leads to vascular compromise
- Richter hernia: a hernia that doesn't involve the entire bowel circumference; only the antimesenteric bowel border is herniated

### URGENT ACTION

Immediate surgical consultation is necessary if signs of bowel obstruction are present, including:

- Persistent pain, even after hernia reduction
- Fever
- Toxic appearance
- Enlarging hernia
- Irreducible hernia
- Signs and symptoms of bowel obstruction

### KEY! DON'T MISS!

Richter's hernia will not involve symptoms of bowel obstruction (such as vomiting) but can lead to perforation and peritonitis.

## BACKGROUND

### ICD9 CODE
- 553.9 Hernia NOS
- 553.0 Hernia, femoral NOS
- 550.9 Hernia, inguinal NOS

### SYNONYMS
Groin hernia.

### CARDINAL FEATURES
- Development of lump or bulge in the groin
- Patient may note sensation of fullness, aching, pain
- Bulge or discomfort may increase in size when patient stands or during periods of increased intra-abdominal pressure
- Unless incarceration has developed, symptoms improve on relaxation or manual manipulation

There are three important types of groin hernias: indirect, direct, and femoral.

Indirect inguinal hernia:
- Passes through internal inguinal ring, which is lateral to the epigastric artery, into the inguinal canal
- Usually remains within inguinal canal; occasionally a large hernial sac passes through the external ring and into the scrotum
- May occur bilaterally
- Accounts for about 60% of all inguinal hernias
- Can affect either sex; indirect hernias are the most common form in younger men and in women
- 5% can eventually strangulate

Direct inguinal hernia:
- Accounts for about 30% of all inguinal hernias
- Passes through external inguinal ring, medial to the epigastric artery in the region of Hesselbach's triangle
- Strangulation is less common than with indirect hernias
- More common in elderly men; uncommon in women
- Direct hernias rarely go into the scrotal sac, unless huge
- Felt as a bulge at the external inguinal ring; however, you cannot establish the type by palpation

Femoral hernia:
- Least common type of hernia; only about 3% of all hernias are femoral
- Involves a loop of bowel slipping through an opening in the femoral triangle, which is inferior to the inguinal canal and medial to the epigastric artery
- Passes through femoral ring, femoral canal, and fossa ovalis
- Right side more commonly affected than left
- Affects females more often than males and older individuals more often than younger ones
- Risk of incarceration, and particularly of strangulation, is especially high (20–30%)
- Rarely occurs in children

## CAUSES
### Common causes
- Failure of obliteration of processus vaginalis (congenital defect)

- Obesity
- Ascites
- Pregnancy
- Chronic cough, including due to chronic obstructive pulmonary disease (COPD)
- Constipation, resulting in straining to defecate
- Straining to urinate, as can occur in prostatism
- Heavy lifting
- Peritoneal dialysis
- Ventriculoperitoneal shunt
- Family history of hernia development
- History of undescended testicle

### Rare causes
- Congenital pelvic abnormality
- Exstrophy of urinary bladder
- Congenital abnormalities of collagen

### Contributory or predisposing factors
Connective tissue may be weakened by:
- Aging
- Cigarette smoking (especially in women)
- Systemic disease
- Prematurity
- Low birthweight
- Chronic steroid use

## EPIDEMIOLOGY
### Incidence and prevalence
PREVALENCE
0.03–0.04/1000.

FREQUENCY
25% of males and 2% of females will suffer from an inguinal hernia at some point during their lifetime.

### Demographics
AGE
- Direct inguinal hernia: predominantly occurs in children, young males
- Indirect inguinal hernia: predominantly affects individuals >30 years of age
- Femoral hernia: very rare in children; more common in older individuals

GENDER
- Indirect inguinal hernias: men are more commonly affected than women (8:1 to 10:1)
- Femoral hernia: more common in women than in men (3:1 to 5:1)

RACE
Hernias are three times more frequent in African-Americans than in Caucasians.

GENETICS
Family tendency noted.

# DIAGNOSIS

## DIFFERENTIAL DIAGNOSIS
### Epididymitis
Epididymitis is characterized by inflammation or infection of the epididymis.

FEATURES
- Pain may begin in the flank or abdomen, progress to scrotum
- Urinary symptoms may include retention, urgency, frequency, dysuria
- Nausea, vomiting
- Fever
- Urethral discharge
- Palpation reveals tender, swollen epididymis
- Scrotum may be inflamed, warm, and erythematous

### Hidradenitis suppurativa
Hidradenitis suppurativa is a chronic acneiform infection of cutaneous apocrine glands, and may involve adjacent tissue, including subcutaneous fat and fascia. Most commonly affects apocrine glands in axillae and groin; less commonly the periareolar, intermammary, pubic, infraumbilical, gluteal, genitofemoral, or perianal regions.

FEATURES
- Women more commonly affected than men
- Nodular lesions in axillae or groin may be firm, tender, painful, erythematous, and fluctuant
- Nodules may spontaneously burst, draining discharge
- Cellulitis of the adjacent tissue is common
- Exacerbations may be prompted by obesity, exposure to excessive heat, propensity to heavy perspiration
- Nodules may fully resolve but tend to recur frequently

### Hydrocele
Hydrocele is the collection of serous fluid in the scrotal tunica vaginalis, spermatic cord, or canal of Nuck.

FEATURES
- Usually asymptomatic
- Scrotal enlargement, without tenderness, pain, or erythema
- May cause minor sensation of heaviness, dragginess
- No fever, genitourinary, gastrointestinal, or systemic symptoms, unless complications (infection) occur
- Enlargement is less notable when patient lies down and increases in the upright position
- May occur bilaterally about 10% of the time

### Lymphogranuloma venereum
Lymphogranuloma venereum is a sexually transmitted lymphatic infection caused by *Chlamydia trachomatis*.

FEATURES
- More commonly affects men than women (6:1)
- Ages 20–40
- Primary stage: painless ulceration at inoculation site
- Secondary (or inguinal) stage: tender lymphadenopathy, usually inguinal, although may involve perirectal or pelvic nodes; progresses to suppurative granulomatous lymphadenitis, perilymphadenitis, and abscess formation

- Tertiary stage: occurs years after initial infection; chlamydial organisms are no longer seen at this stage. Manifested by anogenitorectal syndrome, anorectal stricture, genital elephantiasis, proctocolitis, perirectal and/or ischiorectal abscess, and anal or rectovaginal fistulas

## Testicular torsion

Testicular torsion is a true medical emergency. The testicle twists on the spermatic cord, and venous occlusion can result in engorgement, ischemia, and testicular infarction.

FEATURES
- Usually involves left testicle
- Patients usually under age 30, most commonly 12–18, peak at age 14
- Acute onset
- Severe, unilateral testicular pain
- Other features include scrotal swelling and erythema, fever, nausea, and vomiting
- Testicular palpation is painful
- Affected testicle may appear horizontal, and higher than a normal testicle
- Loss of cremasteric reflex on affected side

## SIGNS & SYMPTOMS
### Signs
- Palpable and/or visible lump in groin
- Lump may be more evident when patient performs Valsalva maneuver

Signs of complications, such as strangulation or incarceration, may include:
- Persistent pain
- Irreducible lump
- Tenderness on palpation
- Fever
- Abdominal distension
- Tympany
- Hyperperistalsis

### Symptoms
- Aching in groin, may radiate into area of hernia
- Femoral hernia may cause pain in medial thigh
- Awareness that lump decreases in size with recumbency, increases in size with standing and with maneuvers that increase intra-abdominal pressure

Symptoms of complications, such as strangulation or incarceration, may include:
- Increase in severity of pain
- Increase in size of groin lump
- No reduction in size with recumbency
- Nausea, vomiting
- Severe constipation or obstipation

## ASSOCIATED DISORDERS
In some rare instances, complete colonic obstruction secondary to herniation may indicate colon cancer in the strangulated intestinal segment.

## KEY! DON'T MISS!
Richter's hernia will not involve symptoms of bowel obstruction (such as vomiting) but can lead to perforation and peritonitis.

## CONSIDER CONSULT
- Irreducible hernia
- Enlarging hernia sac
- Increasing pain or pain even after reduction of hernia sac
- Signs and/or symptoms of bowel obstruction
- Femoral hernia

## INVESTIGATION OF THE PATIENT
### Direct questions to patient
Q How long have you noticed the lump in your groin?
Q Does the lump change in size? What causes the lump to change in size? A lump that enlarges with standing and decreases with recumbency is typical of groin hernia
Q Are you experiencing any pain? Uncomplicated groin hernias may cause some aching or heaviness but don't usually cause acute pain. Severe pain may indicate strangulation or incarceration
Q Have you experienced any change in your bowel habits? Changes in bowel habits could suggest incarceration
Q Have you ever been told that you have a hernia? Hernias can recur, even after surgical treatment
Q Has anyone else in your family ever had a hernia? The tendency to develop a hernia can run in the family
Q Do you have any medical conditions that cause you to cough regularly? Patients with chronic obstructive pulmonary disease (COPD) or chronic bronchitis have a predisposition to the development of hernia
Q Do you have any medical conditions that cause you to strain while urinating or defecating? Prostatism or chronic constipation can predispose to hernia development
Q Do you smoke? Cigarette smoking may cause weakened fascia, predisposing to hernia development

### Contributory or predisposing factors
Q Do you smoke cigarettes? Cigarette smoking (especially in women) may cause weakened fascia, predisposing to hernia development
Q Was your birth premature? Prematurity predisposes to hernia development
Q What was your birthweight? Low birthweight can be a risk factor for hernia development
Q Do you or anyone in your family have any connective tissue disorders? Defects in connective tissue may increase the likelihood of developing a hernia
Q What is your pregnancy history? Pregnancy can weaken the musculature of the pelvic floor, posing an increased risk for hernia development. Multiparity increases the risk

### Family history
Q Do you know of other family members who have had hernias? The tendency to have a hernia can run in families
Q Do you or anyone in your family have any connective tissue disorders? Defects in connective tissue may increase the likelihood of developing a hernia

### Examination
- Examine patient both supine and standing
- Perform baseline resting examination and then again with patient performing the Valsalva maneuver
- Begin by looking carefully at the location of the suspected hernia, observing for any visible lumps, bulges, or asymmetry
- Ask patient to cough or perform Valsalva maneuver, continuing to observe for increase in bulge

- Gently palpate the area, observing for the presence of a lump as well as any tenderness to palpation
- In male patients, use a finger to probe the scrotal sac. Gently advance the finger into the inguinal canal; if the hernia is palpated with the distal tip of the examining finger, it is likely an indirect hernia; if the hernia is palpated with the pad of the finger, it is likely a direct hernia
- A lump below the level of the inguinal ligament is likely a femoral hernia

### Summary of investigative tests
- Diagnosis of a hernia does not require additional testing
- Testing may be ordered by a specialist, if there is evidence that the hernia is strangulated
- Imaging studies may be required prior to surgical repair but will be ordered by the surgical team

### DIAGNOSTIC DECISION
Diagnosis of hernia is nearly always clinical, based on history and examination.

### CLINICAL PEARLS
- Pain is rarely severe or persistent, unless there is a complication. Local pain may suggest incarceration, whereas colicky pain suggests strangulation
- If a hernia is present in the scrotum, it is most likely an indirect hernia
- If a hernia is palpable below the inguinal ligament, it is probably a femoral hernia. The increased risk of complications with femoral hernias dictates early surgical evaluation
- It is frequently not easy to tell if a hernia is direct or indirect by physical examination. You cannot always tell which type it is until operation
- Although the predictive value is not high, in patients who have developed hernias look for a change in bowel habits or any other indications of possible colon cancer. If present, lower endoscopy is indicated, but routine studies (e.g. flexible sigmoidoscopy) do not appear to be cost-effective for every hernia

## TREATMENT

### CONSIDER CONSULT
Immediately if there is evidence of incarceration or strangulation.

### IMMEDIATE ACTION
- Refer immediately to surgeon if patient seems to have any systemic symptoms or suggestions of toxicity, bowel obstruction, or persisting pain
- Begin antibiotic therapy immediately if strangulation or bowel ischemia is suspected

### PATIENT AND CAREGIVER ISSUES
#### Impact on career, dependants, family, friends
Patient should be asked to avoid heavy lifting, which could affect work, recreation, and childcare.

### MANAGEMENT ISSUES
#### Goals
- If possible, reduce hernia sac back through defect in an attempt to prevent incarceration or strangulation
- Immediate surgical treatment is needed for irreducible, incarcerated, or strangulated hernias
- Prompt surgical evaluation and treatment are needed for most hernias, even those that are easily reducible, to prevent enlargement and eventual incarceration/strangulation
- While surgical evaluation and treatment are being completed, efforts should be directed at avoiding an increase in intra-abdominal pressure

#### Management in special circumstances
COEXISTING DISEASE

Most coexisting diseases will not impact on treatment of hernia; only severely debilitated patients may be unable to tolerate hernia repair.

SPECIAL PATIENT GROUPS
- In experienced hands, the risks of operative repair are very low, so that surgical repair is indicated for most patients, especially when the hernia compromises the patient's quality of life
- Severely debilitated patients may need to defer repair of an uncomplicated hernia until their medical condition is stable
- Patients with an uncomplicated hernia in whom watchful waiting is appropriate include the extremely elderly, as well as patients who are suffering from terminal illness or immunosuppression, or whose baseline condition represents an unacceptable surgical risk
- Pregnant women may need to defer repair of an uncomplicated hernia until after delivery
- Note that even debilitated or pregnant patients who appear toxic or who have incarcerated or strangulated hernias will require emergency surgery

### SUMMARY OF THERAPEUTIC OPTIONS
#### Choices
- Reduction of uncomplicated hernia
- Truss, surgical belt or binder
- Herniorrhaphy, including open and laparoscopic herniorrhaphy
- Consider starting a broad-spectrum antibiotic such as cefoxitin if patient appears toxic and bowel ischemia is suspected

#### Clinical pearls
- Emergency surgery is only necessary when strangulation or incarceration is present
- The risk of complications is greatest when hernias first present and the fascial defect is small. Furthermore, hernias that can not be easily reduced are at increased risk. With these

exceptions, it is not possible to reliably predict which hernias are at greatest risk of complication
- The most cautious approach is to refer all hernias for surgical evaluation and to inform patients of what to do if the hernia becomes incarcerated. Waiting for surgical repair does entail some risks of complication, so that surgical consultation for most hernias is indicated
- An argument for early surgery is that hernias tend to enlarge over time and cause more discomfort. Furthermore, large hernias are more difficult to repair than are smaller ones
- Since it is very difficult to distinguish direct from indirect hernias clinically, this is not a good basis for deciding upon referral

### Never
Never delay a surgical referral if there is any suggestion that hernia is incarcerated or strangulated.

### FOLLOW UP
Patient should follow up with surgeon to plan for definitive hernia repair.

### Information for patient or caregiver
- Physician should carefully explain to patient that even though hernia may be asymptomatic, the risk of enlargement and complications is significant, therefore warranting surgical consultation
- Risk of inguinal hernia strangulation is highest in the first 3 months (3%); however, the cumulative risk at 21 months increases to 4.5%
- Femoral hernias in particular carry a very high risk of strangulation (20% at 3 months; 45% at 21 months)

## DRUGS AND OTHER THERAPIES: DETAILS
### Drugs
CEFOXITIN
Consider starting a broad-spectrum antibiotic such as cefoxitin if patient:
- Appears toxic
- May have strangulated hernia with gangrenous bowel
- Has potential contamination of peritoneal cavity

*Dose*
- Adults: 1g intravenously every 8h
- Children: 80mg/kg/day intravenously divided into four equal doses

*Efficacy*
Broad-spectrum antibiotic efficacious for prevention of peritonitis in suspected strangulated/ischemic bowel.

*Risks/benefits*
Risks:
- Use caution in renal disease and history of gastrointestinal disease
- Use caution in pregnancy, breast-feeding, and the elderly
- Use caution in pre-existing coagulopathy
- Use caution with intramuscular injections and hypersensitivity to penicillins

*Side effects and adverse reactions*
- Cardiovascular system: hypotension
- Central nervous system: malaise, headache, dizziness, fever
- Gastrointestinal: nausea, vomiting, diarrhea, pseudomembranous colitis, abdominal pain, liver enzyme disturbances, transient hepatitis and cholestatic jaundice

- Genitourinary: nephrotoxicity, interstitial nephritis
- Hematologic: blood cell dyscrasias
- Musculoskeletal: exacerbation of myasthenia gravis
- Skin: maculopapular rash, urticaria, injection site reaction, rashes, pruritus

*Interactions (other drugs)*
- Aminoglycosides ■ Chloramphenicol ■ Estrogens ■ Loop diuretics ■ Polymyxin B
- Probenecid ■ Oral anticoagulants ■ Typhoid vaccine ■ Vancomycin

*Contraindications*
- Hypersensitivity to cephalosporins ■ Porphyria

## Surgical therapy
HERNIORRHAPHY
- Herniorrhaphy is the only definitive cure for hernia
- All femoral hernias should undergo rapid repair due to very high risk of incarceration and strangulation
- Hernia repair may be elective if hernia is reducible, asymptomatic, and uncomplicated
- Emergency repair is indicated if hernia is incarcerated, very painful, strangulated, or if there is any evidence of toxicity of intestinal obstruction

Approaches to herniorrhaphy include:
- Open nonmesh repair (this traditional approach has a high rate of recurrence because of tension at suture lines, with the exception of experienced hands performing the Shouldice technique)
- Open tension-free mesh repair
- Laparoscopic tension-free mesh repair

*Efficacy*
- Newer tension-free mesh repairs (both open and laparoscopic) have dropped recurrence rates
- Surgical repair greatly lowers the risk of hernia enlargement and eventual incarceration, strangulation, and bowel ischemia, particularly with femoral hernias

*Risks/benefits*
Risks:
- Necessity of general anesthesia for performance of laparoscopic herniorrhaphy increases associated anesthesia risks
- Increased time to perform laparoscopic herniorrhaphy poses an increased risk of certain rare complications
- Laparoscopic herniorrhaphy is limited by greater expense, the need for specially trained operator, and required use of disposable equipment

Benefits:
- Nonlaparoscopic methods may be performed using local or regional anesthesia, eliminating the risks of general anesthesia
- Laparoscopic herniorrhaphy has some advantages because of decrease in pain, faster convalescence, and quicker return to work and other activities, but the advantages are marginal and may not compensate for somewhat higher risk of complications due to bowel obstruction, or injury to nerve, major vessels, bowel and bladder

*Acceptability to patient*
Patient may prefer laparoscopic technique if he or she has read or heard of decreased pain and faster recovery time associated with this technique.

*Follow up plan*
Patient should be monitored after herniorrhaphy due to relatively high recurrence rate (particularly with nonmesh repairs).

*Patient and caregiver information*
After surgical repair, patients should make lifestyle changes aimed at decreasing intra-abdominal pressure or prevent further weakening of the abdominal fascia:
- Achieve and maintain appropriate weight
- Eliminate smoking
- Eat a high-fiber diet and drink eight glasses of water a day to reduce constipation and straining at stool (for more severe constipation, an enema or stool softener may be prescribed)
- Follow instructions regarding heavy lifting

## Other therapies
TRUSS, SURGICAL BELT, OR BINDER
- Devices to attempt to hold a reduced hernia in place are often used, although they do not prevent the continued progression of fascial weakening and defect enlargement
- Use of a truss or other device should not replace prompt surgical evaluation to prevent the eventual incarceration and/or strangulation of a hernia
- Furthermore, a truss or other device should never be used when there is any possibility that a hernia is already incarcerated or strangulated

*Efficacy*
Trusses and other such devices may provide patient with a sense of support but have no efficacy in stopping the natural progression of a hernia.

*Risks/benefits*
- Risk: patient may rely on truss to 'cure' hernia
- Benefit: patient may feel more secure with a truss providing counterpressure to hernia as a temporary measure while awaiting surgical treatment

*Acceptability to patient*
Patient may request truss, thinking that it is a cure.

*Follow up plan*
It is imperative that the primary care physician clarify for the patient that a truss is not a cure and should not replace appropriate surgical management.

*Patient and caregiver information*
- Make sure that patient and caregiver understand that a truss is less a therapy, and more a comfort measure
- Patient and caregiver must understand that a surgical consultation still needs to be obtained

HERNIA REDUCTION
- Appropriate analgesia and/or sedation should be offered as necessary
- Cold pack should be applied to hernia to decrease swelling and blood flow
- Patient is positioned supine, pillow under buttocks
- If reducing an inguinal hernia, tilt patient head down 15–20°
- Ipsilateral leg is externally rotated and flexed prior to hernia reduction
- Guard the hernial ring with two fingers
- Use other hand to guide hernia sac gently but firmly through defect

*Efficacy*
May provide temporary relief of bulging hernia sac.

*Risks/benefits*
Risk: Richter's hernia may be reduced but vasculature to intestine may still be compromised, resulting in gangrene.

*Acceptability to patient*
May provide some relief of aching while awaiting surgical consultation.

*Follow up plan*
Patient should proceed with surgical consultation.

*Patient and caregiver information*
Make sure that patient and caregiver understand that hernia reduction is not a definitive cure but a temporary measure to decrease immediate risk of incarceration and strangulation while awaiting surgical consultation.

## LIFESTYLE
- Achieve and maintain appropriate weight
- Eliminate smoking
- Eat a high-fiber diet and drink eight glasses of water a day to reduce constipation and straining at stool (for more severe constipation, an enema or stool softener may be prescribed)
- Follow safety instructions regarding heavy lifting
- Receive treatment for chronic cough, allergies

### RISKS/BENEFITS
All of the above lifestyle changes have other benefits (e.g. cardiovascular, cancer prevention) aside from helping to prevent worsening of a hernia.

### ACCEPTABILITY TO PATIENT
Lifestyle changes such as smoking cessation and weight loss are some of the hardest to institute and maintain and require regular monitoring and support.

### FOLLOW UP PLAN
- While the patient is instituting lifestyle changes, regular appointments may help provide support
- Many patients benefit from organized weight loss programs
- Patients may require medications to help them break an addiction to tobacco

### PATIENT AND CAREGIVER INFORMATION
- Discuss openly with patient and caregiver the pitfalls of attempting to institute/maintain lifestyle changes
- Help patient and caregiver decide on a realistic plan of action that will provide them with appropriate support to successfully modify risk factors

## OUTCOMES

### EFFICACY OF THERAPIES
- Recurrence ranges estimated to be 5–8% for traditional surgery
- Recurrence is lower for tension-free mesh herniorrhaphy (probably <3%)
- Recurrence after laparoscopic herniorrhaphy is <4%

### PROGNOSIS
- Prognosis depends on hernia size and location, and duration of hernia
- Inguinal hernia: strangulation risk is 3% over first 3 months, 4.5% over first 2 years
- Femoral hernia: strangulation risk is 22% over 3 months, 45% over 2 years
- There is increased strangulation risk with large sac contents and a relatively small fascial defect

#### Clinical pearls
- The greatest variable in success of a surgical procedure is probably the experience of the surgeon, rather than the specific procedure used
- The differences between laparoscopic and open-mesh repair are close enough that the specific choice regarding surgical technique should rest upon the available surgical expertise and whether the patient can tolerate general anesthesia
- If reoperation is necessary for a recurrence, then there is an advantage to being able to take a different surgical approach, rather than operating through a scar. Therefore, some surgeons advise starting with an open, anterior repair, reserving the laproscopic approach for secondary procedures, if necessary
- Surgery for inguinal hernias is well tolerated at all ages and is, therefore, usually appropriate even for elderly patients if the hernia is interfering with quality of life or cannot be reduced easily

#### Therapeutic failure
- Recurrence of hernia constitutes therapeutic failure after surgery
- Recurrence rates are about 2–10%, depending upon surgical methods and expertise

#### Recurrence
Laparoscopic techniques are usually preferred for repair of recurrent hernia.

#### Deterioration
If a patient with known hernia develops more severe pain, enlarging hernia, signs/symptoms of bowel obstruction and/or toxicity, immediate surgical consultation should be obtained.

### COMPLICATIONS
- Incarceration of hernia sac
- Vascular compromise
- Ischemic, gangrenous bowel
- Bowel obstruction

# PREVENTION

- Hernias are thought to be due to pre-existing fascial defects and are therefore not believed to be entirely preventable
- Risk factor modification, however, may prevent a hernia from sliding through an existing defect and may prevent complications such as enlargement, incarceration, and strangulation

## RISK FACTORS
- Failure of obliteration of processus vaginalis (a congenital defect)
- Increased intra-abdominal pressure: this may increase due to a variety of medical conditions, including obesity, ascites, pregnancy, chronic cough (such as due to chronic obstructive pulmonary disease), constipation (or other conditions that result in straining to defecate), straining to urinate (as can occur in prostatism), heavy lifting, peritoneal dialysis, ventriculoperitoneal shunt
- Weakened connective tissue: a variety of conditions can weaken connective tissue, including connective tissue disorders, aging, cigarette smoking, systemic disease, prematurity, low birthweight
- Congenital conditions: hernia is associated with a history of undescended testicle, congenital pelvic abnormality, exstrophy of urinary bladder

## MODIFY RISK FACTORS
- Achieve and maintain appropriate weight
- Eliminate smoking
- Eat a high-fiber diet and drink eight glasses of water a day to reduce constipation and straining at stool (for more severe constipation, an enema or stool softener may be prescribed)
- Follow safety instructions regarding heavy lifting
- Receive treatment for chronic cough, allergies

### Lifestyle and wellness
TOBACCO
Smoking cessation should be encouraged, since cigarette smoking is a known risk factor for weakening connective tissue.

DIET
Diet should be manipulated to ensure easy passage of stool to prevent straining during defecation (increased intra-abdominal pressure can force intestinal contents through a pre-existing fascial defect).

PHYSICAL ACTIVITY
Some clinicians recommend strengthening abdominal musculature.

FAMILY HISTORY
Family history of hernia may increase an individual's risk for development of hernia.

## SCREENING
PHYSICAL EXAMINATION
All complete physical examinations should include screening for the presence of an asymptomatic hernia.

## PREVENT RECURRENCE
- Achieve and maintain appropriate weight
- Eliminate smoking

- Eat a high-fiber diet and drink eight glasses of water a day to reduce constipation and straining at stool (for more severe constipation, an enema or stool softener may be prescribed)
- Follow safety instructions regarding heavy lifting
- Receive treatment for chronic cough, allergies

# RESOURCES

## ASSOCIATIONS
American Gastroenterological Association
7910 Woodmont Ave., Seventh Floor
Bethesda, MD 20814
Tel: (301) 654-2055
Fax: (301) 652-3890
http://www.gastro.org

American Pediatric Surgical Association
60 Revere Drive, Suite 500
Northbrook, IL 60062
Tel: (847) 480-9576
Fax: (847) 480-9282
http://www.eapsa.org

Society for Surgery of the Alimentary Tract, Inc.,
13 Elm Street
Manchester, MA 01944
Tel: (978) 526-8330
Fax: (978) 526-4018
http://www.ssat.com

## KEY REFERENCES
- Approach to the patient with an external hernia. In: Goroll AH, Mulley AG, eds. Primary care medicine, 4th edn. Philadelphia: Lippincott Williams & Wilkins, 2000
- Bax T, Sheppard BC, Crass RA. Surgical options in the management of groin hernias. Am Fam Physician 1999;59(1):143–56
- Surgical options in the management of groin hernias. Available online: American Academy of Family Physicians
- Donohue JH, et al. Laparoscopic herniorrhaphy versus traditional herniorrhaphy. Rochester, MN: Mayo Clinic and Mayo Foundation
- Eubanks WS. In: Townsend CM, Beauchamp RD, Evers BM, eds. Sabiston textbook of surgery, 16th edn. Philadelphia: WB Saunders, 2001
- Marshall KG. Family practice sourcebook: evidence-based emphasis. St. Louis: Mosby-Year Book, 2000
- Scott NW, Webb K, Go PMNYH, et al, on behalf of the EU Hernia Trialists Collaboration. Open mesh versus non-mesh repair of inguinal hernia (Cochrane Review). In: The Cochrane Library, 1, 2002. Oxford: Update Software
- Simons MP. Meta-analysis: Shouldice technique is superior to the Bassini or McVay methods of hernia repair. November/December 1996. Available online: http://www.acponline.org/journals/ebm/novdec96/shouldic.htm
- Society for Surgery of the Alimentary Tract. Surgical repair of groin hernias. Available at the National Guideline Clearinghouse 1998; June 3 (revised January 2000)
- Webb K, Scott NW, Go PMNYH, et al, on behalf of the EU Hernia Trialists Collaboration. Laparoscopic techniques versus open techniques for inguinal hernia repair (Cochrane Review). In: The Cochrane Library, 1, 2002. Oxford: Update Software

## FAQS
### Question 1
When should a patient with a new onset hernia be referred for surgical evaluation?

### ANSWER 1
Since the risk with new onset hernias is greatest in the first few months, early surgical evaluation is the most cautious course.

## Question 2
For elderly patients who are reluctant to undergo surgery, what advice should they be offered?

### ANSWER 2
Surgery is elective, unless the hernia is incarcerated. The impact on their quality of life is the key factor; elderly patients tolerate surgery well. However, there is evidence that rates of mortality and complications are comparable for emergency and elective surgery for incarcerated hernias. Therefore, waiting is a reasonable option if the hernia is not bothering them and if they understand the necessity of seeking medical attention immediately if incarceration develops.

## Question 3
Is there any clinical value to using a truss?

### ANSWER 3
There is no evidence that trusses significantly control symptoms, prevent progression, or reduce the rate of complications. Their use can be driven by patient preferences.

## CONTRIBUTORS
Fred F Ferri, MD, FACP
Andrew H Soll, MD
Jaime Oviedo, MD

# IRRITABLE BOWEL SYNDROME

- Summary Information — 340
- Background — 341
- Diagnosis — 343
- Treatment — 352
- Outcomes — 364
- Prevention — 365
- Resources — 366

## SUMMARY INFORMATION

### DESCRIPTION

- Functional bowel disorder characterized by abdominal discomfort or pain associated with defecation or change in bowel habit and with features of disordered defecation
- Chronic, relapsing course, often overlapping with other functional gastrointestinal disorders
- Diagnosis is by clinical criteria (the Rome II criteria) with exclusion of organic disease
- May be classified as diarrhea-predominant or constipation-predominant irritable bowel syndrome (IBS)
- IBS does not predispose to other chronic or life-threatening disease and does not shorten life; however, it does disrupt the quality of life

### URGENT ACTION

- The presence of 'alarm symptoms,' including persistent nausea and vomiting, melenic stools, weight loss, and anorexia, is not compatible with IBS and denotes a more pressing and sinister diagnosis
- In particular, signs of active bleeding including hematemesis or bright red blood per rectum require urgent or emergency endoscopy by a gastroenterologist

### KEY! DON'T MISS!

- All patients with lower gastrointestinal symptoms should have at least one flexible sigmoidoscopy (diagnostic, not screening) to exclude other diagnoses. A referral to a gastroenterologist for colonoscopy may be preferable in patients at risk for colon cancer
- Abuse of laxatives can cause bloating and chronic diarrhea (or constipation); if patients are not thoroughly queried on this point, the diagnosis may be missed.
- Some other medications, including selective serotonin reuptake inhibitors (SSRIs), thyroid hormone, and certain antiarrhythmics, may mimic diarrhea-predominant IBS and should, therefore, be carefully noted
- Constipation is a common effect of many medication classes as well, especially calcium channel blockers
- Psychosocial problems are common; take time to make patients feel seen and heard
- Organic disease (e.g. inflammatory bowel disease) can mimic or coexist with IBS, justifying the sigmoidoscopy in all symptomatic patients. Coexistent IBS can confound management of inflammatory bowel disease
- Patients whose symptoms develop while the patients are chewing gum may have sorbitol-induced osmotic diarrhea, or so-called chewing gum diarrhea. This condition is easy to diagnose and even easier to treat – by abstaining from the habit

## BACKGROUND

### ICD9 CODE
564.1 Irritable bowel syndrome

### SYNONYMS
Spastic colon, irritable colon, mucous colitis.

### CARDINAL FEATURES
- Chronic, relapsing functional bowel disorder
- Characterized by abdominal discomfort or pain associated with defecation or change in bowel habit and with features of disordered defecation
- May be classified as diarrhea-predominant irritable bowel syndrome (IBS) or constipation-predominant IBS
- Diagnosis is by symptom-based criteria (Rome II criteria) along with cost-effective exclusion of organic disease
- Symptoms must have been present for 12 weeks or more within the past 12 months; the 12 weeks need not be consecutive
- Psychologic stress exacerbates gastrointestinal distress in patients with IBS to a greater degree than in the normal population
- Treatment is symptomatic; there is no cure

### CAUSES
#### Common causes
- Cause unknown, but symptoms are thought to result from disturbed intestinal motility and enhanced visceral sensitivity
- IBS is 10 times more likely to occur after acute infectious diarrhea
- Other postulated (but unproven) causes include inflammation, food sensitivity, lack of dietary fiber, and antibiotics
- Genetic factors may play a role in development of IBS, since clustering within families has been well described

#### Contributory or predisposing factors
Psychosocial trauma, e.g. a history of physical or sexual abuse, major loss (death or divorce), or other major trauma, is more common in patients presenting with IBS than in those without the disorder.

### EPIDEMIOLOGY
#### Incidence and prevalence
INCIDENCE
0.1–0.2/1000.

PREVALENCE
1.5–2.0/1000.

FREQUENCY
- In the US, IBS affects 14–24% of women and 5–9% of men
- IBS is the most common reason for referral to gastroenterologists, accounting for 20–50% of referred patients

#### Demographics
AGE
- Presentation is most common between the ages 30 and 50 years
- Onset in old age is rare

GENDER
Female:male ratio = 2:1, but this may reflect patterns of care seeking rather than actual incidence.

RACE
Prevalence is similar in Caucasians and African-Americans but may be lower in people of Hispanic origin.

GENETICS
Unknown but more common in families of patients.

# DIAGNOSIS

## DIFFERENTIAL DIAGNOSIS
### Ulcerative colitis
FEATURES
- Peak onset is at 15–35 years
- Bloody diarrhea with mucus is common, along with fever, abdominal pain, and tenesmus
- Patients often report weight loss
- Sigmoidoscopy or colonoscopy usually reveals mucosal erythema, granularity, hemorrhage, and pseudopolyps
- Barium enema film usually shows loss of haustrations, mucosal irregularity, and ulceration

### Crohn's disease
FEATURES
- Onset is biphasic, at 15–35 years and 70–80 years of age
- Fever, abdominal pain, and diarrhea (often without blood) are common presenting symptoms
- Fatigue and weight loss are common
- Anorectal fissures, fistulas, and abscesses may be present
- Sigmoidoscopy, colonoscopy, or barium enema films usually reveal nodularity, rigidity, ulcers, cobblestoning, skip lesions (segmental defects), strictures, and fistulas

### Infectious diarrhea
FEATURES
- Chronic diarrhea with cramps is the most common presenting symptom
- Blood and mucus often present in stool in *Entamoeba histolytica* infection
- Malaise and weight loss common in *E. histolytica* infection and can be seen in *Giardia lamblia* infection
- History may reveal recent travel to endemic areas (especially with *E. histolytica* or *G. lamblia*)
- Stool examination reveals cysts and ova of *E. histolytica* or *G. lamblia*
- Stool culture reveals presence of *Clostridium difficile*
- Sigmoidoscopy may show pseudomembrane formation in severe cases of *C. difficile* infection

### Diverticulitis
FEATURES
- Pain, fever, and altered bowel habit are usual presenting symptoms
- Left lower abdominal pain may be found on physical examination
- Leukocytosis is common (but absent in up to 45%)
- Computed tomography (CT) and barium enema both will detect diverticula (mucosal outpouchings), usually in the sigmoid colon. However, CT has become the test of choice to detect diverticulitis
- Increased soft tissue density within pericolic fat as result of inflammation, bowel wall thickening, pericolic fluid formation, and soft tissue inflammatory masses

### Colorectal malignancy
FEATURES
- Most common in patients over 50 years of age
- Left-sided cancers usually present with rectal bleeding, altered bowel habit (constipation, intermittent diarrhea, and tenesmus), and abdominal or back pain
- Cecal and ascending colon cancers usually present with anemia, occult blood in stool, and weight loss
- Diagnosis is confirmed by flexible sigmoidoscopy or, preferably, colonoscopy

### Lactose intolerence
**FEATURES**
- Abdominal distension and bloating are common
- Diarrhea and occasionally constipation are usual presenting symptoms
- Symptoms are exacerbated by intake of dairy products
- Trial of lactose-free diet for 2 weeks produces marked improvement in symptoms
- Positive lactose hydrogen breath test confirms diagnosis
- Lactose intolerance often presents with irritable bowel syndrome (IBS), exacerbating symptoms presumably by causing abdominal distension that provokes pain and adding an osmotic element to the diarrhea

### Medications
**FEATURES**
- A concordance of symptoms with starting or taking of the medication provides helpful data
- A trial of stopping medication or reducing dose will confirm the impression
- A rechallenge provides confirmation of the cause
- Some medications exacerbate or mimic diarrhea-predominant IBS; the most common of these are antacids, laxatives, selective serotonin reuptake inhibitors, thyroid hormone, and metformin.
- Other medications, such as narcotics, calcium channel blockers, and anticholinergic agents, exacerbate or mimic constipation-predominant IBS

### Malabsorption syndromes
**FEATURES**
- Present with diarrhea, sometimes marked by large volume, foul stool
- Weight loss is frequent
- Bacterial overgrowth is an important complicating factor, especially in older patients or patients with bowel dysmotility

### Endocrinopathies
**FEATURES**
- Hyperthyroidism and hypothyroidism can produce diarrhea. Characteristic features may be subtle, and laboratory confirmation is essential, especially in older patients
- Diabetes mellitus type 1 and type 2: several mechanisms produce diarrhea, including autonomic neuropathy and bacterial overgrowth. Metformin may produce diarrhea

### Dietary factors
**FEATURES**
Ingestion of large amounts of nonabsorbable 'diet' sweeteners can produce diarrhea that may mimic IBS.

### Painless diarrhea
**FEATURES**
- Although painless diarrhea may be functional, if pain is lacking, the diagnosis of IBS should not be made
- There are usually no distinctive features of painless diarrhea. As noted, the cause may be idiopathic (no diagnosis identified), but often specific entities are found, such as collagenous or lymphocytic colitis

## SIGNS & SYMPTOMS
### Signs
- A normal physical examination is most common
- Abdominal distension may be visible. This can be a rather dramatic feature
- Tender sigmoid colon may be palpable

- Radiography is often normal, but exaggerated haustral contractions may be seen in barium enema and marked contractions may be seen on sigmoidoscopy
- Patients may be generally tense and anxious
- Patients with constipation-predominant IBS may have a rectocele, rectal prolapse, or internal and external hemorrhoids apparent on examination

## Symptoms

- History of at least 12 weeks in the preceding 12 months of abdominal pain or discomfort that is relieved with defecation, has an onset associated with change in frequency of stool, or has an onset associated with change in appearance of stool (pain must have at least two of these features to meet criteria for diagnosis of IBS)
- Patients with diarrhea-predominant IBS usually report more than three bowel movements per day, loose or watery stools, and urgency
- Patients with constipation-predominant IBS usually report fewer than three bowel movements per week, hard and lumpy stools, and straining during bowel movement
- Some patients may report alternating diarrhea and constipation
- Patients may report feelings of incomplete evacuation and abdominal fullness, bloating, or swelling
- Clear or white mucus is often passed with stool
- Occasionally, incontinence and tenesmus occur
- Symptoms are commonly exacerbated by stress

## ASSOCIATED DISORDERS

- Psychiatric illnesses – depression, anxiety, panic disorder – have a higher than normal prevalence in patients presenting with IBS
- Migraine occurs more frequently in patients with IBS than in the general population
- Patients with IBS frequently experience urinary dysfunction, most commonly increased bladder frequency, urgency, and nocturia
- Sexual dysfunction, including inhibited sexual desire, is more common in persons with IBS than in those with organic bowel disease
- Altered sleep patterns are common, especially among patients with diarrhea-predominant IBS

## KEY! DON'T MISS!

- All patients with lower gastrointestinal symptoms should have at least one flexible sigmoidoscopy (diagnostic, not screening) to exclude other diagnoses. A referral to a gastroenterologist for colonoscopy may be preferable in patients at risk for colon cancer
- Abuse of laxatives can cause bloating and chronic diarrhea (or constipation); if patients are not thoroughly queried on this point, the diagnosis may be missed.
- Some other medications, including selective serotonin reuptake inhibitors (SSRIs), thyroid hormone, and certain antiarrhythmics, may mimic diarrhea-predominant IBS and should, therefore, be carefully noted
- Constipation is a common effect of many medication classes as well, especially calcium channel blockers
- Psychosocial problems are common; take time to make patients feel seen and heard
- Organic disease (e.g. inflammatory bowel disease) can mimic or coexist with IBS, justifying the sigmoidoscopy in all symptomatic patients. Coexistent IBS can confound management of inflammatory bowel disease
- Patients whose symptoms develop while the patients are chewing gum may have sorbitol-induced osmotic diarrhea, or so-called chewing gum diarrhea. This condition is easy to diagnose and even easier to treat – by abstaining from the habit

## CONSIDER CONSULT

- Patients with alarm symptoms or signs (gastrointestinal bleeding, anemia, anorexia, weight loss, etc) should be referred to a gastroenterologist for flexible sigmoidoscopy (at least) and,

preferably, colonoscopy
- Patients with refractory symptoms also deserve a gastroenterologic evaluation

## INVESTIGATION OF THE PATIENT
### Direct questions to patient

Q How long have you been experiencing symptoms? To qualify as having IBS, patients must have had symptoms for at least 12 weeks (not necessarily consecutive) in the preceding 12 months; more recent onset of shorter duration should suggest a different diagnosis, although it may represent early and evolving IBS

Q Are symptoms relieved by defecation? This is characteristic of IBS

Q Are symptoms exacerbated after food or during menses? Both are common in IBS

Q Are symptoms exacerbated by stress? Very common finding in persons with IBS

Q Do you ever use laxatives? Careful questioning is required to elucidate possible laxative abuse, which can cause chronic diarrhea or constipation

### Contributory or predisposing factors
Is there any history of psychosocial trauma? History of physical or sexual abuse is common in patients presenting with IBS

### Family history

Q Do any family members have IBS? Incidence is higher among family members, although the genetics of the syndrome is not known

Q Is there any family history of colon or rectal malignancy? Consider this as differential diagnosis in persons with appropriate symptoms and history

### Examination
- Palpate the abdomen. Usually normal, but a tender left lower quadrant may be palpable; tenderness or guarding in any other area should suggest a different diagnosis
- Perform a digital rectal examination if rectal obstruction is suspected. Patients with IBS often experience pain on rectal examination but no obstruction or palpable masses are found. Examination may reveal signs of straining, including a rectocele, prolapse, and internal or external hemorrhoids. Stool should be guaiac negative

### Summary of investigative tests
The majority of investigative tests are normal in patients with IBS; they are ordered to exclude other diagnoses, depending on presenting symptoms and history.
- Hematologic evaluation, including complete blood count (CBC) and erythrocyte sedimentation rate (ESR), will help exclude IBD (ulcerative colitis and Crohn's disease), colorectal malignancy and diverticulitis
- Stool for occult blood and fecal leukocytes may give a clue to inflammation or neoplasia
- Lactose hydrogen breath test should be performed if there is a high index of suspicion of parasitic infection, and stool testing will usually confirm *Clostridium difficile* infection
- *Giardia* antigen test of stool may be more sensitive or available than direct examination of stool
- Stool examination test should be considered in patients with diarrhea-predominant symptoms, especially if a lactose-free diet trial shows equivocal results. Lactose intolerance can mimic or complicate management of IBS
- Flexible sigmoidoscopy or colonoscopy should be performed in patients with recent onset of symptoms suggestive of IBS and in those with suspected colorectal malignancy; the procedure may be performed by a gastroenterologist or primary care physician, depending on experience
- For diarrhea-predominant IBS, an evaluation might also include stool fat, to evaluate for malabsorption
- Stool weight provides a useful clue to another mechanism for diarrhea; stool weight is rarely greater than 300g daily in IBS

## DIAGNOSTIC DECISION

Formal diagnosis is made by symptom assessment (according to the Rome II criteria). (Thompson WG, Longstreth GF, Drossman DA, et al. Functional bowel disorders and functional abdominal pain [1]

These criteria require at least 12 weeks (not necessarily consecutive) in the preceding 12 months of abdominal discomfort or pain that has two of three features:
- Relieved with defecation
- Onset associated with change in frequency of bowel movement
- Onset associated with change in form of stool

Supportive symptoms for a diagnosis of irritable bowel syndrome include:
- Abnormal stool frequency (>3/day or <3/week)
- Abnormal stool form
- Abnormal stool passage (straining, urgency, feeling of incomplete evacuation)
- Passage of mucus
- Bloating and abdominal distension

A positive symptom assessment combined with a cost-effective diagnostic screen (hematology, stool examination, flexible sigmoidoscopy) to exclude organic disease is the basis for diagnosis of irritable bowel syndrome.

Some patients who do not meet formal criteria may still have irritable bowel syndrome.

The American Gastroenterological Association has produced position statements on irritable bowel syndrome:
- American Gastroenterological Association medical position statement: irritable bowel syndrome [2]
- Drossman DA, Whitehead WE, Camilleri M. Irritable bowel syndrome: a technical review for practice guideline development [3]

The American Academy of Family Physicians has published an article and statement about irritable bowel syndrome:
- Dalton CB, Drossman DA. Diagnosis and treatment of irritable bowel syndrome [4]

## CLINICAL PEARLS
- Consider lactose intolerance because it can confound and mimic IBS. A clinical assessment and therapeutic trial may be sufficient
- Symptoms of IBS suggest an irritable or inflamed lower gastrointestinal tract; a thoughtful clinical assessment is necessary to make a diagnosis. A reasonably confident diagnosis of IBS can be made based upon the history; this is the value of the Rome criteria. However, some patients with an irritable bowel will not meet formal criteria, usually because their IBS is less frequent or is precipitated mainly by stressful events
- Occasional surprises warrant performing a minimal evaluation in patients with persistent symptoms. The risk of organic disease is low, but a high level of suspicion for the rather obvious clues is important: fever, anorexia, weight loss, gastrointestinal blood loss, anemia, etc.
- In patients over 50 years of age or with any risk factors for colon cancer, a sigmoidoscopy or colonoscopy is routine; symptoms of IBS are only another reason to do one of these tests properly once
- IBS is usually a disorder that comes and goes, varying in intensity. Persistent, progressive symptoms warrant a work-up
- When diarrhea is the predominant problem, additional tests are indicated, such as thyroid function studies, and three stools for fecal leukocytes and ova and parasites

- Persistent diarrhea without pain is not IBS
- Persistent diarrhea warrants a work-up, as do symptoms that are progressive or awaken the patient from sleep
- IBS cannot be implicated in cases with anorexia, malnutrition, and weight loss unless there is concurrent psychologic illness. Even then, the cause is not the IBS per se

## THE TESTS
### Body fluids
COMPLETE BLOOD COUNT (CBC)
*Description*
Venous blood.

*Advantages/Disadvantages*
Quick, inexpensive test for anemia and leukocytosis.

*Normal*
- Hemoglobin – women: 12–16g/dL (7.4–9.9mmol/L)
- Hemoglobin – men: 13–18g/dL (8.1–11.2mmol/L)
- Total leukocytes: 4300–10,800/mcL (4.3–10.8x10$^9$/L)

*Abnormal*
- Hemoglobin – women: <12g/dL (<7.4mmol/L)
- Hemoglobin – men: <13g/dL (<8.1mmol/L)
- Total leukocytes: >10,800/mcL (>10.8x10$^9$/L)

*Cause of abnormal result*
- Anemia may be a sign of colorectal malignancy, IBD, or diverticulitis
- May also occur from underlying endocrinopathies, including thyroid disorders and diabetes, or other chronic disorders
- An elevated mean corpuscular volume may be a sign of Crohn's disease with terminal ileitis
- Eosinophilia on the differential cell count may denote underlying parasitic infection
- Leukocytosis may be a sign of diverticulitis or pancreatitis

ERYTHROCYTE SEDIMENTATION RATE (ESR)
*Description*
Venous blood.

*Advantages/Disadvantages*
Quick, inexpensive test that helps rule out ulcerative colitis.

*Normal*
Men: 0–15mm/h
Women: 0–20mm/h
(The upper limit of normal is a function of age. It can generally be figured as half of the patient's age. For example, an ESR of 40 may be perfectly normal for an 84-year-old patient.)

*Abnormal*
Men: >15mm/h
Women: >20mm/h

*Cause of abnormal result*
Elevated ESR may be a sign of ulcerative colitis but is nonspecific and may be elevated in a multitude of other inflammatory disorders.

*Drugs, disorders and other factors that may alter results*
Corticosteroids can cause low ESR measurement.

## MICROSCOPIC EXAMINATION OF STOOL
*Description*
Stool samples (preferably three separate samples taken on three separate days) are used to provide inoculum for wet mount slides, which are examined for the presence of cysts of parasites and of occult blood. Can also be examined for presence of stool leukocytes.

*Advantages/Disadvantages*
- Cysts can be missed if fewer than three samples are examined
- Quick, inexpensive test

*Normal*
- No cysts seen
- No blood cells seen
- Occasional stool leukocytes

*Abnormal*
- Cysts of *Gardia lamblia* or *Entamoeba histolytica* identified
- Blood cells visible
- Sheets of stool leukocytes

*Cause of abnormal result*
- Presence of cysts indicates amebiasis or giardiasis
- Presence of occult blood may indicate colorectal malignancy

*Drugs, disorders and other factors that may alter results*
- Test is not very sensitive or specific for colorectal malignancy
- False-positive results can occur with ingestion of red meat, horseradish, turnips, iron, or aspirin
- False-negative results can occur with vitamin C ingestion
- Results may be affected by sampling and laboratory technique

## STOOL CULTURE
*Description*
Stool sample grown in tissue culture to detect *C. difficile* toxin, the presence of which is confirmed by neutralization with specific antitoxin.

*Advantages/Disadvantages*
- Test is highly specific for *C. difficile* infection with good laboratory technique, but in some patient populations only 75% of isolates carry toxin
- Other tests, including cytotoxic, enzyme-linked immunosorbent assay (ELISA), and latex agglutination studies, all have imperfect sensitivity and specificity

*Normal*
*C. difficile* toxin not detected.

*Abnormal*
*C. difficile* toxin detected. May remain positive for up to 8 weeks after successful treatment.

*Cause of abnormal result*
*C. difficile* present in stool.

*Drugs, disorders and other factors that may alter results*
Sampling and laboratory technique may affect results.

## Imaging
### FLEXIBLE SIGMOIDOSCOPY
*Advantages/Disadvantages*
- The test is normal in patients with IBS; it is performed to exclude pathologic conditions
- Will miss any lesion proximal to the splenic flexure

*Normal*
Sigmoid colon appears normal.

*Abnormal*
- Strong, painful spasms on insertion of the sigmoidoscope may be seen in patients with IBS, but the test is certainly not diagnostic
- Polyps or carcinoma may be seen in patients with colorectal malignancy
- Mucosal erythema, granularity, friability, exudate, hemorrhage, ulcers, and pseudopolyps are characteristic of ulcerative colitis, Crohn's disease
- Mucosal nodularity, deep ulceration, cobblestoning, skip lesions, strictures, and fistulas are typical of Crohn's disease

*Cause of abnormal result*
- Colorectal malignancy
- Ulcerative colitis
- Crohn's disease

*Drugs, disorders and other factors that may alter results*
Enema preceding sigmoidoscopy can initiate mucus production and edema of mucosa, so that normal vessel pattern is obscured. However, unless diarrhea is marked, enemas are usually necessary.

### COLONOSCOPY
*Advantages/Disadvantages*
- Ability to visualize the entire colon and possibly the terminal ileum
- Ability to take biopsy specimens or remove polyps
- The test should be normal in patients with IBS, since it is performed to exclude other pathologic conditions
- The test is performed by a specialist
- The bowel preparation is occasionally inadequate, making the test difficult to perform
- There is a slight risk of perforation of the bowel, or bowel hemorrhage
- The procedure requires the use of analgesia and sedative medication

*Normal*
Colon and terminal ileum appear normal.

*Abnormal*
- Strong, painful spasms on insertion of the sigmoidoscope may be seen in patients with IBS, but the test is certainly not diagnostic
- Polyps or carcinoma may be seen in patients with colorectal malignancy
- Mucosal erythema, granularity, friability, exudate, hemorrhage, ulcers, and pseudopolyps are characteristic of ulcerative colitis, Crohn's disease
- Mucosal nodularity, deep ulceration, cobblestoning, skip lesions, strictures, and fistulas are typical of Crohn's disease

- Outpouchings of the mucosa are seen in diverticular disease, and inflammation is visualized in diverticulitis

*Cause of abnormal result*
- Colorectal malignancy
- Ulcerative colitis
- Crohn's disease
- Diverticular disease

*Drugs, disorders and other factors that may alter results*
Enemas are usually not used, since orally ingested bowel preparation is required. If the bowel preparation is inadequate, this may alter the efficacy of the test. If an enema is used, it can initiate mucus production and edema of mucosa, so that normal vessel pattern is obscured.

## Special tests
LACTOSE HYDROGEN BREATH TEST
*Description*
Hydrogen in breath is measured at start of test and every 30min for 3h after ingestion of 25g lactose or 2g/kg.

*Advantages/Disadvantages*
Test is highly specific for lactose intolerance.

*Normal*
Change in breath hydrogen <20ppm.

*Abnormal*
Change in breath hydrogen >20ppm.

*Cause of abnormal result*
Lactase deficiency, leading to fermentation of malabsorbed lactose by intestinal bacteria, with subsequent production of intestinal gas.

*Drugs, disorders and other factors that may alter results*
- False-positive results can occur if patient does not fast before the test, or if the patient has been smoking
- False-negative results can occur with recent antibiotic use

# TREATMENT

## CONSIDER CONSULT

- Patients in whom the diagnosis is in doubt, who do not respond to therapy, and whose symptoms become progressively worse, become incapacitating, interfere with daily activities, or are associated with any alarm symptoms, should be referred to a gastroenterologist for further assessment and treatment
- Patients with psychosocial problems that are not responding to initial therapy may be referred to a psychiatrist for co-management
- Patients with a suspected diagnosis of colorectal malignancy should be referred immediately to a gastroenterologist

## PATIENT AND CAREGIVER ISSUES

### Patient or caregiver request

- Reassure patients that irritable bowel syndrome (IBS) does not predispose to gastrointestinal malignancy or inflammatory bowel disease
- Emphasize to patients that the symptoms are not just 'in their mind' but can be explained by a physical phenomenon and are definitely real

### Health-seeking behavior

Has the patient been taking laxatives or antidiarrheal medications? Use of these medications may obscure the symptom pattern of IBS; also, be aware that laxative abuse can present as chronic diarrhea or constipation.

## MANAGEMENT ISSUES

### Goals

- Control of gastrointestinal symptoms
- Identification and management of any coexisting psychiatric illness
- Establishment of a good physcan-patient relationship, educating and reassuring the patient that symptoms of IBS are very real

### Management in special circumstances

COEXISTING DISEASE

Coexisting psychiatric illness can usually be managed in the primary care setting; referral to a psychiatrist is necessary only if psychiatric symptoms are refractory to treatment.

COEXISTING MEDICATION

Patients self-administering laxatives or antidiarrheal medication should be advised to stop before commencing the prescribed regimen. Should also minimize if possible other medications that may affect motility, including selective serotonin reuptake inhibitors (SSRIs), anticholinergics, narcotics, calcium channel blockers, thyroid hormone, nonsteroidal anti-inflammatory drugs, antiarrhythmics, etc.

SPECIAL PATIENT GROUPS

Anecdotal information suggests that IBS is worse in pregnancy, but there is no increased risk to mother or fetus.

PATIENT SATISFACTION/LIFESTYLE PRIORITIES

Patients should be informed that IBS is a chronic condition and all treatments will need to be taken long term; at the same time, patients should be reassured that recurrences decrease with age.

# SUMMARY OF THERAPEUTIC OPTIONS
## Choices
Treatment strategy is based on the predominant symptoms and their severity, the degree of functional impairment, and the presence of psychologic difficulties.
- All patients should be given advice on diet and other lifestyle modifications that affect symptoms of IBS; patients with mild symptoms may need nothing more than this and reassurance
- Tricyclic antidepressants are well known to improve neuropathic pain and are efficacious at least in a subset of IBS patients. Doses lower than the antidepressant range are effective (e.g. amitriptyline 10–25mg or imipramine 25–50mg before bedtime). The dose can be increased, depending upon the responsiveness. Responses take 2–3 weeks to develop
- Especially if depression is present, SSRIs (paroxetine, fluoxetine, or sertraline) may be quite effective in also treating the IBS. However, SSRIs may cause diarrhea, particularly in the elderly
- For patients with abdominal pain as their main symptom antispasmodic agents such as dicyclomine or hyoscyamine can be effective. Intermittent use as needed is preferable to a regular scheduled dose
- Patients with chronic diarrhea as their main symptom should be given an antimotility drug such as loperamide to be used as circumstances require, rather than on a regular schedule
- Patients with chronic constipation as their main symptom should be given a bulking agent such as psyllium, a natural insoluble fiber, or methylcellulose, a synthetic and partially soluble fiber, along with appropriate advice to increase water consumption
- Psychologic treatments, e.g. cognitive-behavioural therapy or hypnotherapy, may be beneficial for patients with moderate to severe symptoms; patients are usually referred by a gastroenterologist
- Peppermint oil and dietary changes may also help to improve symptoms

## Guidelines
The American Gastroenterological Association has produced position statements on irritable bowel syndrome:
- American Gastroenterological Association medical position statement: irritable bowel syndrome [2]
- Drossman DA, Whitehead WE, Camilleri M. Irritable bowel syndrome: a technical review for practice guideline development [3]

The American Academy of Family Physicians has published an article and statement about irritable bowel syndrome:
- Dalton CB, Drossman DA. Diagnosis and treatment of irritable bowel syndrome [4]

## Clinical pearls
- There is no specific therapy for IBS. Since it is a chronic disorder, focusing on education and lifestyle changes is preferable
- Graduating therapy for the severity of symptoms is a useful approach. Mild to moderate cases warrant a focus on lifestyle changes, education, and stress management, with intermittent use of pharmacologic agents for periods of increased symptoms. In moderate to severe cases, illness behavior often dominates the picture. A supportive physician-patient relationship is most important. Psychotherapy or behavioral modifications can frequently be quite effective
- Low-dose tricyclic antidepressants are certainly worth trying, since they can be quite effective and are safe and inexpensive

## Never
Never assume a diagnosis of IBS in a patient at risk from colon cancer or with signs or symptoms suggesting other serious diagnoses.

## FOLLOW UP
### Plan for review
Re-evaluate the patient's condition 3–6 weeks after starting treatment. If treatment is unsuccessful, additional studies based on subtype may be performed; referral to a gastroenterologist is sometimes necessary at this stage.

### Information for patient or caregiver
- Patients should be reassured that IBS is not a purely psychologic illness and that symptoms are very real
- Inform patients that IBS is a chronic illness with no cure, but treatments do improve symptoms and acute attacks decrease with age
- Reinforce the importance of a healthy diet and regular exercise

## DRUGS AND OTHER THERAPIES: DETAILS
### Drugs
LOPERAMIDE
Antidiarrheal suitable for IBS patients with diarrhea as predominant symptom.

*Dose*
Adult: 2–4mg orally up to four times daily.

*Efficacy*
Effective treatment for diarrhea-predominant IBS.

*Risks/benefits*
Risks:
- Use caution in liver disease, dehydration, and severe ulcerative colitis
- Not recommmended for children

Benefit: improves symptoms of diarrhea, urgency, and fecal soiling.

*Side effects and adverse reactions*
- Central nervous system: fatigue, dizziness, drowsiness
- Gastrointestinal: nausea, constipation, toxic megacolon, abdominal cramps and bloating, paralytic ileus, vomiting
- Genitourinary: nephrotoxicity
- Respiratory: respiratory depression
- Skin: rash

*Interactions (other drugs)*
No known interactions.

*Contraindications*
- Acute diarrhea caused by infectious microorganisms – enteroinvasive *Escherichia coli*, *Salmonella*, *Shigella* ▪ Development of abdominal distension or inhibition of peristalsis
- Pseudomembranous colitis associated with broad-spectrum antibiotics

*Evidence*
- A double-blind cross-over trial in 28 patients found that loperamide produced significantly increased gastric emptying time and delayed both small bowel and whole gut transit time as well as improving symptoms of diarrhea, urgency, and borborygmi; 18 of the patients reported feeling better while taking loperamide than they did on placebo treatment [5] *Level P*
- A multicenter, double-blind, randomized controlled trial of 90 patients compared loperamide

with placebo and found that treatment with loperamide significantly improved stool consistency and reduced the frequency of defecation and the intensity of pain [6] *Level P*

*Acceptability to patient*
Generally good.

*Follow up plan*
Review after 3 weeks.

*Patient and caregiver information*
Advise patient that combination with diet and lifestyle modifications will produce the best outcome.

## PSYLLIUM
Natural insoluble bulk laxative suitable for constipation-predominant IBS.

*Dose*
- Adult: 1–2 rounded teaspoons (2.5–4.03g/rounded teaspoon) orally one to three times per day, or
- 1 rounded teaspoon effervescent powder consisting of 50% psyllium and 50% dextrose solution (3.4–6.0g drug) in 8oz glass of liquid one to three times per day, or
- Child aged 6–12 years: 1 teaspoon (2.0g of drug) in an empty glass and add 8oz of cool water; stir for 3–5s. May be taken one to three times per day.
- The patient should follow all forms with up to 8 glasses of water a day to ensure the psyllium works as a 'slurry' rather than as 'cement', or constipation may be worsened.

*Efficacy*
Widely prescribed but of unproven efficacy for constipation-predominant IBS.

*Risks/benefits*
- Not suitable for use in persons with acute abdominal pain, nausea, or vomiting
- Sugar-free preparations may contain aspartame and are not suitable for phenylketonurics

*Side effects and adverse reactions*
Gastrointestinal: anorexia, nausea, vomiting, abdominal pains, diarrhea, constipation, bloating, bowel obstruction.

*Interactions (other drugs)*
**No significant interactions noted.**

*Contraindications*
- **Intestinal obstruction**
- **Fecal impaction**

*Acceptability to patient*
Patients may be highly sensitive to intestinal gas produced by bacterial fermentation of fiber, which can cause compliance problems.

*Follow up plan*
Review after 3 weeks.

*Patient and caregiver information*
- Reassure patients that any increase in intestinal gas will usually disappear with time
- Patients must maintain adequate fluid intake

- Inform patients that inhalation of dust from powder can cause wheezing and runny eyes and nose, or more severe allergic reactions
- Combination with diet and other lifestyle recommendations will produce the best outcome

## DICYCLOMINE
Antispamodic suitable for patients with abdominal pain as main symptom.

### Dose
- Adult: 160mg/day orally (in four equally divided doses)
- Adult intramuscular dosage (should only be used temporarily when the patient cannot take oral medication, and should not be used for periods longer than 1 or 2 days): 80mg/day (in four equally divided doses).

### Efficacy
- Effective treatment for abdominal pain, but should not be used long term
- Only dose with documented efficacy is 40mg four times a day

### Risks/benefits
- Suitable for men and women with abdominal pain as the predominant symptom
- Anticholinergic side effects are common, especially among elderly
- Use caution in hepatic and renal disease, ulcerative colitis, hyperthyroidism, and cardiac conditions
- Use caution in small children

### Side effects and adverse reactions
- Cardiovascular system: palpitations, tachycardia
- Central nervous system: coma in children less than 3 months old, confusion, seizures, stimulation in elderly
- Eyes, ears, nose, and throat: blurred vision
- Gastrointestinal: constipation, nausea, dry mouth, vomiting
- Genitourinary: urinary retention
- Skin: rashes, fever

### Interactions (other drugs)
- Amantadine - Antihistamines - Levodopa - Ketoconazole - Monoamine oxidase inhibitors (MAOIs) - Phenothiazines - Tricyclic antidepressants

### Contraindications
- Narrow-angle glaucoma - Gastrointestinal disorders: gastrointestinal obstruction, gastrointestinal atony, toxic megacolon, paralytic ileus - Myasthenia gravis - Pregnancy – there are no studies documenting safety in pregnancy

### Evidence
A randomized, double-blind, placebo-controlled study of dicyclomine in patients with recent irritable bowel syndrome concluded that 2 weeks' treatment was better than placebo in improving the overall condition of the patient, decreasing abdominal pain, decreasing abdominal tenderness, and improving bowel habits [7] *Level P*

### Acceptability to patient
Anticholinergic side effects may cause compliance problems.

### Follow up plan
Review after 3 weeks.

*Patient and caregiver information*
Combining dicyclomine with diet and other lifestyle modifications will produce the best outcome.

## HYOSCYAMINE
Antimuscarinic suitable for IBS patients with pain as predominant symptom.

*Dose*
Sublingual tablets:
- Adult: 0.125–0.25mg sublingual tablet every 4h, or as needed before meals and at bedtime, or
- Child: 2–12 years of age: half to one sublingual tablet (0.0625–0.125mg) every 4h, or as needed. Do not exceed 6 tablets in 24h

Tablets:
- Adults and patients 12 years of age and older: 1–2 tablets every 12h. Do not exceed 12 tablets in 24h
- Child 2–12 years of age: Half to one tablet every 4h or as needed. Do not exceed 6 tablets in 24h

Elixir:
- Adults and patients 12 years of age and older: 1–2 teaspoonfuls every 4h or as needed. Do not exceed 12 teaspoonfuls in 24h
- Child 2–12 years of age weighing:

10kg (22lb): a quarter of a teaspoon
20kg (44lb): half a teaspoon
40kg (88lb): three-quarters of a teaspoon
50kg (110lb): one teaspoon
The doses may be repeated every 4h or as needed. Do not exceed 6 teaspoonfuls in 24h

Injection:
- Adult: 0.5–1.0mL (0.25–0.5mg) subcutaneously, intramuscularly, or intravenously without dilution. Some patients may require only a single dose; others may require administration two, three, or four times a day at 4h intervals

*Efficacy*
- Effective treatment for acute episodes of abdominal pain
- No documentation of effectiveness in patients with symptoms of constipation or bloating

*Risks/benefits*
- Suitable for acute episodes only: can lose effect if given as chronic treatment
- Can cause constipation
- Not suitable for use in pregnancy or lactation
- Sublingual preparation has a rapid onset of action and so is good for acute pain
- Use caution in cardiac disorders, hyperthyroidism, renal and hepatic disease, and ulcerative colitis

*Side effects and adverse reactions*
- Cardiovascular system: palpitations, tachycardia
- Central nervous system: confusion, headache, stimulation in the elderly
- Eyes, ears, nose, and throat: visual disturbances
- Gastrointestinal: constipation, nausea, dry mouth, vomiting
- Genitourinary: urinary difficulties
- Skin: allergic reactions

*Interactions (other drugs)*
- Antihistamines ■ Antimuscarinics ■ Amantadine ■ Atenolol ■ Digoxin ■ Haloperidol
- MAOIs ■ Phenothiazines ■ Tricyclic antidepressants

*Contraindications*
- Narrow-angle glaucoma ■ Obstructive uropathy ■ Tachycardia, unstable cardiovascular status, myocardial ischemia ■ Gastrointestinal obstructive disease, paralytic ileus, gastrointestinal atony, toxic megacolon ■ Myasthenia gravis

*Acceptability to patient*
Generally good.

*Follow up plan*
Review after 3 weeks. Do not use as long-term therapy.

*Patient and caregiver information*
Advise patient that combination with diet and other lifestyle modifications will provide the best outcome.

AMITRIPTYLINE
Tricyclic antidepressant suitable for IBS patients with coexisting depression.

*Dose*
10–100mg/day, orally.

*Efficacy*
At doses below antidepressive levels, it can be quite effective treatment for pain in IBS.

*Risks/benefits*
- Can cause constipation, especially at higher doses, so it needs to be used cautiously or not at all in constipation-predominant IBS
- Analgesic and anticholinergic effects may improve symptoms of pain and discomfort in IBS, as well as treating depression
- Since antidepressants are needed on a continual basis, drug should be used only in patients with chronic or recurring symptoms
- Broad side effect profile, especially at higher doses
- May have withdrawal if stopped abruptly
- May cause significant drowsiness, so the patient must adapt to dosage schedule and daytime 'hangover' drowsiness
- Patients often gain significant weight, even on low doses
- Can achieve symptom relief in lower doses than when used to treat depression; this can help reduce side effects and enhance compliance
- Use caution in narrow-angle glaucoma and hepatic and renal disease

*Side effects and adverse reactions*
- Cardiovascular system: ventricular tachycardia, orthostatic hypotension, palpitations, hypertension, myocardial infarction, stroke, congestive heart failure, PR and/or QT prolongation
- Central nervous system: drowsiness, sedation, dizziness, anxiety, confusion, tremor, pseudoparkinsonism, seizures, EEG changes, neuroleptic malignant syndrome
- Eyes, ears, nose, and throat: visual disturbances, mydriasis, dry mouth
- Gastrointestinal: nausea, vomiting, diarrhea, constipation, abdominal pain, dry mouth, jaundice, anorexia
- Genitourinary: sexual dysfunction, breast enlargement, galactorrhea, gynecomastia

*Interactions (other drugs)*
- Anticonvulsants (barbiturates, carbamazepine) ■ Antimuscarinics (atropine, phenothiazines, H1 antagonists, other tricyclic antidepressants, clozapine, cyclobenzaprine disopyramide)
- Cimetidine ■ Cisapride ■ Clonidine ■ Cocaine ■ Central nervous system depressants (entacapone, hypnotics, anxiolytics, ethanol, sedatives, etc) ■ Disulfiram ■ Dofeltilide
- Guanabenz, guanfacine ■ Levodopa ■ Opiate agonists ■ MAOIs ■ SSRIs ■ St Johns Wort, Valerian ■ Sympathomimetics ■ Thyroid hormone ■ Tramadol

*Contraindications*
- Weigh risk and benefits of use in pregnant women or in women wishing to become pregnant ■ Acute recovery phase of myocardial infarction ■ Avoid using together with MAOI

*Evidence*
A randomized, double-blind placebo-controlled trial of 40 patients with irritable bowel syndrome found that 12 weeks' treatment with amitriptyline was significantly more effective than placebo in producing global improvement, increasing feelings of wellbeing, reducing abdominal pain, and increasing satisfaction with bowel movements [8] *Level P*

*Acceptability to patient*
Patients may not feel antidepressant effects for 2–3 weeks, and side effects are common, which can cause problems with compliance.

*Follow up plan*
Review at 3 weeks.

*Patient and caregiver information*
- Use caution when driving
- Avoid rising quickly from sitting to standing
- Increase fluid intake to avoid constipation
- Avoid alcohol and other central nervous system depressants
- Do not discontinue abruptly after long-term use
- Wear sunscreen or a large hat to avoid photosensitivity reactions

## FLUOXETINE
SSRI suitable for IBS patients with coexisting depression or panic disorder.

*Dose*
10–20mg/day, orally.

*Efficacy*
Effective treatment for depression and panic disorder coexisting with IBS.

*Risks/benefits*
- Not suitable as sole, first-line treatment for IBS
- In addition to psychotropic effects, fluoxetine has neuromodulatory and analgesic effects
- Diarrhea is a common side effect, so drug is better used in patients with constipation-predominant IBS. Should not use concurrently with alosetron as they have competing mechanisms of action
- Lower side effect profile makes fluoxetine preferable to tricyclic antidepressants for many patients
- Use with caution in the elderly and children
- Use caution in renal and hepatic disease, cardiac disease, and bipolar disorder and suicidal tendencies

- Use caution in seizure disorders, diabetes, and anorexia nervosa
- Use caution with pregnancy and breast-feeding
- Risk of serious cutaneous systemic illness and events
- Anaphylactoid events have been reported
- Possibility of interactions with highly protein-bound drugs
- Advise caution with driving and operating machinery

*Side effects and adverse reactions*
- Cardiovascular system: sinus bradycardia, orthostatic hypotension
- Central nervous system: anxiety, nervousness, insomnia, drowsiness, fatigue, dizziness, tremor, headache, mania, seizures, extrapyramidal symptoms, somnolence
- Chest pain and chills
- Eyes, ears, nose, and throat: visual disturbances, altered taste, ear pain, tinnitus
- Gastrointestinal: nausea, vomiting, anorexia, diarrhea, dry mouth, dyspepsia, weight loss, weight gain
- Genitourinary: sexual dysfunction
- Metabolic: hyperglycemia, hypothyroidism, hyponatremia
- Musculoskeletal: myalgia
- Respiratory: respiratory infection
- Skin: rash, pruritus, urticaria, sweating

*Interactions (other drugs)*
- Alosetron
- Amphetamine, dextroamphetamine
- Anticonvulsants (benzodiazepines, carbamazepine, phenytoin)
- Antidepressants (tricyclic, tryptophan and especially MAOIs)
- Antihistamines (nonsedating, cyproheptadine)
- Antipsychotics (haloperidol, lithium)
- Beta-blockers
- Buspirone
- Calcium channel blockers
- Cyproheptadine
- Dexfenfluramine, fenfluramine
- Dextromethorphan
- Diuretics
- Statins
- St Johns Wort
- Selegiline
- Warfarin

*Contraindications*
- Use of MAOI within 14 days
- Do not use if patient enters a manic phase

*Evidence*
Trials of antidepressant agents in irritable bowel syndrome to date have examined tricyclic agents rather than selective serotonin reuptake inhibitors (SSRIs), which have not been evaluated for use in irritable bowel syndrome. However, SSRIs are now in common use because of their low side effect profile and their better safety than the tricyclic antidepressants, and anecdotal evidence suggests that they may be as effective as the tricyclic agents [2] *Level C*

*Acceptability to patient*
Therapeutic response may take 4–6 weeks, which can cause compliance problems.

*Follow up plan*
Review at 6 weeks.

*Patient and caregiver information*
- Advise patient to take in mornings, to avoid insomnia
- Inform patient that therapeutic response may take 4–6 weeks

## Complementary therapy
DIETARY CHANGES
- Decreasing dietary sugar, increasing fiber, eliminating food allergens

- Meals high in sugar can contribute to IBS symptoms by causing slowing of peristalsis as well as promoting bacterial overgrowth in the small intestine. Dietary fiber seems to benefit those IBS sufferers who experience constipation more than those with predominant diarrhea symptoms. Certain foods may serve more as irritants than as direct allergies, and therefore trials of food group elimination should be considered. The most common food group irritants for people with IBS are dairy and grains

*Risks/benefits*
Virtually no known risks of dietary manipulation to control symptoms.

*Evidence*
An uncontrolled study examined the effect of dietary exclusion in women with irritable bowel syndrome. Symptomatic improvement was noted in 48.2% of patients after 3 weeks. 79% of these patients remained well on a modified diet during the follow-up period [9] *This study does not meet the criteria for level P*

*Acceptability to patient*
Dietary changes are often difficult for patients to implement.

*Follow up plan*
Usual care.

*Patient and caregiver information*
Food elimination trials require complete abstinence from the target food group for at least 2 weeks, with reintroduction to determine if symptoms recur.

## PEPPERMINT OIL
*Efficacy*
Enteric coated volatile oils, such as peppermint oil, inhibit gastrointestinal smooth muscle action, and therefore improve pain/discomfort from intestinal spasm. Enteric coating is important to avoid the rapid absorption of menthol (the primary active ingredient in peppermint oil) in the upper intestine.

*Risks/benefits*
Peppermint oil is essentially risk-free. Occasional patients will notice heartburn. Rarely a transient skin rash occurs. Nonenteric coated peppermint oil can cause rectal burning, gastroesophageal reflux and heartburn.

*Evidence*
An RCT compared enteric-coated peppermint oil for one month vs placebo in patients with symptoms of irritable bowel syndrome. Symptoms of abdominal pain, distension, stool frequency, borborygmi and flatulence were all significantly improved with peppermint oil [10] *Level P*

*Acceptability to patient*
Generally well tolerated.

*Follow up plan*
Regular follow-up as for any chronic condition.

*Patient and caregiver information*
Be sure to use enteric coated oil to avoid reflux, heartburn, rectal burning and potential lack of efficacy.

## Other therapies

COGNITIVE-BEHAVIORAL THERAPY

*Efficacy*
Effective treatment for anxiety and other psychologic symptoms associated with IBS; may also improve gastrointestinal symptoms.

*Risks/benefits*
- Symptoms most likely to show favorable response are abdominal pain and diarrhea
- Positive response most likely in patients who experience symptom exacerbations with stress
- No risks associated with this treatment

*Evidence*
A randomized clinical trial (not blinded) compared behavioral psychotherapy with medical treatment in 42 patients with irritable bowel syndrome. Behavioral therapy produced improved gastrointestinal and psychologic scores at 4 and 9 months, and improvement in gastrointestinal symptoms correlated with improved psychologic scores [11] *Level P*

*Acceptability to patient*
Some patients have difficulty accepting psychologic treatment, which can lead to compliance problems.

*Follow up plan*
Review after 6 weeks.

*Patient and caregiver information*
Combination with diet and other lifestyle modifications will produce the best outcome.

HYPNOTHERAPY

*Efficacy*
Effective treatment for psychologic and gastrointestinal symptoms in patients with IBS.

*Risks/benefits*
- Symptoms most likely to show favorable response are abdominal pain and diarrhea
- Positive response most likely in patients who experience symptom exacerbations with stress
- No risks associated with this treatment

*Evidence*
A randomized controlled trial (not blinded) compared treatment with hypnotherapy with treatment with psychotherapy in 30 patients with irritable bowel syndrome. Hypnotherapy was found to improve abdominal pain, abdominal distension, bowel habit, and general wellbeing. No relapses were reported in the hypnotherapy group during 3 months of follow up [12] *Level P*

*Acceptability to patient*
Some patients have difficulty accepting psychologic treatment, which can lead to compliance problems.

*Follow up plan*
Review at 6 weeks.

*Patient and caregiver information*
Combination of hypnotherapy with diet and other lifestyle modifications will produce the best outcome.

## LIFESTYLE

### Diet:
- High-fiber diets for constipation-predominant IBS are often recommended but their efficacy is not proven; ensure patients' fluid intake is adequate
- Fatty foods, beans and legumes, and cruciferous vegetables can aggravate IBS symptoms in some persons and should be avoided
- Patients with lactose intolerance should limit intake of milk and other dairy products
- Sorbitol, mannitol, and fructose can exacerbate diarrhea and should be avoided by persons with diarrhea-predominant IBS. In particular, patients should be advised to refrain from using chewing gum containing sorbitol
- Reducing intake of apple and grape juice, bananas, nuts, and raisins may lessen incidence of flatulence
- Patients may find that keeping a food diary helps identify foods that can worsen symptoms
- Patients should avoid alcohol and caffeine, both of which can exacerbate symptoms

### Exercise:
- Regular exercise helps maintain regular bowel habit

### Stress avoidance:
- Learning relaxation techniques will help patients whose symptoms are aggravated by stress

## RISKS/BENEFITS
There are no risks associated with these lifestyle modifications.

## ACCEPTABILITY TO PATIENT
- Increasing dietary fiber can cause a transient increase in gas and abdominal bloating, but patients should be informed that any worsening of symptoms will resolve after a few weeks
- IBS is a chronic condition, and patients need to maintain lifestyle modifications long term; some persons have difficulty complying with this, especially when symptoms abate

## FOLLOW UP PLAN
Review after 6 weeks.

## PATIENT AND CAREGIVER INFORMATION
Remind patients that long-term adherence to diet and other lifestyle modifications will produce the best outcome.

## OUTCOMES

### EFFICACY OF THERAPIES
More than 60% of patients respond successfully to treatment over the initial 12 months.

### Evidence
Evidence from 70 randomized, double-blind, placebo-controlled parallel or cross-over trials of pharmacologic interventions in adults with irritable bowel syndrome found strong evidence for the efficacy of antispasmodics in patients with abdominal pain as the predominant symptom, good evidence that loperamide improves diarrhea, and evidence that antidepressant agents produce global improvement, although this was based on a small number of suboptimal studies; similarly, the 5-hydroxytryptamine receptor antagonists require further investigation [13] *Level M*

### Review period
Review after 3–6 weeks.

### PROGNOSIS
Prognosis for patients with IBS is excellent. There is no evidence that the syndrome shortens life expectancy or predisposes to other disease.

### Clinical pearls
Establishing a positive physician-patient relation is a central feature of therapy. Once a reasonably confident diagnosis is made, seeing the patient back for discussion and follow up is probably more useful than expensive testing or pharmacotherapy.

### Therapeutic failure
Patients with refractory symptoms should be referred to a gastroenterologist for further evaluation and treatment.

### Recurrence
Symptoms of IBS usually recur and can be managed with the same treatments used for a previous attack, where these proved effective.

### Deterioration
Patients with severe symptoms that do not respond to first-line therapies should be referred to a gastroenterologist for further assessment and treatment.

## PREVENTION

Prevention of IBS is difficult because the cause in unknown and the main risk factor is psychosocial trauma, which is not modifiable by patients.

### RISK FACTORS
Psychosocial trauma: a history of physical or sexual abuse is more common among patients with IBS than those who do not have the syndrome.

### SCREENING
Screening for IBS is unnecessary.

### PREVENT RECURRENCE
Recurrence of symptoms is best prevented by maintaining a healthy diet, exercising regularly, and avoiding stress.

# RESOURCES

## ASSOCIATIONS

American Academy of Family Physicians
11400 Tomahawk Creek Parkway
Leawood, KS 66211-2672
Tel: (913) 906-6000
http://www.aafp.org

American Gastroenterological Association
7910 Woodmount Ave., 7th Floor
Bethesda, MD 20814
Tel: (301) 654-2055
Fax: (301) 652-3890
http://www.gastro.org

American College of Gastroenterologists
4900 B South 31st Street
Arlington, VA 22206
Tel: (703) 820-7400
Fax: (703) 931-4520
http://www.acg.gi.org

## KEY REFERENCES

- American Family Physicians. Clinical briefs: new drug for IBS in women http://www.aafp.org/afp/20000715/clinical.html.
- Camilleri M. Therapeutic approach to the patient with irritable bowel syndrome. Am J Med 1999;107(suppl 5A):27S–32S
- Farthing MJ. Irritable bowel syndrome: new pharmaceutical approaches to treatment. Best Pract Res Clin Gastroenterol 1999;13:461–71
- Fauci AS, et al, eds. Harrison's principles of internal medicine: companion handbook, 14th edn. New York: McGraw-Hill; 1998, p831–2
- Feldman M, et al, eds. Sleisenger and Fordtran's gastrointestinal and liver disease:pathophysiology/diagnosis/management, 6th edn. Philadelphia: WB Saunders, 1997
- Goldman L, Bennett JC. Cecil textbook of medicine, 21st edn. Philadelphia: WB Saunders, 2000: p1672
- Hammer J, Talley N. Diagnostic criteria for the irritable bowel syndrome. Am J Med 1999;107(suppl. 5A):5S–11S
- Maxwell PR, et al. Irritable bowel syndrome. Lancet 1997;350:1691–4
- Schmulson M, Chang L. Diagnostic approach to the patient with irritable bowel syndrome. Am J Med 1999;107(suppl 5A):20S–26S
- Whitehead WE. Patient subgroups in irritable bowel syndrome that can be defined by symptom evaluation and physical examination. Am J Med 1999;107(suppl 5A):33S–40S

### Evidence references and guidelines

1. Thompson WG, Longstreth GF, Drossman DA, et al. Functional bowel disorders and functional abdominal pain. Gut 1999;45(suppl 2):II43–7
2. Anonymous. American Gastroenterological Association medical position statement: irritable bowel syndrome. Gastroenterology 1997;112:2118–9. Available online from the National Guidelines Clearinghouse
3. Drossman DA, Whitehead WE, Camilleri M. Irritable bowel syndrome: a technical review for practice guideline development. Gastroenterology 1997;112:2120–37
4. Dalton CB, Drossman DA. Diagnosis and treatment of irritable bowel syndrome. Am Fam Physician 1997;55:875–87
5. Cann PA, Read NW, Holdsworth CD, Barends D. Role of loperamide and placebo in management of irritable bowel sydrome (IBS). Dig Dis Sci 1984;29:239–47

6  Efskind PS, Bernklev T, Vatn MH. A double-blind placebo controlled trial with loperamide in IBS. Scand J Gastroenterol 1996;31:436–8
7  Page JG, Dirnberger GM. Treatment of the irritable bowel syndrome with Bentyl (dicyclomine hydrochloride). J Clin Gastroenterol 1981;3:153–6
8  Rajagopaln M, Kurian G, John J. Symptom relief with amitriptyline in the irritable bowel syndrome. J Gastroenterol Hepatol 1998;13:738–41
9  Nanda R, James R, Smith H, et al. Food intolerance and the irritable bowel syndrome. Gut 1989;30:1099–1104. Medline
10 Liu JH, Chen GH, Yeh HZ, et al. Enteric-coated peppermint oil capsules in the treatment of irritable bowel syndrome: a prospective randomized trial. J Gastroenterol 1997;32:765–8
11 Corney RH, Stanton R, Newell R, at al. Behavioural psychotherapy in the treatment of IBS. J Psychosom Res 1991;35:461–9
12 Whorwell PJ, Prior A, Faragher EB. Controlled trial of hypnotherapy in treatment of severe refractory IBS. Lancet 1984;2(8414):1232–3
13 Jailwala J, Imperiale TF, Kroenke K, et al. Pharmacologic treatment of the irritable bowel syndrome: a systematic review of randomized controlled trials. Ann Intern Med 2000;113:136–47

# FAQS
## Question 1
When is flexible sigmoidoscopy indicated in the evaluation of a patient with suspected IBS?

### ANSWER 1
Flexible sigmoidoscopy is indicated particularly where the diagnosis is in doubt or when there is any question about colonic neoplasia. In younger patients, an argument can be made that the test is not cost-effective, although it may have benefit in assuring an anxious patient.

## Question 2
Why is alosetron indicated only for women? How seriously should I consider the risk of ischemic colitis and severe impaction for an otherwise well-tolerated and effective treatment? Finally, is alosetron worth its cost?

### ANSWER 2
The reason that alosetron is not effective in men is unclear. Further trials are under way. The magnitude of the risk from ischemic colitis has not been established. This risk plus the chronic nature of this disorder makes one cautious about continuous use of the drug.

# CONTRIBUTORS
Russell C Jones, MD, MPH
Jane L Murray, MD
Andrew H Soll, MD
Brennan Spiegel, MD

# LACTOSE INTOLERANCE

| | | |
|---|---|---|
| ■ | Summary Information | 370 |
| ■ | Background | 371 |
| ■ | Diagnosis | 373 |
| ■ | Treatment | 379 |
| ■ | Outcomes | 383 |
| ■ | Prevention | 384 |
| ■ | Resources | 385 |

## SUMMARY INFORMATION

### DESCRIPTION
- Inability to process lactose usually due to decreased amounts of lactase in the intestines, but other causes include small intestine mucosal disease, infections and inherited lactase deficiency
- Symptoms include flatulence, bloating, nausea, cramps, abdominal pain and diarrhea usually within 0.5–2h after intake of lactose-containing food or drinks (dairy products and milk)
- Diagnostic tests include a careful history, hydrogen breath test, stool acidity test, and very rarely small bowel biopsy
- Treatment is simple and straightforward: avoidance of lactose-containing products usually results in symptom relief

### URGENT ACTION
No urgent action is required

### KEY! DON'T MISS!
- Assess for malnutrition and malabsorption in patients with lactase deficiency
- Consider celiac disease in patients who present with symptoms of lactose intolerance late in life and who are in an ethnic group with a low occurrence rate of lactose intolerance
- Lactose intolerance frequently presents and exacerbates irritable bowel syndrome. It is very helpful to make this distinction, since the patient can be educated and better taught to deal with their dual disorders

## BACKGROUND

### ICD9 CODE
271.3 Lactose intolerance

### SYNONYMS
- Lactase deficiency
- Milk intolerance

### CARDINAL FEATURES
- Symptoms include flatulence, bloating, nausea, cramps, and diarrhea, starting within 0.5–2h after ingestion of lactose-containing products (milk, dairy products, etc.)
- Avoidance of lactose-containing products usually results in symptom relief
- Three forms of lactose intolerance are recognized: congenital lactose intolerance, primary lactose intolerance, and secondary lactose intolerance
- Congenital lactose intolerance is very rare
- Primary lactose intolerance is common in adults, varies among individuals, and appears to be a natural occurrence depending on ethnicity
- Secondary lactose intolerance occurs with intestinal disease that impairs absorption or speeds up transit (celiac disease, acute or chronic infections associated with malabsorption, or reduction in the mucosal surface resulting from surgical resection)

### CAUSES
#### Common causes
- Primary lactose intolerance is common among adults of susceptible races, but usually starts within 2–5 years after birth, appears to be a natural occurrence of decreasing lactase enzyme
- Secondary lactose intolerance is usually transient in nature and results from injury to the intestinal mucosa (diarrhea), reduction in mucosal surface (surgical resection), or another digestive tract indication (rotavirus disease, giardiasis, ascariasis, inflammatory bowel disease), and other malabsorptive conditions

#### Rare causes
Congenital lactose deficiency is more common in premature infants than full-term infants.

#### Contributory or predisposing factors
- Race
- Age

### EPIDEMIOLOGY
#### Incidence and prevalence
- Approximately 50 million people in the US have some level of lactose intolerance
- Approximately 1/3–1/5 of the people with lactose intolerance exhibit symptoms
- At least 50% of infants with diarrhea (acute or chronic) are lactose intolerant

INCIDENCE
- 3/10 (30/1000) non-Caucasian people
- 1/10 (10/1000) Caucasian people

PREVALENCE
- 3/10 (30/1000) non-Caucasian people
- 1/10 (10/1000) Caucasian people

## Demographics

### AGE
- Primary lactose intolerance is more prevalent among teenagers and adults, but lactase activity appears to decline between 2 and 5 years of age in non-Caucasian people
- Secondary lactose intolerance can occur at any age and is dependent on the causative condition
- Congenital lactose intolerance is usually obvious from birth

### GENDER
- Similar frequencies of lactose intolerance are observed between males and females
- 44% of women with lactose intolerance are able to digest lactose during pregnancy

### RACE
- 5–12% of American Caucasians
- 60–75% of African-Americans, Mexican-Americans, and American Jewish
- 90% Asian-Americans
- 75–100% Native Americans

### GENETICS
Congenital lactose intolerance is very rare, but is reported more frequently among premature infants than full-term infants.

# DIAGNOSIS

## DIFFERENTIAL DIAGNOSIS
### Irritable bowel syndrome
FEATURES
- Abdominal cramps
- Diarrhea, constipation or an alternating pattern

### Crohn's disease
FEATURES
- Bloody diarrhea
- Abdominal distension
- Hyperactive bowel sounds
- Abdominal tenderness
- Abnormal development with delayed growth in children
- Abscesses in the perianal or rectal areas
- Mouth ulcers
- Atrophic glossitis
- Joint swelling, joint tenderness, hepatosplenomegaly, erythema nodosum, clubbing

### Ulcerative colitis
FEATURES
- Bloody diarrhea
- Abdominal distension
- Abdominal tenderness
- Fever
- Dehydration
- Liver disease, sclerosing cholangitis, iritis, uveitis, episcleritis, arthritis, erythema nodosum, pyoderma gangrenosum, and aphthous stomatitis

### Pancreatic insufficiency
FEATURES
- Fat malabsorption
- Chronic abdominal pain
- Weight loss
- Fatty or greasy stools
- Diarrhea
- Epigastric mass
- Jaundice
- Diabetes

### Sprue (celiac disease)
FEATURES
- Sensitivity to gluten
- Familial history
- Abdominal tenderness
- Abdominal distension
- Fever
- Glossitis
- Cheilosis
- Hyperkeratosis
- Hyperpigmentation
- Weight loss

- Fatigue
- Diarrhea
- Anemia
- Delayed growth
- Nutrient malabsorption
- Osteoporosis

### Cystic fibrosis
FEATURES
- Failure to thrive in children
- Increased chest diameter
- Digital clubbing
- Chronic cough
- Abdominal distension
- Greasy, foul-smelling feces
- Chest sounds

## SIGNS & SYMPTOMS
### Signs
- Symptoms usually appear within 0.5–2h after ingesting lactose-containing drinks or food
- Physical examination results may be normal

### Symptoms
- Abdominal cramping
- Abdominal bloating
- Flatulence
- Diarrhea

## ASSOCIATED DISORDERS
It is important to distinguish primary lactose intolerance due to a genetic cause in the absence of mucosal disease from secondary lactase insufficiency due to associated mucosal disease. These associated disorders reflect mucosal disease or other factors that compromise digestion and absorption of nutrients.
- Malabsorption disorders including carbohydrate, nutrient, mucosal, and lactose malabsorption
- Malnutrition
- Gastroenteritis
- Alcoholism
- Osteoporosis
- Calcium deficiency
- Sprue (tropical, nontropical, or celiac)
- Giardiasis
- Immunoglobulin deficiencies
- Crohn's disease
- Cystic fibrosis

## KEY! DON'T MISS!
- Assess for malnutrition and malabsorption in patients with lactase deficiency
- Consider celiac disease in patients who present with symptoms of lactose intolerance late in life and who are in an ethnic group with a low occurrence rate of lactose intolerance
- Lactose intolerance frequently presents and exacerbates irritable bowel syndrome. It is very helpful to make this distinction, since the patient can be educated and better taught to deal with their dual disorders.

## CONSIDER CONSULT
- Refer patients with other gastrointestinal (GI) disorders to an endoscopist for further diagnostic procedures
- Refer patients to a dietitian for proper dietary modifications

## INVESTIGATION OF THE PATIENT
### Direct questions to patient
- **Q** When do you experience the symptoms? Lactase deficiency is variable among patients but usually occurs within 0.5–2h after ingesting lactose-containing products
- **Q** When did you first start experiencing symptoms? Lactose intolerance usually starts during teenage years or adulthood. However, lactase production decreases 2–5 years after birth in many individuals with primary lactose intolerance
- **Q** Have you had any other GI disorders recently? Secondary lactose intolerance is associated with other conditions
- **Q** How severe are the symptoms? Symptoms are variable among patients, and based on the severity of symptoms diet modification can usually be prescribed

### Contributory or predisposing factors
- **Q** Is there a history of predisposing factors? Race other than Caucasian
- **Q** How long have you had these symptoms? Primary lactose intolerance usually starts during the teenage years or adulthood, but some patients start to experience symptoms when the level of lactase enzyme decreases between ages 2 and 5 years
- **Q** Have you had a surgical procedure that reduced the mucosal surface of your intestines? Resection? Removal of lactase-producing mucosa can cause lactose intolerance
- **Q** What medications or treatments have you had? Certain drugs and treatments are associated with lactose intolerance including broad-spectrum antibiotics, colchicine, some chemotherapeutic agents and radiation therapy

### Family history
Is there a familial history of lactose intolerance? Genetics appears to be heavily involved in lactose intolerance.

### Examination
- Is the patient within normal weight ranges for height, age, sex, and race? Lactose intolerance can rarely result in weight loss due to decreased food intake
- Assess the patient's diet for lactose-containing products
- Assess the pattern of diarrhea experienced by the patient
- Assess the patient for dehydration, an uncommon side effect of the diarrhea associated with lactose intolerance
- Consider celiac disease if the patient has symptoms of lactose intolerance relatively late in life and the patient is from an ethnic group with a low occurrence rate of lactose intolerance
- Assess patient's history of symptoms carefully and determine likelihood of lactose intolerance based on duration of symptoms, severity of symptoms, dietary history, ethnic background, and familial history

### Summary of investigative tests
- Lactose-free diet test: a diet without lactose-containing products can eliminate symptoms thereby affirming diagnosis of lactose intolerance. This is certainly the most cost-effective approach and points to one important treatment
- Hydrogen breath test: used to confirm lactose intolerance. Typically not required when lactose-free diet test has been performed. Considerable false negatives and false positives
- Lactose tolerance test: a useful test used in patients with concurrent disorders such as celiac disease or gastroenteritis to determine the level of lactose intolerance (not for use in infants or

young children). Patients are given a lactose load, and blood glucose and symptoms are monitored. Disorders of gastric emptying and diabetes alter the results
- Stool acidity test: pH testing of stool samples (<6) can indicate lactose intolerance
- Small bowel biopsy: not indicated unless there is evidence of malabsorption or other GI disease
- Small bowel series: not indicated unless there is evidence of malabsorption or other GI disease

## DIAGNOSTIC DECISION
- Avoidance of lactose-containing products with a concomitant resolution and decreased occurrence of symptoms indicates lactose intolerance
- Lactose intolerance is indicated by an increase in breath hydrogen of at least 20ppm within 90min of initiation of the test (50g of lactose in liquid form)
- Stool acidity less than 6.5 pH is indicative of osmotic diarrhea and lactose intolerance
- Lactose intolerance is indicated by a clinically relevant, lower than expected increase of blood sugar levels within 30–50min of initiation of test (at least 50g of lactose according to body weight)
- The American Academy of Family Physicians has published relevant clinical information: Lake AM. Chronic abdominal pain in childhood: diagnosis and management. Am Fam Phys 1999;59:1823–30

## CLINICAL PEARLS
- There is a huge variation of visceral sensation among individuals. If lactose intolerance presents in individuals with low visceral sensation, symptoms will be diarrhea and gas, with little abdominal pain. In contrast, in subjects with an irritable gut that is sensitive to distension, pain will be an early symptom
- Lactose that is not absorbed by the small bowel passes into the colon where it is converted to short-chain fatty acids and hydrogen gas by the bacterial flora. Short-chain fatty acids are absorbed by the colonic mucosa, decreasing the consequences of lactase insufficiency. This is one reason why lactose intolerance is highly variable in its presentation among individuals. The production of hydrogen by colonic bacteria serves as the basis for the lactose breath hydrogen test used to diagnose lactose maldigestion (see below)

Several other factors account for the variability of symptoms among subjects with lactose intolerance:
- Meals with higher osmolality and fat content slow gastric emptying and reduce the severity of lactose-induced symptoms
- The rate of intestinal transit is highly variable among people. Those with more rapid transit will be more symptomatic
- The bacterial flora and degree of colonic salvage makes a big difference on the load of unabsorbed lactose persisting in the colon

## THE TESTS
### Body fluids
STOOL ACIDITY
*Description*
Obtain fresh stool samples and test immediately for pH value. This test is rarely used.

*Advantages/Disadvantages*
- Especially useful in infants and young children who are not able to have the hydrogen breath test or the lactose tolerance or challenge tests
- Simple test, but moderately insensitive
- Results are only valid when the samples are collected fresh and the assay is performed immediately

*Abnormal*
pH values less than 6.5 indicate lactose intolerance.

*Cause of abnormal result*
Undigested lactose ferments and creates lactic acid present in the stool.

## Tests of function
HYDROGEN BREATH TEST
*Advantages/Disadvantages*
- Especially useful in children
- Not for use in infants or young children who may experience dehydration from the diarrhea associated with a lactose load
- Inexpensive, safe for use in children and adults, and sensitive
- Considerable false-negatives and false-positives

*Abnormal*
An increase of at least 20ppm in breath hydrogen within 90min of initiation of the test indicates lactose intolerance.

*Cause of abnormal result*
An increase in breath hydrogen resulting from undigested lactose that is fermented and produces gas.

*Drugs, disorders and other factors that may alter results*
Avoid certain foods, certain medications, and smoking before taking the test. Disorders of gastric emptying and bacterial overgrowth will alter results.

## Biopsy
SMALL BOWEL BIOPSY
*Description*
Obtain a biopsy sample of the small bowel.

*Advantages/Disadvantages*
- Generally not indicated for lactose intolerance and it will not make the diagnosis. It will only serve to evaluate for other disease.
- Invasive nature makes this procedure unacceptable, especially considering the easier, safer, and less invasive nature of the more preferred procedures
- May help determine whether lactose intolerance is primary or secondary in nature

## Imaging
SMALL BOWEL SERIES
*Advantages/Disadvantages*
Useful only when there is significant malabsorption present.

## Special tests
LACTOSE TOLERANCE TEST
*Description*
Used in patients with other disorders such as celiac disease or gastroenteritis.

*Advantages/Disadvantages*
- Provides supporting evidence for diagnosis
- Blood samples are collected and analyzed for serum glucose levels after a lactose load is ingested and symptoms are monitored
- Reasonably sensitive and specific, but cumbersome and largely replaced by the breath hydrogen test where available

*Abnormal*
Increases in serum glucose levels less than 20mg/dL with other symptoms of lactose intolerance indicate lactase deficiency.

## LACTOSE-FREE DIET TEST
*Advantages/Disadvantages*
- Elimination of all lactose-containing products from diet should resolve symptoms of lactose intolerance
- Simple and cost-free way to confirm the diagnosis
- May not work for all patients

*Normal*
Symptoms of lactose intolerance resolve and are not present during lactose-free period.

# TREATMENT

## CONSIDER CONSULT
- Refer patients with other gastrointestinal (GI) disorders to a gastroenterologist for further evaluation
- Refer patients to a dietitian for proper dietary modifications

## IMMEDIATE ACTION
Carefully evaluate patients with obvious severe malnutrition. Lactose intolerance is not the problem, but is probably reflecting a more serious process. Depending upon the degree of malnutrition, rapid assessment and nutritional intervention are indicated.

## PATIENT AND CAREGIVER ISSUES
### Patient or caregiver request
**Q** How severely must I limit my lactose consumption? This depends upon the response. Patients only need to reduce intake enough to reduce symptoms to an acceptable level

**Q** How do I know which products contain lactose? This question is important to answer and provides an opportunity to educate patients on how to read food labels. Patients with a family or cultural history may naturally avoid lactose-containing products, but may need to be further educated about how inclusive lactose is in many products, including some medications

**Q** Is there a medicine or product that I can take that will allow me to consume lactose? Some people experience symptomatic relief with the use of oral lactase

**Q** If I eat yogurt every day, can I consume lactose-containing products? This is an important issue as some research has indicated that despite the high amount of lactose in yogurt, patients are able to tolerate yogurt because the cultures used to make yogurt produce lactase

### Health-seeking behavior
- Does the patient avoid all lactose consumption or just particular food or drink items? Severity of lactose intolerance varies widely among patients
- Can the patient consume any lactose at all? Some patients can consume small amounts of lactose-containing products
- Does the patient exhibit symptoms of lactose intolerance? Some patients may show lactose intolerance based on laboratory tests, but not have active symptoms
- Has the patient tried some of the lactase additives? If so, did the product resolve or prevent the symptoms? Lactase replacement does not work for all patients with lactose intolerance

## MANAGEMENT ISSUES
### Goals
- Relieve symptoms
- Educate patients about dietary modifications

### Management in special circumstances
COEXISTING DISEASE
- Broad-spectrum antibiotics are associated with lactose intolerance
- Other GI disorders are commonly diagnosed in lactose intolerant patients
- Secondary lactose intolerance is commonly caused by concurrent GI disorders (viral gastroenteritis, bacterial infections, celiac disease, giardiasis, antibiotic use, etc.)
- Patients with celiac disease or dermatitis herpetiformis who are lactose intolerant should not ingest any dairy products and are usually not effectively treated with lactose reducing agents

COEXISTING MEDICATION
- Lactose is used in the production of 20% of all prescription drugs and 6% of all over-the-counter drugs, including birth control pills, gas-reducing agents, and stomach acid reducing agents

- Medications that are associated with GI effects can cause or exacerbate lactose intolerance (broad-spectrum antibiotics, colchicine, chemotherapeutic agents such as antimetabolites, and radiation therapy)

SPECIAL PATIENT GROUPS
- Although 44% of all women with lactose intolerance achieve normal lactose tolerance during pregnancy, assess dietary needs of mother and fetus carefully to ensure proper nutrient intake
- Infants may require a soy-based infant formula to replace breast milk
- Calcium and vitamin D supplements may be necessary, especially in severely affected patients, children, and elderly patients
- Do not feed any lactose-containing product to infants or small children with congenital lactase deficiency
- Frequency of lactose intolerance is higher in some ethnic groups than others, therefore, consider potential for lactose intolerance and cultural issues when diagnosing and treating patients in those ethnic groups

PATIENT SATISFACTION/LIFESTYLE PRIORITIES
- Patient must modify dietary habits to prevent future occurrence of symptoms
- Dietary modifications may create a potential compliance problem, but many patients have lactose intolerance temporarily and recover their ability to consume lactose-containing products
- Elderly patients require calcium and vitamin D supplements to avoid osteoporosis

## SUMMARY OF THERAPEUTIC OPTIONS
### Choices
- First choice of treatment is avoidance of lactose-containing products and dietary modification to ensure proper nutritional intake
- Lactase additives such as LactAid, Pregestimil, and Lidalac
- Lactose-reduced food items, such as lactose-free milk
- Patient education about dietary modification and food with hidden lactose

### Guidelines
- The American Academy of Family Physicians has published relevant clinical information: Lake AM. Chronic abdominal pain in childhood: diagnosis and management. Am Fam Phys 1999;59:1823–30
- The American Academy of Pediatrics has published a relevant policy statement: Anon. The practical significance of lactose intolerance in children. Pediatrics 1978;62:240–5
- The American Academy of Pediatrics has also published a supplement to this policy statement: American Academy of Pediatrics Committee on Nutrition. Practical significance of lactose intolerance in children: supplement. Pediatrics 1990;86:643–4

### Clinical pearls
- Live culture yogurts may be well tolerated by many lactose-intolerant patients and provide a source of calcium and nutrition. However, if dairy products have been added back after fermentation, symptoms may develop
- Intolerance to lactose gets worse with low intake. A slow increase in lactose exposure may increase tolerance, probably due to increased colonic salvage

### Never
Do not allow infants or small children born with lactase deficiency to consume lactose-containing products.

## FOLLOW UP
### Plan for review
- Prescribe a lactose-free diet and monitor patient for symptoms after approximately 3 weeks
- Patient may add lactose-containing products back into the diet slowly until the threshold for tolerance is achieved
- Monitor patients for dehydration and other nutritional deficiencies, such as calcium and vitamin D deficiencies

### Information for patient or caregiver
- Acquired or secondary lactose intolerance may be a temporary condition
- Severity of lactose intolerance varies among patients and some intake of dairy products may be possible
- Yogurt appears to be well tolerated by lactose-intolerant patients
- Whole milk or chocolate milk may be easier to drink than skim milk
- Yogurt and hard cheeses may be better tolerated than milk
- Lactose intolerance is relatively easy to treat and is usually controlled by avoidance of lactose-containing foods
- Lactose-reducing agents may not work for all patients
- Lactose is used as a base in many prescription and over-the-counter medications
- Patients should learn how to read all food labels to identify hidden lactose
- Patients should take calcium and vitamin D supplements to ensure proper dietary intake of nutrients and to meet the recommended daily allowances for these nutrients

## DRUGS AND OTHER THERAPIES: DETAILS
### Drugs
LACTASE
*Dose*
- 1–2 tablets before consumption of lactose-containing food or drink
- Alternatively, add capsules to milk

*Efficacy*
- Lactase is a 'digestive supplement which aids milk digestion'
- Efficacy is unproven and varies among patients, some patients may not experience symptom relief

*Risks/benefits*
- Risk: not effective for all patients with lactose intolerance
- Benefit: reduces potential for symptoms

*Side effects and adverse reactions*
None are reported.

*Interactions (other drugs)*
No interactions are reported.

*Contraindications*
No contraindications are reported.

*Acceptability to patient*
Patients may forget to take the medication and experience symptoms of lactose intolerance.

### Other therapies
LACTOSE-FREE DIET
Elimination of all lactose-containing products from diet.

*Efficacy*
May not work for all patients.

## LIFESTYLE
Avoiding lactose in the diet is the most effective form of treatment for lactose intolerance.

RISKS/BENEFITS
- There is an increased risk for calcium and vitamin D deficiencies in a lactose-free diet
- Symptoms are usually resolved without further need of treatment.

ACCEPTABILITY TO PATIENT
Dietary modifications may be difficult for the patient to adhere to and may increase the potential for compliance problems.

FOLLOW UP PLAN
Follow-up monitoring should occur approximately 3 weeks after the start of lactose-free diet to determine effectiveness and to assess potential for other concomitant GI disorders

PATIENT AND CAREGIVER INFORMATION
- Patients must be educated to read food labels for hidden lactose
- Patients must ask their pharmacists about lactose content before taking any prescribed or over-the-counter medications
- Patients must know their level of lactose intolerance

## OUTCOMES

### EFFICACY OF THERAPIES
- Lactose avoidance and lactose-free diets are very successful treatments for lactose-intolerant patients within 3 weeks
- Lactase additives and lactose-free products may not work for all patients

#### Review period
Patients should experience relief within 3 weeks of starting a lactose-free diet.

### PROGNOSIS
- Prognosis for successful suppression of symptoms is very high if the patient adheres to lactose avoidance
- Lactose additives or lactose-free foods do not work for all patients
- For patients with primary lactose intolerance, lactose avoidance will be necessary for the remainder of their life
- For patients with secondary lactose intolerance, lactose avoidance may be necessary for only a few months or until the causative condition is resolved

#### Clinical pearls
Most patients rapidly take control of their own management for simple lactose intolerance. There are no consequences in the large majority of cases, as long as calcium intake is maintained.

### COMPLICATIONS
Calcium and vitamin D deficiency are possible with lactose-free diets; therefore, encourage patients to eat foods high in calcium and vitamin D and to use supplements as needed.

### CONSIDER CONSULT
Lactose intolerance is rarely the cause for referral.

# PREVENTION

## RISK FACTORS
- Race: specific ethnic groups are more susceptible than others
- Age: teenagers and adults are more likely to experience symptoms of primary lactose intolerance; symptoms of secondary lactose intolerance can occur at any age; and premature infants are more likely to have congenital lactose intolerance than full-term infants

## MODIFY RISK FACTORS
### Lifestyle and wellness
ALCOHOL AND DRUGS
- Limit consumption of alcohol; alcohol is a gastrointestinal (GI) irritant and may increase the potential for secondary lactose intolerance
- Patient should consult their physician about the potential for GI irritation from specific medications such as broad-spectrum antibiotics, chemotherapeutic agents, radiation therapy
- Patient should consult their physician and their pharmacist about the amount of lactose in all prescription and over-the-counter medications

DIET
- Reduce intake or avoid lactose-containing products permanently for primary lactose intolerance and as long as necessary for secondary lactose intolerance
- Patients with congenital lactose intolerance should not consume lactose
- Reduce intake or avoid all food products with 'hidden' lactose such as breads, baked goods, processed foods, instant foods, lunch meat, salad dressings, and candy
- Avoid food products with whey, curds, dry milk, milk solids, and nonfat dry milk
- Eat foods high in calcium and vitamin D to meet recommended daily allowances and to avoid deficiencies or take other forms of calcium replacement.

FAMILY HISTORY
- Certain races are more susceptible to primary lactose intolerance
- Familial history increases the potential for lactose intolerance

## SCREENING
ENDOSCOPY
Endoscopy is usually reserved for those patients with lactose intolerance and concurrent GI disorders.

## PREVENT RECURRENCE
Avoid lactose-containing products.

### Reassess coexisting disease
GI disorders commonly cause or are associated with lactose intolerance, therefore, carefully assess patients with a history of lactose intolerance.

INTERACTION ALERT
Broad-spectrum antibiotics, colchicine, chemotherapeutic agents, and radiation therapy are associated with GI effects and may increase the potential for secondary lactose intolerance.

PATIENT SATISFACTION/LIFESTYLE PRIORITIES
Patients must be aware of their condition, including severity and avoid all potential causative.

# RESOURCES

## ASSOCIATIONS

American College of Gastroenterology
4900 B South 31st Street
Arlington, VA 22206
Tel: (703) 820-7400
Fax: (703) 931-4520
http://www.acg.gi.org

American Gastroenterological Association
Seventh Floor
7910 Woodmont Avenue
Bethesda, MD 20814
Tel: (301) 654-2055
Fax: (301) 652-3890
http://www.gastro.org

Digestive Disease National Coalition
Suite 200
507 Capitol Court NE
Washington, DC 20003
Tel: (202) 544-7497
Fax: (202) 546-7105

National Institutes of Diabetes and Digestive and Kidney Diseases (NIDDK)
National Institutes of Health (NIH)
Bethesda, MD 20892
Tel: (301) 496-4000 (
http://www.niddk.nih.gov

## KEY REFERENCES

- Rakel: Conn's current therapy 2000, 52nd edn. Philadelphia: WB Saunders, 2000, p507–14
- Goldman L, Bennett JC. Cecil textbook of medicine, 21st edn. Philadelphia: WB Saunders, 2000, p712–22
- Lactose intolerance, http://www.gastro.org/public/lactose.html
- Lactose intolerance, http://www.niddk.nih.gov/health/digest/pubs/lactose/lactose.htm
- Engstrom PF, Goosenberg EB. Diagnosis and management of bowel disease. Professional Communications, 1999, chapter 15

## CONTRIBUTORS

Eric F Pollak, MD, MPH
Andrew H Soll, MD

# MALLORY–WEISS SYNDROME

- Summary Information — 388
- Background — 389
- Diagnosis — 391
- Treatment — 397
- Outcomes — 402
- Prevention — 404
- Resources — 405

## SUMMARY INFORMATION

### DESCRIPTION

- Linear mucosal tears at the gastroesophageal junction
- Typically, tears occur following episodes of retching or nonbloody vomiting
- Mucosal tears can cause upper gastrointestinal bleeding, most likely hematemesis. Isolated melena or hematochezia is less common
- A history of excessive alcohol intake preceding the episode of bleeding is often found in patients with Mallory–Weiss tears
- Mallory–Weiss syndrome is an endoscopic diagnosis and should be considered in the differential diagnosis of all patients with upper gastrointestinal bleeding

### URGENT ACTION

- Immediate action is the same as for any cause of acute upper gastrointestinal hemorrhage and includes appropriate initial resuscitation
- Establish intravenous access with fluid replacement, including blood transfusion if indicated
- If patient appears shocked, then central venous access is indicated
- Insert nasogastric tube and lavage with water or saline to see if 'coffee ground' material or fresh blood is aspirated
- Blood should be taken for complete blood count, prothrombin time, and cross-match
- $H_2$ receptor antagonists or an intravenous or oral proton pump inhibitor may be administered, but these have no appreciable effect on mortality rate
- Upper gastrointestinal endoscopy should be carried out as soon as possible to confirm the diagnosis and exclude other causes

## BACKGROUND

### ICD9 CODE
530.7 Mallory–Weiss syndrome

### SYNONYMS
- Gastroesophageal laceration-hemorrhage syndrome
- Mucosal lacerations of the cardioesophageal junction
- Emetogenic mucosal laceration

### CARDINAL FEATURES
- Accounts for 5–15% of all cases of upper gastrointestinal bleeding
- Characterized by esophagogastric mucosal tears, which are most commonly linear
- 30–50% of patients report retching or vomiting preceding the onset of bleeding
- 5–10% of patients will only have melena or hematochezia. 2–5% of patients present with syncope without initial evidence of overt bleeding
- May occur following episode of heavy retching after excessive consumption of alcohol
- May also be associated with hiatus hernia, esophagitis, coughing, Valsalva maneuver, or ingestion of aspirin or other nonsteroidal anti-inflammatory drugs (NSAIDs)
- 90% of cases will settle spontaneously with conservative management
- Can occur in any age group

### CAUSES
#### Common causes
Sudden increase of intra-abdominal pressure leading to mucosal tears at the esophagogastric junction. Usually, but not exclusively, from vomiting or violent retching.

#### Contributory or predisposing factors
- Excessive alcohol intake, especially binge drinking
- Pre-existing hiatus hernia
- Respiratory disease leading to violent coughing
- Valsalva maneuver during defecation when constipated
- Disorders of coagulation
- Anticoagulant or antiplatelet medication (e.g. warfarin)
- Eating disorders with self-induced vomiting
- Seizures
- Trauma
- Heavy lifting

Rare:
- Retching during esophagogastroduodenoscopy
- Hiccups under anesthesia

### EPIDEMIOLOGY
#### Incidence and prevalence
INCIDENCE
0.04/1000.

FREQUENCY
Accounts for 5–15% of all acute upper gastrointestinal hemorrhage.

#### Demographics
AGE
Can occur at any age but is more common in adults.

### GENDER
Most series report male predominance, likely related to greater forces generated by abdominal muscles or higher incidence of alcohol abuse in men.

# DIAGNOSIS

## DIFFERENTIAL DIAGNOSIS

- Differential diagnosis of Mallory–Weiss syndrome includes any possible cause of acute upper gastrointestinal bleeding
- It may be distinguished from other causes on the basis of preceding symptomatology and/or physical findings, but final diagnosis relies on esophagogastroduodenoscopy

### Peptic ulceration of esophagus, stomach, or duodenum

Peptic ulcers are caused by the action of the acid gastric juice.

FEATURES

- A history of epigastric or upper abdominal pain may be given
- Preceding dyspeptic symptoms may be present
- *Helicobacter* serology is positive in 50% of patients

### Reflux esophagitis

Reflux esophagitis is an inflammatory response secondary to gastroesophageal reflux.

FEATURES

- Common during pregnancy and may be associated with hiatus hernia; other etiologic factors include anything that lowers the esophageal sphincter pressure (e.g. certain foods, smoking, some drugs)
- Heartburn and regurgitation, which may be aggravated by lying down, bending over, or raising intra-abdominal pressure

### Acute gastritis

Gastritis is associated with nonsteroidal anti-inflammatory drugs (NSAIDs), alcohol, and renal failure.

FEATURES

Inflamed, red, edematous mucosa seen on endoscopy.

### Erosive gastropathy

Erosive gastropathy is usually caused by aspirin or other NSAIDs, or portal hypertension.

### Duodenitis

Duodenitis may occur on its own or in association with duodenal ulceration.

FEATURES

- Inflamed, reddened mucosa
- Etiology includes smoking, alcohol, and NSAIDs

### Esophageal varices

Esophageal varices are associated with portal hypertension most commonly secondary to alcohol-induced cirrhosis of the liver.

FEATURES

- Other signs of portal hypertension may be present on initial examination
- Can produce life-threatening hematemesis

### Swallowed blood

- Physical examination of oropharynx, nose, or respiratory tract may reveal the source, or there may be a clear history of preceding trauma or underlying respiratory disease
- Esophagogastroduodenoscopy will be negative for an upper gastrointestinal source

### Esophageal or gastric neoplasms
Additional typical symptoms of esophageal tumors and gastric malignancy are dysphagia, weight loss, anorexia, nausea, and abdominal pain.

### Arteriovenous malformations
Includes hereditary telangiectasia, Dieulafoy's lesions, and angiodysplasias.

FEATURES
- There may be evidence of arteriovenous malformations at other sites or a family history of such lesions
- Angiography may be required to make diagnosis

### Boerhaave's syndrome
Boerhaave's syndrome refers to esophageal rupture associated with forceful vomiting, classically after overeating or excessive drinking.

FEATURES
- Spontaneous esophageal rupture
- May be associated with a history of acute chest pain preceding vomiting
- Bleeding is rare
- Endoscopy is contraindicated
- Chest X-ray may show free air or pleural effusion
- Computed tomography (CT) scanning with water-soluble contrast will identify the perforation
- High mortality rate due to mediastinitis and pleural effusion
- Requires immediate surgical repair

## SIGNS & SYMPTOMS
### Signs
- Evidence of alcohol consumption with intoxication or signs of chronic alcohol abuse
- Hypovolemic shock, with low blood pressure, rapid pulse, and peripheral vasoconstriction
- Fresh or altered blood around patient's mouth or on clothing

### Symptoms
- Vomiting of bright red blood or coffee-ground material, or passage of melena which may or may not be preceded by retching, nonbloody vomiting, violent coughing, or hiccuping
- Dyspepsia or retrosternal discomfort is possible

## ASSOCIATED DISORDERS
Esophagitis (peptic or infectious).

## CONSIDER CONSULT
Referral for endoscopy is indicated in all cases of acute upper gastrointestinal bleeding, even if the patient appears hemodynamically stable.

## INVESTIGATION OF THE PATIENT
### Direct questions to patient
- Q Do you have a history of previous gastrointestinal bleeding? Mallory–Weiss syndrome recurrence is relatively uncommon, so a history of previous upper gastrointestinal bleeding may indicate another diagnosis
- Q Do you have a history of peptic ulceration? If such a history is present, then it is a more likely cause of the bleeding
- Q How much alcohol do you drink? Mallory–Weiss syndrome is often associated with binge alcohol drinking

Q Were you retching before you vomited blood? This is a common, but not invariable, feature of Mallory–Weiss syndrome
Q Were you coughing violently before vomiting blood? Preceding violent coughing would tend to support the diagnosis of Mallory–Weiss syndrome
Q Are you taking any prescribed or over-the-counter (OTC) medication? The most relevant drugs are aspirin or other NSAIDs, anticoagulants, and antiplatelet drugs. Also ask about use of antacids and $H_2$ receptor antagonists because they may indicate long-standing dyspeptic symptoms
Q Have you lost weight recently? Gastric or esophageal malignancies may be associated with bleeding and weight loss

## Contributory or predisposing factors
Q Do you have a history of bleeding problems? Any coagulopathy may complicate upper gastrointestinal bleeding and cause more profuse hemorrhage from even a fairly minor Mallory–Weiss tear, even though it is not the actual cause
Q Do you have liver disease? Liver disease may suggest an alternative diagnosis, such as esophageal varices, although liver disease in an alcoholic would not preclude Mallory–Weiss syndrome
Q Do you have a hiatus hernia? Hiatus hernia is a predisposing factor in Mallory–Weiss syndrome

## Examination
- Assess hemodynamic status through pulse, blood pressure, orthostatic changes, and central venous pressure: in cases of massive blood loss the patient will be in shock and will require ABC (airway, breathing, circulation) management
- Examine for signs of alcoholism and liver disease: alcoholism and liver disease predispose to clotting disorders and can exacerbate blood loss
- Palpate the abdomen for rebound, guarding, tenderness, masses, or organomegaly: check for signs of acute abdomen or visceral perforation – a large liver mass may indicate liver disease or malignancy
- Examine for signs of bleeding disorder: reduced ability to clot will exacerbate blood loss
- Rectal examination to look for signs of melena or fresh rectal bleeding: bright red blood per rectum usually indicates a lower gastrointestinal cause of bleeding but is seen in up to 10% of upper gastrointestinal bleeds

## Summary of investigative tests
- Complete blood count: including hemoglobin, hematocrit, and platelet levels. In the early stages the hematocrit will be more useful than hemoglobin level in determining extent of hemorrhage because the latter may appear normal until hemodilution has occurred
- Prothrombin time: particularly important in patients receiving anticoagulant medication and for diagnosis of liver disease
- Urea and electrolytes: raised urea suggests ingestion of blood
- Liver function tests: may reveal significant liver disease, which is a potentially complicating factor
- Esophagogastroduodenoscopy: a gastroenterologist should be consulted and an endoscopy should be performed as soon as the patient is hemodynamically stable or at least within the first 24h
- Angiography: this will be ordered and carried out by an interventional radiologist in cases where the bleeding site cannot be identified or controlled by endoscopy
- Chest X-ray: will not identify source of bleeding but is indicated if there is a history of chest pain preceding the hematemesis in order to exclude esophageal rupture (Boerhaave's syndrome)

## DIAGNOSTIC DECISION
In most cases diagnosis is made on endoscopy by visualization of the tear.

## CLINICAL PEARLS
- Mallory–Weiss tears often present as hematemesis acutely without other symptoms
- History of antecedent vomiting, retching, or paroxysmal coughing is strongly suggestive of Mallory–Weiss tears

## THE TESTS
### Body fluids
COMPLETE BLOOD COUNT
*Description*
Cuffed venous blood sample.

*Advantages/Disadvantages*
- Advantage: easy to take sample in the clinic setting
- Disadvantage: not specific for Mallory–Weiss syndrome; may not reflect severity of bleed in early stage

*Normal*
- Hemoglobin: male 13.6–17.7g/dL (8.4–11.0mmol/L); female 12.0–15.0g/dL (7.4–9.3mmol/L)
- Hematocrit: male 39–49%; female 33–43%
- Platelet count: 130–400x10$^9$/L

*Abnormal*
- Hemoglobin: male <13.6g/dL (<8.4mmol/L); female <12.0g/dL (<7.4mmol/L); hemoglobin may initially appear normal and may not drop until fluid replacement and hence hemodilution occur
- Hematocrit: male <39%; female <33%
- Platelet count: <130x10$^9$/L

*Cause of abnormal result*
Significant blood loss.

*Drugs, disorders and other factors that may alter results*
Pre-existing anemia, common in chronic alcoholics, may make it difficult to assess degree of blood loss.

PROTHROMBIN TIME
*Description*
Cuffed venous blood sample.

*Advantages/Disadvantages*
- Advantage: easy to take sample in the clinic setting
- Disadvantage: not specific for Mallory-Weiss syndrome

*Normal*
10–12s.

*Abnormal*
- >12s
- Keep in mind the possibility of a false-positive result

*Cause of abnormal result*
- Liver disease or anticoagulant medication
- Consumption coagulopathy in cases of severe uncontrolled bleeding

*Drugs, disorders and other factors that may alter results*
Oral anticoagulant medication.

## UREA AND ELECTROLYTES
*Description*
Cuffed venous blood sample.

*Normal*
- Blood urea nitrogen: 8–18mg/dL (3–6.5mmol/L)
- Sodium: 135–147mEq/L (135–147mmol/L)
- Potassium: 3.5–5mEq/L (3.5–5mmol/L)

*Abnormal*
- Blood urea nitrogen: >18mg/dL (>6.5mmol/L)
- Sodium: >147mEq/L (>147mmol/L)
- Potassium: <3.5mEq/L (<3.5mmol/L)

*Cause of abnormal result*
- Ingestion of blood, as would occur with gastrointestinal bleeding, may result in a raised blood urea nitrogen
- Vomiting can give rise to hypernatremia and hypokalemia
- Hypovolemia and renal hypoperfusion
- Keep in mind the possibility of a false-positive result

*Drugs, disorders and other factors that may alter results*
- Blood urea nitrogen may be raised if renal blood flow is impaired due to blood loss or if there is coexisting renal disease or dehydration secondary to the vomiting
- Drugs such as aminoglycosides, diuretics, lithium, and corticosteroids may also be the cause of raised blood urea nitrogen
- Coexisting renal disease or vomiting may affect sodium and potassium levels

## LIVER FUNCTION TEST
*Description*
Cuffed venous blood sample.

*Advantages/Disadvantages*
Disadvantage: not specific for liver disease – abnormal liver function test results may occur in a number of nonliver-related diseases.

*Normal*
- Alanine aminotransferase (ALT): 0–35U/L
- Alkaline phosphatase: 30–120U/L
- Aspartate aminotransferase (AST): 0–35U/L
- Gamma-glutamyl transferase: 0–30U/L

*Abnormal*
- ALT: >35U/L
- Alkaline phosphatase: >120U/L
- AST: >35U/L
- Gamma-glutamyl transferase: >30U/L
- Keep in mind the possibility of false-positive results

*Cause of abnormal result*
- Hepatitis
- Cirrhosis
- Excess alcohol
- Drug-induced (e.g. NSAIDs)

*Drugs, disorders and other factors that may alter results*
- Myocardial infarction and congestive heart failure
- Severe muscle trauma
- Malignancy
- Antibiotics, antihypertensive agents, NSAIDs
- Bone tumors and Paget's disease of bone
- Thyrotoxicosis
- Acute pancreatitis

## Imaging
CHEST X-RAY
*Description*
Indicated if there is high degree of suspicion that an esophageal perforation may have occurred.

*Advantages/Disadvantages*
Advantage: useful in the diagnosis of aspiration pneumonia.

*Normal*
Mallory–Weiss syndrome should not produce any radiographic abnormalities.

## Other tests
ESOPHAGOGASTRODUODENOSCOPY

*Description*
- Involves passing a double-channel, therapeutic videoendoscope into the oropharynx, and then the esophagus, stomach, and duodenum
- Procedure can be used as both a diagnostic test to visualize the source of bleeding and a therapeutic measure to administer appropriate treatment
- Patient should be medically resuscitated before endoscopy and hemodynamically stable
- Airway must be protected during the procedure, if necessary by intubation if bleeding is very active or if the patient is particularly uncooperative or restless
- Patient will generally need to be sedated during the procedure

*Advantages/Disadvantages*
- Advantage: can confirm or exclude Mallory–Weiss tear

Disadvantages:
- Endoscopy carries a small risk (1/1000) of causing tears or perforations, especially in a restless patient
- Can be technically difficult to perform, especially in the presence of active bleeding

*Abnormal*
Linear mucosal laceration with or without active bleeding is most commonly seen at the gastroesophageal junction.

# TREATMENT

## CONSIDER CONSULT
Unless the bleeding is clinically insignificant (e.g. in the absence of even mild hypovolemic shock), cases of suspected Mallory-Weiss syndrome should be referred for endoscopy by an experienced gastroenterologist for treatment.

## IMMEDIATE ACTION
- Initial medical resuscitation with intravenous fluids and blood products as required
- Correct any coagulopathies (e.g. prolonged prothrombin time, decreased platelets)

## PATIENT AND CAREGIVER ISSUES
### Patient or caregiver request
Q **Will this happen to me again?** Recurrence is uncommon unless the conditions that led to the first episode are repeated

Q **Is there any medication I should take to prevent it from recurring?** Not really. Antacids, $H_2$ receptor antagonists, or proton pump inhibitors may be given but will not specifically protect against recurrences

### Health-seeking behavior
Q **Have you waited too long?** If this is the case and bleeding is severe and/or prolonged, then the patient is more likely to present with significant hypovolemic shock

Q **Have you self-medicated?** The patient may have tried antacids, $H_2$ receptor antagonists, or antiemetics before presenting

Q **Have you visited the emergency room?** The patient is likely to present to the emergency room, especially if bleeding is very active. The patient may become significantly hypovolemic over a short time and present in a state of collapse

## MANAGEMENT ISSUES
### Goals
- Correct hypovolemia if present
- Correct coagulopathies if present
- Identify source of bleeding
- Stop bleeding if not already ceased spontaneously

### Management in special circumstances
Airway should be protected, by intubation if necessary, during endoscopy in patients with active bleeding or altered mental state.

### COEXISTING DISEASE
- A coagulopathy may increase the severity of the bleeding and will need to be corrected
- Coagulation in patients with liver disease (alcoholic or nonalcoholic) may be problematic and difficult to correct
- Alcoholic patients who are intoxicated at the time of presentation may be more difficult to assess and manage due to lack of cooperation or altered mental state. They may need intubation and mechanical ventilation in cases of severe bleeding

### COEXISTING MEDICATION
Any medication that can prolong bleeding time (e.g. aspirin, anticoagulants, antiplatelet drugs) will need to be stopped, if possible, because they may reduce the efficacy of treatment for Mallory–Weiss syndrome.

PATIENT SATISFACTION/LIFESTYLE PRIORITIES
Recurrence is rare (0–5%), and in 80–90% of cases no active treatment is required to correct the acute episode, nor is any long-term therapy indicated.

## SUMMARY OF THERAPEUTIC OPTIONS
### Choices
The choice of therapeutic options depends on the presence or absence of active bleeding at the time of endoscopy.

It is a common practice to treat Mallory–Weiss tears that are still bleeding at the time of endoscopy. Injection and/or coagulation are the preferred modalities. Other endoscopic techniques are not standard treatments. Angiography should be performed if the bleeding cannot be controlled at endoscopy, and surgery if angiography fails.

- Conservative management: in the absence of active bleeding, the first choice of therapy is conservative or supportive only, with adequate resuscitation as required
- Endoscopic thermal coagulation: carried out at the time of endoscopy if site of bleeding can be identified. A variety of methods is available, including heater probes and bipolar electrocoagulation
- Endoscopic injection therapy, most commonly using epinephrine at site of bleeding. May be used as a precursor to thermal coagulation in order to better visualize the site or on its own as a first line of treatment. Ethanolamine may also be used
- Other modalities of endoscopic therapy, such as clips, sutures, or band ligation, are available but are less commonly used than either thermal or injection therapy
- Vasopressin, coils, or Gelfoam may be injected into arterial tree to occlude bleeding vessel during angiography in cases where endoscopic treatment has failed to identify or control the source of bleeding
- Laparotomy with gastrostomy and oversewing of tear: a last resort and rarely indicated, but a possible option if all other treatments fail and bleeding persists
- Lifestyle changes may be beneficial

### Clinical pearls
A nasogastric tube should not be inserted after diagnosis of a Mallory–Weiss tear since it may aggravate the bleeding site.

## FOLLOW UP
- Recurrence of Mallory–Weiss syndrome is uncommon except in patients with intrinsic or drug-induced coagulopathies, or in alcoholics
- Repeat endoscopy is only indicated if bleeding recurs
- Follow-up is only required if a blood transfusion has been given and the hemoglobin level needs to be rechecked, or if anticoagulant medication is stopped and/or reversed during the acute stage and needs to be restarted and monitored

### Plan for review
If hemoglobin is low in the acute stage and blood transfusion or oral iron therapy is used, then recheck hemoglobin level at 4-week intervals until stabilized in the normal range.

### Information for patient or caregiver
- Excessive alcohol intake should be avoided
- Use of aspirin or other nonsteroidal anti-inflammatory drugs (NSAIDs) should be limited
- Patients with bleeding disorders or liver disease or those taking anticoagulants/antiplatelet drugs are at greater risk of recurrence

# DRUGS AND OTHER THERAPIES: DETAILS
## Drugs
EPINEPHRINE

*Dose*
0.5–1.0mL of 1:10,000 solution injected submucosally around lesion. Can inject a total of 2–6mL.

*Efficacy*
May not be sufficient alone to stop bleeding completely and is most commonly used in conjunction with thermal coagulation.

*Risks/benefits*
Risks:
- Excessive activity from epinephrine can cause other life-threatening cardiac reactions (tachydysrhythmia, hypertension, myocardial ischemia, stunned heart syndrome)
- Use caution in elderly and nursing mothers
- Use caution in cardiovascular disease, hypertension, thyrotoxicosis and hyperthyroidism
- Effects on vasculature are dose-dependent

Benefit: minimal risk of systemic absorption.

*Side effects and adverse reactions*
Only occur if drug is systemically absorbed.
- Cardiovascular system: hypertension, palpitations, myocardial ischemia, myocardial infarction, tachydysrhythmia
- Central nervous system: headache, tremor, subarachnoid hemorrhage (in overdosage), anxiety, dizziness, cold extremities
- Gastrointestinal: nausea and vomiting

*Interactions (other drugs)*
- Alpha2-adrenoceptor stimulants
- Antidepressants (monoamine oxidase inhibitors (MAOIs) and tricyclics)
- Antipsychotics
- Beta-blockers
- Doxapram
- Oxytocin

*Contraindications*
- Local anesthesia of fingers and toes
- General anesthesia with halogenated hydrocarbons or cyclopane
- Labor
- Cardiac dysrhythmias
- Coronary insufficiency
- Angle-closure glaucoma
- Organic brain damage

*Follow up plan*
Patient will need to be monitored for at least 24h following this therapy because there is always a risk of rebleeding.

VASOPRESSIN

*Dose*
Selective intra-arterial injection of 0.2–0.4U/min until bleeding stops.

*Efficacy*
Successful in up to 70% of patients who require this treatment.

*Risks/benefits*
Risks:
- Use caution in thyroid, cardiac, vascular, or renal disease
- Use caution in epilepsy, migraine, asthma, or polyuria

- Use caution in the elderly, children, pregnancy, and breast-feeding
- Can cause water intoxication

*Side effects and adverse reactions*
- Cardiovascular system: hypertension, sinus bradycardia, myocardial infarction, angina, dysrhythmias, atrioventricular block
- Central nervous system: headache, dizziness, confusion, flushing, tremor
- Gastrointestinal: nausea, vomiting, abdominal pain, diarrhea, flatulence
- Genitourinary: uterine contractions
- Metabolic: hyponatremia
- Skin: sweating, pallor, urticaria, injection site reaction

*Interactions (other drugs)*
- Antidepressants (tricyclic) ▪ Carbamazepine ▪ Chlorpropamide ▪ Clofibrate ▪ Epinephrine
- Ethanol ▪ Fludrocortisone ▪ Heparin ▪ Lithium ▪ Morphine

*Contraindications*
- Peripheral vascular disease ▪ Chronic nephritis ▪ Coronary artery disease

*Follow up plan*
Patient will need to be monitored for at least 24h following this therapy because there is always a risk of rebleeding.

## Surgical therapy
LAPAROTOMY WITH GASTROSTOMY AND OVERSEWING OF TEAR
Rarely indicated except in severe hemorrhage when other treatments have failed or are inappropriate.

*Efficacy*
Highly effective.

*Risks/benefits*
Risk: major operative procedure requiring general anesthetic with usual attendant risks.

*Acceptability to patient*
May be only remaining life-saving option to stop bleeding if other treatments fail and hemorrhage persists.

*Follow up plan*
Normal postoperative care following abdominal surgery.

## Endoscopic therapy
ENDOSCOPIC THERMAL COAGULATION
*Efficacy*
Very effective for bleeding from vessels up to 2.5mm in diameter.

*Risks/benefits*
Risks:
- Perforation
- Deep thermal damage to surrounding tissue
- Retching during endoscopy may cause or extend a Mallory–Weiss tear
- Chest pain, transient dysphagia, sore throat

*Follow up plan*
Repeat endoscopy with further treatment if bleeding does not stop.

### ENDOSCOPIC INJECTION THERAPY
*Efficacy*
- A single treatment stops bleeding in >90% of cases that require active intervention
- More than one treatment may be required in some patients
- Commonly used prior to thermal coagulation to allow better visualization of lesion

*Risks/benefits*
Risk: systemic absorption of sclerosing agent, chest pain, transient dysphagia, sore throat.

*Acceptability to patient*
Morbidity rate is low with this form of treatment, and because it can be carried out at the time of the diagnostic endoscopy, no additional procedure is required.

*Follow up plan*
A second course of treatment may be necessary if bleeding persists.

## LIFESTYLE
- Recurrence is uncommon but is more likely in alcoholic patients, who should therefore be encouraged to reduce their alcohol intake
- Ingestion of aspirin or other NSAIDs should also be discouraged or limited where this has been identified as a probable risk factor

### ACCEPTABILITY TO PATIENT
Abstaining from alcohol or reducing alcohol intake may be unacceptable or very difficult for some patients to achieve.

### PATIENT AND CAREGIVER INFORMATION
Need to stress benefits of reducing alcohol intake and highlight risks of increased alcohol consumption.

## OUTCOMES

### EFFICACY OF THERAPIES
- Once diagnosis has been confirmed, 80–90% of patients with Mallory-Weiss syndrome respond rapidly to conservative management with healing of the lesion within 10 days
- Endoscopy with injection and/or thermal coagulation is usually effective in >90% of patients requiring intervention, with immediate cessation of bleeding
- Angiography with intra-arterial vasopressin is effective in up to 70% of cases in whom it is used

### Review period
- Rebleeding in Mallory–Weiss is uncommon, but if it does occur it is usually during the first 24h after initial onset
- Repeat endoscopy with or without therapy is necessary if rebleeding occurs
- Low-risk patients without active bleeding at time of endoscopy may not require >24h of observation, with no further follow up required
- Low-risk patients who respond well to endoscopic treatment may only require 48h of inpatient care

### PROGNOSIS
- Prognosis is good in low-risk patients with recurrence rare after the initial period of observation and/or treatment (0–5%)
- Patients with portal hypertension, cirrhosis, or underlying coagulopathy are most at risk of significant morbidity or even death from Mallory–Weiss syndrome

### Clinical pearls
- Bleeding due to a Mallory–Weiss tear is usually self-limited
- Endoscopic therapy if needed is generally successful
- Recurrence is uncommon

### Therapeutic failure
Failure of endoscopic injection therapy with or without thermal coagulation may be followed by intra-arterial vasopressin or in extreme cases by oversewing of the lesion either laparoscopically or following laparotomy.

### Recurrence
- Repeat endoscopy is indicated if rebleeding occurs with further injection therapy with or without thermal coagulation as indicated
- If endoscopic therapy fails to stop recurrent bleeding, then surgical treatment may be necessary

### Deterioration
Persistent or recurrent bleeding, particularly in patients with pre-existing portal hypertension or a coagulopathy, may lead to deterioration in the patient's condition.

### COMPLICATIONS
- Hypovolemic shock: characterized by low blood pressure, rapid pulse, and low central venous pressure – requires rapid correction with intravenous fluids and blood transfusion if necessary
- Renal hypoperfusion secondary to hypovolemia: characterized by oliguria and deterioration in renal function
- Disseminated intravascular coagulation: if hemorrhage is severe enough, this may occur with rebleeding or failure to respond to hemostatic measures; may only be apparent from laboratory investigations

- Exsanguination and death
- Complications may arise from investigation and/or therapy rather than from the condition itself (e.g. endoscopic perforation or rebleeding due to endoscopic trauma)

# PREVENTION

- Prevention is more relevant to recurrence than to the first episode, which may be totally unpredictable
- Some groups of patients may be more at risk for Mallory–Weiss syndrome but only if they first experience a symptom such as vomiting or coughing
- Prevention needs to be aimed at the symptoms leading up to a Mallory–Weiss tear

## RISK FACTORS

- **Alcoholic binge drinking (with or without pre-existing liver disease):** accounts for <50% of patients presenting with Mallory–Weiss syndrome
- **Hiatus hernia:** not specifically a cause of Mallory–Weiss syndrome, but a frequently occurring coexisting/predisposing feature
- **Ingestion of aspirin or other nonsteroidal anti-inflammatory drugs (NSAIDs):** may predispose patient to vomiting and/or esophagitis or gastritis, which are associated with a greater risk of Mallory–Weiss
- **Abrupt increase in gastric transmural pressure:** can occur as a result of, e.g., vomiting, coughing, pregnancy, Valsalva maneuver, or hiccuping; hence constipation or lifting heavy objects could be risk factors

## MODIFY RISK FACTORS
### Lifestyle and wellness
ALCOHOL AND DRUGS
- Discourage binge drinking of alcohol
- Advise caution in the unprescribed use of aspirin or other NSAIDs

## PREVENT RECURRENCE

- Mainly aimed at modifying risk factors
- No medication or other therapy will specifically prevent recurrence, but hiatus hernia, esophagitis, gastritis, or other predisposing coexisting disease should be treated

### Reassess coexisting disease
- Treat coexisting hiatus hernia, esophagitis, or gastritis if these are known to have precipitated an episode of Mallory–Weiss syndrome
- Respiratory disease should be adequately managed to prevent violent or prolonged coughing attacks
- Severe retching/vomiting in patients with known portal hypertension or a coagulopathy should be rapidly controlled to prevent Mallory–Weiss syndrome from occurring

# RESOURCES

## KEY REFERENCES
- The Merck manual of diagnosis and therapy, 17th edn. New Jersey: Merck Publications, 1997, chapter 20: Esophageal laceration and rupture
- Cook DJ, Guyatt GH, Salena BJ, Laine LA. Endoscopic therapy for acute nonvariceal upper gastrointestinal hemorrhage: a meta-analysis. Gastroenterology 1992;102:139–48
- Harris JM, DiPalma JA. Clinical significance of Mallory–Weiss tears. Am J Gastroenterol 1993;88(12):2056–8
- Sleisinger and Fordtran's gastrointestinal and liver disease, 6th edn. Philadelphia: WB Saunders, 1998, p204
- Hixson SD, Burns RP, Britt LG. Mallory–Weiss syndrome: retrospective review of eight years' experience. South Med J 1979;72(10):1249–51
- Hastings PR, Peters KW, Cohn I Jr. Mallory–Weiss syndrome. Review of 69 cases. Am J Surg 1981;142(5):560–2

## FAQS
### Question 1
When should endoscopy be done?

ANSWER 1
Patients should undergo endoscopy as soon as they are hemodynamically stable.

### Question 2
Should antiacid secretory medication be prescribed?

ANSWER 2
Yes. The drug of choice is an oral proton pump inhibitor given for 4–6 weeks to ensure adequate healing.

### Question 3
When can aspirin or another nonsteroidal anti-inflammatory drug be prescribed?

ANSWER 3
It should be safe to administer those drugs 10–14 days after the acute bleeding.

## CONTRIBUTORS
Gordon H Baustian, MD
Andrew F Ippoliti, MD
Jaime Oviedo, MD

# PANCREATITIS

| | | |
|---|---|---|
| ■ | Summary Information | 408 |
| ■ | Background | 409 |
| ■ | Diagnosis | 411 |
| ■ | Treatment | 422 |
| ■ | Outcomes | 426 |
| ■ | Prevention | 428 |
| ■ | Resources | 430 |

## SUMMARY INFORMATION

### DESCRIPTION

- Inflammation of the pancreas
- Symptomatology and complications are due to autodigestion of the pancreas and surrounding tissue, caused by leaking pancreatic enzymes
- Severe cases may result in necrosis of areas of the pancreas (necrotizing pancreatitis)
- 80% of all cases caused by either obstructive gallstone pathology or heavy alcohol use
- May be acute or chronic
- Recurrence rate up to 50% without resolution of precipitating factors

### URGENT ACTION

- Severe acute necrotizing pancreatitis necessitates surgical consultation
- Severe pancreatitis necessitates hospitalization in an intensive care unit
- Be aware that third-space fluid losses will require aggressive fluid
- If fluids do not reverse a shock state, consider using pressors
- Be alert to concomitant coagulopathy or hypoalbuminemia, which requires fresh frozen plasma and/or serum albumin infusion
- Hypocalcemia with tetany will require intravenous calcium gluconate administration
- Be alert to the development of adult respiratory distress syndrome
- Be sure to ask patients whether they have HIV infection/AIDS. If so, ascertain their drug regimen. Patients being treated with antiretroviral therapy (various cocktails using the nucleoside reverse transcriptase inhibitor drugs such as stavudine, didanosine, hydroxyurea) have a high risk of very severe pancreatitis

### KEY! DON'T MISS!

Be alert to the development of:

- Tetany secondary to hypocalcemia
- Adult respiratory distress syndrome
- Infection secondary to necrotizing pancreatitis
- Shock, requiring more aggressive intravascular fluid replacement, possible pressors
- Coagulopathy and/or hypoalbuminemia, requiring administration of fresh frozen plasma, serum albumin, and/or intravascular fluids

## BACKGROUND

### ICD9 CODE
577.0 Acute pancreatitis

### CARDINAL FEATURES
- Inflammation of the pancreas
- Moderate to severe midepigastric pain, radiating to the back
- Anorexia, nausea, and vomiting
- Symptomatology and complications are due to autodigestion of the pancreas and surrounding tissue, caused by leaking pancreatic enzymes
- Blood levels of pancreatic enzymes are elevated
- 80% of all cases are caused by either choledocholithiasis or heavy alcohol use
- Recurrence rate of up to 50% without resolution of precipitating factors

Ranson's criteria of severity of acute pancreatitis:
- Used to assess the prognosis of the patient
- Patients with three or four Ranson's criteria have a 15% mortality; those with seven or eight criteria have a reported 100% mortality
- Patients who present with more than three Ranson's criteria should be considered to have severe acute pancreatitis, and should be referred to a surgeon and monitored in an intensive care unit

Ranson's criteria are as follows.
Ranson's criteria on admission:
- Age >55 years
- White blood cell count >16,000x10$^9$
- Serum glucose >200mg/dL (>11mmol/L)
- Serum lactate dehydrogenase >350 IU/L
- Aspartate aminotransferase >60 IU/L

Ranson's criteria within first 48h:
- Hematocrit drop >10%
- Blood urea nitrogen rise >2mg/dL
- $p_aO_2$ <60mmHg (<8kPa)
- Serum calcium <8mg/dL (<2mmol/L)
- Base deficit >-4
- Fluid sequestration estimated to be >6L

### CAUSES
#### Common causes
- 30–75% of all cases are due to biliary tract disease (gallstone obstructing sphincter of Oddi or ampulla of Vater, sludge)
- Over 30% of pancreatitis is due to complications of heavy alcohol use (usually >100g/day over several years); areas of increased alcohol use have high rates of alcohol-related pancreatitis
- 10–30% are idiopathic

#### Rare causes
- Hereditary pancreatitis
- Medications (including thiazide diuretics, furosemide, corticosteroids, tetracycline, estrogen, valproic acid, metronidazole, azathioprine, methyldopa, pentamidine, ethacrynic acid, procainamide, sulindac, nitrofurantoin, angiotensin-converting enzyme inhibitors, danazol,

cimetidine, piroxicam, gold, ranitidine, sulfasalazine, isoniazid, acetaminophen, cisplatin, opiates, erythromycin)
- Chemical exposure (methanol, cobalt, zinc, mercuric chloride, creosol, lead, organophosphates, chlorinated naphthalenes)
- Pregnancy
- Organ damage after abdominal or back injury (blunt or penetrating)
- Complications after surgery or after endoscopic retrograde cholangiopancreatography
- Viral infections (including mumps, Coxsackievirus, HIV, Epstein–Barr)
- Parasites (including ascariasis, clonorchiasis)
- Carcinoma (duodenal, pancreatic)
- Structural abnormalities, such as pancreas divisum or abnormalities of the duodenum/ampulla, bile ducts, sphincter of Oddi, main pancreatic duct, or accessory pancreatic duct
- Penetrating duodenal ulcer disease
- Vascular disease (ischemic or vasculitic disorders, severe hypotension)
- Metabolic disorders (such as hyperparathyroidism with concomitant hypercalcemia, hyperlipoproteinemia)
- Renal failure

### Contributory or predisposing factors
- AIDS: HIV-positive patients have a high rate of severe, rapidly fatal necrotizing pancreatitis, particularly as a result of antiretroviral use
- Alcoholism: chronic heavy drinking damages the pancreas and may result in pancreatitis
- Biliary disease: obstruction or edema of the ampulla of Vater can allow bile to reflux into the pancreatic ducts or may cause direct damage to the acinar cells, which may lead to pancreatitis
- Vitamin D poisoning and cardiopulmonary bypass: may trigger acute hypercalcemia with subsequent acute pancreatitis

## EPIDEMIOLOGY
### Incidence and prevalence
INCIDENCE
Acute pancreatitis: 0.195/1000.

### Demographics
AGE
Pancreatitis increases with age.

GENDER
Males are twice as commonly affected as females.

RACE
- Caucasians: annual incidence is 0.057/1000
- African-Americans: annual incidence is 0.207/1000

GEOGRAPHY
City areas have twice the incidence of rural areas.

## DIAGNOSIS

### DIFFERENTIAL DIAGNOSIS
#### Abdominal aortic aneurysm
Abdominal aortic aneurysm is a localized dilation of the abdominal aorta with an increase in diameter of at least 50%.

FEATURES
- Sudden-onset severe abdominal pain
- 30–50% of patients present classically, with pain, hypotension, tachycardia, and a pulsatile abdominal mass
- An abdominal bruit and lateral propagation of aortic pulse wave may be noted
- Typical patient is >65 years of age
- Commonly associated conditions include smoking, chronic obstructive pulmonary disease, atherosclerotic vascular disease, and hypertension
- Less commonly associated conditions include Marfan's syndrome, Ehlers–Danlos syndrome, collagen vascular diseases, and mycotic aneurysm
- Familial association

#### Cholangitis
Cholangitis (infection of the biliary tree) can be associated with pancreatitis, especially if caused by an impacted stone.

FEATURES
- May occur following endoscopic retrograde cholangiopancreatography
- Increased incidence in patients with history of gallstones, recent cholecystectomy, previous cholangitis, or HIV/AIDS
- May be associated with parasitic infestation in endemic areas
- Increased incidence in Asians and African-Americans who have concomitant sickle cell disease
- Charcot's triad: right upper quadrant pain, fever, jaundice
- Reynold's pentad: right upper quadrant pain, fever, jaundice, sepsis, mental status dysfunction
- May present with pruritus and acholic or hypocholic stools

#### Cholelithiasis, cholecystitis, and biliary colic
Gallstones can impact in the bile system leading to cholecystitis and other complications, including pancreatitis.

FEATURES
- Increased incidence in people of Hispanic or northern European origin, and in Pima Indians
- Uncommon in African-Americans, except those with sickle cell disease
- Gallstones: women are more often affected than men
- Cholecystitis: men are more often affected than women
- Pain is located in right upper quadrant and is constant, boring in quality, and referred to scapular region
- Onset frequently within hours of eating
- Nausea, vomiting, fever common
- Murphy's sign is common (inspiratory pause during palpation of right upper quadrant)

#### Gastroenteritis
An acute inflammation of the lining of the stomach and intestines.

FEATURES
- Primary symptom is diarrhea
- May include nausea, vomiting

- Fever may be present
- Abdominal pain usually crampy, intermittent
- Dehydration common complication
- May be viral, bacterial, parasitic, drug-induced, food-borne, secondary to medications, or associated with recent chemotherapy or radiation treatment

### Hepatitis
Inflammation of the liver.

FEATURES
- Right upper quadrant pain
- Prominent hepatomegaly
- Nausea, vomiting
- May note acholic stools, dark urine
- Scleral icterus, jaundice may be more prominent
- Pruritus
- There may be risks for infection, e.g. occupational exposure to infected body fluids (in healthcare workers), multiple sexual partners, homosexual behavior (in males), intravenous drug use, previous blood transfusions, dialysis, travel to developing countries, ingestion of contaminated shellfish, maternal transmission, amebic infestation

### Mesenteric ischemia
Mesenteric ischemia is occlusion of the mesenteric artery by thrombus or (rarely) embolus.

FEATURES
- Severe abdominal pain
- Few abdominal signs upon examination
- Nausea, vomiting
- Diarrhea common
- Rapidly progressing abdominal distension
- Ileus
- Peritonitis
- Shock
- High incidence of concomitant cardiovascular disease (e.g. congestive heart failure, cardiac arrhythmias, recent past history of myocardial infarction, atherosclerotic disease, previous history of deep vein thrombosis, digoxin administration)

## SIGNS & SYMPTOMS
### Signs
Acute pancreatitis:
- Pallor
- Diaphoresis
- Tender upper abdomen
- Fever may reach 101–103°F (38.4–39.5°C)
- Distension may be present
- Intestinal ileus common
- Initial hypertension

Severe acute pancreatitis:
- Severe cases may demonstrate guarding, percussion tenderness, tenderness with motion
- Grey-Turner's sign (flank ecchymosis)
- Cullen's sign (periumbilical ecchymosis)
- Shallow respirations caused by splinting secondary to abdominal pain

- Increased heart rate, usually 100–150 beats/min
- Hypotension supervenes secondary to third-space fluid losses, hypovolemia

## Symptoms
- Diffuse moderate to severe upper abdominal pain
- Pain described as boring and constant
- Radiation of pain straight through or around to the back
- Pain often unaffected by positional change, although it is sometimes improved by leaning forward
- Pain often rapidly escalates in intensity, peaking within about 10–20min of onset
- Pain may be intractable even after narcotic administration
- Nausea, vomiting
- Dyspnea due to diaphragmatic splinting secondary to pain

## KEY! DON'T MISS!
Be alert to the development of:
- Tetany secondary to hypocalcemia
- Adult respiratory distress syndrome
- Infection secondary to necrotizing pancreatitis
- Shock, requiring more aggressive intravascular fluid replacement, possible pressors
- Coagulopathy and/or hypoalbuminemia, requiring administration of fresh frozen plasma, serum albumin, and/or intravascular fluids

## CONSIDER CONSULT
Refer patients who have signs of:
- Pancreatic ascites (absent abdominal pain, increasing abdominal girth, elevated serum amylase)
- A suspected biliary etiology for their pancreatitis

Ranson's crieteria of severity of acute peritonitis:
- Patients who present with more than three Ranson's criteria should be considered to have severe acute pancreatitis, and should be referred to a surgeon and monitored in an intensive care unit

Ranson's criteria are as follows.
Ranson's criteria on admission:
- Age >55 years
- White blood cell count >16,000x10$^9$
- Serum glucose >200mg/dL (>11mmol/L)
- Serum lactate dehydrogenase >350 IU/L
- Aspartate aminotransferase >60 IU/L

Ranson's criteria within first 48h:
- Hematocrit drop >10%
- Blood urea nitrogen rise >2mg/dL
- $p_aO_2$ <60mmHg (<8kPa)
- Serum calcium <8mg/dL (<2mmol/L)
- Base deficit >-4
- Fluid sequestration estimated to be >6L

## INVESTIGATION OF THE PATIENT
### Direct questions to patient
Q Do you have a history of gallbladder disease? Biliary tract disease is responsible for between 30% and 75% of all cases of pancreatitis

- **Q** How much alcohol do you drink? Chronic heavy drinking is responsible for >30% of all cases of pancreatitis
- **Q** Have you recently drunk a large amount of alcohol? A recent drinking binge may precede an episode of pancreatitis
- **Q** Have you had any recent medical procedures or diagnostic tests? Pancreatitis can occur following endoscopic retrograde cholangiopancreatography
- **Q** Have you had any changes in your bowel habits? When was the last time you passed a bowel movement? Intestinal gas? Ask investigative questions to disclose signs of ileus, obstruction, carcinoma

## Contributory or predisposing factors
Have you recently suffered from mumps? Mumps is associated with pancreatitis.

## Family history
- **Q** Has anyone else in your family had pancreatitis? Certain genetic factors can cause a familial pancreatitis, including a defect in the trypsinogen gene or a variant mutation of the cystic fibrosis transmembrane conductance regulator gene
- **Q** Do you have a family history of gallstone disease? Gallstone disease is a major cause of pancreatitis and may be familial
- **Q** Has anyone in your family had a drinking problem? Alcoholism is a major cause of pancreatitis, and is often familial. A patient may be in denial about his or her drinking but may be able to identify other family members who have had drinking problems

## Examination
Acute pancreatitis:
- **Record temperature** – temperature is often elevated in acute pancreatitis, registering around 101–103°F (38.4–39.5°C)
- **Examine the skin for stigmata of chronic alcohol use** – look for caput medusae, spider angiomas; also look for signs of jaundice, erythematous skin nodules
- **Auscultate lungs** – 10–20% of patients with pancreatitis have pulmonary findings, most commonly left-sided. These findings may include basilar rales, atelectasis, pleural effusion
- **Examine the abdomen for distension** - pancreatitis (as well as other abdominal pathology) often results in abdominal distension
- **Auscultate abdomen** – are the bowel sounds hypoactive? Absent? Is there an abdominal bruit? Ileus is common in pancreatitis, although it is also common in other abdominal pathologies
- **Percuss abdomen** – dullness may suggest ascites; hyper-resonance may suggest pneumoperitoneum. Ascites is suggestive of pancreatitis, whereas pneumoperitoneum may suggest intestinal perforation
- **Palpate abdomen** – Is there hepatomegaly? What is the location of any tenderness? Murphy's sign? Pulsatile abdominal mass? Peritoneal signs? Rigidity? Guarding? Pancreatitis may present with hepatomegaly

Severe pancreatitis:
- **Check vital signs** – including respirations, heart rate, and blood pressure. Pancreatitis often presents with tachypnea, tachycardia, and hypertension (early in the course). Hypotension generally supervenes within short order, due to third-space losses
- **Examine the abdomen** – pancreatitis may result in peritoneal signs. Murphy's sign is common in biliary disease and, therefore, may accompany pancreatitis. Look for Cullen's sign (bluish area around the umbilicus, signifying hemoperitoneum) and Turner's sign (flank discoloration signifying tissue catabolism of hemoglobin)

## Summary of investigative tests

- Complete blood count: it is important to evaluate presence of infection. White blood cell count is also among Ranson's criteria, which are used to assess severity of acute pancreatitis and to predict prognosis
- Serum amylase: damage to pancreatic acinar cells results in leakage of pancreatic enzymes, significantly increasing blood levels
- Urine amylase: may offer improved diagnostic aid in face of normal or equivocal serum amylase elevation; also useful for discriminating elevated serum amylase levels caused by pancreatitis from those caused by macroamylasemia, a benign inherited condition that gives a falsely elevated serum amylase in otherwise healthy people
- Serum lipase: damage to pancreatic acinar cells results in leakage of pancreatic enzymes, significantly increasing blood levels
- Serum calcium: hypocalcemia suggests saponification. Serum calcium also evaluated as part of Ranson's criteria
- Serum glucose: damage to pancreas interferes with insulin production and release, causing hyperglycemia. The degree of hyperglycemia is also evaluated as part of Ranson's criteria
- Liver function tests: can help assess cause of pancreatitis
- Plain abdominal X-rays: evaluate for gallstones, sentinel loop, colon cutoff sign
- Plain chest X-rays: evaluate for atelectasis and pleural effusion
- Abdominal ultrasound: may be used to assess the gallbladder for stones and the biliary tree for dilation
- Abdominal computed tomography (CT) is generally not necessary unless necrosis is suspected; performed with contrast for optimal diagnostic information. Acutely, CT may reveal enlargement of the pancreas. Later in illness, CT may be used to identify necrotizing pancreatitis or fluid collection within the pancreas. CT may be used as guidance for needle aspiration of fluid in the evaluation of infection

## CLINICAL PEARLS

- The combination of serum amylase and lipase determinations is more accurate than either test alone
- Liver function tests may help identify gallstone-induced pancreatitis
- Radiologic studies are of diagnostic, prognostic, and therapeutic value in managing pancreatitis

## THE TESTS
### Body fluids
COMPLETE BLOOD COUNT
*Description*
Venous blood sample.

*Advantages/Disadvantages*
Advantages:
- Simple, widely available, inexpensive test
- Can give results rapidly

Disadvantage: nonspecific; indicates presence of infection/inflammation, but not source.

*Normal*
Hemoglobin:
- Males – 13.6–17.7g/dL
- Females – 12.0–15.0g/dL

White blood cell profile:
- Total – 3200–9800/mm$^3$ (3.2–9.8x10$^9$/L)
- Lymphocytes – 1200–3300/mm$^3$ (1.2–3.3x10$^9$/L)
- Mononuclear cells – 200–700/mm$^3$ (0.2–0.7x10$^9$/L)
- Granulocytes – 1800–6600/mm$^3$ (1.8–6.6x10$^9$/L)

Platelet count:
- 130,000–400,000/mm$^3$ (130–400x10$^9$/L)

*Abnormal*
- Leucocytosis (total white cell count >9800/mm$^3$ (>9.8x10$^9$/L)
- Keep in mind the possibility of a false-positive result

*Cause of abnormal result*
Inflammation/infection of the pancreas.

*Drugs, disorders and other factors that may alter results*
- Other infections or inflammatory disorders may elevate the white cell count
- Steroid medications, lithium, and nonsteroidal anti-inflammatory drugs (NSAIDs) may falsely elevate leukocyte count

### SERUM AMYLASE
*Description*
- Venous blood sample
- Levels begin to rise within about 2–12h of episode onset; 85–90% of patients have increased values within 24h
- Levels peak at about 24h, returning to normal within 48–72h

*Advantages/Disadvantages*
- Advantage: simple, easy to obtain
- Disadvantage: a false low or normal value may occur in the scenario of acute on chronic relapsing pancreatitis

*Normal*
0–130U/dL.

*Abnormal*
In acute pancreatitis, serum amylase levels are increased to more than three times the upper limit of normal.

*Cause of abnormal result*
- Acute pancreatitis
- Chronic relapsing pancreatitis

*Drugs, disorders and other factors that may alter results*
Serum amylase may also be elevated in patients with:
- Biliary tract disease
- Perforated abdominal viscus
- Peritonitis
- Diabetic ketoacidosis
- Chronic renal insufficiency
- Macroamylasemia

## SERUM LIPASE
*Description*
- Venous blood sample
- Levels begin to rise within about 3–6h of episode onset
- Levels peak at about 24h, returning to normal within 7–10 days

*Advantages/Disadvantages*
Advantages:
- Simple, easy to obtain
- More specific for pancreatic damage than serum amylase, although somewhat less sensitive

*Normal*
0–160U/L.

*Abnormal*
- In acute pancreatitis, serum lipase levels are more than three times the upper limit of normal
- Note, however, that a false low or normal value may occur in lipemia

*Cause of abnormal result*
- Acute pancreatitis
- Chronic relapsing pancreatitis

*Drugs, disorders and other factors that may alter results*
Serum lipase may also be elevated in patients with:
- Biliary tract disease
- Perforated abdominal viscus
- Intra-abdominal hemorrhage
- Intestinal obstruction or ischemia
- Renal failure
- Pregnancy
- Mumps
- Peptic ulcer
- Pancreatic carcinoma

## URINE AMYLASE
*Description*
- Urine collection over one hour, 2h, or 24h
- Urinary amylase becomes elevated about 24h after serum amylase
- Urinary amylase stays elevated for about 7–10 days after the serum levels have already returned to normal
- It is crucial that the urinary amylase level is interpreted as units/h rather than units/100mL, to avoid a reading artifact due to urine volume

*Advantages/Disadvantages*
Advantages:
- May offer improved diagnostic aid in face of normal or equivocal serum amylase elevation
- Also useful for discriminating serum amylase elevation caused by pancreatitis from that caused by macroamylasemia, a benign inherited condition that gives a falsely elevated serum amylase in otherwise healthy people

Disadvantages:
- May be difficult to fully collect a 24h urine
- Urinary amylase levels (unlike serum amylase levels) may be artificially reduced in the face of renal failure

*Normal*
2.6–21.2 IU/h.

*Abnormal*
>21.2 IU/h.

*Cause of abnormal result*
May be elevated in pancreatitis, owing to elevated serum levels resulting in increased renal clearance of amylase.

*Drugs, disorders and other factors that may alter results*
Other disorders that may result in elevated urinary amylase levels include:
- Carcinoma of the pancreas, ovary, or lung
- Cholecystitis
- Ectopic pregnancy
- Mumps or other salivary gland infection
- Heavy alcohol ingestion
- Obstruction of intestine or pancreatic duct
- Perforated ulcer
- Urinary amylase levels may be artificially reduced in renal failure

Medications that can artificially elevate urinary amylase levels include:
- Asparaginase
- Aspirin
- Cholinergics
- Corticosteroids
- Indomethacin
- Loop and thiazide diuretics
- Methyldopa
- Codeine
- Morphine
- Oral contraceptives
- Pentazocine

## SERUM CALCIUM
*Description*
- Venous blood sample
- May be used to predict prognosis as part of Ranson's criteria

*Advantages/Disadvantages*
Advantages:
- Simple, widely available, inexpensive test
- Can give results rapidly

Disadvantage: nonspecific; abnormality may indicate a wide range of problems.

*Normal*
8.6–10.0mg/dL (2.1–2.5mmol/L).

*Abnormal*
- <8mg/dL (2mmol/L)
- Be aware of false-positive results

*Cause of abnormal result*
- Hypocalcemia may suggest saponification, precipitation of calcium in areas affected by fat necrosis
- Hypocalcemia may also reflect hypoalbuminemia

*Drugs, disorders and other factors that may alter results*
- Falsely normal results may occur if patient was previously hypercalcemic
- Lowered serum calcium secondary to pancreatitis may drop high calcium level into normal range

## FASTING SERUM GLUCOSE
*Description*
- Venous blood sample, taken while patient is in fasting state
- May be used to predict prognosis as part of Ranson's criteria

*Advantages/Disadvantages*
Advantages:
- Simple, widely available, inexpensive test
- Can give results rapidly

Disadvantage: nonspecific; abnormality may indicate a wide range of problems.

*Normal*
Fasting glucose: 60–100mg/dL (3.5–5.5mmol/L).

*Abnormal*
- Fasting glucose: >100mg/dL (>5.5mmol/L)
- Be aware of false-positive results

*Cause of abnormal result*
Hyperglycemia reflects abnormality of pancreatic function.

*Drugs, disorders and other factors that may alter results*
Other causes of pancreatic dysfunction can cause hyperglycemia (e.g. pre-existing diabetes mellitus, cystic fibrosis).

## LIVER FUNCTION TESTS
*Description*
Venous blood sample.

*Advantages/Disadvantages*
Advantages:
- Simple, widely available, inexpensive test
- Can give results rapidly

Disadvantage: nonspecific; abnormality may indicate a wide range of problems.

*Normal*
- Alkaline phosphatase: 30–300 IU/L
- Alanine aminotransferase (ALT): 5–35 IU/L
- Aspartate aminotransferase (AST): 5–35 IU/L
- Bilirubin: 0–1.0mg/dL (2-18mcmol/L)

*Abnormal*
Values above the normal range.

*Cause of abnormal result*
Elevated liver function tests may be secondary to biliary tract or hepatic disease, which may be causative factors for pancreatitis.

*Drugs, disorders and other factors that may alter results*
- Infectious mononucleosis
- Severe muscle trauma and inflammation
- Pregnancy

## Imaging
PLAIN ABDOMINAL AND CHEST X-RAYS
*Advantages/Disadvantages*
Advantages:
- Fast, noninvasive, routine tests
- Require no preparation or use of contrast media
- Inexpensive

Disadvantage: radiation exposure.

*Abnormal*
Findings in pancreatitis may include:
- Sentinel loop of bowel
- Calcifications
- Gallstones
- Atelectasis in lower lobes of the lungs
- Pleural effusion

Findings in differential diagnoses of pancreatitis include:
- Air-fluid level seen in bowel obstruction
- Free air under the diaphragm due to bowel perforation

*Cause of abnormal result*
- Sentinel loop: denotes localized ileus of jejunal loop
- Calcifications: suggests chronic pancreatitis
- Visualized gallstones: may prompt further diagnostic efforts to demonstrate biliary obstruction
- Atelectasis, pleural effusion: may denote diaphragmatic involvement secondary to acute pancreatitis

ABDOMINAL ULTRASOUND
*Description*
Used to assess the gallbladder for stones and the biliary tree for dilation suggesting recent stone passage.

*Advantages/Disadvantages*
Advantages:
- Images the gallbladder for stones and the biliary tree for dilation, which would suggest recent stone passage; it is more sensitive than computed tomography (CT) scanning for this purpose
- No radiation exposure
- Generally easy to assess and may be more readily available than CT scanning
- Less expensive than CT scanning

Disadvantages:
- Does not visualize the pancreas well, although this is not required unless there is suspicion of necrosis
- Requires an experienced radiographer and specialized equipment

*Normal*
Normal images of the gallbladder and the biliary tree.

*Abnormal*
- Gallstones in the gallbladder
- Dilation of the biliary tree, suggesting recent gallstone passage

## ABDOMINAL COMPUTED TOMOGRAPHY (CT)
*Description*
- Provides images of liver, biliary tree, and pancreas
- Unnecessary in uncomplicated pancreatitis; generally not necessary unless necrosis suspected
- Optimal information obtained by giving a rapid bolus dose of contrast, with immediate imaging providing dynamic information

*Advantages/Disadvantages*
Advantages:
- CT images of pancreas and liver are optimal
- Noninvasive
- Can be used for CT-guided fine-needle aspiration of a pancreatic inflammatory mass

Disadvantages:
- Requires CT scanner and experienced operator
- Expensive and not always readily available
- Involves radiation exposure
- Allergic reaction to contrast material can occur

*Normal*
Normal images of liver, biliary tree, and pancreas.

*Abnormal*
The following may be present:
- Pancreatic and/or peripancreatic inflammation
- Involvement of neighboring organs
- Fluid collections
- Venous thrombosis
- Intrapancreatic or peripancreatic gas

*Cause of abnormal result*
CT scan can reveal pancreatic pathology, as well as many other forms of intra-abdominal pathology.

# TREATMENT

## CONSIDER CONSULT
Refer patients who have:
- Signs of shock or impending acute respiratory distress syndrome, with or without cardiac dysfunction
- Necrotizing pancreatitis (fever, leukocytosis, organ failure, including gastrointestinal bleeding or impending acute respiratory distress syndrome)
- Pancreatic abscess (6 weeks or so into the course of acute pancreatitis, patient presents with rising fever, leukocytosis, localized tenderness, and an epigastric mass)

## IMMEDIATE ACTION
Patients who present with more than three Ranson's criteria should be considered to have severe acute pancreatitis, and should be referred to a surgeon and monitored in an intensive care unit.

## PATIENT AND CAREGIVER ISSUES
### Forensic and legal issues
Care may be complicated legally if patient presents with acute pancreatitis while still intoxicated from a recent drinking binge.

### Impact on career, dependants, family, friends
- Pancreatitis secondary to general medical problems will have the same impact as many other acute medical conditions
- Pancreatitis secondary to alcohol use may present extra complexities, necessitating the help of specialists in addiction medicine (including psychiatrists, psychologists, and social workers)
- Chronic or recurrent pancreatitis may result in disruption to relationships and to job performance

### Patient or caregiver request
- Patients who have pancreatitis secondary to medical problems other than alcohol use may know that alcohol use is a common cause of pancreatitis, and may feel concerned that healthcare personnel are 'suspicious' of the etiology of their illness
- Patients who have pancreatitis secondary to alcohol use may be in denial about their drinking and its relationship to their medical illness

## MANAGEMENT ISSUES
### Goals
- To provide a multidisciplinary approach to the management of acute pancreatitis
- To provide supportive management, including parenterally administered analgesia, intravenous fluids, nutritional support, and prevention and treatment of complications
- To avoid the onset of infection and organ failure, and delaying surgery
- To diagnose and treat any treatable underlying etiologies of pancreatitis to reduce recurrent bouts of pancreatitis and long-term sequelae secondary to pancreatic failure

### Management in special circumstances
COEXISTING DISEASE
Be sure to ask patients whether they have HIV infection/AIDS. If so, ascertain their drug regimen. Patients being treated with antiretroviral therapy (various cocktails using the nucleoside reverse transcriptase inhibitor drugs such as stavudine, didanosine, hydroxyurea) have a high risk of very severe pancreatitis.

PATIENT SATISFACTION/LIFESTYLE PRIORITIES
Patients who have pancreatitis secondary to heavy alcohol use may need intervention to help

them understand the necessity of abstinence from alcohol use. Consider involving specialists in alcohol rehabilitation.

## SUMMARY OF THERAPEUTIC OPTIONS
### Choices
- Intravenous fluids and electrolytes: maintaining hemodynamic stability is paramount in the management of pancreatitis and may require placement of a central line, as well as accurate assessment of intake and output (including a urinary catheter)
- Nil by mouth until nausea and vomiting cease and bowel sounds return, usually within 48h
- Consider nasogastric suction to decrease gastric gastrin secretion, and to prevent gastric contents from entering the duodenum; while nasogastric suctioning was once standard treatment, it is now reserved for patients with intractable nausea and vomiting
- Analgesic treatment to control pain: generally requires parenteral narcotic analgesia for sufficient pain relief. Meperidine is the drug of choice over morphine because of the tendency for morphine to increase spasm of sphincter of Oddi
- Enteral or parenteral nutrition may be required for those patients who cannot tolerate oral feeding for a prolonged period of time (over 4 days). Although parenteral nutrition was once thought to be best, recent studies suggest that enteral nutrition (administered beyond the ligament of Treitz) may be equally efficacious. When begun within 48h of admission, enteral feedings have proven to decrease infectious and necrotic complications in severe acute pancreatitis. This is a specialist treatment
- Infection is common, and the use of antibiotic treatment should be considered in patients with pancreatic necrosis, biliary pancreatitis with cholangitis. Prophylactic intravenous broad-spectrum antibiotics should also be considered in patients whose Ranson's score predicts severe pancreatitis. Prophylactic antibiotics are not recommended in mild pancreatitis because of the risk of multiresistant bacteria and fungal infections
- Surgical therapy has a limited role in the following scenarios: gallstone-induced pancreatitis (endoscopic retrograde cholangiopancreatography or a cholecystectomy when acute pancreatitis subsides); perforate peptic ulcer; and excision or drainage of necrotic tissue or infected foci. These are specialist treatments
- Certain lifestyle changes, notably reduction in alcohol intake (if relevant), may be needed

### Never
- Never undervalue conservative management in the majority of cases of acute pancreatitis
- Never rush in to surgery: surgery should be delayed for as long as possible, owing to its high morbidity and mortality. The main absolute indication for surgery is infected pancreatic necrosis

## FOLLOW UP
### Plan for review
- The patient should be observed closely for signs of clinical improvement or deterioration
- Ranson's criteria should be rechecked at 48h after admission and throughout hospitalization, to ensure that the patient is improving and to identify complications early
- In particular, careful surveillance for the development of infection should be maintained
- Continuous pulse oximetry is necessary to identify and correct ensuing acute respiratory distress syndrome quickly
- Serial amylase or lipase measurements are not useful for tracking improvement
- Restarting feeds does not require normalization of pancreatic enzymes and normally occurs after 48h in uncomplicated pancreatitis
- Computed tomography scanning is required if the patient's clinical status does not improve or if it deteriorates, to identify a pancreatic abscess or necrosis
- Surgical consult should be obtained if necrosis or abscess is identified, in biliary pancreatitis, in hemorrhagic pancreatitis, or if Ranson's score continues to worsen despite careful medical management

- The presence of gallstones must be investigated to exclude them as a cause of pancreatitis
- If a biliary source is suspected, a surgeon should be consulted for assessment of cholecystectomy and/or endoscopic retrograde cholangiopancreatography

### Information for patient or caregiver
- The patient should be made aware of the chances of complications occurring relatively late in the course of pancreatitis
- The patient should be aware that underlying conditions as well as the acute condition will require treatment

## DRUGS AND OTHER THERAPIES: DETAILS
### Drugs
MEPERIDINE
Analgesic agent.

*Dose*
- Adult: 50–100mg intravenously or intramuscularly every 3–4h as required
- Child: 0.5–0.8mg/lb intramuscularly, subcutaneously, or orally up to the adult dose, every 3 or 4h as necessary. Each dose of the syrup should be taken in half a glass of water

*Efficacy*
Similar analgesic effect to that of morphine, but with less chance of spasm of sphincter of Oddi.

*Risks/benefits*
Risks:
- Use caution in respiratory conditions including asthma, renal or hepatic impairment, hypothyroidism, and Addison's disease
- Use caution in the elderly
- Use caution in patients with supraventricular tachycardias

Benefits:
- Decreased pain
- Sedation

*Side effects and adverse reactions*
- Cardiovascular system: tachycardia, bradycardia, palpitations, postural hypotension
- Central nervous system: drowsiness, sedation, seizures, dizziness, tremors
- Gastrointestinal: nausea, vomiting, constipation, anorexia
- Respiratory: respiratory depression
- Skin: rash

*Interactions (other drugs)*
- Antihistamines ▪ Anxiolytics/hypnotics (chloral hydrate, glutethimide) ▪ Barbiturates
- Cimetidine ▪ Ciprofloxacin ▪ Ethanol ▪ Monoamine oxidase inhibitors ▪ Methocarbamol
- Metoclopramide ▪ Mexiletine ▪ Neuroleptics ▪ Phenytoin ▪ Ritonavir ▪ Selegine
- Tricyclic antidepressants

*Contraindications*
▪ Existing central nervous system depression ▪ Alcohol abuse ▪ Monoamine oxidase inhibitor therapy (within 14 days) ▪ Severe renal impairment ▪ Severe or acute bronchial asthma ▪ Respiratory depression ▪ Pregnancy category B

*Acceptability to patient*
Generally acceptable to patient, because degree of pain is great enough to require analgesia.

*Follow up plan*
Monitor for respiratory depression, and adjust dosage/frequency of administration accordingly.

*Patient and caregiver information*
This medication is not addictive when used for analgesia.

## Other therapies
FLUID REPLACEMENT
Fluid replacement with normal saline and/or a colloid solution, and maintenance of hemodynamic stability is a crucial aspect of the management of pancreatitis.

*Risks/benefits*
Risk: careful monitoring is mandatory to prevent fluid overload, particularly in elderly, debilitated, and pediatric patients.

*Follow up plan*
- Careful monitoring of fluid input and output is required
- Patients can sequester >6L fluid in severe acute pancreatitis, and fluid balance may need to be monitored through central venous pressure monitoring

## LIFESTYLE
Recommend:
- Discontinuation of alcohol use, with rehabilitation, if necessary
- Institution of healthy, low-fat diet, if indicated

RISKS/BENEFITS
Risk: truly alcoholic patients will require detoxification, which may complicate management of acute illness.

ACCEPTABILITY TO PATIENT
- Alcoholism is difficult to conquer and may require the intervention of other professionals, such as psychiatrists, psychologists, social workers, support and/or 12-step groups
- Patients may find a change of diet difficult

FOLLOW UP PLAN
Alcoholic patients need close follow up and monitoring to prevent/identify relapse.

## OUTCOMES

### EFFICACY OF THERAPIES
#### Review period
Patients should be reviewed for at least 6 months after an acute episode of acute pancreatitis.

### PROGNOSIS
Prognosis can be predicted from Ranson's scores as follows:
- Score of 0–2 represents an extremely low mortality rate
- Score of 3–5 represents a mortality rate ranging from 10–20%
- Score >5 represents a mortality rate above 50%, as well as a high rate of complications; up to 20% of patients have severe disease with significant morbidity and mortality

Ranson's criteria of severity of acute pancreatitis:
- Used to assess the prognosis of the patient
- Patients with three or four Ranson's criteria have a 15% mortality; those with seven or eight criteria have a reported 100% mortality
- Patients who present with more than three Ranson's criteria should be considered to have severe acute pancreatitis, and should be referred to a surgeon and monitored in an intensive care unit

Ranson's criteria are as follows.
Ranson's criteria on admission:
- Age >55 years
- White blood cell count >16,000x10$^9$
- Serum glucose >200mg/dL (>11mmol/L)
- Serum lactate dehydrogenase >350 IU/L
- Aspartate aminotransferase >60 IU/L

Ranson's criteria within first 48h:
- Hematocrit drop >10%
- Blood urea nitrogen rise >2mg/dL
- $p_aO_2$ <60mmHg (<8kPa)
- Serum calcium <8mg/dL (<2mmol/L)
- Base deficit >-4
- Fluid sequestration estimated to be >6L

#### Clinical pearls
- Prognostic indicators are useful but must be individualized to each patient
- 80% of patients with an acute attack of pancreatitis will have a mild episode that subsides within 7 days, and only 1–3% will progress to more severe involvement or develop complications
- 20% of patients with an acute attack will have an attack that may be categorized as severe by one of the criteria for grading of severity (e.g. Ranson's criteria). Of these patients, 2–3% will die within 72h of multiple organ failure
- Hemoconcentration at admission and at 24h have been found to be strong risk factors for the development of pancreatic necrosis
- Approx. 30–50% of patients with pancreatic necrosis develop secondary infection

#### Therapeutic failure
In the case of failure of medical management:
- Look for complications including necrosis, abscess, pseudocyst, or stone impaction
- Consider adding antibiotics if signs of infection supervene

Surgical referral for:
- Possible surgical debridement of pancreas
- Drainage of abscesses, phlegmon
- Postoperative lavage of pancreatic bed
- Surgery to repair eroded major vessels in hemorrhagic pancreatitis
- Sphincterotomy or cholecystectomy may be necessary if biliary stones are obstructing
- Endoscopic retrograde cholangiopancreatography to remove gallstone from the common duct

## Recurrence

Recurrence of nonalcoholic pancreatitis necessitates a search for predispositions to acute pancreatitis, including common bile duct stones, covert alcohol use, drugs, HIV infection, congenital ductal abnormalities, or an obstructing ampullary or ductal cancer.

Surgical consultation may be required for:
- Pseudocyst decompression
- Excision of infected necrotic pancreatic tissue
- Ductal decompression
- Pancreatic resection (distal pancreatectomy or Whipple procedure)
- Endoscopic sphincterotomy
- Stent placement in major pancreatic duct or pancreatic pseudocyst
- Extracorporeal shock wave lithotripsy for biliary stones

## Deterioration

Failure of medical management points to necessity for surgical consult.

## Terminal illness
- The patient's clinical condition can continue to deteriorate, indicating terminal disease
- Palliation of pain is paramount in these circumstances
- A minimum of invasive procedures are used in these circumstances

## COMPLICATIONS
- Infected pancreatic necrosis
- Pancreatic abscess, pseudocyst, phlegmon
- Pseudoaneurysm formation may lead to bleeding into a pseudocyst cavity or ductal system
- Intestinal obstruction
- Common bile duct obstruction
- Internal pancreatic fistula
- Continued pancreatic dysfunction, resulting in diabetes, steatorrhea
- Shock
- Renal failure
- Adult respiratory distress syndrome

## CONSIDER CONSULT

Always refer to a surgeon when:
- Infections or surgical complications (pancreatic pseudocyst, abscess, phlegmon) supervene
- Medical management does not result in improvement in the patient's condition

# PREVENTION

## RISK FACTORS
- **Heavy drinking:** binge drinking in particular puts a person at high risk of developing pancreatitis
- **Abdominal trauma:** injuries due to athletic or recreational activities, or to being unrestrained during a motor vehicle accident, can cause pancreatic injury that leads to pancreatitis

## MODIFY RISK FACTORS
- Avoid heavy drinking, particularly binge drinking
- Protect against abdominal trauma (during athletic and recreational activities, as well as by always using a seatbelt in a motor vehicle)

### Lifestyle and wellness
ALCOHOL AND DRUGS
Binge drinking and heavy alcohol use can be a risk factor for pancreatitis.

DIET
Large fatty meals can exacerbate biliary disease, resulting in pancreatitis.

PHYSICAL ACTIVITY
Athletic and recreational activities that may result in abdominal trauma can increase risk for pancreatitis.

ENVIRONMENT
Chemical exposures that can prompt pancreatitis include:
- Methanol
- Cobalt
- Zinc
- Mercuric chloride
- Creosol
- Lead
- Organophosphates
- Chlorinated naphthalenes

FAMILY HISTORY
Increased risk of pancreatitis with family history of:
- Biliary disease
- Defect in trypsinogen gene
- Variant mutation of cystic fibrosis transmembrane conductance regulator gene
- Hyperlipidemia
- Alcoholism

DRUG HISTORY
Causative medications may include:
- Thiazide diuretics
- Furosemide
- Corticosteroids
- Tetracycline
- Estrogen
- Valproic acid
- Metronidazole
- Azathioprine

- Methyldopa
- Pentamidine
- Ethacryinic acid
- Procainamide
- Sulindac
- Nitrofurantoin
- Angiotensin-converting enzyme inhibitors
- Danazol
- Cimetidine
- Piroxicam
- Gold
- Ranitidine
- Sulfasalazine
- Isoniazid
- Acetaminophen
- Cisplatin
- Opiates
- Erythromycin

## PREVENT RECURRENCE
Underlying conditions should be treated, including:
- Biliary disease
- Alcoholism

### Reassess coexisting disease
INTERACTION ALERT
Patients who are HIV-positive or are being treated for AIDS with antiretroviral therapy (various cocktails using the nucleoside reverse transcriptase inhibitor drugs such as stavudine, didanosine, hydroxyurea) have a high risk of very severe pancreatitis.

PATIENT SATISFACTION/LIFESTYLE PRIORITIES
Patients who must give up alcohol use may find the lifestyle change very difficult and may benefit from supportive therapy.

# RESOURCES

## ASSOCIATIONS
American Society for Gastrointestinal Endoscopy
13 Elm Street
Manchester, MA 01944-1314
Tel: (978) 526-8330
Fax: (978) 526-4018
E-mail: asge@shore.net
http://www.asge.org

## KEY REFERENCES
- Delcenserie R, Yzet T, Ducroix JP. Prophylactic antibiotics in treatment of severe acute alcoholic pancreatitis. Pancreas 1996;13:198–201
- Kalfarentzos F, Kehagias J, Mead N, et al. Enteral nutrition is superior to parenteral nutrition in severe acute pancreatitis: results of a randomized prospective trial. Br J Surg 1997;84:1665–9
- Munoz A, Katerndahl DA. Diagnosis and management of acute pancreatitis. Am Fam Physician 2000;62:164–74
- Sainio V, Kemppainen E, Puolakkainen P, et al. Early antibiotic treatment in acute necrotising pancreatitis. Lancet 1995;346:663–7
- American Gastroenterological Association Medical Position Statement: treatment of pain in chronic pancreatitis. Gastroenterology 1998;115:763–4

## FAQS
### Question 1
When should an abdominal computed tomography scan be performed?

### ANSWER 1
In patients with suspected severe disease and clinical deterioration. Patients with over 50% necrosis have a poor prognosis.

### Question 2
When should I refer for endoscopic retrograde cholangiogram?

### ANSWER 2
In patients who are considered to have severe pancreatitis as assessed by grading criteria within 72h of onset in the setting of abnormal liver function tests.

### Question 3
What can be expected after successful treatment?

### ANSWER 3
Patients usually recover fully from acute pancreatitis and do not experience recurrence if the cause is removed. Alcohol consumption should be eliminated even if it is not the determined cause of the disease. Smoking, which stresses the body's defenses against inflammation, should be stopped. A trial and error approach to specific foods is usually indicated. Patients often find high-fat foods difficult to digest.

### Question 4
What is the treatment for acute pancreatitis?

### ANSWER 4
Treatment for acute pancreatitis depends on the severity of the condition. Sometimes the patient needs hospitalization with administration of intravenous fluids to help restore blood volume.

Antibiotics are often prescribed if infection occurs, and pain medications are often used to provide relief. Surgery is sometimes needed when complications such as infection, cysts, or bleeding occur.

## CONTRIBUTORS
Gordon H Baustian, MD
Rudolph A Bedford, MD
Laura Targownik, MD, FRCP(C)
Brennan Spiegal, MD

# PEPTIC ULCER

| | | |
|---|---|---|
| ■ | Summary Information | 434 |
| ■ | Background | 435 |
| ■ | Diagnosis | 438 |
| ■ | Treatment | 447 |
| ■ | Outcomes | 458 |
| ■ | Prevention | 460 |
| ■ | Resources | 462 |

## SUMMARY INFORMATION

### DESCRIPTION

- Chronic ulceration in the gastrointestinal tract lining of the duodenum and stomach
- Gnawing, burning, epigastric pain typically 2–4h after meals, relieved by food, antacids, or antisecretory agents
- Duodenal ulcers: classically nocturnal pain, causing early morning awakening. Symptomatic periods appearing in clusters followed by symptom-free periods
- Nonsteroidal anti-inflammatory drug-induced ulcers are often silent; initial presentation may be gastrointestinal perforation or bleeding

### URGENT ACTION

- If the physician finds evidence of acute gastrointestinal bleeding, emergency endoscopy and hospitalization are indicated. If patient is experiencing severe hemorrhage, refer immediately to hospital for emergency care. However, even bleeding that starts slowly can accelerate rapidly, thereby requiring all patients with acute bleeding to be evaluated as rapidly as possible
- Perforation usually presents with sudden abdominal pain and signs of an acute abdomen
- Obstruction presents with protracted nausea and vomiting

## BACKGROUND

### ICD9 CODE
- 538.6 Peptic ulcer disease
- 531.3 Peptic ulcer, stomach, acute
- 531.7 Peptic ulcer, stomach, chronic
- 532.3 Peptic ulcer, duodenum, acute
- 532.7 Peptic ulcer, duodenum, chronic
- 532.9 Duodenal ulcer
- 531.9 Peptic ulcer

### SYNONYMS
- PUD
- Duodenal ulcer
- Gastric ulcer

### CARDINAL FEATURES
Duodenal ulcers:
- Gnawing, burning, epigastric pain typically 2–3h after meals, relieved by food, antacids, or antisecretory agents
- Nocturnal pain, causing early morning awakening
- Symptomatic periods appearing in clusters followed by symptom-free periods

Gastric ulcers:
- Symptoms similar to those seen with duodenal ulcers, although gastric ulcer symptoms have been said to get worse with eating. However, there is no precision to the clinical discrimination between gastric and duodenal ulcers

Although the above symptoms are classic for peptic ulcer, they are nonspecific; the large majority of patients with these classic symptoms do not have peptic ulcers. Furthermore, many peptic ulcers are silent:
- Nonsteroidal anti-inflammatory drug (NSAID)-induced ulcers are even more likely to be clinically silent; initial presentation may be gastrointestinal perforation or bleeding

### CAUSES
#### Common causes
There are two common specific causes of peptic ulcers:
- Infection with *Helicobacter pylori*, which was initially found in more than 90% of duodenal ulcers, and more than 80% of gastric ulcer cases (*H. pylori* is found much less commonly in peptic ulcer in the US)
- Use of nonsteroidal anti-inflammatory medications

There are several less common forms of peptic ulcer:
- Zollinger–Ellison syndrome, and other hypersecretory syndromes such as mastocytosis and possibly antral G cell hyperplasia
- Stress ulcer: occurring in physiologically stressed patients, usually in an intensive care unit, and usually with prolonged, multisystem failure including respiratory compromise, sepsis, and/or coagulopathy. Although superficial damage, usually in the gastric mucosa, is common in patients after major surgery or with stress, complications can result from gastric or duodenal ulcers
- 'Idiopathic' duodenal ulcer (often occurring in younger males and associated with robust acid hypersecretion)

Several cofactors that hasten the development of peptic ulcer disease have been identified:
- Regional impairment of healing: the gastroduodenal mucosa frequently breaks down in response to trauma or exposure to endogenous and exogenous noxious agents such as gastric acid, pepsin, bile salts, or NSAIDs. Endogenous defenses such as prostaglandins and growth factors regulate mucus and bicarbonate secretion, gastric tight junctions, and blood flow to minimize damage; however, rapid repair prevents ulcer formation. Even in ulcer patients mucosal biopsies rapidly heal, but ulcers persist and recur, often in the same region. The local factors that prevent ulcer healing and cause persistence have not been defined; candidate mechanisms include increased fibrosis and scarring, and decreased regional blood flow
- Cigarette smoking is a risk factor for *H. pylori* ulcer before, but not after, cure of the infection
- Use of corticosteroids, when added to NSAIDs

In the case of gastric ulceration, other etiologies should be considered:
- Gastric neoplasms, most commonly gastric adenocarcinoma
- Crohn's disease, which may present with aphthous ulcerations anywhere along the gastrointestinal tract, including the stomach

### Serious causes
All gastric ulcerations must be biopsied at the time of endoscopy to rule out a gastric malignancy masquerading as a benign peptic ulcer. Adequate biopsies (usually a minimum of four biopsies of the margin and one of the base, each with good tissue and not blood or mucus) appropriately interpreted by an expert pathologist are essential.

### Contributory or predisposing factors
- NSAID use and infection with *H. pylori*
- Cigarette smoking (greater than half a pack/day)
- Probable association with corticosteroid use, primarily in a setting of NSAID use
- No association with consumption of dietary spices, alcohol, caffeine, or acetaminophen has been established
- Family elements have not been defined in common forms of peptic ulcer. The obvious familiar association that had been recognized was a correct observation; however, the primary cause was not genetic elements, but clustering of *H. pylori* infection. It is likely there are other familiar elements, but these remain to be defined
- Even with the defined factors, such as *H. pylori* and NSAIDs, there is only a 1% yearly incidence (new cases) of clinical peptic ulcer; it is unknown why only a small subset of subjects at risk develop ulcers

## EPIDEMIOLOGY
### Incidence and prevalence
Duodenal ulcer to gastric ulcer ratio is 2:1, although this is changing.

INCIDENCE
- Duodenal ulcer: 200,000–400,000 new cases annually
- Gastric ulcer: 50,000–100,000 new cases annually, incidence in adults is 50/100,000
- These numbers are likely to fall dramatically with the decreased incidence of *H. pylori*, and decreased use of gastrointestinal toxic NSAIDs

PREVALENCE
Duodenal ulcer lifetime prevalence: 10% for men, 5% for women, though rates are highly dependent upon local prevalence of *H. pylori*; the prevalence of both *H. pylori* and peptic ulcer are rapidly decreasing in the US.

## Demographics

### AGE
- Duodenal ulcer: 25–75 years of age, uncommon before age 15
- Gastric ulcer: 55–65 years of age, rare before age 40
- Peptic ulcer disease is uncommon before puberty, although hemorrhage and perforation are important complications for pediatric patients

### GENDER
- Duodenal ulcer seen slightly more frequently in men than in women
- Gastric ulcer seen equally between the sexes, but female predominance among NSAID users

### GENETICS
Higher incidence with HLA-B12, B5, Bw35 phenotypes, and with identical twins. There is some association between these markers and *H. pylori* infection.

### SOCIOECONOMIC STATUS
- Possible association with lower socioeconomic status and manual labor
- More common among individuals living in close quarters
- These factors are probably due to more prevalent *H. pylori* infection

## DIAGNOSIS

### DIFFERENTIAL DIAGNOSIS
#### Nonulcer dyspepsia
Nonulcer dyspepsia is a generalized stomach upset (a sensitive or irritable stomach) in the absence of mucosal breaks seen on endoscopy. Unknown cause, though may be associated with stress or diet. The relationship to *Helicobacter pylori* infection is highly controversial. Available data indicate that benefit from cure of *H. pylori* is marginal in most subjects; however, many specialists will still treat *H. pylori*-positive dyspeptic patients with antibiotics because there are few other satisfying options and some patients do 'seem' to benefit.

FEATURES
- Diffuse abdominal pain or discomfort
- Pain not usually relieved by antacids

#### Carcinoma
Including gastric carcinoma, pancreatic carcinoma, lymphoma.

FEATURES
- Epigastric or abdominal mass
- Supraclavicular lymphadenopathy ('Virchow's node')
- Periumbilical mass ('Sister Mary Joseph node')
- Ridge along rectal cul-de-sac ('Blummer's shelf')
- Skin pallor secondary to anemia
- Hemoccult-positive stools
- Identified by endoscopy
- Definitive identification by evaluation of biopsy specimens (pinch biopsies of ulcer margin are greatly superior to cytology)

#### Helicobacter pylori-associated gastritis
Specifically identified as stomach inflammation without accompanying ulceration.

FEATURES
- Erythema and nodularity
- No reliable association with symptoms or epigastric tenderness

#### Superficial gastropathy due to nonsteroidal anti-inflammatory drugs (NSAIDs) or alcohol
Associated with use of NSAIDs, and with excessive alcohol ingestion.

FEATURES
- Erosions
- Subepithelial hemorrhages
- Gastritis (inflammation of the gastric lining) is not seen with NSAIDs or alcohol per se
- There is no reliable association with symptoms

#### Gastroesophageal reflux
Gastroesophageal reflux (GERD) is a disorder characterized by heartburn caused by gastric content reflux into the esophagus.

FEATURES
- Physical examination generally unremarkable
- Three patterns of heartburn are noted: 'supine' reflux that occurs lying down, 'stress' reflux

occurring with increased abdominal pressure (e.g. bending over, gardening), and 'upright' reflux that occurs postprandially
- Dysphagia occurs with esophageal spasm, irritation, or stricture due to fibrosis
- Regurgitation of stomach contents into mouth
- Respiratory complications can be seen: chronic cough, bronchospasm, laryngitis
- Noncardiac chest pain
- Abdominal fullness, bloating with belching

### Crohn's disease

Crohn's disease is a chronic inflammatory bowel disease, affecting any part of the gastrointestinal tract, but usually the terminal ileum and/or colon. May also present with aphthous ulcerations in the stomach, thereby mimicking classic peptic ulcer disease on endoscopic evaluation.

FEATURES
- Fever
- Abdominal pain
- Diarrhea
- Fatigue, weight loss, growth retardation (in children)
- Acute ileitis
- Anorectal fissures, abscesses

### Pancreatitis

Pancreatitis is an inflammatory process (acute or chronic) of the pancreas.

FEATURES
Acute:
- Epigastric tenderness and guarding
- Fever
- Tachycardia, decreased breath sounds
- Jaundice
- Hypoactive bowel sounds
- Ascites
- Abdominal mass
- Evidence of intra-abdominal bleeding

Chronic:
- Epigastric and left upper quadrant pain in some cases
- Significant weight loss
- Bulky, foul-smelling stools with pancreatic insufficiency
- Epigastric mass
- Jaundice

### Cardiac-associated conditions

Including variant angina, myocardial infarction, pericarditis.

### Dissecting aneurysm

Aortic dissection occurring when an internal tear occurs, allowing blood to infiltrate between medial layers of the aorta.

FEATURES
- Hypertension or hypotension
- Unequal or absent peripheral pulses
- Murmur of aortic insufficiency

- Hemiplegia or paraplegia
- Hoarseness, dysphagia, airway compromise (due to mass effect)
- Cardiac tamponade (due to dissection into pericardial sac)

### Biliary colic
Caused by gallstones obstructing the cystic duct or common bile duct.

FEATURES
- Severe, cramping pain usually in the right upper quadrant or epigastrium, may radiate to back or right shoulder
- Pain typically occurs at night, usually lasting for several hours
- Called 'colic,' but usually undulates rather than occurring in sharp waves like intestinal colic

### Acute cholecystitis
Acute cholecystitis is a right upper quadrant pain, usually associated with fever and leukocytosis that develops in association with inflammation of the gallbladder, gallstones, and often with obstruction of the cystic duct by stones or edema.

FEATURES
- Pain in the right upper quadrant, which may radiate to back or right shoulder
- Pain usually occurs at night, lasting from a few minutes to several hours

### Other upper and lower gastrointestinal conditions
Including pneumonia, high small bowel obstruction, subphrenic abscess, early appendicitis, hepatitis.

## SIGNS & SYMPTOMS
### Signs
Duodenal and gastric ulcer:
- Epigastric tenderness (not a specific or sensitive sign)
- Stool guaiac-positive, gross gastrointestinal bleeding, or anemia (presenting signs in a very small percentage of cases with complicated ulcer)

### Symptoms
- Symptomatic periods occur in clusters lasting a few weeks, followed by symptom-free periods
- Nocturnal pain can cause early morning awakening
- Nonspecific dyspeptic complaints (belching, bloating, abdominal distension)
- NSAID-induced ulcers are often silent
- Weight loss can occur with benign or malignant gastric ulcers, and sometimes with duodenal ulcers
- Epigastric pain, classically occurring 2–4h after a meal (when food buffer has emptied, but acid secretion remains high), relieved by food, antacids, or antisecretory agents
- Symptoms of gastrointestinal bleeding including melena, bright-red blood per rectum, or hematemesis

## ASSOCIATED DISORDERS
- Zollinger–Ellison syndrome
- Systemic mastocytosis
- Chronic obstructive pulmonary disease
- Chronic renal failure
- Cirrhosis
- Hyperparathyroidism
- Carcinoid syndrome
- Polycythemia rubra vera

- Basophilic leukemia
- Porphyria cutanea tarda

## CONSIDER CONSULT
- Epigastric pain in the presence of sinister symptoms, including progressive nausea and vomiting, anorexia, hematemesis, bright-red blood per rectum, melena, or weight loss should prompt referral to a gastroenterologist for upper endoscopy
- Prolonged nausea, especially with vomiting, requires endoscopic evaluation before a firm diagnosis is made

## INVESTIGATION OF THE PATIENT
### Direct questions to patient
**Q** Have you developed any alarm symptoms in association with dyspepsia? Determine whether the patient has experienced progressive nausea or vomiting, anorexia, hematemesis, bright-red blood per rectum, melena, or weight loss. These may be signs of a more sinister underlying diagnosis, including gastric cancer, and should always prompt referral to a gastroenterologist for possible endoscopy

**Q** Have you been experiencing epigastric pain shortly after meal consumption? Determine whether there are specific foods or food groups that are triggering this pain, as patient may have food allergies or lactose intolerance

**Q** Have you found relief for abdominal pain by taking over-the-counter medications? Determine which medications have been effective; patient may be treated with these rather than prescribing expensive and stronger medications

**Q** Have you experienced epigastric pain during stressful periods without a correlation to food intake? Patient may need a work-up for stress-related emotional disorders rather than (or in addition to) an evaluation for a possible ulcer

**Q** Have you noticed that the painful periods cycle with pain-free periods? This is typical for peptic ulcer disease, but may also be correlated with stressful periods in the patient's life. Get further clarification on what else may be happening in patient's life during these cycles

### Contributory or predisposing factors
**Q** Are you taking NSAIDs or corticosteroids in high doses over long periods of time? Chronic use of these drugs is associated with ulcer occurrence (but the incidence of clinically relevant ulcers in NSAID users is low – 0.5–4%/year of NSAID use). Furthermore, some patients get complicated ulcers after only a few days of NSAID use

**Q** Are you a cigarette smoker? Cigarette smoking (more than half a pack/day) is a risk factor for peptic ulcer disease, its recurrence, and complications

### Family history
**Q** Is there a family history of ulcers or other stomach problems? A family history of duodenal ulcer has been reported, but most cases are due to familial clustering of *Helicobacter pylori* infection

**Q** Is there a family history of polyendocrine adenomatosis? Zollinger–Ellison syndrome is a noted cause of peptic ulceration. Rare, but interesting, and important in these patients

### Examination
There are no reliable signs of peptic ulcer.

### Summary of investigative tests
- Urea breath test to verify presence of *Helicobacter pylori*
- Blood antibody test to verify presence of *H. pylori* infection
- Serum amylase level to rule out suspected pancreatitis
- Fasting serum gastrin level to rule out suspected Zollinger–Ellison syndrome

- Endoscopy to confirm or rule out presence of ulcers (normally performed by a specialist)
- Upper gastrointestinal barium series to confirm or rule out presence of ulcers, although this is considerably less sensitive and specific than endoscopy
- Fecal occult blood to rule out intraluminal source of bleeding, including underlying peptic ulcer disease
- Mucosal biopsy and cytology to confirm or rule out *H. pylori* infection (normally performed by a specialist)
- *H. pylori* stool antigen test to confirm or rule out *H. pylori* infection

## DIAGNOSTIC DECISION

Classic peptic ulcer disease is suspected through evaluation of location of the pain, relationship of the pain to eating, and relation to *H. pylori* infection or NSAID use. Confirmation of an ulcer diagnosis requires endoscopy or occasionally upper gastrointestinal tract radiography.

## CLINICAL PEARL(S)

- Alarm symptoms (e.g. gastrointestinal bleeding, weight loss) must be looked for, since these can provide early evidence of serious underlying disease
- The symptoms of peptic ulcer are nonspecific, and most patients with classic ulcer symptoms do not have ulcer disease
- The symptoms of peptic ulcer are insensitive; many patients have silent peptic ulcers, some of which may complicate without ever producing heralding symptoms
- Persistent, refractory, or recurrent dyspepsia always warrants at least one endoscopy
- Even though the rate of *H. pylori* in peptic ulcer is falling in the US, the pretest prevalence remains high, especially in individuals growing up in an impoverished environment. Therefore, when one encounters a single negative test in the presence of an established ulcer diagnosis, the chance of a false-negative test is 10% at a pretest prevalence of 50%, and 50% at a pretest prevalence of 90%. Additional testing for *H. pylori* is essential, especially in the setting of a complicated ulcer
- The most common cause of non-*H. pylori*, non-NSAID ulcers are a false-negative history that fails to detect occult NSAID use, and false-negative testing that fails to reveal underlying *H. pylori* infection

## THE TESTS
### Body fluids
BLOOD ANTIBODY TEST FOR HELICOBACTER PYLORI
*Description*
Whole blood is collected via fingerstick, with results obtained within 10min if the primary care physician has a laboratory onsite.

*Advantages/Disadvantages*
Advantages:
- Small specimen needed
- Relatively noninvasive procedure

Disadvantages:
- Not practical in the primary care setting that doesn't have a laboratory available
- Somewhat less accurate than breath test

*Normal*
Immunoglobulin (Ig) G and IgA antibodies specific for *H. pylori* typically not seen.

*Abnormal*
- IgG- and IgA-specific antibodies for *H. pylori* present
- Keep in mind the possibility of a false-positive result (reported to be as high as 7%) or a false-

negative result (reported to be as high as 40%, depending upon the characteristics of the test and the pretest prevalence of *H. pylori* infection)

*Cause of abnormal result*
Abnormal result indicates *H. pylori* infection.

## SERUM AMYLASE
*Description*
Whole blood is collected via venipuncture, serum is isolated by centrifugation. Serum amylase test is performed immediately if PCP has laboratory onsite, or can be performed at a central testing facility.

*Advantages/Disadvantages*
- Advantage: small specimen needed, relatively noninvasive procedure
- Disadvantage: test decreases the likelihood of diagnosis of pancreatitis, but does not serve to confirm peptic ulcer disease

*Normal*
- 0–130 IU/L, by enzymatic methods
- 50–150 IU/L

*Abnormal*
- >130 IU/L
- Keep in mind the possibility of a false-positive result

*Cause of abnormal result*
The most common cause of elevated serum amylase is pancreatitis; however, it could indicate a perforated peptic ulcer.

Elevated serum amylase can be seen in, for example:
- Acute nonhemorrhagic pancreatitis (elevation noted early in the course of the disease, 3-6h after the onset of pain)
- Acute exacerbation of chronic pancreatitis
- Partial gastrectomy
- Pancreatic duct obstruction
- Intestinal obstruction with strangulation
- Ruptured tubal pregnancy
- Ruptured aortic aneurysm
- Acute cholecystitis

## SERUM GASTRIN
*Description*
Whole blood is collected from a fasting patient via venipuncture, serum is isolated by centrifugation. Serum gastrin test can be performed immediately if physician has a laboratory onsite, or can be performed at a central testing facility.

*Advantages/Disadvantages*
- Advantage: small specimen needed, relatively noninvasive procedure
- Disadvantage: negative test decreases the likelihood of diagnosis of Zollinger–Ellison syndrome, but is not useful for a positive diagnosis of peptic ulcer

*Normal*
- Under age 65: <300pg/mL
- Over age 65: 200–800pg/mL

*Abnormal*
- Under age 65: >300pg/mL
- Over age 65: <200pg/mL or >800pg/mL
- Keep in mind the possibility of a false-positive result

*Cause of abnormal result*
Serum gastrin elevated in:
- States with reduced acid secretion, such as advanced gastritis
- Stomach cancer
- *Helicobacter pylori* infection
- Zollinger–Ellison syndrome
- Pernicious anemia

*Drugs, disorders and other factors that may alter results*
Values will be falsely increased in nonfasting patients, diabetics taking insulin, and after gastroscopy.

## FECAL OCCULT BLOOD
*Description*
Patients are instructed to have a meat-free diet for at least 3 days before the test. Over three separate days, the patient collects a stool sample, and then thinly smears a small part of the feces from two separate areas of the stool onto two spaces on the Hemoccult test pad. The specimen does not have to be refrigerated, and the sample can be mailed or brought into the physician's office when collection is completed.

*Advantages/Disadvantages*
Advantage: relatively simple, noninvasive procedure.

Disadvantages:
- Patients may find collection procedure distasteful
- Only confirms blood in gastrointestinal tract; does not confirm peptic ulcer disease
- Generally less sensitive for detecting blood from an upper gastrointestinal source vs lower gastrointestinal source

*Normal*
Negative.

*Abnormal*
Test sensitivity is adjusted to detect blood loss >5–10mL/day, which is considered positive for blood in the stool.

*Cause of abnormal result*
Occult blood may be present from any intraluminal break in the mucosa, including peptic ulcer disease.

*Drugs, disorders and other factors that may alter results*
False-positive results:
- Iron tablets
- Meat in the diet within 4 days of the test
- Foods high in peroxidase activity, including turnips, fish, and horseradish

False-negative results:
- Vitamin C, when taken in quantities >500mg/day, may cause false-negative results

## UREA BREATH TEST FOR HELICOBACTER PYLORI
*Description*
Patient ingests 75mg of 13C-urea dissolved in 200mL of orange juice. Breath samples are taken at baseline (preingestion) and at 30min postingestion. Samples are measured by isotope ratio mass spectrometry.

*Advantages/Disadvantages*
- Advantage: noninvasive procedure, very sensitive and specific, very reproducible. Special kits can be obtained in the primary care setting
- Disadvantage: more expensive than standard enzyme-linked immunosorbent assay (ELISA) or antibody assays

*Abnormal*
Isotope-labeled carbon dioxide seen in postingestion specimen.

*Cause of abnormal result*
- *Helicobacter pylori* infection
- Keep in mind the possibility of a false-negative or -positive result

*Drugs, disorders and other factors that may alter results*
False-negative findings seen in patients taking proton pump inhibitors (PPIs), high-dose histamine receptor antagonists, antimicrobial agents, or bismuth-containing compounds.

## Biopsy
### GASTRIC MUCOSAL BIOPSY
*Description*
Gastric biopsy performed during endoscopic examination, allowing collection of specimens for testing of urease activity, histology, and occasional culture for *H. pylori* (culture for *H. pylori* is generally only performed in specialty laboratories for establishing resistance to clarithromycin or metronidazole).

*Advantages/Disadvantages*
Advantages:
- Endoscopic examination of the gastrointestinal tract is the gold standard for accurate diagnosis of peptic ulcer, and can diagnose malignancy
- More accurate than radiography (accuracy >95% in diagnosing peptic ulcer disease, excludes malignancy in >99% of cases)

Disadvantages:
- Invasive procedure
- Routinely performed by a gastroenterologist, requiring referral

*Abnormal*
- Biopsy specimens test positive for urease, culture positive for *H. pylori*
- Biopsy specimens of ulcer margin display pathology positive for malignancy
- Keep in mind the possibility of a false-positive result for urease

*Cause of abnormal result*
- *H. pylori* infection
- Gastric malignancy

*Drugs, disorders and other factors that may alter results*
If a PPI (omeprazole, lansoprazole, rabeprazole, and pantoprazole) has been prescribed before biopsy, sensitivity of histologic examination and rapid urease tissue test for *H. pylori* are reduced.

## Imaging
UPPER GASTROINTESTINAL X-RAY SERIES WITH BARIUM CONTRAST
*Advantages/Disadvantages*
Advantages:
- Noninvasive procedure, helps to confirm or rule out malignancy
- 70–90% accurate in diagnosing peptic ulcer disease

Disadvantages:
- Low sensitivity for duodenal ulcer with single-contrast study; air-contrast study should be performed if duodenal ulcer suspected
- Not specific for confirmation of malignancy; endoscopy and biopsy are always required to confirm the diagnosis
- Routinely requires referral to gastroenterologist

*Abnormal*
- Ulcer(s) detected projecting beyond the lumen, with folds radiating from margins, radiolucent band (Hampton line) paralleling ulcer base
- Possible malignancy noted (ulcer within a mass, folds that do not radiate from ulcer margin, ulcer >2.5–3cm diameter)

*Cause of abnormal result*
- Presence of ulcer
- Presence of gastric malignancy

## Special tests
HELICOBACTER PYLORI STOOL ANTIGEN TEST
*Description*
Stool samples collected and stored for up to 72h at 35.6–46.4°F (2–8°C), or frozen at -4°F (-20°C) until analysis. The antigen test is performed using a sandwich enzyme immunoassay with antigen detection.

*Advantages/Disadvantages*
Advantages:
- Not time consuming
- More inexpensive than breath test
- Can be performed even in newborn children
- Test can be performed at any laboratory
- May be useful to prove success of eradication therapy, with a negative predictive value of 98% (a rate that is comparable to urea breath testing)

Disadvantage: retesting must be delayed at least 4 weeks after cessation of antibiotic therapy.

*Normal*
Optical density OD450 <0.140 indicates the absence of *H. pylori* infection.

*Abnormal*
- Optical density OD450 >0.160 indicates the presence of *H. pylori* infection
- Keep in mind the possibility of a false-positive result; an optical density from 0.140–0.159 is considered equivocal and should be repeated

*Cause of abnormal result*
*H. pylori* infection.

## TREATMENT

### CONSIDER CONSULT
If the patient requires biopsy via endoscopy, upper gastrointestinal series with barium, or exploratory laparotomy, refer to gastroenterologist for procedure.

### IMMEDIATE ACTION
If the patient is experiencing symptoms of active bleeding, including hematemesis, bright-red blood per rectum, or new-onset melena, refer to a gastroenterologist immediately.

### PATIENT AND CAREGIVER ISSUES
#### Patient or caregiver request
Q If I just change my diet will the ulcer go away? The association between foods and ulcer occurrence is nebulous, at best. Dietary changes may affect symptoms, but will not heal or prevent ulcers

Q I had an *Helicobacter pylori* test done when I had an ulcer before, but the results were negative, why do I still have an ulcer? A substantial percentage of ulcers are not associated with *H. pylori* infection. Likewise, false-negative results may occur in up to 20% of cases, depending on which assay was used to detect infection in the first place

#### Health-seeking behavior
- Are recurrent symptoms due to recurrent ulceration? Especially after cure of *H. pylori* infection, recurrent symptoms are often not due to recurrent ulceration. Refractory symptoms, especially with health-seeking behavior, warrants a thorough psychosocial assessment
- Has the patient been self-medicating with over-the-counter (OTC) medications? Antacids may have become ineffective, necessitating this visit. Also, if patient was taking nonsteroidal anti-inflammatory drugs (NSAIDs) for stomach pain, these may have exacerbated this flare-up

### MANAGEMENT ISSUES
#### Goals
- Eradication of *H. pylori* infection, if present
- Reduce exposure to NSAIDs
- Reduction of severity or elimination of epigastric pain
- Prevent further ulcer flare-ups

#### Management in special circumstances
Special patient groups include children, the elderly, patients undergoing chronic treatment with NSAIDs or glucocorticoids, those with aggressive or complicated ulcer disease, and asymptomatic bleeders.

COEXISTING DISEASE
Aggressive or complicated ulcer disease (perforation or hemorrhagic conditions) requires more aggressive treatment than would normally be indicated in typical peptic ulcer disease.

COEXISTING MEDICATION
Patients requiring NSAID or glucocorticoid treatment for coexisting disease may experience more frequent flare-ups of their ulcer disease. Consider modifying treatment regimen for these patients.

SPECIAL PATIENT GROUPS
- Recent guidelines have been published for treatment of children with *H. pylori*. Recommended regimens for *H. pylori* in children exclude bismuth (amoxicillin, clarithromycin, and proton pump inhibitor – PPI; amoxicillin, metronidazole, and PPI; clarithromycin, metronidazole, and PPI)

- In the elderly population, triple therapy with bismuth combined with two antibiotics for 14 days is associated with failure to eradicate, poor compliance because of side effects, the need for frequent dose administration, and relatively long duration of treatment. Short-term, low-dose treatment regimens may be more effective in the *H. pylori*-positive older patient
- Any patient with bleeding requires referral to a gastroenterologist for definitive diagnosis and endoscopic therapy, if indicated

PATIENT SATISFACTION/LIFESTYLE PRIORITIES
Patients should be warned in advance that successful eradication of *H. pylori* in the setting of peptic ulcer disease does not automatically eliminate symptoms. Some patients will continue to have dyspepsia. Therefore, while eradication of *H. pylori* is safe and effective in treating peptic ulcer, it may not always meet the patients' expectations and satisfaction.

## SUMMARY OF THERAPEUTIC OPTIONS
### Choices
- Choice if *H. pylori* infection is present: eradication therapy is required. Quadruple therapy consists of dual antibiotics plus PPI and bismuth
- In general, if the ulcer is small (<1cm), uncomplicated, and lacking a prior refractory course, additional therapy with antisecretory agents is optional
- Choice for *H. pylori*-negative ulcer: antisecretory agents. Histamine-2 receptor antagonists ($H_2$ blockers) are an acceptable choice and are less expensive than PPIs, especially with use of generic preparations
- PPIs are somewhat more effective than $H_2$ receptor antagonists, especially when PPIs are used in higher dose. All of these drugs are safe. Antacids and sucralfate, although effective, have little role in current therapy
- For NSAID ulcers, treatment is the same as for non-NSAID ulcers. NSAIDs should be discontinued if possible as healing will be improved
- For prevention of NSAID ulcers, cotherapy with misoprostol reduces ulcer complications. However, use of cyclo-oxygenase-2 specific anti-inflammatory medications appears equally effective in reducing the rate of ulcer complications, and is better tolerated than the NSAID-misoprostol combination
- Surgical intervention may still be rarely required for complicated ulcers that do not respond to conventional therapy: vagotomy is indicated for surgery of duodenal ulcers; subtotal gastrectomy is indicated for complicated gastric ulcers that have not responded to aggressive medical management
- Lifestyle changes that may benefit patients include cessation of cigarette smoking, avoidance of aspirin and NSAID use, avoidance of excessive alcohol use

### Guidelines
The American College of Gastroenterology have produced the following guidelines:
- Practice guidelines: Medical treatment of peptic ulcer disaease. Practice Parameters Committee of the American College of Gastroenterology [1]
- ACG treatment guideline: treatment and prevention of NSAID-induced ulcers. Committee on Practice Parameters of the American College of Gastroenterology [2]

### Clinical pearl(s)
- For *H. pylori*-positive patients with ulcer disease, effective management requires antibiotic therapy. The challenge is to treat once, since metronidazole and clarithromycin both have a high risk of inducing resistance if *H. pylori* is not eradicated
- Success in curing *H. pylori* requires both selecting an effective regimen and educating the patient so that they are compliant with the regimen
- Careful follow-up to assure *H. pylori* eradication is essential in patients who have had complicated or refractory ulcers. The breath test or stool antigen test are the best methods;

testing should be conducted at least 4 weeks after antibiotic therapy, bismuth, and PPI have been stopped
- Recurrent symptoms may or may not reflect recurrent *H. pylori* infection. Re-evaluation with endoscopy may be necessary to assure cure of *H. pylori* infection and healing of ulcers
- All gastric ulcers deserve at least one careful endoscopy and biopsy run. If the gastric ulcer appears grossly benign and biopsies (at least four jumbo biopsies at the ulcer edge or seven conventional biopsies) are negative, the chances of missing underlying malignancy are very low. Repeat endoscopy to assure healing is not always essential, but only if one is confident about negative results from the initial endoscopy

## FOLLOW UP
### Plan for review
- Confirm eradication of *H. pylori* by biopsy, urea breath test, or stool antigen test in patients who had complicated, refractory, or recurrent ulcers, or who remain symptomatic. If *H. pylori* infection persists, the antibiotic regimen requires careful consideration
- Present guidelines suggest urea breath test confirmation for asymptomatic patients as well, though the cost effectiveness of this recommendation is not well defined
- Serology can also be used for confirmation, comparing pretreatment to 6-month post-treatment titers. However, a carefully performed quantitative assay performed simultaneously on both samples is essential for reliability. Therefore, this approach is hard to apply in practice settings
- Monitor clinical response for patients with acute duodenal ulcer. Follow-up endoscopy is not indicated unless the ulcer was large or complicated or if symptoms persist
- Confirm healing of gastric ulcers. Appropriately performed and interpreted biopsies are essential, at the outset, after 8–12 weeks, or both, to exclude gastric malignancy. Repeat endoscopy and biopsy is essential for patients with a poor clinical response or with persisting ulcers
- For all patients, symptomatic relief does not preclude malignancy. Likewise, persistence of symptoms does not exclude successful healing of the ulcer, with symptoms persisting due to a functional disorder (i.e. a sensitized upper gastrointestinal tract) or some other etiology

### Information for patient or caregiver
- Patients must be instructed on correct dose administration procedures for these complex antibiotic regimens. In particular, patients should be warned that missing even one or two pills significantly reduces the effectiveness of therapy. Patients should be informed regarding minor and major side effects and instructed to continue therapy for minor effects and call or come in for major side effects
- Patients should be instructed regarding the impact of NSAIDs on their condition, and should be encouraged to refrain from their use if possible
- Patients should be provided information on reducing or eliminating cigarette smoking
- Patients should be encouraged to monitor any recurrence of symptoms

## DRUGS AND OTHER THERAPIES: DETAILS
### Drugs
HELICOBACTER PYLORI ERADICATION THERAPY
PPI regimens for *H. pylori* infection:
- Although several regimens have been used for *H. pylori* infection, only those few with superior efficacy should be used
- PPIs enhance antibiotic action and can be used with two of three antibiotics: clarithromycin, amoxicillin, and metronidazole
- Regimens combining a PPI with a single antibiotic (amoxicillin or clarithromycin) were popular because of simplicity, but are not advised because cure rates are below 70%. Regimens with two of these antibiotics work much better than one; the addition of metronidazole or ampicillin

to omeprazole and clarithromycin boosts cure rates to above 85% in compliant patients over 7–10 days
- Although shorter periods may be successful, a 14-day therapy period is still advised
- All five PPIs appear to be equally effective in enhancing antibiotic action, especially if used in twice-daily doses

Bismuth regimens including quadruple therapy:
- The same three antibiotics (amoxicillin, metronidazole, and clarithromycin) are useful in combination with bismuth; however, with bismuth, tetracycline can also be combined with either clarithromycin or metronidazole
- Although one-week therapy with bismuth-metronidazole-tetracycline (BMT) works reasonably well with good compliance and *H. pylori* that is sensitive to metronidazole, 14-day therapy is advised because of frequent metronidazole resistance
- Adding a PPI to bismuth plus two antibiotics is called quadruple therapy. Adding a PPI to BMT improves cure rates, especially for metronidazole-resistant *H. pylori*. Use of higher dose metronidazole (500mg three times a day) also improves effectiveness, especially with metronidazole-resistant *H. pylori*
- Since bismuth in the subsalicylate form available in the US (Pepto-Bismol) has not been demonstrated to share the ulcer-healing properties of bismuth subcitrate, antisecretory agents need to be added to the bismuth therapies to assure ulcer healing. Therefore, BMT plus PPI is the optimal bismuth regimen

Recommended regimens for *H. pylori*
First-line choices:
- PPI plus clarithromycin plus amoxicillin (this regimen is a first choice because failures will only develop resistance to one antibiotic). Note that ampicillin cannot be substituted for amoxicillin
- Bismuth subsalicylate plus tetracycline, metronidazole, and PPI (this regimen is also a first-line choice). The improved efficacy obtained with adding a PPI to BMT probably justifies the added costs. Note that doxycycline cannot be substituted for tetracycline

Second-line choices:
- PPI plus clarithromycin and metronidazole: a second-line choice only because failures will likely be resistant to both metronidazole and clarithromycin. Otherwise, this is a good regimen
- Omeprazole plus metronidazole plus amoxicillin: efficacy is compromised by metronidazole resistance to a greater extent than with metronidazole plus clarithromycin

*Dose*
Doses of the individual agents comprising the above regimens:
- PPI: full dose, twice daily (e.g. omeprazole 20mg twice daily)
- Amoxicillin: 500mg twice daily
- Metronidazole: 500mg twice daily if combined with PPI or 500mg three times daily when combined with bismuth (although a 250mg four times daily regimen is often used in combination with bismuth, the higher dose appears to be more effective)
- Bismuth subsalicylate: two tablets, four times daily
- Tetracycline: 500mg twice daily when combined with bismuth (tetracycline cannot be combined with PPI in the absence of bismuth)
- Ideal length of therapy is 14 days

*Efficacy*
For eradication of *H. pylori* infection, clarithromycin plus metronidazole plus PPI, clarithromycin plus amoxicillin plus PPI, and BMT-PPI are the combinations that produce the best results.

*Risks/benefits*
Risks:
- Complex regimens are cumbersome for patients, side effects are annoying, and cost may be a factor in whether patients continue therapy for full dosage period
- Risk of bacterial resistance to metronidazole or clarithromycin
- Avoid alcohol while taking metronidazole

Benefit: eradication of *H. pylori* promotes healing and markedly reduces ulcer recurrence.

*Side effects and adverse reactions*
- Gastrointestinal: pseudomembranous colitis (treat with metronidazole), diarrhea due to antibiotics (may resolve by changing amoxicillin to tetracycline in bismuth regimens), nausea/vomiting
- Skin: Stevens–Johnson syndrome (rare), rash

*Interactions (other drugs)*
- Diazepam (omeprazole may prolong elimination time of diazepam) - Warfarin (omeprazole may prolong elimination time of warfarin) - Phenytoin (omeprazole may prolong elimination time of phenytoin) - Drugs metabolized by the cytochrome 3A4 pathway (clarithromycin can interact with these)

*Contraindications*
Hypersensitivity to any component of the therapy.

*Evidence*
- A systematic review found that gastric ulcer recurrence rates were significantly reduced in patients receiving eradication therapy, compared with antisecretory treatment (4–6 weeks), at one year after treatment [3] *Level M*
- This review also found that triple therapy achieved higher healing rates than antisecretory therapy for patients with a duodenal ulcer [3] *Level M*
- Another systematic review found that most patients with peptic ulcers and *H. pylori* infection were effectively treated 6 weeks after the start of eradication therapy [4] *Level M*

*Acceptability to patient*
- Patients may find a multiple drug regimen complicated and hard to follow
- Price of medications may be an issue for the uninsured patient

*Follow up plan*
- Monitor patient response to treatment. If any adverse response to treatment, consider modifying treatment plan to deal with reactions. If treatment is ineffective, revise therapeutic plan or consider referral to gastroenterologist. Culture and sensitivity of resistant *H. pylori* may be useful in planning additional therapy for difficult to eradicate strains
- Monitor treatment regimen acceptability/ease of use. If patient isn't comfortable with dose regimen, consider modifying treatment plan

*Patient and caregiver information*
- Provide patient with information regarding why triple therapy regimen must be strictly followed
- Provide patient with information on dosage schedule (i.e. take tablets with meal, before meals)
- Provide patient with information on possible side effects or adverse events to look out for during treatment

## HISTAMINE-2 RECEPTOR ANTAGONISTS (H2 BLOCKERS)
Cimetidine, ranitidine, famotidine, and nizatidine are all used to treat peptic ulcers that are not related to *H. pylori* infection or continuing NSAID use.

### Dose
- Cimetidine: 800mg/day
- Ranitidine: 300mg/day
- Famotidine: 40mg/day
- Nizatidine: 300mg/day

### Efficacy
These drugs have all been shown to be effective antisecretory agents for use in treating gastric and duodenal ulcers. However, used alone they are inadequate therapy for *H. pylori* ulcers (*H. pylori* must be cured) or for NSAID ulcers, if NSAIDs cannot be stopped.

### Risks/benefits
Risks:
- Drug interactions are greater with $H_2$ receptor antagonists than with other forms of treatment for peptic ulcer disease, therefore patients may have limited choices due to concomitant drug issues
- Symptomatic response does not preclude possible gastric malignancy

Benefits:
- Less difficult dosage regimen than use of multiple drug program
- Several of these drugs are available as OTC medications and may be less costly than prescription products

### Side effects and adverse reactions
- Central nervous system: lethargy, confusion, headache, depression, hallucinations
- Genitourinary (cimetidine): reversible impotence, gynecomastia
- Hematologic: thrombocytopenia, leukopenia, hepatitis

### Interactions (other drugs)
- Cimetidine interacts with theophylline, warfarin, phenytoin, and lidocaine via inhibition of cytochrome P450 isozymes (leading to reduced drug clearance)
- Ranitidine and famotidine have rarely been associated with increased theophylline levels
- Magnesium-containing antacids

### Contraindications
If patients have known renal insufficiency (glomerular filtration rate <30mL/min), $H_2$ receptor antagonists use should be discouraged or the dose reduced.

### Acceptability to patient
- Patients may find single-drug regimen easy to deal with
- Costs of drugs (OTC vs prescription) may be an issue for the uninsured patient

### Follow up plan
- Monitor patient response to treatment. If any adverse response to treatment, consider modifying treatment plan to deal with reactions. If treatment is ineffective, revise therapeutic plan or consider referral to gastroenterologist
- Monitor treatment regimen acceptability/ease of use. If patient isn't comfortable with dosage regimen, consider modifying treatment plan

*Patient and caregiver information*
- Provide patient with information on dosage schedule (i.e. take tablets with meal, before meals)
- Provide patient with information on possible side effects or adverse events to look out for during treatment

## PROTON PUMP INHIBITORS
- The PPIs, omeprazole, lansoprazole, rabeprazole, and pantoprazole, decrease gastric acid secretion by inhibiting hydrogen-potassium adenosine triphosphate
- This is an off-label indication if the drugs are being used to treat an NSAID-induced ulcer

*Dose*
- Omeprazole: 20–40mg/day
- Lansoprazole: 15–30mg/day
- Rabeprazole: 20mg/day
- Pantoprazole: 40mg/day

*Efficacy*
These drugs induce more rapid healing of peptic ulcer than $H_2$ receptor antagonists, especially at higher doses. There is very little difference in their efficacy in inhibiting acid secretion.

*Risks/benefits*
Risks:
- Symptomatic response does not preclude possible gastric malignancy
- Costs are high

Benefits:
- Simple treatment regimen and more rapid healing
- Cure of *H. pylori* infection is enhanced more effectively by these agents than by $H_2$ receptor antagonists

*Side effects and adverse reactions*
- Serious side effects are rare
- Central nervous system: headache, dizziness
- Gastrointestinal: nausea, vomiting, diarrhea, constipation, flatulence, abdominal pain, hepatitis, pancreatitis
- Genitourinary: interstitial nephritis, gynecomastia, urinary problems, urinary infections
- Hematologic: agranulocytosis, thrombocytopenia, anemia, neutropenia, and other blood cell disorders
- Skin: purpura, Stevens–Johnson syndrome, alopecia, erythema multiforme, rash

*Interactions (other drugs)*
Omeprazole:
- Calcium channel antagonists (nifedipine, nimodipine, nisoldipine, nitrendipine)
- Carbamazepine
- Cefpodoxime, cefuroxime
- Clarithromycin
- Diazepam
- Digoxin
- Enoxacin
- Glipizide, glyburide
- Itraconazole, ketoconazole
- Methotrexate
- Phenytoin
- Sucralfate
- Tacrolimus
- Tolbutamide
- Warfarin

Lansoprazole:
- Theophylline
- Glipizide
- Glyburide
- Ketoconazole
- Iron

Rabeprazole:
- Digoxin
- Itraconzaole
- Ketoconazole

Pantoprazole:
- Digoxin ■ Itraconzaole ■ Ketoconazole

*Contraindications*
- Pregnancy and breast-feeding ■ Gastric carcinoma ■ Hepatic impairment

*Evidence*
A RCT compared omeprazole and ranitidine in patients with a peptic ulcer (or more than 10 erosions) requiring continuous NSAID therapy. Omeprazole was significantly more effective for healing than ranitidine after 8 weeks of treatment [5] *Level P*

*Acceptability to patient*
Simple dosage regimen may make this a more acceptable treatment option.

*Patient and caregiver information*
- All PPIs should be taken 30–60min before meals because the parietal cells must be actively secreting acid for PPIs to cause maximal inhibition. Lansoprazole, in particular, may be less effective if taken after meals. However, careful comparison studies have not been performed. Provide patient with information on dosage schedule (i.e. take tablets with meal, before meals)
- Provide patient with information on possible side effects or adverse events to look out for during treatment

## MISOPROSTOL
This prostaglandin E1 analog inhibits gastric acid secretion and may protect gastric mucosa. However, its only indication is for concurrent use with NSAIDs to prevent development of ulcers; these agents are not indicated for peptic ulcer in the absence of NSAID use. Furthermore, efficacy has not been established for healing ulcers induced by NSAIDs.

*Dose*
200–600mcg/day with food.

*Efficacy*
When administered to patients receiving concomitant NSAIDs, misoprostol reduces ulcer complications by about 50%.

*Risks/benefits*
- Risk: high-dose misoprostol has serious side effect profile, should be reserved for patients at high risk for NSAID-induced ulcers
- Benefit: suppression of ulcer complications induced by NSAID use

*Side effects and adverse reactions*
- Central nervous system: headache
- Gastrointestinal: abdominal pain, constipation, diarrhea, dyspepsia, flatulence, nausea, vomiting
- Genitourinary: cramps, spotting, vaginal bleeding

*Interactions (other drugs)*
When taken with phenylbutazone, increased adverse effects (headache, flushes, dizziness, nausea).

*Contraindications*
- Use of this drug by pregnant women is contraindicated due to its abortifacient effects
- Breast-feeding women should not use this drug ■ This drug is contraindicated for women of child-bearing age due to the uterine contraction side effects

*Acceptability to patient*
Patient tolerance is often a problem, especially at higher doses.

*Follow up plan*
- Monitor patient response to treatment. If any adverse response to treatment, consider modifying treatment plan to deal with reactions. If treatment is ineffective, revise therapeutic plan or consider referral to gastroenterologist
- Monitor treatment regimen acceptability/ease of use. If patient is not comfortable with dosage regimen, consider modifying treatment plan

*Patient and caregiver information*
- Misoprostol must be taken with food for duration of NSAID therapy. Provide patient with information on dosage schedule
- Provide patient with information on possible side effects or adverse events to look out for during treatment
- Provide patient with caution regarding abortifacient effects and possible plans to become pregnant

## Surgical therapy
Surgery for refractory ulcers is rarely performed. For duodenal ulcers, patients undergo highly selective vagotomy. For gastric ulcers, patients undergo ulcer removal with antrectomy or hemigastrectomy without vagotomy.

VAGOTOMY
Indicated for surgery of duodenal ulcers.

*Efficacy*
Highly selective vagotomy provides a safe and effective treatment for duodenal ulcers.

*Risks/benefits*
Risk:
- Mortality rate of 0.3% and recurrence rate of 3–30%

Benefits:
- Low recurrence rate when compared with medical treatment alone. However, in *H. pylori*-positive subjects, elective surgery has absolutely no role, compared with antibiotic therapy
- Furthermore, surgery has no role for elective management of NSAID ulcers; continued use of NSAIDs is a risk factor for ulcer recurrence after surgery

*Acceptability to patient*
Most common patient complaint after surgery is abdominal discomfort or vomiting after meals, which may be secondary to recurrent ulcer, afferent loop obstruction, bile reflux gastritis, gastric outlet obstruction, or stump carcinoma. However, many of these symptoms can be explained by dumping syndrome rather than concomitant or secondary illness. Other complications include postvagotomy diarrhea, bezoar, anemia, and osteomalacia and osteoporosis due to vitamin D and calcium malabsorption.

*Follow up plan*
- Monitor patient's abdominal complaints postsurgery. Many may be due to dumping syndrome, but could possibly be controlled with diet modification and medication. Diarrhea is a common problem postvagotomy; patient should be evaluated for treatable conditions (lactose intolerance or fat malabsorption) before providing symptomatic therapy
- Monitor patient's overall health. Malabsorption may produce steatorrhea, bacterial overgrowth

- Monitor patient's hematology profile. Deficiencies of folate, vitamin B12, or iron can lead to anemia

*Patient and caregiver information*
Patient may need to change diet or eating style after surgery. Modifying diet to treat symptoms of dumping syndrome may be indicated, including changes to six meals per day and avoidance of liquids with meals.

### SUBTOTAL GASTRECTOMY
Indicated for complicated gastric ulcers that have not responded to aggressive medical management.

*Efficacy*
Subtotal gastrectomy is effective for gastric ulcers, in the absence of duodenal ulcers.

*Risks/benefits*
- Risk: morbidity and mortality are always possible with surgical procedures
- Benefit: low recurrence rate, but there are no benefits compared with effective cure of *H. pylori* infection or discontinuation of NSAIDs, if either were the causative factors

*Acceptability to patient*
Most common patient complaint after surgery is abdominal discomfort or vomiting after meals, which may be secondary to recurrent ulcer, afferent loop obstruction, bile reflux gastritis, gastric outlet obstruction, or stump carcinoma. However, many of these symptoms can be explained by dumping syndrome rather than concomitant or secondary illness. Other complications include postvagotomy diarrhea, bezoar, anemia, and osteomalacia and osteoporosis due to vitamin D and calcium malabsorption.

*Follow up plan*
- Monitor patient's abdominal complaints postsurgery. Many may be due to dumping syndrome, but could possibly be controlled with diet modification and medication. Diarrhea is a common problem postvagotomy; patient should be evaluated for treatable conditions (lactose intolerance or fat malabsorption) before providing symptomatic therapy
- Monitor patient's overall health. Malabsorption may produce steatorrhea, bacterial overgrowth
- Monitor patient's hematology profile. Deficiencies of folate, vitamin B12, or iron can lead to anemia

*Patient and caregiver information*
Patient may need to change diet or eating style after surgery. Modifying diet to treat symptoms of dumping syndrome may be indicated, including changes to six meals/day and avoidance of liquids with meals.

## LIFESTYLE
Lifestyle changes that may benefit patients with peptic ulcer disease include cessation of cigarette smoking, avoidance of aspirin and NSAID use, avoidance of excessive alcohol use.

### RISKS/BENEFITS
Benefits:
- Cessation of cigarette smoking is associated with a decreased risk of peptic ulcer development, faster ulcer healing, and lower risk of ulcer recurrence
- Discontinuation of aspirin and NSAID use is associated with decreased incidence of gastritis and gastric ulcer. Dyspepsia and mucosal irritation decrease with NSAID discontinuation
- Alcohol-related gastritis will decrease with avoidance of excessive use

ACCEPTABILITY TO PATIENT
These lifestyle changes may not be as acceptable to patients as would medication to treat their symptoms of peptic ulcer disease. Patients may need help with modifying these behaviors.

FOLLOW UP PLAN
Monitor patient's success with smoking cessation goals, and prescribe medical treatment if needed.

PATIENT AND CAREGIVER INFORMATION
Information on the positive effects of discontinuing these behaviors should be provided.

## OUTCOMES

### EFFICACY OF THERAPIES

- Patients who do not exhibit anemia, gastrointestinal bleeding, anorexia, early satiety, or weight loss with their first reported severe dyspepsia should respond to empiric antiulcer therapy within 2 weeks
- Eradication of *Helicobacter pylori* with triple or quadruple therapies usually takes up to 2 weeks. For patients who do not have *H. pylori*, acute therapy can last several weeks (4–12 weeks) before relief is seen
- In up to 50% of patients there is no significant improvement of symptoms, despite successful eradication of *H. pylori* and ulcer healing. This may be due to additional underlying causes of dyspepsia harbored by the patient, including concurrent gastroesophageal reflux, which will not respond to *H. pylori* eradication

### Evidence

- A systematic review found that gastric ulcer recurrence rates were significantly reduced in patients receiving eradication therapy, compared with antisecretory treatment (4–6 weeks), at one year after treatment [3] *Level M*
- Triple therapy achieved higher healing rates than antisecretory therapy for patients with duodenal ulcers [3] *Level M*
- A systematic review found that most patients with peptic ulcers and *H. pylori* infection were effectively treated 6 weeks after the start of eradication therapy [4] *Level M*
- A randomized controlled trial (RCT) compared omeprazole and ranitidine in patients with a peptic ulcer (or more than 10 erosions), requiring continuous nonsteroidal anti-inflammatory drug (NSAID) therapy. Omeprazole was significantly more effective for healing than ranitidine after 8 weeks of treatment [5] *Level P*

### PROGNOSIS

- Ulcer relapse rates after *H. pylori* eradication are reduced compared with patients with persisting infection. However, recent meta-analysis indicated that up to 20% recurrence within 6 months of successful eradication [4]
- The true rate of ulcer recurrence varies by location and regional *H. pylori* prevalence
- Reinfection rates are less than 1% per year. However, the risk of rebleeding after *H. pylori* therapy is markedly reduced, unless continued use of NSAIDs is a factor
- NSAID-related ulcers may occur independent of *H. pylori* infection status

### Clinical pearl(s)

- Because *H. pylori* resistance to metronidazole and, to a lesser extent for clarithromycin, is common, one of the two most effective regimens should be used initially. When treating *H. pylori*, do not reserve the best for last
- Treatment of *H. pylori* infection is problematic because of the frequent development of resistance following use of metronidazole or clarithromycin. Therefore, plan treatment so that it is successful the first time. Patient education is essential. Proton pump inhibitors (PPIs), rather than $H_2$ receptor antagonists, should be used with antibiotics
- With any refractory ulcer, consider persisting, often surreptitious use of NSAIDs, especially aspirin
- Refractory ulcers should also prompt consideration of hypersecretory states, such as the Zollinger–Ellison syndrome
- Patients need to be carefully educated regarding the necessity to take the complex regimens required to cure *H. pylori*; taking a partial course can create resistant organisms. Make sure that the patient starts off taking the full dose; even after 5–7 days, the chance of success exceeds 70 or 80%, especially if antibiotic resistance is not present. Patients should be

informed about the minor (e.g. nausea, loose stools) and major (severe skin rash or diarrhea) side effects and what to do if they do develop them

### Therapeutic failure

- If the patient has confirmed persisting *H. pylori* infection after antibiotic therapy, then the second regimen should be selected either based the initial regimen or upon culture and sensitivity of *H. pylori*. In general, the second treatment should utilize antibiotics not used the first time. If the patient was not treated with clarithromycin, then PPI, clarithromycin, and amoxicillin regimen would be the first choice. If the patient failed a clarithromycin regimen, then high-dose quadruple therapy (PPI, bismuth, metronidazole, and tetracycline) is the best option
- Rarely, failure to resolve non-*H. pylori* ulcers with drug treatment may require surgical intervention. It is almost always possible to control ulcer disease with antisecretory therapy. The only exception is persisting NSAID use; surreptitious use is an important factor

### Recurrence

- Treatment of recurrence of *H. pylori* infection requires careful thought since resistance is likely to develop if the patient has been treated in the past with either metronidazole or clarithromycin
- Recurrence of non-*H. pylori* ulcers can be treated with alternative therapy ($H_2$ receptor antagonists vs PPI)
- Recurrence that does not respond to treatment may require referral for surgical intervention

### Deterioration

- If the patient presents with ulcer complications and their condition deteriorates despite medical treatment, referral for surgical intervention may be indicated. Delay in referral of patients for bleeding ulcers creates an increased risk
- If persisting symptoms are the problem, the first step is to determine if an ulcer accounts for the persisting symptoms. Often, symptoms persisting after ulcers heal probably indicates that the symptoms results from a sensitized upper gastrointestinal tract

## COMPLICATIONS

- Gastrointestinal bleeding occurs with deep ulcers
- Gastric outlet obstruction occurs in a small subset of patients with peptic ulcer disease with ulcers near the pyloric channel
- Perforation occurs in a small percentage of peptic ulcer patients
- Penetration of ulceration into the pancreas is a rare complication associated with ulcers in the posterior wall of the duodenal bulb

## CONSIDER CONSULT

If the patient has a nonhealing ulcer despite appropriate medical treatment, refer to surgeon for evaluation of possible surgical treatment plan.

## PREVENTION

### RISK FACTORS

- **Nonsteroidal anti-inflammatory drug (NSAID) use:** chronic use is strongly associated with peptic ulcer disease
- **Cigarette smoking:** smoking more than half a pack of cigarettes per day correlates with peptic ulcer disease, but data only show this association with *Helicobacter pylori*-positive ulcers
- **Family history of ulcers:** there appears to be a higher incidence of peptic ulcer disease with identical twins and specific phenotypes (HLA-B12, B5, Bw35). However, a strong familial clustering of ulcer disease reflects familial clustering of *H. pylori* infection that is largely independent of genetic factors
- **Zollinger–Ellison syndrome:** patients with this condition frequently suffer from peptic ulcer disease

### MODIFY RISK FACTORS

#### Lifestyle and wellness

An overall healthy lifestyle, with regular physical examinations for patients with familial tendencies to gastrointestinal disease, is recommended.

#### TOBACCO

Discontinuation of smoking is considered beneficial, even without diagnosed disease states.

#### ALCOHOL AND DRUGS

Limiting alcohol use and discontinuing the use of drugs is considered beneficial, even without diagnosed disease states.

#### DIET

A low-fat diet, with emphasis on three regular meals daily, is considered beneficial.

#### FAMILY HISTORY

If there is a history of peptic ulcer disease (or other gastrointestinal diseases) in the family, an education program should make the patient aware of all risk factors for disease. The presence of *H. pylori* infection should be sought.

#### DRUG HISTORY

If the patient is currently taking NSAIDs or glucocorticoids for other conditions, an education program is recommended to make the patient aware of the risks of chronic NSAID use.

### SCREENING

- General population screening for peptic ulcer disease is not indicated. Screening for *H. pylori* infection is not thought to be appropriate in the absence of symptoms. However, some physicians elect to screen for *H. pylori* infection, noting positive infection in the patient's records. If an *H. pylori*-positive patient requires antibiotics, then it would advisable to give a regimen that cures *H. pylori* infection
- Patients presenting at the physician's office with chronic dyspepsia should be evaluated for *H. pylori* infection

### PREVENT RECURRENCE

Patients should be instructed that changes in lifestyle can help reduce recurrence. However, these changes may not totally prevent recurrence of ulcer attacks, as there may be other underlying causes of disease.

## Reassess coexisting disease

- Critically ill patients who require prolonged mechanical ventilation are at high risk for gastrointestinal bleeding if they also have *H. pylori* infection
- Patients with osteoarthritis or other conditions requiring chronic NSAID or glucocorticoid use should be monitored for possible recurrence of ulcer due to the effects of the NSAIDs

INTERACTION ALERT

Patients with conditions requiring chronic NSAID use should be monitored for possible recurrence of ulcer due to the effects of the NSAIDs.

# RESOURCES

## ASSOCIATIONS
National Digestive Diseases Information Clearinghouse
2 Information Way
Bethesda, MD 20892-3570
Toll-free: (800) 891-5389
Tel: (301) 654-3810
Fax: (301) 907-8906
E-mail: nddic@info.niddk.nih.gov
http://www.niddk.nih.gov

## KEY REFERENCES
- Braden B, Posselt H-G, Ahrens P, et al. New immunoassay in stool provides an accurate noninvasive diagnostic method for *Helicobacter pylori* screening in children. Pediatrics 2000;106:115–7
- Chan FK, Hawkey CJ, Lanas Al. *Helicobacter pylori* and nonsteroidal anti-inflammatory drugs: a three way debate. Am J Med 2001;110:55S–57S
- Peterson WL, Fendrick AM, Cave DR, et al. *Helicobacter pylori*-related disease: guidelines for testing and treatment. Arch Intern Med 2000;160:1285–91
- NIH Consensus Development Panel on *Helicobacter pylori* in peptic ulcer disease. JAMA 1994;272:65–9
- Bujanover Y, Reif S, Yahav J. *Helicobacter pylori* and peptic disease in the pediatric patient. Pediatr Clin North Am 1996;43:213–34
- Salcedo JA, Al-Kawas F. Treatment of *Helicobacter pylori* infection. Arch Intern Med 1998;158:842–51
- Schwartz H, Krause R, Sahba B, et al. Triple versus dual therapy for eradicating *Helicobacter pylori* and prevention ulcer recurrence: a randomized, double-blind, multicenter study of lansoprazole, clarithromycin, and/or amoxicillin in different dosing regimens. Am J Gastroenterol 1998;93:584–90
- Kuipers EJ, Klinkenberg-Knol EC, Meuwissen SG. *Helicobacter pylori*, proton pump inhibitors and gastroesophageal reflux disease. Yale J Biol Med 1999;72:211–8
- Agrawal NM, Aziz K. Prevention of gastrointestinal complications associated with nonsteroidal anti-inflammatory drugs. J Rheumatol Suppl 1998;51:17–20
- Greenall MJ, Lehnert T. Vagotomy or gastrectomy for elective treatment of benign gastric ulceration? Dig Dis Sci 1985;30:53–61
- Reid DA, Duthie HL, Ransom CJ, Johnson AG. Late follow-up of highly selective vagotomy with excision of the ulcer compared with Billroth I gastrectomy for treatment of benign gastric ulcer. Br J Surg 1982;69:605–7

### Evidence references and guidelines
1. Practice guidelines: Medical treatment of peptic ulcer disaease. Practice Parameters Committee of the American College of Gastroenterology. JAMA 1996;275:622–9
2. ACG treatment guideline: treatment and prevention of NSAID-induced ulcers. Committee on Practice Parameters of the American College of Gastroenterology. Am J Gastroenterology 1998;93:2037–46
3. Penston JG. Review article: Clinical aspects of *Helicobacter pylori* eradication therapy in peptic ulcer disease. Aliment Pharmacol Ther 1996;10:469–86. Reviewed in: Clinical Evidence 2001;6:364–77
4. Laine L, Hopkins RJ, Girardi LS. Has the impact of *Helicobacter pylori* therapy on ulcer recurrence in the United States been overstated? A meta-analysis of rigorously designed trials. Am J Gastroenterol 1998;93:1409–15. Reviewed in: Clinical Evidence 2001;6:364–77
5. Yeomans ND, Tulassay Z, Juhasz L, et al. A comparison of omeprazole with ranitidine for ulcers associated with nonsteroidal anti-inflammatory drugs. Acid Suppression Trial: Ranitidine versus Omeprazole for NSAID-associated Ulcer Treatment (ASTRONAUT) Study Group. N Engl J Med 1998;338:719–26. Medline

## FAQS
### Question 1
How often do patients with *Helicobacter pylori*-positive peptic ulcer disease get symptomatic improvement after successful *H. pylori* eradication?

### ANSWER 1
Symptomatic improvement is found in the majority of patients with *H. pylori*-positive ulcers following successful cure of the infection. However, roughly 30% have some persistent symptoms,

which often take the form of heartburn, functional dyspepsia, or irritable bowel syndrome. Of interest, when patients with ulcers undergo surgery (highly selectively vagotomy) for refractory ulcers or symptoms, about 40% still have persisting symptoms, but <10% have persisting ulcers. In contrast, <10% of patients who were responsive to medical therapy before surgery presented with recurrent symptoms. Furthermore, in patients presenting with peptic ulcer, about 30% also have symptoms suggestive of irritable bowel syndrome and acid reflux. The conclusion is that ulcers are commonly associated with functional gastrointestinal disorders; therefore, after curing the *H. pylori* and healing ulcers, anticipate the necessity to continue treatment for persisting functional symptoms in some patients.

## Question 2
Do I really need to confirm cure of *Helicobacter pylori* in patients with peptic ulcer disease if they remain asymptomatic after antibiotic treatment?

### ANSWER 2
If the patient had complicated or troublesome ulcer disease, then confirming cure is important. However, if the ulcer disease was a mild, short-lived condition, then confirmation of cure is optional, as long as the patient remains asymptomatic. However, with the advent of simple, noninvasive tests to establish cure, confirming cure on all patients is a reasonable option. Regardless, the choice should be discussed with the patient and their views considered in the decision.

## Question 3
When is culture for *Helicobacter pylori* necessary?

### ANSWER 3
Culture for *H. pylori* requires special expertise by laboratories dedicated to studying this problem. Sensitivities play no role, since *H. pylori* is sensitive to numerous antibiotics in culture that are ineffective in vivo. The primary reason to culture *H. pylori* is to identify resistance to metronidazole and clarithromycin; this is appropriate when the patient has failed therapy.

## Question 4
How do I choose the best therapy for *Helicobacter pylori*?

### ANSWER 4
Once *H. pylori* infection has been confirmed, the strategy should be to prepare the patient for one successful course of antibiotics, because failure creates resistance. First establish whether the patient has a history of untoward antibiotic reactions, and whether they recall being treated with clarithromycin or metronidazole. If so, you can assume a >50% chance of resistance to that antibiotic; therefore, choose a regimen without that antibiotic. The first-line choices are a proton pump inhibitor (PPI), amoxicillin, and clarithromycin, or quadruple therapy (a PPI, bismuth, metronidazole, and tetracycline). Higher doses of metronidazole are recommended for the latter, and a 14-day course is advised for both regimens to provide the best chances for cure.

## Question 5
Does *Helicobacter pylori* infection increase the risk from nonsteroidal anti-inflammatory drugs (NSAIDs)? Should patients be tested for *H. pylori* before starting NSAIDs?

### ANSWER 5
This is a controversial area. Much of the available data in the literature were obtained studying endoscopic ulcers; these studies were done by endoscoping all patients taking NSAIDs. Since <4% of patients taking NSAIDs develop ulcers during the course of a year on NSAIDs, and 10–20% of patients taking NSAIDs have things that look like ulcers at endoscopy, most of what you see at endoscopy never becomes a clinically significant ulcer. Furthermore, many patients

who enroll on NSAID studies come from arthritis clinics where they have been on NSAIDs for a long time. This is a very different population from the patient in your office who you want to start on NSAIDs for the first time. In patients with a known ulcer history, NSAIDs exacerbate the underlying ulcer diathesis and frequently result in complications. However, in adults without an ulcer history, about 1–3% of the asymptomatic adult population have active, subclinical ulcer disease (silent, asymptomatic ulcers, or scars found upon surveillance endoscopy or X-ray); this subclinical ulcer disease is largely due to *H. pylori* infection.

Ulcer risk is highest in the first month or two after starting NSAID therapy; it is a reasonable hypothesis that some of the early ulcer risk with NSAIDs is due to precipitation of bleeding or complications in patients with subclinical peptic ulcer. Curing *H. pylori* before the start of NSAID therapy may reduce ulcer formation and new guidelines support curing *H. pylori*, if present, before starting NSAIDs.

## CONTRIBUTORS
Gordon H Baustian, MD
Andrew H Soll, MD
Brennan Spiegel, MD

# ACUTE PERITONITIS

| | | |
|---|---|---|
| ■ | Summary Information | 466 |
| ■ | Background | 467 |
| ■ | Diagnosis | 468 |
| ■ | Treatment | 477 |
| ■ | Outcomes | 486 |
| ■ | Prevention | 487 |
| ■ | Resources | 488 |

## SUMMARY INFORMATION

### DESCRIPTION
- Inflammation of the peritoneal lining or the peritoneal fluid
- Commonly caused by bacterial infection or chemical irritation
- May be localized or generalized
- May be primary or secondary to perforated viscus

### URGENT ACTION
Assess rapidly for presence of perforated viscus, which is a surgical emergency.

### KEY! DON'T MISS!
It is crucial to assess for the presence of a surgical abdomen, and refer immediately to a surgeon for assessment.

## BACKGROUND

### ICD9 CODE
567.2 Peritonitis.

### CARDINAL FEATURES
- Pain, guarding, abdominal rigidity
- Fever
- Absent bowel sounds
- Hypotension, tachycardia, acidosis
- Untreated, may quickly lead to multiorgan failure due to septic shock

### CAUSES
#### Common causes
Primary peritonitis:
- Refers to spontaneous infection of ascites (spontaneous bacterial peritonitis) that was previously present secondary to an underlying condition, most commonly cirrhosis
- Spontaneous bacterial infection, with no predisposing condition
- Also may refer to a less common condition of primary inflammation of the peritoneal lining that occurs in the absence of infection, as in familial Mediterranean fever or systemic lupus erythematosus
- May be seen when ascites is from other causes, including metastatic malignancy, congestive heart failure, or nephrotic syndrome, though this is far less common
- Common organisms include *Escherichia coli*, *Klebsiella pneumoniae*, *Streptococcus pneumoniae*, and other streptococcal species
- Other pathogens implicated in primary peritonitis include *Mycobacterium tuberculosis*, *Neisseria gonorrhoeae*, *Chlamydia trachomatis*, and *Coccidioides immitis*

Secondary peritonitis:
- Bacterial infection due to a perforated viscus, such as a perforated appendix, ruptured peptic ulcer, ruptured ectopic pregnancy, Crohn's disease, cholecystitis, diverticulitis, pancreatitis; bowel obstruction, acute salpingitis, pelvic inflammatory disease, abdominal trauma (including peritonitis presenting after abdominal surgery)
- Common pathogens usually reflect endogenous micro-organisms which are normally found in the gut, such as *E. coli*, *Bacteroides fragilis*, various enterococci and *Bacteroides* species, *Fusobacterium*, various *Clostridium* species, *Peptococcus*, *Peptostreptococcus*, and *Eubacterium*
- Infection with multiple organisms is common

#### Serious causes
- It is crucial to assess quickly whether acute peritonitis is secondary to a perforated viscus (surgical abdomen), so that appropriate surgical intervention can be undertaken in a timely fashion
- Spontaneous bacterial peritonitis also requires urgent treatment

## DIAGNOSIS

### DIFFERENTIAL DIAGNOSIS
#### Pneumonia (bacterial, viral)
FEATURES
- Sudden onset
- Fever and chills
- Pleuritic chest pain
- Shortness of breath, shallow inspiratory effort
- Tachypnea, tachycardia
- Cough, sputum production
- Abdominal pain

#### Sickle cell anemia
FEATURES
- Pain crises, affecting bones, joints, abdomen, viscera, back
- Increased risk of infection, especially with encapsulated organisms due to functional asplenia

#### Herpes zoster
FEATURES
- Low-grade fever
- Prodromal phase occurs prior to eruption of vesicular rash, involves dermatomal distribution of tingling, paresthesia, pain
- Eruption of erythematous, macropapular rash along involved dermatomal distribution, with characteristic evolution to pustular/hemorrhagic vesicles
- Postherpetic neuralgia

#### Tabes dorsalis
FEATURES
- Characteristic lancinating lightning pains, may initially affect limbs, but may also cause severe, sudden abdominal pain
- Visceral crisis involves severe abdominal pain and vomiting
- Ataxia, hypotonia, hyporeflexia, impaired kinesthesia
- Bilateral Argyll Robertson pupils
- Romberg's sign

#### Diabetic ketoacidsis
FEATURES
- Abdominal pain, tenderness to palpation
- Nausea, vomiting, decreased bowel sounds
- Tachycardia, tachypnea, may have fever
- Acetone breath
- Dehydration
- Acidosis

#### Porphyria
FEATURES
- Neurovisceral symptoms include severe abdominal pain and tenderness, nausea, vomiting, ileus, decreased bowel sounds
- Afebrile
- Hypotension, tachycardia
- Pain in limbs, muscle weakness
- Dysuria and urinary retention

- Dark red or brown urine
- May have psychiatric and neurologic symptoms, including sensory and motor impairment, psychosis, hallucinations, depression, and seizures

## Plumbism
### FEATURES
Three potential clinical syndromes are distinguished:
- Alimentary: anorexia, constipation, severe abdominal spasms, colicky pain, abdominal rigidity
- Neuromuscular: painless peripheral neuritis, primarily of extensors
- Cerebral type (lead encephalopathy): seizures, coma, long-term neurological sequelae, including retarded cognition, hyperactivity

## Uremia
### FEATURES
- Anorexia, vomiting
- Abdominal pain
- Muscle cramps and twitching, neuropathy
- Nocturia, polyuria
- Confusion, depression, seizures

## SIGNS & SYMPTOMS
### Signs
- Patient tends to lie still, supine, knees flexed
- Fever
- Tachycardia, hypotension
- Hypoactive bowel sounds
- Diffuse abdominal tenderness, rebound tenderness
- Abdominal distension, with percussive hyper-resonance
- Board-like rigidity of abdomen
- Involuntary guarding
- Shallow, rapid inspiratory effort
- Signs and symptoms may be subtle or absent in spontaneous bacterial peritonitis

### Symptoms
- Abdominal pain (may be sudden and severe in case of ruptured viscus), increased with movement, inspiration
- Nausea, vomiting
- Constipation, absent flatus

## KEY! DON'T MISS!
It is crucial to assess for the presence of a surgical abdomen, and refer immediately to a surgeon for assessment.

## CONSIDER CONSULT
- Referral is required for patients with severe, sudden onset of abdominal pain, which may be due to a ruptured viscus
- Paracentesis or peritoneal lavage with aspiration may be helpful adjuncts to an exploration to help differentiate primary peritonitis from secondary peritonitis

## INVESTIGATION OF THE PATIENT
### Direct questions to patient
Q When did your pain begin? What things seem to improve or worsen your pain?
Understanding duration, progression, and issues of amelioration vs exacerbation are important

for developing differential diagnosis
- **Q Have you had a fever?** Bacterial peritonitis often presents with fever
- **Q Have you recently suffered any injuries?** Recent abdominal trauma is a predisposing factor for peritonitis
- **Q Have you had any recent surgery?** Recent abdominal surgery is a predisposing factor for peritonitis, as are many surgical conditions (i.e. bowel perforation, appendicitis)
- **Q Are you taking any medications?** Patients receiving immunosuppressive medications may have masked symptoms; therefore, high level of suspicion for peritonitis must be maintained

### Contributory or predisposing factors
**Is there a history of predisposing factors?** A number of conditions have peritonitis as a complication, including: peptic ulcer disease, diverticulosis, Crohn's disease, systemic lupus erythematosus, familial Mediterranean fever, cirrhosis, hepatitis, congestive heart failure, a history of malignancy, lymphedema, nephrotic syndrome, HIV infection, porphyria

### Examination
- **General examination.** Patients with peritonitis tend to lie still, and appear very unwell
- **Check temperature.** Patients with peritonitis are usually febrile
- **Check heart rate, blood pressure.** Patients with peritonitis are usually tachycardic; hypotension may supervene if patient is becoming septic
- **Observe pattern of breathing.** Patients with peritonitis are usually tachypneic
- **Survey mucous membranes, skin turgor for signs of dehydration.** Patients with peritonitis are often dehydrated, owing to associated nausea and vomiting
- **Check eyes for scleral icterus, skin for jaundice.** Certain liver and gallbladder conditions predisposing to peritonitis may cause icterus, jaundice
- **Visually assess abdomen for signs of distension.** Ascites is a common condition predisposing to peritonitis
- **Auscultate abdomen using light pressure, observing for signs of tenderness, noting presence/absence/hypoactivity of bowel sounds.** Specific abdominal pathology leading to peritonitis will present with specific patterns of tenderness, possible ileus
- **Percuss abdomen gently, listening intently for hyper-resonance of an air-filled abdomen or dullness of fluid-filled abdomen.** Examine carefully to determine possible perforation of an intestinal viscus (resulting in air-filled abdomen) or presence of ascites (resulting in fluid-filled abdomen)
- **Palpate abdomen gently, beginning in quadrant furthest from area of maximal tenderness; observe for guarding, note referred or rebound tenderness, rigidity.** Board-like rigidity is a sign of severe peritonitis; begin away from area of maximal tenderness in order to be able to perform the most complete examination possible
- **Perform a rectal examination.** Rectal examination may reveal presence of an abscess, may add to information regarding abdominal tenderness/pain

### Summary of investigative tests
If peritonitis is suspected clinically:
- Urgent transfer to the emergency department is indicated
- No initial testing would need to be carried out by the primary care physician in this situation

In case of diagnostic doubt, the following tests may be useful:
- Complete blood count
- Electrolyte studies
- Arterial blood gases
- Blood culture
- Serum amylase may help determine the cause of peritonitis. Amylase is most commonly raised with pancreatitis, but may also be high with perforated viscus

- Ascitic fluid analysis: consider paracentesis and/or peritoneal lavage with Ringer's lactate; examine aspirated fluid for blood, pus, bile, digested fat, amylase content, and Gram stain for presence/identification of bacteria
- Plain abdominal radiographs can provide useful information about patterns of bowel gas and the presence of free air in the abdominal cavity
- Chest X-ray may reveal air under the diaphragm in the case of perforated viscus
- Consider computed tomography (CT) scanning with oral and intravenous contrast, which is particularly useful in patients with fever; abdominal X-rays are not likely to reveal pathology that CT scanning cannot
- Consider ultrasound scan, which may be able to provide useful information in cholecystitis and cholangitis, hepatic abscess, small bowel inflammation (e.g. in Crohn's disease), and the presence of ascitic fluid; however, many areas of the abdomen are not well visualized, and increased bowel gas or intra-abdominal free air reduces its usefulness

## DIAGNOSTIC DECISION
- The most important decision to make in a patient with suspected peritonitis is the differentiation of primary peritonitis from secondary peritonitis
- Primary peritonitis can generally be treated medically, while secondary peritonitis generally will require a surgical intervention
- Factors which make primary peritonitis more likely include (1) less severe or no pain; (2) gradual onset; (3) the absence of peritoneal signs (rebound, guarding); and (4) the presence of predisposing condition causing ascites, most commonly cirrhosis
- Factors which make secondary peritonitis more likely include (1) severe pain of relatively sudden onset; (2) peritoneal signs; and (3) the absence of cirrhosis
- The two most useful tests to differentiate between primary and secondary peritonitis are (1) peritoneal tap and (2) radiographic imaging of the abdomen for free air
- The presence of multiple organisms in culture or Gram stain of peritoneal fluid is highly suggestive of a perforated viscus and secondary peritonitis
- The presence of free air on an upright or lateral decubitus abdominal film is specific for perforated viscus, unless there has been recent abdominal surgery or peritoneal manipulation
- If free air is not seen and perforated viscus is still strongly suspected, a CT scan may be more sensitive to finding free air from a perforated viscus and assessing underlying disease process

## CLINICAL PEARL(S)
- If caught early, spontaneous bacterial peritonitis (SBP) is often subtle in its presentation. The most common early symptoms are fever, abdominal pain or tenderness, and altered mental status. Some patients are asymptomatic
- SBP rarely develops without obvious, large volume ascites
- In patients with ascites, peritoneal taps are indicated for any sign of infection, unless obviously due to a viral syndrome
- Almost all patients with SBP have portal hypertension. The serum-ascitic fluid albumin gradient is almost invariably >1.1g/L. Patients with ascites due to nephrotic syndrome also seem at risk for SBP. Low protein in the ascitic fluid (<1g/L) seems to play an important role in predisposing to spontaneous infection probably due to the low level of bacterial opsonins

## THE TESTS
### Body fluids
COMPLETE BLOOD COUNT
*Description*
Venous blood sample.

*Advantages/Disadvantages*
Advantages: fast, easy, inexpensive test that can give virtually immediate results.

*Normal*
- Hemoglobin: 13.6–17.7g/dL (males); 12.0–15.0g/dL (females)
- Red blood cells: 4.3–5.9x10$^6$/mm$^3$ (males); 3.5–5.0x10$^6$/mm$^3$ (females)
- White blood cells (WBC): 3.8–11.0x10$^3$/mm$^3$
- Neutrophils: 1.94–7.78x10$^3$/mm$^3$
- Lymphocytes: 1.08–3.10x10$^3$/mm$^3$
- Monocytes: 0.240–0.870x10$^3$/mm$^3$
- Eosinophils: 0.028–0.531x10$^3$/mm$^3$
- Basophils: 0.011–0.106x10$^3$/mm$^3$
- Platelets: 156–352x10$^3$/mm$^3$

*Abnormal*
- Leukocytosis with left shift is indicative of infection, but not specific to peritonitis
- Hematocrit level may also help give an indication of hydration status

*Cause of abnormal result*
Systemic infection.

*Drugs, disorders and other factors that may alter results*
- Immunosuppressed patients may have low WBC in the setting of infection, while patients on corticosteroid medications may have high WBC (up to 20,000) in the absence of infection
- Sepsis or severe infection can sometimes not cause leukocytosis, but only a shift to the left
- A myriad of other disorders are reflected in blood count abnormalities, including anemia, leukemia, platelet disorders, allergic phenomena; complete blood count results must be carefully correlated with clinical condition

ELECTROLYTE STUDIES
*Description*
Venous blood sample.

*Advantages/Disadvantages*
Advantages: fast, inexpensive, can be performed immediately.

*Normal*
- Sodium: 135–147mEq/L
- Potassium: 3–5mEq/L
- Blood urea nitrogen (BUN): 8–18mg/dL
- Creatinine: 0.6–1.2mg/dL
- Phosphate: 2.5–5mg/dL
- Magnesium: 1.8–3.0mg/dL
- Calcium: 8.8–10.3mg/dL
- Albumin: 4–6g/dL

*Abnormal*
- Examine results for signs of dehydration (increased BUN), other electrolyte derangements caused by vomiting
- Keep in mind the possibility of a false-positive result

*Cause of abnormal result*
Dehydration resulting from vomiting or inadequate oral intake in a patient with peritonitis.

*Drugs, disorders and other factors that may alter results*
Many situations can alter results of electrolyte studies; results must be carefully correlated with patient's clinical condition.

## ARTERIAL BLOOD GAS
*Description*
Arterial blood sample.

*Advantages/Disadvantages*
- Advantages: Simple test with rapid results
- Disadvantage: painful

*Normal*
- pH: 7.35–7.45
- $pO_2$: 100–105mmHg
- $pCO_2$: 35–45mmHg

*Abnormal*
- Values outside the normal range
- Use values to determine presence of metabolic and/or respiratory acidosis

*Cause of abnormal result*
Metabolic acidosis may result from lactic acid production in ischemic tissue.

*Drugs, disorders and other factors that may alter results*
Be aware that smokers will often have abnormal results, as will patients with pulmonary conditions.

## BLOOD CULTURE
*Description*
- Try to draw blood during fever spike
- Aseptic technique essential
- Preferred method involves three culture sets drawn 3h apart; some practitioners suggest drawing from more than one site
- Best to draw prior to starting antibiotics, but if antibiotics must be started prior to culture draw, note on laboratory request form

*Advantages/Disadvantages*
- Advantage: may reveal presence of causative micro-organism, as well as identifying that micro-organism's antibiotic sensitivities
- Disavantage: may be negative if infection is sequestered in abdomen, or if peritonitis is due to chemical irritation of peritoneum

*Normal*
No growth after 72h; may choose to continue running plate for up to one week to ensure no growth.

*Abnormal*
- Positive culture growth
- Keep in mind the possibility of a false-positive result, often due to surface skin contaminants

*Cause of abnormal result*
True bacteremia.

*Drugs, disorders and other factors that may alter results*
Verify whether or not patient has been started on antibiotics, or whether patient has recently completed a course of antibiotics, as antibiotic usage could result in a false-negative result.

### SERUM AMYLASE
*Description*
Venous blood sample.

*Advantages/Disadvantages*
Advantages: easily obtained, rapid results.

*Normal*
60–180U/L.

*Abnormal*
- Value above normal limits
- Keep in mind the possibility of a false-positive result

*Cause of abnormal result*
Most commonly from pancreatitis, though elevation also seen in biliary tract disease and perforated viscus, particularly with perforated ulcer.

*Drugs, disorders and other factors that may alter results*
- Amylase values are often abnormally elevated in chronic renal insufficiency due to decreased amylase clearance
- Macroamylasemia occurs when an abnormal serum protein binds to normal serum amylase producing a macroamylase complex that is not cleared by normal kidneys, thereby elevating serum amylase

### ASCITIC FLUID ANALYSIS
*Description*
- Performed through paracentesis if ascites is present
- If no ascitic fluid found, consider performing peritoneal lavage and testing aspirated lavage fluid
- Ascitic fluid should be analyzed for (1) cell count with differential; (2) protein and albumin; and (3) Gram stain and culture. A matching serum albumin is helpful in determining if the ascitic fluid is due to cirrhosis
- Optional tests include (1) cytology for malignant cells and (2) glucose and lactate dehydrogenase (LDH)

*Advantages/Disadvantages*
Advantages:
- Test can be rapidly performed; fluid can be rapidly analyzed
- Can be diagnostic of peritonitis, and may help differentiate between primary and secondary causes of peritonitis

Disadvantages:
- Slightly painful
- Slight risk of causing pneumothorax, bowel perforation, or intraperitoneal bleeding

*Normal*
Normally no ascites in the abdomen. Patients with uninfected ascites from an underlying condition will have fewer than 250 cells(PMNs)/mm$^3$.

*Abnormal*
- Examine aspirated fluid for presence of blood, pus, digested fat, amylase level
- Polymorphonuclear cell count >250 cells/mm$^3$ suggests spontaneous bacterial peritonitis
- Greatly elevated polymorphonuclear cell count (5000 cells/mm$^3$ suggests a secondary cause of peritonitis
- Increased amylase suggests a perforated viscus or pancreatitis
- Gram stain positive

*Cause of abnormal result*
- May indicate perforated viscus, infection, chemical irritation due to presence of spilled pancreatic juices and/or bile
- May help distinguish between peritonitis secondary to perforation and spontaneous bacterial peritonitis

## Imaging
PLAIN ABDOMINAL RADIOGRAPHS
*Description*
- Will generally include supine and upright films
- In situations when the patient cannot be positioned upright (severe pain, mechanically ventilated), the left lateral decubitus position may be useful for identifying free intra-abdominal air

*Advantages/Disadvantages*
Advantages:
- Noninvasive
- Widely available, relatively inexpensive
- Easily obtained

Disadvantages: exposes the patient to small amounts of ionizing radiation; not ideal for pregnant patients (or patients who may be pregnant).

*Abnormal*
- Free air in abdomen, under diaphragm, indicating likely ruptured viscus
- Signs of other abdominal pathology, including ileus, bowel dilation, intestinal edema, volvulus, intussusception, vascular occlusion

*Cause of abnormal result*
May see features characteristic of specific forms of abdominal pathology which could be causing secondary peritonitis.

*Drugs, disorders and other factors that may alter results*
Other abdominal pathology may be revealed.

CHEST X-RAY
*Advantages/Disadvantages*
Advantages:
- Can help clarify differential diagnosis
- Safe, quick, provides information regarding chest pathology, or presence of air under the diaphragm which could suggest perforation of abdominal viscus

*Abnormal*
- Presence of chest pathology which could account for shallow inspiration, referred pain
- Presence of subdiaphragmatic air

*Cause of abnormal result*
- Ruptured viscus could result in collection of subdiaphragmatic air
- Chest, lung pathology could be revealed

### CT SCAN OF ABDOMEN, WITH ORAL AND INTRAVENOUS CONTRAST
*Advantages/Disadvantages*
Advantages:
- May reveal presence of abdominal pathology, thereby helping to distinguish between causes of peritonitis best served by medical management, versus those requiring immediate laparotomy
- May also be helpful to guide paracentesis
- Generally provides more information than plain abdominal X-rays
- Sensitive to very small volumes of intra-abdominal free air (more so than plain abdominal radiographs)
- Very useful for identifying bowel obstruction (especially high-grade bowel obstruction), including closed-loop obstruction with strangulation
- Sensitive to intestinal ischemia and infarction
- Procedure of choice for diagnosing abscess and revealing its location and extent, including postoperative abscess
- Reveals the extent of abscess-related sinus tracts and fistulas
- More useful than plain radiographs for clarifying diagnostic doubt about a diagnosis of appendicitis in patients without a clear clinical picture

Disadvantages:
- More expensive and less readily available than plain radiographs
- Risk of adverse reaction to the contrast medium

*Abnormal*
CT scanning can point to numerous intra-abdominal pathologies that can cause peritonitis.

### ABDOMINAL ULTRASOUND
*Advantages/Disadvantages*
Advantages:
- Often useful for providing clues about a gynecological cause of pain
- Does not expose the patient to ionizing radiation, and therefore particularly useful in pregnant patients (or patients who may be pregnant)
- Especially useful in right upper quadrant pain
- Useful for determining presence of gallbladder and bile duct pathology
- Useful in detecting a small amount of ascitic fluid

Disadvantages:
- Useful information derived from this test may be limited by patient's pain from pressure of transducer
- Not as useful in overweight and obese patients
- Operator-dependent

*Abnormal*
Abdominal ultrasound scanning can point to various intra-abdominal pathologies that can cause peritonitis.

# TREATMENT

## CONSIDER CONSULT
Refer immediately if surgical abdomen is suspected.

## IMMEDIATE ACTION
- Intravenous fluid and electrolyte therapy to correct dehydration, metabolic, and electrolyte derangements
- If a perforated viscus is suspected: (1) obtain surgical consultation immediately and (2) start on broad-spectrum antibiotics to cover aerobic and anaerobic gut organisms
- If primary bacterial peritonitis is suspected: (1) perform blood cultures and peritoneal tap and (2) start broad-spectrum antibiotics aimed at aerobic organisms, generally a third-generation cephalosporin or a fluoroquinolone

## PATIENT AND CAREGIVER ISSUES
### Health-seeking behavior
**Is the patient on antibiotics or has the patient recently been on antibiotics?** This information can affect results of laboratory testing on blood and ascitic fluid samples.

## MANAGEMENT ISSUES
### Goals
- Quickly assess need for emergency surgery
- Correct fluid, electrolyte, and metabolic disturbances
- Begin appropriate intravenous antibiotics in a timely fashion to prevent spread of infection
- Reduce patient's pain

### Management in special circumstances
Some patients may reveal more minimal pain symptomatology, requiring a higher degree of suspicion:
- Very young patients
- Elderly patients
- Patients taking corticosteroids or other immunosuppressive agents
- Patients with ascites

### COEXISTING DISEASE
Patients with pre-existing conditions which suggest the development of ascites will benefit from both diagnostic and possibly therapeutic paracentesis.

### COEXISTING MEDICATION
Remember that patients on immunosuppressive regimens may have less intense pain, but a greater chance of perforation.

### SPECIAL PATIENT GROUPS
Treatment will remain the same, but a higher degree of suspicion regarding serious abdominal pathology must be maintained when considering diagnosis in the very young, the elderly, and patients who are on immunosuppressive regimens.

## SUMMARY OF THERAPEUTIC OPTIONS
### Choices
- Intravenous antibiotic therapy, to be determined by specific setting of peritonitis and by sensitivities as determined through laboratory testing
- For presumed spontaneous bacterial peritonitis awaiting cultures, monotherapy is appropriate with cefotaxime or ceftriaxone

- For presumed secondary bacterial peritonitis awaiting cultures, several antibiotic combination regimens can be used to cover aerobic and anaerobic bowel flora: ampicillin plus gentamicin (or another aminoglycoside) plus clindamycin or metronidazole; gentamicin (or another aminoglycoside) plus clindamycin; gentamicin (or another aminoglycoside) plus cefoxitin, cefotetan, clindamycin, or chloramphenicol
- Infusion of antibiotics through abdominal peritoneal dialysis (e.g. intraperitoneal gentamicin plus vancomycin or intraperitoneal ceftazidime); this therapy would normally be instigated by a specialist
- May require surgery, depending on existence of intra-abdominal pathology
- Fluid, electrolyte, and metabolic derangements must be resolved through appropriate fluid resuscitation
- Ileus or obstruction may require nasogastric intubation, suction
- Pain will probably require treatment with intravenous or intramuscular analgesics such as morphine or meperidine

### Clinical pearl(s)
- If fever, abdominal pain or tenderness, or altered mental status are present, treatment of presumed bacterial peritonitis should begin as soon as ascitic fluid, blood, and urine have been obtained for culture and analysis. If patients lack these findings, treatment can await results of the ascitic fluid polymorphonuclear neutrophil leukocyte count
- In spontaneous bacterial peritonitis, the likely organisms are *Escherichia coli*, *Streptococcus pneumoniae*, and *Enterobacteriaceae*. Infection rarely occurs with anaerobic bacteria and *Mycobacterium tuberculosis*. Appropriate initial therapy is a third generation cephalosporin with good antistreptococcal activity
- In secondary peritonitis, infection with *Enterobacteriaceae*, obligate anaerobes, and *Enterococci* are most common, thereby justifying the two- and three-drug regimens. However, *Staphylococci*, *M. tuberculosis*, and *Neisseria gonorrhoeae* are also occasionally found
- For spontaneous bacterial peritonitis, nephrotoxic antibiotics should be avoided because of a high risk of renal failure in the face of cirrhosis, ascites, and peritonitis
- Recent studies have indicated that infusion of albumin reduces the risks of renal failure and improves survival in patients with spontaneous bacterial peritonitis

## FOLLOW UP
### Plan for review
- Most patients with primary bacterial peritonitis will respond to appropriate therapy within 48h
- If there is no response or condition is worsening, repeat paracentesis may be necessary
- If cell count is increasing, this suggests the initial antibiotic choice is ineffective, or that there is actually an unrecognized perforated viscus
- Repeat paracentesis is generally not necessary in patients responding appropriately to therapy

### Information for patient or caregiver
To reduce risk of future episodes, patients with one episode of primary peritonitis should take either one double-strength trimethoprim-sulfamethoxazole daily or a quinolone antibiotic once a week (e.g. ciprofloxacin).

## DRUGS AND OTHER THERAPIES: DETAILS
### Drugs
CEFOTAXIME
*Dose*
Adult dose: 2g intravenously every 8h for 5 days.

*Efficacy*
Good efficacy against Gram-positive and Gram-negative organisms.

*Risks/benefits*
Risks:
- Use caution with hypersensitivity to penicillins
- Use caution with renal impairment
- Risk of pseudomembranous colitis
- Potentially life-threatening arrhymias following rapid (less than 60s) bolus administration via central venous catheter have been observed

Benefit: preferable to many other regimens, owing to its lack of nephrotoxic effects.

*Side effects and adverse reactions*
- Central nervous system: headache, sleep disturbance, confusion, dizziness
- Gastrointestinal: anorexia, nausea, diarrhea, abdominal pain, bleeding, raised liver enzymes, vomiting, pseudomembranous colitis
- Genitourinary: moniliasis, vaginitis
- Hematologic: neutropenia, transient leukopenia, eosinophilia, thrombocytopenia, agranulocytosis
- Hypersensitivity manifestations: pruritus, fever, eosinophilia, urticaria, and (rarely) anaphylaxis (2.4%)
- Skin: rash, dermatitis, injection site reaction
- Other: interstitial nephritis and transient elevations of blood urea nitrogen and creatinine have been occasionally observed with cefotaxime sodium, transient elevations in serum glutamic pyruvic transminase, serum glutamic oxaloacetic transaminase, serum lactate dehydrogenase, and serum alkaline phosphatase levels have been reported

*Interactions (other drugs)*
- Aminoglycosides
- Chloramphenicol
- Oral anticoagulants
- Probenecid
- Vancomycin
- Polymyxin B

*Contraindications*
- Hypersensitivity to cefotaxime
- Age less than one month

*Acceptability to patient*
Acute, severe nature of illness makes treatment highly acceptable to patient.

CEFTRIAXONE
*Dose*
Adult dose: 1–2g intravenously every 24h for 5 days.

*Efficacy*
Effective against a wide spectrum of bacteria, including many Gram-positive and Gram-negative organisms; not effective against anaerobes.

*Risks/benefits*
Risks:
- Use caution in patients with penicillin hypersensitivity
- Use caution in renal disease
- Risk of pseudomembranous colitis

Benefits:
- Good choice in elderly patients
- Provides sustained, high bactericidal levels in blood

*Side effects and adverse reactions*
- Central nervous system: headache, sleep disturbance, confusion, dizziness
- Gastrointestinal: anorexia, nausea, diarrhea, abdominal pain, bleeding, raised liver enzymes
- Genitourinary: nephrotoxicity
- Hematologic: bone marrow suppression
- Skin: rash

*Interactions (other drugs)*
- Aminoglycosides
- Chloramphenicol
- Oral anticoagulants
- Probenecid
- Vancomycin
- Polymyxin B

*Contraindications*
- Hypersensitivity
- Infants less than one month

*Acceptability to patient*
Acute, severe nature of illness makes treatment highly acceptable to patient.

AMPICILLIN
*Dose*
Adult dose: 500mg every 6h intravenously.

*Efficacy*
- Effective, particularly against mixed infections, as part of combination therapy (e.g. combined with gentamicin plus clindamycin or with gentamicin plus metronidazole)
- Effective against many Gram-positive and Gram-negative organisms

*Risks/benefits*
Risks:
- Use caution in renal disease mononucleosis
- Use caution in neonates or the elderly
- Do not administer for prolonged or repeated treatment

Benefit: generally well-tolerated.

*Side effects and adverse reactions*
- Central nervous system: seizures, hallucinations, anxiety
- Gastrointestinal: nausea, diarrhea, vomiting, altered liver function tests, pseudomembranous colitis
- Genitourinary: urinary problems, renal damage, moniliasis, vaginitis
- Hematologic: bleeding disorders, bone marrow depression
- Hypersensitivity reactions

*Interactions (other drugs)*
- Allopurinol (may increase incidence of rash)
- Atenolol
- Chloramphenicol (inhibits effect of ampicillin)
- Macrolide and tetracycline antibiotics (inhibit effect of ampicillin)
- Methotrexate
- Oral contraceptives
- Phenindione
- Probenecid (decreases renal tubular secretion of ampicillin)
- Warfarin

*Contraindications*
Hypersensitivity.

*Acceptability to patient*
Acute, severe nature of illness makes treatment highly acceptable to patient.

*Follow up plan*
Monitor stool for change in frequency and consistency, especially in elderly patients.

*Patient and caregiver information*
Educate patient to inform healthcare personnel about stool changes.

## GENTAMICIN

*Dose*
Dose is calculated according to body weight: adults: 3mg/kg/day diluted in 50–100mL normal saline or 5% dextrose in water and infused intravenously over 30–60min in divided doses every 8h.

*Efficacy*
- Effective against broad spectrum of Gram-negative bacteria
- Useful against mixed infections
- Particularly efficacious as part of antibiotic combination (e.g. with clindamycin, with ampicillin plus clindamycin, or with ampicillin plus metronidazole)

*Risks/benefits*
Risks:
- Use caution in prolonged use (may lead to overgrowth of resistant organisms)
- Use caution in pregnancy and lactation, and in neonates and the elderly
- Use caution in Parkinson's disease, renal disease and hypokalemia, and in hearing deficit
- Potentially toxic
- Blood levels need monitoring for safety

*Side effects and adverse reactions*
- Cardiovascular system: changes in blood pressure, palpitations
- Central nervous system: neurotoxicity, dizziness, confusion, convulsions
- Eyes, ears, nose, and throat: irritation, tinnitus, deafness, ototoxicity, visual disturbances
- Gastrointestinal: altered liver function tests, anorexia, nausea, vomiting
- Genitourinary: nephrotoxicity
- Hematologic: blood cell disorders
- Respiratory: respiratory depression
- Skin: rash

*Interactions (other drugs)*
- Amphotericin B ■ Anticholinesterases (neostigmine, pyridostigmine) ■ Antibiotics (penicillins, cephalosporins, polymixins, vancomycin) ■ Anticholinesterases (neostigmine, pyridostigmine) ■ Cyclosporine ■ Loop diuretics ■ Neuromuscular blocking agents (atracurium, vecuronium) ■ Nonsteroidal anti-inflammatory drugs ■ Platinum compounds (carboplatin, cisplatin) ■ Succinylcholine

*Contraindications*
- Hypersensitivity to gentamicin or other aminoglycosides ■ Myasthenia gravis
- Pre-existing deafness ■ Renal impairment

*Acceptability to patient*
Acute, severe nature of illness generally makes treatment highly acceptable to patient.

*Follow up plan*
- Carefully monitor renal and eighth cranial nerve function throughout therapy
- Monitor aminoglycoside serum levels to avoid toxicity
- Monitor stool for change in frequency and consistency, especially in elderly patients

*Patient and caregiver information*
Educate patient to inform healthcare personnel about stool changes.

## CLINDAMYCIN
*Dose*
Adult doses:
- Serious infections: 150–300mg every 6h, orally
- More severe infections: 300–450mg every 6h, orally

*Efficacy*
- Effective against a broad range of Gram-positive and anaerobic bacteria
- Combination therapy (e.g. with gentamicin or with ampicillin plus gentamicin) is efficacious, particularly against mixed infections

*Risks/benefits*
Risks:
- Risk of pseudomembranous enterocolitis higher with clindamycin than with other antibiotics, patients developing diarrhea should be instructed to stop treatment immediately
- Use caution in hepatic or renal disease
- Use caution in the elderly
- Use caution in history of gastrointestinal disease
- Use caution in tartrazine dye hypersensitivity
- Treatment failure can occur due to compliance problems

Benefit: efficacious against anaerobic intra-abdominal infections.

*Side effects and adverse reactions*
- Gastrointestinal: pseudomembranous enterocolitis, abdominal pain, diarrhea, nausea, vomiting
- Genitourinary: vaginitis
- Hematologic: agranulocytosis
- General: hypersensitivity reactions (most commonly rashes)

*Interactions (other drugs)*
- **Erythromycin** ■ **Neuromuscular blocking agents** ■ **Neostigmine, pyridostigmine**

*Contraindications*
- **Hypersensitivity to clindamycin** ■ **Enteritis** ■ **Colitis**

*Acceptability to patient*
Acute, severe nature of illness makes treatment highly acceptable to patient.

*Follow up plan*
Monitor stool for change in frequency, consistency, especially in elderly patients.

*Patient and caregiver information*
Educate patient to inform healthcare personnel about stool changes.

## METRONIDAZOLE
*Dose*
Recommended dosage schedule for adults:
- Loading dose: 15mg/kg infused over 1h (approximately 1g for a 70kg adult)
- Maintenance dose: 7.5mg/kg infused over 1h every 6h (approximately 500mg for a 70kg adult)
- Maximum daily dose: 4g

*Efficacy*
- Effective against trichomoniasis, amebiasis, giardiasis, anaerobic bacteria (both Gram-positive and Gram-negative), and protozoa
- Combination antibiotic therapy (e.g. with ampicillin plus gentamicin) is efficacious, particularly against mixed infections

*Risks/benefits*
Risks:
- Nausea and vomiting likely if alcohol is taken
- Caution in hepatic and renal impairment
- Caution in central nervous system disease or history of seizures

Benefit: effective when used as part of combination therapy for anaerobic coverage.

*Side effects and adverse reactions*
- Central nervous system: dizziness, headache, seizures, ataxia, peripheral neuropathy
- Gastrointestinal: nausea, vomiting, taste disturbance, diarrhea, abdominal pain, dry mouth, anorexia, constipation
- Genitourinary: urination difficulties, cystitis, vaginal dryness
- Hematologic: blood cell disorders
- Skin: rashes, itching, flushing

*Interactions (other drugs)*
- Alcohol
- Antiepileptics
- Anticoagulants
- Barbiturates
- Carbamazepine
- Cholestyramine
- Cimetidine
- Colestipol
- Disulfiram
- Fluorouracil
- Lithium

*Contraindications*
- **Pregnancy and breast-feeding**
- Blood dyscrasias

*Acceptability to patient*
Acute, severe nature of illness makes treatment highly acceptable to patient.

*Follow up plan*
- Monitor for candidiasis and treat with additional candidacidal agents if necessary
- Monitor stool for change in frequency and consistency, especially in elderly patients

*Patient and caregiver information*
Educate patient to inform healthcare personnel about stool changes.

## MORPHINE
*Dose*
Adult dose: 2–10mg intravenously or intramuscularly every 4h as required for pain.

*Efficacy*
Effective against severe pain.

*Risks/benefits*
Risks:
- Use caution in the elderly and patients under 18 years of age
- Use caution in hepatic and renal disease, hypothryoidism, Addison's disease, abdominal disorders, and prostatic hypertrophy
- Nausea may be aggravated, and thus morphine should be given with an antiemetic

*Side effects and adverse reactions*
- Cardiovascular system: bradycardia, tachycardia, palpitations, hypotension, hypertension, syncope
- Central nervous system: drowsiness, sedation, headache, vertigo, hallucinations, dysphoria, euphoria, mood changes, dependence, anxiety, restlessness
- Eyes, ears, nose, and throat: dry mouth, miosis, blurred vision
- Gastrointestinal: constipation, nausea, vomiting, abdominal pain, biliary spasm
- Genitourinary: urinary difficulties, decreased libido
- Respiratory: respiratory depression
- Skin: rashes, pruritus, urticaria, sweating, flushing

*Interactions (other drugs)*
- Alcohol
- Anticoagulants
- Antidepressants (tricyclic)
- Antihistamines
- Antihypertensives
- Antipsychotics
- Anxiolytics and hypnotics
- Cimetidine
- Ciprofloxacin
- Domperidone
- Esmolol
- Monoamine oxidase inhibitors (MAOIs)
- Metoclopramide
- Mexiletine
- Moclobemide
- Opiate antagonists
- Rifamycins
- Ritonavir

*Contraindications*
- Hypersensitivity to morphine
- Morphine sulfate injection contains sodium bisulfite, which may cause allergic-type reactions including anaphylactic symptoms and life-threatening or less severe asthmatic episodes in certain susceptible people
- Heart failure secondary to chronic lung disease
- Cardiac arrhythmias
- Brain tumor
- Acute alcoholism
- Delerium tremens
- Convulsive states
- Respiratory depression
- Hemorrhage
- Acute asthma attack
- Paralytic ileus
- Head injury or raised intracranial pressure
- Injection in pheochromocytoma
- Pregnancy category C
- Breast-feeding

*Acceptability to patient*
Patients may find impairment of mental faculties unpleasant.

*Follow up plan*
Depending on length of use, consider weaning patient incrementally, rather than abruptly discontinuing use.

## MEPERIDINE

*Dose*
Adults: 50–150mg intramuscularly every 3–4h as required for pain.

*Efficacy*
Known to be effective against moderate to severe pain.

*Risks/benefits*
Risks:
- Use caution in head injury, respiratory conditions including asthma, renal or hepatic impairment, hypothyroidism, and Addison's disease
- Use caution in the elderly
- Use caution in patients with supraventricular tachycardias

Benefit: provides rapid analgesia (within 30min or so) after parenteral administration.

*Side effects and adverse reactions*
- Cardiovascular system: tachycardia, bradycardia, palpitations, postural hypotension
- Central nervous system: drowsiness, sedation, seizures, dizziness, tremors

- Gastrointestinal: nausea, vomiting, constipation, anorexia
- Respiratory: respiratory depression
- Skin: rash

*Interactions (other drugs)*
- Antihistamines
- Anxiolytics/hypnotics (chloral hydrate, glutethimide)
- Barbiturates
- Cimetidine
- Ciprofloxacin
- Ethanol
- MAOIs
- Methocarbamol
- Metoclopramide
- Mexiletine
- Neuroleptics
- Phenytoin
- Ritonavir
- Selegiline
- Tricyclic antidepressants

*Contraindications*
- Existing central nervous system depression
- Alcohol abuse
- MAOI therapy (within 14 days)
- Severe renal impairment
- Severe or acute bronchial asthma
- Respiratory depression

*Acceptability to patient*
Patients may find impairment of mental faculties and gastrointestinal effects unpleasant.

*Follow up plan*
Depending on length of use, consider weaning patient incrementally, rather than abruptly discontinuing use.

# OUTCOMES

## PROGNOSIS

Prognosis will depend on the cause of peritonitis, the individual patient's previous state of health, pre-existing conditions, and the time between the onset of the peritonitis and diagnosis and treatment.

### Clinical pearl(s)

- Early recognition is essential for all forms of bacterial peritonitis. Spontaneous bacterial peritonitis is universally fatal once the patient develops shock. Likewise, fatality will occur with an unoperated perforated viscus, unless it spontaneously seals or is walled off
- Antibiotic prophylaxis should be considered for patients with a history of spontaneous bacterial peritonitis and persisting ascites
- For spontaneous bacterial peritonitis, follow-up analysis of ascitic fluid should reveal a sterile culture and a marked decrease in polymorphonuclear neutrophil leukocyte counts. However, if the presentation is typical (advanced cirrhosis, infection with a single organism, high glucose concentration >50mg/dL, lactate dehydrogenase within the range of normal serum concentrations and low ascitic total protein concentration <1g/dL) and the response to therapy is good, then repeat is not necessary
- Repeat paracentesis is necessary if any features are atypical. A lack of resolution also warrants a consideration of secondary bacterial peritonitis and possibly surgical intervention. The risks of surgery are very high in cirrhosis with spontaneous bacterial peritonitis, so that surgery must be cautiously pursued

## COMPLICATIONS

- Abscess formation
- Hypovolemia
- Sepsis, progressing to septic shock
- Organ failure (kidneys, liver)
- Acute respiratory distress syndrome

## PREVENTION

### RISK FACTORS
- Recent surgery
- Recent abdominal trauma
- Alcoholic or postnecrotic cirrhosis
- Hepatitis
- Congestive heart failure
- Metastatic malignancy
- Systemic lupus erythematosus
- Lymphedema
- Nephrotic syndrome
- Porphyria
- Familial Mediterranean fever
- Peptic ulcer disease
- Crohn's disease
- Cholecystitis
- Cholangitis
- Diverticular disease
- Pancreatitis
- Pelvic inflammatory disease
- Peritoneal dialysis
- Use of prednisone or other immunosuppressive agents

## RESOURCES

### KEY REFERENCES
- Sort P, Navasa M, Arroyo V, et al. Effect of intravenous albumin on renal impairment and mortality in patients with cirrhosis and spontaneous bacterial peritonitis. N Engl J Med 1999;341:403–9
- Peritoneum. In: Cotran RS, ed. Robbins pathologic basis of disease. Philadelphia: WB Saunders, 2000
- Peritonitis. In: Mandell GL, et al, eds. Principles and practice of infectious diseases. New York: Churchill Livingstone, 2000
- Peritonitis of other causes. In: Feldman M, et al, eds. Sleisenger & Fordtran's gastrointestinal and liver disease. Philadelphia: WB Saunders, 1998
- Surgical peritonitis. In: Feldman M, et al, eds. Sleisenger & Fordtran's gastrointestinal and liver disease. Philadelphia: WB Saunders, 1998

### FAQS

**Question 1**
In a patient with cirrhosis and ascites, how can I differentiate spontaneous from secondary peritonitis?

ANSWER 1
The same rules apply, except that it is even more important to be accurate because performing laparotomy in the face of ascites and spontaneous bacterial peritonitis carries a very high mortality. The differentiation rests on ascitic fluid analysis, imaging studies, and the response to therapy.

**Question 2**
What are the risk factors for spontaneous bacterial peritonitis?

ANSWER 2
There are three major risk factors: a total ascitic protein <1g/L, variceal hemorrhage, and a prior episode of spontaneous bacterial peritonitis.

**Question 3**
Is there any place for antibiotics in patients with ascites, but no history of spontaneous bacterial peritonitis?

ANSWER 3
There is some evidence that there may be some benefit for patients with a high risk profile, but the issue remains controversial and no clear guidelines have been defined.

### CONTRIBUTORS
Joseph E Scherger, MD, MPH
Andrew H Soll, MD
Laura Targownik, MD, FRCP(C)

# PROCTITIS

- Summary Information — 490
- Background — 491
- Diagnosis — 493
- Treatment — 498
- Outcomes — 505
- Prevention — 506
- Resources — 507

## SUMMARY INFORMATION

### DESCRIPTION

- Relatively common condition
- Bleeding, mucus per rectum
- Tenesmus
- May be associated with ulcerative colitis
- Often because of a sexually transmitted pathogen

### URGENT ACTION

- Usually not an emergency unless associated with acute pancolitis
- This may require urgent gastrointestinal/surgical referral and admission to hospital

### KEY! DON'T MISS!

- Important to distinguish perianal Crohn's disease from other causes of proctitis
- Critical to distinguish anorectal carcinoma from simple proctitis

## BACKGROUND

### ICD9 CODE
569.49 Acute proctitis
556.2 Ulcerative proctitis (nonspecific)
556.3 Ulcerative proctitis with ulcerative sigmoiditis
K62.7 Radiation proctitis
098.7 Gonococcal proctitis
099.52 Chlamydial proctitis
556.2 Idiopathic proctitis
006.8 Amebic proctitis

### SYNONYMS
Ulcerative proctitis

### CARDINAL FEATURES
- Rectal bleeding
- May be painful or painless
- May be associated with mucus
- Diarrhea and frequency of bowel habit
- Tenesmus

### CAUSES
#### Common causes
- Idiopathic ulcerative proctitis
- Crohn's proctitis
- Irradiation proctitis
- Infective proctitis (*Neisseria gonnorrhoea*, herpes simplex virus)

#### Rare causes
- Hemolytic-uremic syndrome
- Connective tissue disease
- Vasculitis
- Amyloidosis
- Behçet's syndrome
- Chronic lymphocytic leukemia
- Lymphoma
- Lipid proctocolitis
- Allergic proctocolitis
- Tuberculosis/syphilis
- *Entamoeba histolytica* and *Giardia lamblia*, most often in patients with AIDS

#### Serious causes
- Chemical proctitis
- Panproctocolitis

#### Contributory or predisposing factors
- Diarrhea secondary to food poisoning exacerbates proctitis
- Anal intercourse predisposes to infective etiologies

### EPIDEMIOLOGY
#### Incidence and prevalence
INCIDENCE
15/1000 in the US.

PREVALENCE
40/1000 in the US.

## Demographics
AGE
- Peak incidence in third and fourth decades but can affect any age
- Entirely dependent upon etiology of proctitis

GENDER
Male:female equal incidence.

RACE
More common in Caucasians in western Europe and North America.

GEOGRAPHY
More common in North America and western Europe.

SOCIOECONOMIC STATUS
- More common in higher socioeconomic groups
- Immigrants to western countries appear to develop the risk ratio of the host country

# DIAGNOSIS

## DIFFERENTIAL DIAGNOSIS
### Rectal carcinoma
Rectal and anal carcinoma may be mistaken for proctitis and vice versa.

FEATURES
- Tenesmus
- Weight loss
- Dark red bleeding
- Positive family history
- Rectal examination may reveal 'Blummers shelf' or frank mass, which should indicate a diagnosis other than simple proctitis

### Perianal abscess
FEATURES
- Fluctuant swelling
- Perianal cellulitis
- In some instances may indicate underlying inflammatory bowel disease, which in turn may cause proctitis

### Hemorrhoids
May be internal or external prolapsed piles.

FEATURES
- Itching
- Perianal discharge
- Bright red rectal bleeding

### Anal fissure
FEATURES
- Bright red blood on defecation
- Pain on defecation

### Fistula
Either anorectal or rectovaginal.

FEATURES
- May present with recurrent abscesses and discharge
- Rectovaginal fistula may be a complication of childbirth
- Fecal matter passed through the vagina

### Food poisoning/dysentery
FEATURES
- May present with rectal bleeding, bloody diarrhea
- Common organisms *Campylobacter*, *Shigella*, *Salmonella* and *Escherichia coli*

### Anal abuse/rape
FEATURES
- History may be difficult to elicit but is of great importance for diagnosis

## SIGNS & SYMPTOMS
### Signs
- Anemia may be present if there is significant blood loss
- Anal inflammation, erythema, or ulceration may be present
- Proctoscopy may reveal edema, erythema, or ulceration
- Bleeding or pus from anus
- Pain or discomfort on rectal examination with spasm
- Abdominal tenderness if colitis is present

### Symptoms
- Change in bowel habit, diarrhea
- Weight loss
- Bleeding per rectum
- Pus or mucus per rectum
- Pain on defecation

## ASSOCIATED DISORDERS
Main association is with proctocolitis (ulcerative colitis and Crohn's disease).

## KEY! DON'T MISS!
- Important to distinguish perianal Crohn's disease from other causes of proctitis
- Critical to distinguish anorectal carcinoma from simple proctitis

## CONSIDER CONSULT
- Failure to resolve with simple medical measures
- Uncertainty of diagnosis
- Perianal Crohn's disease
- Presence of pancolitis
- Suspicion of anorectal carcinoma

## INVESTIGATION OF THE PATIENT
### Direct questions to patient
- **Q** How long have the symptoms been present? A complete history is essential since it can often lead to the specific diagnosis or at least focus the work-up
- **Q** Change in bowel habit, blood mixed with feces, bowel frequency? The signs and symptoms of patients with acute proctitis are variable and may include abdominal cramping, diarrhea with or without blood, mucorrhea, and dehydration
- **Q** Any symptoms indicating severity? The clinical course usually varies from mild to moderate but on occasion, patients may present with severe colitis with perforation requiring urgent operative intervention
- **Q** Additional factors in history? Inquiring about the timing and onset of symptoms as they relate to possible recent foreign travel history, antibiotic use, addition of new pets to the household, and similar symptoms in others in close contact may all provide clues to the etiologic factor

### Contributory or predisposing factors
- **Q** What illnesses have you had in the past? Any other medical problems? Coexistent cardiac or peripheral vascular disease is often related to ischemic colitis and patients that have undergone radiation therapy to the abdomen and pelvis may develop colitis several years later. Psoriasis and seronegative spondyloarthropathy are also associated with proctitis
- **Q** What medicines are you taking? Current medications such as new drugs, antibiotics, cardiac medications, and immunosuppressive agents may all provide insight into the etiology of the colitis
- **Q** Do you ever engage in anorectal intercourse? This predisposes to common sexually transmitted pathogens that may induce proctitis

**Q** Have you had a lot of stress in your life recently? Stress may cause frequent bowel movements and worsen proctitis

## Family history
Any positive family history? A detailed family history of gastrointestinal disorders, including inflammatory bowel disease and colorectal cancer, should be obtained.

## Examination
- What are the findings on rectal examination? Rectal examination, consisting of a digital examination and proctoscopic evaluation is mandatory
- Any abnormalities in the stool? Examination of the stool will reveal its consistency and the presence of occult or gross blood
- Does the mucosa look normal? Inspection of the mucosa may identify edema, ulcerations, and inflammation, as well as specific findings that are pathognomonic for certain disease processes. The mucosa may easily bleed with minimal pressure ('wipe test')
- What is the extent of proctitis? The pattern and level of the mucosal involvement are also important and should be noted
- Can you see the proximal margin complete? If mucosal involvement is too proximal to visualize the limiting edge consider proctocolitis

## Summary of investigative tests
- Stool microscopy and culture: useful to evaluate for infectious proctocolitis. Invasive organisms, including *Campylobacter*, *Shigella*, and *Salmonella*, may present with sheets of leukocytes in a stool specimen. Microscopy is additionally useful for an assessment of ova and parasites, which may help diagnose *Entamoeba histolytica* and other parasitic pathogens. Culture is useful both to identify a specific pathogen, and to determine sensitivity to antibiotics
- Serology for identification of potential causative microorganisms: most useful for herpes simplex virus (HSV), in which an anti-HSV-II IgM may indicate recent exposure, and for syphilis, in which a rapid plasma reagin/venereal disease report may be positive. Bacterial pathogens are generally not diagnosed by serum studies
- Endoscopy and histopathology: most direct diagnostic modality, as proctitis is a histopathologic diagnosis by definition. Can confirm clinical suspicion that symptoms are because of underlying anorectal inflammation
- Plain and contrast radiology: useful if proctocolitis is considered, rather than simple proctitis. May help to evaluate the sigmoid and descending colonic mucosa. Lack of haustra may be seen with ulcerative colitis (pipe-stem colon), and mucosal irregularities may be seen with mucosal edema and ulcerations

## DIAGNOSTIC DECISION
Guidelines have been produced by the American Society for Colon and Rectal Surgeons and published under Core Subjects 2000.

## THE TESTS
### Body fluids
SEROLOGY
*Description*
In particular cases serologic testing can be useful in identifying serum antibodies to organisms such as syphilis, *Chlamydia*, cytomegalovirus, and others.

*Advantages/Disadvantages*
- These tests are expensive and although rising serum titers may imply a systemic infection, they are not specific for gastrointestinal involvement
- Genetic probes, polymerase chain reaction technology, and DNA hybridization techniques are

becoming available to identify several pathogens in the stool but their expense prohibits their widespread use at this time

*Abnormal*
Keep in mind the possibility of a falsely abnormal result.

## STOOL ANALYSIS AND CULTURES
*Description*
- Several organisms produce variable findings on microscopic stool examination including *Salmonella*, *Yersinia*, and *Clostridium difficile*. Although fecal microscopic examination is neither infallible nor even helpful in all cases, it is inexpensive and yields immediate information that can often guide therapy
- A Gram stain should be performed to identify *Neisseria gonorrhea*, *Campylobacter*, and ova and parasites (O&P). At least three specimens may be required for O&P analysis because of the intermittent shedding of ova cysts

*Advantages/Disadvantages*
- Because of the relatively low yield of stool cultures, testing should be performed when there are signs of systemic illness, fever, bloody diarrhea, dehydration, or a prolonged course of the diarrhea
- Routine blood agar cultures are sufficient for the identification of most causes of acute colitis
- If *N. gonorrhea* is suspected, immediate plating on Thayer-Martin medium should be performed
- Cultures to isolate chlamydial infections require the use of a plastic or metal cotton swab because wood interferes with the assay
- Viral cultures should be considered in immunosuppressed patients and may require several weeks to complete. With all cultures, multiple specimens may be necessary to increase the yield of a positive result

*Abnormal*
Keep in mind the possibility of a falsely abnormal result.

*Cause of abnormal result*
- The presence of a large number of leukocytes in the stool indicates an inflammatory process characteristic of certain invasive organisms such as *Shigella*, *Campylobacter*, and certain strains of *E. coli* (EIEC, EHEC)
- The absence of fecal leukocytes is typical of colitides caused by enterotoxins secreted by rotavirus, parasites (*Entameba histolytica*, *Giardia lamblia*), certain strains of *E. coli* (ETEC, APEC, EAEC), *Vibrio cholerae* and food poisoning bacteria (*Staphylococcus aureus*, *Clostridium perfringens*, *Bacillus cereus*)

## Biopsy
### HISTOPATHOLOGY
*Description*
Histopathologic examination of rectal mucosa obtained by endoscopic biopsy can be helpful if obtained within 4 days of the onset of symptoms.

*Advantages/Disadvantages*
- In the acute setting, distinguishing between infectious proctitis and idiopathic ulcerative proctitis may be difficult since both will show edema, neutrophils in the lamina propria, and superficial cryptitis with preservation of the normal crypt pattern
- In lymphogranuloma venereum, often see crypt abscesses and granulomas. Syphilis may produce granulomatous changes as well
- HSV may produce giant cells with inclusion bodies

*Abnormal*
Keep in mind the possibility of a falsely abnormal result.

## Imaging
BARIUM ENEMA
*Advantages/Disadvantages*
Unprepared barium enema may show extent of disease and enough gross mucosal changes to establish diagnosis of ulcerative colitis or Crohn's colitis.

*Abnormal*
- Loss of mucosal pattern, thumbprinting, etc. will only be seen in associated colitis rather than proctitis
- Keep in mind the possibility of a falsely abnormal result

## Special tests
ENDOSCOPY
*Description*
Evaluation of the rectal and colonic mucosa utilizing flexible sigmoidoscopy and/or colonoscopy can be very useful in establishing the diagnosis and determining the extent of the disease.

*Advantages/Disadvantages*
- Endoscopic evaluation is contraindicated in acutely ill patients with severe colitis for fear of perforation
- Flexible sigmoidoscopy can be performed in the office setting with or without bowel preparation
- Colonoscopy may add additional information especially in situations where the inflammatory changes are proximal to the sigmoid colon; it also allows for inspection of the terminal ileum
- Biopsies of inflamed and normal mucosa should be obtained for histopathologic evaluation

*Abnormal*
Positive biopsy would be considered an abnormal finding. Unaffected by drugs although attenuation of biopsy findings may be found if patient already on therapy.

# TREATMENT

## IMMEDIATE ACTION
- Usually not an emergency except when associated with acute pancolitis
- This may require urgent referral to coloproctologist/gastroenterologist and admission to hospital

## PATIENT AND CAREGIVER ISSUES
### Patient or caregiver request
- Sexually transmitted disease aspects
- May be worried about anal/rectal carcinoma

### Health-seeking behavior
Patient may have attempted self-medication with proprietary hemorrhoidal creams/ointments.

## MANAGEMENT ISSUES
### Goals
- Symptom control
- Relief of tenesmus/pain
- Confirmation of diagnosis
- Treatment of infection with appropriate antibiotics

### Management in special circumstances
Special circumstances if proctitis is thought to be related to sexually transmitted disease.

COEXISTING DISEASE
Specific management needed if colitis also present.

COEXISTING MEDICATION
Care may be needed if other medication is being administered in suppository format.

SPECIAL PATIENT GROUPS
Elderly and disabled patients may find use of suppositories difficult.

PATIENT SATISFACTION/LIFESTYLE PRIORITIES
- Use of enema based preparations may be difficult
- Use of condoms must be stressed for patients with sexually transmitted proctitis

## SUMMARY OF THERAPEUTIC OPTIONS
### Choices
- Topical steroids and sytemic steroids form the mainstay of the management of refractory proctitis. Mild proctitis will respond to topical steroids
- Antidiarrheals useful symptomatic treatment in primary care setting
- Aminosalicylates mainstay of second line treatment
- Metronidazole specific therapy in infective proctitis and combination therapy of Crohn's disease
- Ciprofloxacin effective antibiotic in most cases of infective proctitis
- Immunosuppressives third line therapy, usually under supervision of gastroenterologist
- Restorative proctocolectomy and ileal pouch anal anastomosis may have a selective role in treatment of chronic refractory distal proctocolitis that has not responded to steroids. Decision to be made in conjunction with colorectal surgeon

## Clinical pearls
In severe acute proctitis patients may be unable to discriminate between liquid, gas, and solid feces because of 'stiff rectum', which occurs secondary to inflammation. Returning ability to discriminate implies clinical improvement.

## Never
Avoid treating for an infectious proctitis without microbiological evidence.

## FOLLOW UP
Recommendations will differ between infectious and idiopathic forms of proctitis.

## Plan for review
- Infectious forms may need two negative culutures and cessation of symptoms prior to discharge
- Idiopathic forms may need symptom control plus quiescence of disease

## DRUGS AND OTHER THERAPIES: DETAILS
### Drugs
TOPICAL STEROIDS
Corticosteroid-containing suppositories or enemas.

*Dose*
- Hydrocortisone suppository: insert one suppository (25mg) in rectum daily (morning and night) for 2 weeks; in more severe cases insert one suppository three times daily or two suppositories twice daily
- Hydrocortisone enema: 100mg rectal retention enema, nightly, as required for 21 days

*Efficacy*
- Topical preparations used in mild proctitis
- Systemic therapy indicated in more severe, intractable disease particularly when associated with panproctocolitis

*Risks/benefits*
- Good first line treatment
- Will not treat severe systemic disease
- Some systemic absorption will occur with rectal preparations
- Simple dosing regimen allows for better patient compliance, also allows for application directly to area affected
- Use caution in elderly due to risk of diabetes and osteoporosis
- Use caution in patients with psychosis, seizure disorders or myasthenia gravis
- Use caution in congestive heart failure, hypertension
- Use caution in ulcerative colitis, peptic ulcer or esophagitis

*Side effects and adverse reactions*
- Cardiovascular system: hypertension, thromboembolism
- Central nervous system: insomnia, euphoria, depression, psychosis, seizures
- Endocrine: adrenal suppression, impaired glucose tolerance, growth suppression in children
- Eyes, ears, nose, and throat: cataract, glaucoma, blurred vision
- Gastrointestinal: dyspepsia, peptic ulceration, esophagitis, oral candidiasis, nausea, vomiting
- Musculoskeletal: proximal myopathy, osteoporosis
- Skin: rash, dermatitis, pruritus, atrophy, hypopigmentation, striae, xerosis, burning, stinging upon application, alopecia, conjunctivitis, delayed healing, acne, striae
- Systemic side effects: systemic absorption of hydrocortisone is minimal but theoretical

*Interactions (other drugs)*
- No known interactions with topical hydrocortisone although systemic absorption theoretically means that drug interactions can occur ■ Adrenergic neurone blockers, alpha blockers, beta blockers, beta 2 agonists ■ Aminoglutethamide ■ Anticonvulsants (carbamazepine, phenytoin, barbiturates) ■ Antidiabetics ■ Antidysrhythmics (calcium channel blockers, cardiac glycosides) ■ Antifungals (amphotericin, ketoconazole) ■ Antihypertensives (angiotensin-converting enzyme (ACE) inhibitors, diuretics: loop and thiazide, acetazolamide; angiotensin II receptor antagonists, clonidine, diazoxide, hydralazine, methyldopa, minoxidil) ■ Cyclosporine ■ Erythromycin ■ Methotrexate ■ Nonsteroidal anti-inflammatory drugs (NSAIDs) ■ Nitrates ■ Nitroprusside ■ Oral contraceptives ■ Rifampin ■ Ritonavir ■ Somatropin ■ Vaccines

*Contraindications*
- Systemic infection ■ Poor circulation ■ History of tuberculosis ■ Cushing's syndrome
- Recent myocardial infarction

*Acceptability to patient*
Simple and effective. Suppository and enema format disliked by some patients.

*Follow up plan*
None in particular. Can be self-treated.

*Patient and caregiver information*
If self-treating, need to be aware if symptoms worsen.

### ANTIDIARRHEALS
- Useful in modulating the symptoms of diarrhea
- Loperamide hydrochloride

*Dose*
Loperamide hydrochloride: initially 4mg orally, followed by 2mg after each loose stool, maximum dose of 16mg/day.

*Efficacy*
Useful only if underlying diarrhea.

*Risks/benefits*
- Patient needs to be told that the antidiarrheal therapy is not treating the underlying disease
- Use caution in liver disease, dehydration, and severe ulcerative colitis
- Not recommmended in children

*Side effects and adverse reactions*
- Central nervous system: fatigue, dizziness, drowsiness
- Gastrointestinal: nausea, constipation, toxic megacolon, abdominal cramps and bloating, paralytic ileus, vomiting
- Genitourinary: nephrotoxicity
- Respiratory: respiratory depression
- Skin: rash

*Interactions (other drugs)*
- Bethanechol ■ Cholestyramine ■ Cisapride ■ Metoclopramide ■ Erythromycin

*Contraindications*
- Development of abdominal distension or inhibition of peristalsis ■ Acute diarrhea owing to

infectious organisms such as *Escherichia coli, Salmonella, Shigella* ■ Pseudomembranous colitis associated with broad-spectrum antibiotics ■ Acute dysentery

*Acceptability to patient*
Simple and effective for minor symptomatic disease.

*Follow up plan*
No specific follow up needed.

## AMINOSALICYLATES
Various preparations. Various forms and differing bioavailability. Drugs useful in proctitis must reach the distal colon in active format: alternatively they may be administered in enema form. Olsalazine is effective maintenance therapy.

*Dose*
- Olsalazine: 1g orally in divided doses daily
- Sulfasalazine: initially 1g three to four times daily; maintenance dose is 2g/day in divided doses every 6h

*Efficacy*
Most effective for proctocolitis related to inflammatory bowel disease. Infectious proctitis unlikely to resolve with this treatment alone.

*Risks/benefits*
- Should be used with caution during pregnancy and breast-feeding
- Use caution in renal disease
- Use caution in children

*Side effects and adverse reactions*
- Central nervous system: fever, depression, dizziness, headache
- Gastrointestinal: nausea, vomiting, diarrhea, abdominal pain, anorexia, bloating, raised liver enzymes, hepatitis
- Hematologic: blood cell dyscrasias
- Musculoskeletal: arthralgia
- Skin: rash, pruritus

*Interactions (other drugs)*
**Digoxin.**

*Contraindications*
■ Hypersenstivity to salicylates ■ Severe renal impairment

*Acceptability to patient*
Usually quite simple, safe treatment. For long-term patients, periodic checking of the white cell count may be appropriate.

*Follow up plan*
Periodic monitoring of complete blood count, creatinine, alanine aminotransferase for long-term patients.

*Patient and caregiver information*
Warn about common side effects.

## METRONIDAZOLE
Useful in antibiotic associated proctocolitis (*Clostridium difficile* toxin) but also useful in conditions like giardiasis.

*Dose*
250–500mg three-times daily for 7–14 days.

*Efficacy*
In infectious causes, rapid efficacy.

*Risks/benefits*
- May have neuropathy
- Good for combination therapy for anaerobic coverage
- Nausea and vomiting likely if alcohol is taken
- Avoid in pregnancy and nursing
- Caution in hepatic and renal impairment, central nervous system disease, or history of seizures

*Side effects and adverse reactions*
- Central nervous system: dizziness, headache, siezures, ataxia, peripheral neuropathy
- Gastrointestinal: nausea, vomiting, taste disturbance, diarrhea, abdominal pain, dry mouth, anorexia, constipation
- Genitourinary: urination difficulties, cystitis, vaginal dryness
- Hematological: blood cell disorders
- Skin: rashes, itching, flushing

*Interactions (other drugs)*
- Alcohol ■ Antiepileptics ■ Anticoagulants ■ Barbiturates ■ Carbamazepine
- Cholestyramine ■ Cimetidine ■ Colestipol ■ Disulfiram ■ Fluorouracil ■ Lithium ■ Warfarin

*Contraindications*
First trimester of pregnancy, as it is a known carcinogen in rats.

*Acceptability to patient*
May leave metallic taste in mouth. Interaction with alcohol may be problematic.

*Follow up plan*
Need repeat stool cultures if for infective indication.

*Patient and caregiver information*
Mention interaction with alcohol.

## CIPROFLOXACIN
Quinolone antibiotic useful in infectious proctitis.

*Dose*
Ciprofloxacin 500mg orally, twice daily.

*Efficacy*
Most useful for Gram-negative infectious colidities, including *Campylobacter, Yersinia, Shigella,* and *Salmonella.*

*Risks/benefits*
- Not suitable for children or growing adolescents

- Caution in adolescents, pregnancy, epilepsy, glucose-6-phosphate dehydrogenase deficiency, renal disease

*Side effects and adverse reactions*
- Central nervous system: anxiety, depression, dizziness, headache, seizures
- Eyes, ears, nose, and throat: visual disturbances
- Gastrointestinal: abdominal pain, altered liver function, anorexia, diarrhoea, heartburn, vomiting
- Skin: photosensitivity, pruritus, rash

*Interactions (other drugs)*
- Antacids
- Beta-blockers
- Cyclosporine
- Caffeine
- Didanosine
- Diazepam
- Mineral supplements (zinc, magnesium, calcium, aluminium, iron)
- NSAIDs
- Opiates
- Oral anticoagulants
- Phenytoin
- Theophylline
- Warfarin

*Contraindications*
Contraindicated in children less than 18 years of age as it may produce a transient arthropathy in this group.

*Acceptability to patient*
- Generally well tolerated, mild and infrequent side effects
- Many drug interactions
- Clinically important drug interaction between ciprofloxacin and theophylline in asthmatics

*Follow up plan*
Follow up stool culture.

## IMMUNOSUPPRESSIVES
- Azathioprine
- Cyclosporine
- Usually initiated in secondary care, may be useful in cases of intractable proctitis. Azathioprine may be used as a steroid sparing agent

*Dose*
- Azathioprine: 50mg–150mg orally three times a day
- Cyclosporine: 10mg/kg

*Efficacy*
Useful for ulcerative colitis or Crohn's that has not responded to preparations.

*Risks/benefits*
- Potent drug, very close monitoring needed
- Has no depressant effects on bone marrow
- Increased susceptibility to infection and possible development of neoplasia
- Bacterial, fungal, viral and protozoal infections often occur and can be fatal
- Avoid excessive sunlight
- Use caution in hypertension
- Use caution in children and the elderly
- Use caution in hepatic or biliary tract disease
- Recent vaccinations will be rendered ineffective

*Side effects and adverse reactions*
- Gastrointestinal: nausea, vomiting, diarrhea, abdominal pain, hepatic failure, jaundice
- Genitourinary: depression of spermatogenesis

- Hematologic: anemia, leukopenia, pancytopenia, thrombocytopenia
- Musculoskeletal: arthralgia, myalgia, malaise
- Skin: rash, alopecia
- Miscellaneous: fungal, bacterial, protozoal and viral infections, may increase risk of neoplasm (skin cancer, reticulocyte or lymphomatous tumors)

*Interactions (other drugs)*
- ACE inhibitors ■ Allopurinol ■ Anticoagulants ■ Carbamazepine ■ Clozapine ■ Co-trimoxazole (TMP-SMX) ■ Cyclosporine ■ Methotrexate ■ Nondepolarizing muscle blockers ■ Vaccines ■ Warfarin

*Contraindications*
- Intramuscular injections ■ Pregnancy or breast-feeding ■ Vaccines

*Acceptability to patient*
High side effect profile. May be acceptable as an alternative to surgery, particularly with stoma formation.

*Follow up plan*
Close follow up with monthly complete blood count and renal function tests.

*Patient and caregiver information*
Side effect profile must be mentioned.

### Surgical therapy
Intractable distal proctocolitis/proctitis refractory to steroids and possibly immunosuppressive therapy, surgical intervention may have a role.

RESTORATIVE PROCTOCOLECTOMY AND ILEAL POUCH ANAL ANASTOMOSIS
This is a major procedure and should only be used for occasional cases of refractory proctitis.

*Efficacy*
Sphincter saving surgery if performed by experts and with careful case selection may improve symptoms and quality of life.

*Risks/benefits*
Pouch surgery may have a considerable number of potential complications:
- Fistula
- Recurrent abscess
- Anastomotic stricture/stenosis
- Sexual/bladder dysfunction
- General complications of major surgery

*Acceptability to patient*
- Major aggressive surgery. Patient needs to be fully counseled
- If outcome less than ideal, patient may be dissatisfied

*Follow up plan*
Careful follow up essential after surgery for at least 3–5 years.

*Patient and caregiver information*
Careful counseling and information about results and complications essential.

# OUTCOMES

## EFFICACY OF THERAPIES
- Simple topical therapies will lead to a resolution of proctitis in 50% of patients within 2–6 weeks, unless there is an underlying infectious etiology which, in turn, must be treated with the appropriate antibiotics
- Of the remaining 50%, half will be controlled by second-line treatments, e.g. mesalamine. However, half of this group will relapse
- The last 25% may need systemic steroids or immunosuppressants
- 75% of this last group will relapse
- Fewer than 5% of all patients require maintenance systemic steroids and/or surgery
- Of infective etiologies, >90% will improve within one week and completely resolve within 6 weeks with appropriate antibiotic therapy

### Review period
6 weeks to 6 months depending on etiology.

## PROGNOSIS
- Simple topical therapies (e.g. corticosteroid suppositories) will lead to a resolution of proctitis in 50% of patients within 2–6 weeks unless there is an underlying infectious etiology which, in turn, must be treated with the appropriate antibiotics
- Of the remaining 50%, half will be controlled by second line treatments, e.g. mesalamine. However, half of this group will relapse
- The last 25% may need systemic steroids or immunosuppressants
- 75% of this last group will relapse
- Fewer than 5% of all patients require maintenance systemic steroids and/or surgery
- Of infective etiologies, 90%+ will improve within one week and completely resolve in 6 weeks

### Clinical pearls
- Advise patients to avoid stressful life events which may precipitate a relapse
- Lidocaine ointment or gel applied per rectum may be used to help with fecal urgency

### Therapeutic failure
- Up to 50% of patients will require second-line therapy
- However, over 90% will have resolution of symptoms with appropriate drug treatment

### Recurrence
25% of patients will relapse.

### Deterioration
Fewer than 10% will have deterioration to panproctocolitis.

## COMPLICATIONS
Progression to pancolitis is the main concern.

## PREVENTION

### RISK FACTORS
Smoking: weak evidence for positive correlation between ulcerative proctitis and smoking and inverse correlation between Crohn's proctitis and smoking.

### MODIFY RISK FACTORS
**Lifestyle and wellness**

TOBACCO
Weak evidence for positive correlation between ulcerative proctitis and smoking, and inverse correlation between Crohn's proctitis and smoking.

DIET
Weak relationship between diet (e.g. spicy food, onions) and exacerbation of proctitis in some patients.

SEXUAL BEHAVIOR
Strong risk with unprotected promiscuous anal intercourse and infective proctitis.

FAMILY HISTORY
Weak correlation between Crohn's and ulcerative colitis and family history.

### PREVENT RECURRENCE
- Olsalazine suppositories. 500mg twice daily is effective at maintaining remission
- Avoid risk factors

# RESOURCES

## ASSOCIATIONS
American Society of Colon and Rectal Surgeons
85 W. Algonquin Road, Suite 550
Arlington Heights, IL 60005
Tel: (847) 290-9184
Fax: (847) 290-9203
http://www.fascrs.org

## KEY REFERENCES
- Marvin L, Corman MD, eds. Colon and rectal surgery, 3rd edn. Philadelphia: JB Lippincott, 1993 chapters 16, 20
- Marvin H, Sleisenger MD, John S, Fordtran MD, eds. Gastrointestinal disease, 5th edn. Philadelphia: WB Saunders, 1993, chapters 10, 55, 56, 57, 58, 62, 75, 76
- Bockus, Haubrich, Schaftner, Berk, eds. Gastroenterology, 5th edn. Philadelphia: WB Saunders, 1995, chapters 69, 89
- Yamada, et al, eds. Gastroenterology, 2nd edn. Philadelphia: JP Lippincott, 1995, chapters 80, 84
- Sutherland LR, May GR, Shaffer EA. Sulphasalazine revisited: a meta analysis of 5-aminosalicylic acid in the treatment of ulcerative colitis. Ann Intern Med 1993;118:540–49
- Singleton JW, Hanauer SB, Gitnick GL. Mesalazine capsules for the treatment of active Crohn's disease: results of a 16 week trial. Gastroenterology 1993;104:1293–1301
- Marshall JK, Irvine EJ. Rectal aminosalicylate therapy for distal ulcerative colitis: a meta analysis. Aliment Pharmacol & Ther 1995;9:293–300
- Jewell DP. Corticosteroids for the management of ulcerative colitis and Crohn's disease. Gastroenterol Clin N Am 1989;18:21–33
- Lichtiger S, Present DH, Kornbluth A, Gelernt I. Cyclosporine in severe ulcerative colitis refractory to steroid therapy. NEJM 1994;330:1841–5
- Vernia P, Fracasso PL, Casale V, et al. Topical butyrate for acute radiation proctitis: randomized, crossover trial. Lancet 2000;356:1232–35

## FAQS
### Question 1
Does proctitis resolve with no therapy?

### ANSWER 1
Some mild cases may resolve without therapy; however, the time to resolution will be reduced in infectious proctitis by a course of antibiotics.

### Question 2
How does one manage irradiation proctitis?

### ANSWER 2
Irradiation proctitis is a difficult condition to treat. Mesalamine enemas, topical steroids, and short chain fatty acid enemas have all been used with variable success. Vernia P, Fracasso PL, Casale V, et al. Topical butyrate for acute radiation proctitis: randomized, crossover trial. Lancet 2000;356:1232–35.

### Question 3
Can diversion of the fecal stream help treat intractable proctitis?

### ANSWER 3
Probably not. In addition, stoma formation, even temporary, is a radical measure for a benign condition. Diversion can itself produce diversion colitis and/or proctitis.

### Question 4
Does long-standing ulcerative proctitis have premalignant potential?

### ANSWER 4
Predisposition to severe dysplasia, and hence cancer, is related to extent of disease, duration, and severity. Hence, it is unlikely that proctitis confined to the rectum would be a high risk situation. Serial biopsies should help to settle the situation: if severe dysplasia was present pouch surgery might be an option.

### Question 5
Can gonococcal proctitis develop from direct spread from the patient's own genitalia?

### ANSWER 5
Not usually. Anoreceptive intercourse is the usual precondition.

## CONTRIBUTORS
Fred F Ferri, MD, FACP
Andrew H Soll, MD
Brennan Spiegel, MD

# PSEUDOMEMBRANOUS COLITIS

| | | |
|---|---|---|
| ■ | Summary Information | 510 |
| ■ | Background | 511 |
| ■ | Diagnosis | 512 |
| ■ | Treatment | 518 |
| ■ | Outcomes | 525 |
| ■ | Prevention | 527 |
| ■ | Resources | 528 |

## SUMMARY INFORMATION

### DESCRIPTION
- An infection of the colon caused by *Clostridium difficile*
- Overgrowth of *C. difficile* is a result of broad-spectrum antibiotic use
- Clinically, *C. difficile* causes a wide range of disease severity ranging, at one end, from severe pseudomembranous colitis, through antibiotic-associated colitis without pseudomembranes, through antibiotic-associated diarrhea without colitis, to asymptomatic carrier state at the other end

### URGENT ACTION
- In immunocompromised patients, the concern for toxic megacolon must remain high in the primary care physician's mind
- Any question of a surgical abdomen requires immediate surgical intervention
- In cases of severe diarrhea and/or dehydration, refer to hospital for rehydration therapy

### KEY! DON'T MISS!
Fulminant pseudomembranous colitis with distended, compromised full-thickness bowel wall carries a dismal prognosis, even with surgical intervention.

## BACKGROUND

### ICD9 CODE
008.45 *C. difficile*, pseudomembranous colitis

### SYNONYMS
- Antibiotic-associated diarrhea
- Antibiotic-induced colitis
- Antibiotic-induced enterocolitis

### CARDINAL FEATURES
- Caused by exotoxins of *Clostridium difficile*
- Fibrinous pseudomembrane forms over colonic mucosa
- Associated with previous antibiotic use in most cases
- Treatment is with metronidazole or vancomycin

### CAUSES
#### Common causes
Caused by *C. difficile* exotoxins A and B.

#### Contributory or predisposing factors
- Antibiotic exposure: can occur with any antibiotic, but is most frequently seen with amoxicillin, ampicillin, and cephalosporins. Historically, most classically associated with clindamycin and lincomycin. These antibiotics are currently less frequently used
- Recent surgery, specifically bowel surgery, may leave patient in vulnerable condition for infection while hospitalized
- Shock: severe impairment of tissue perfusion may lead to irreversible organ damage
- Alteration of endogenous intestinal microflora by immunosuppression with cancer chemotherapy or infection by other pathogens such as *Salmonella* or *Shigella* spp.
- Immunocompromised conditions (low CD4+ count) can enable bacterial overgrowth. More commonly, however, it is the frequent use of antibiotics that provides the most potent risk factor in these patients
- Prolonged hospitalization: nosocomial infection is common
- Advanced age: elderly immune systems are more vulnerable

### EPIDEMIOLOGY
#### Incidence and prevalence
PREVALENCE
0.067/1000 patients treated with antibiotics.

FREQUENCY
Epidemic or endemic in hospitals (7–15%) or nursing homes (2–8%).

#### Demographics
AGE
40–75 years, but does occur in children. Neonates tend to be asymptomatic carriers.

GENDER
Same in males and females.

SOCIOECONOMIC STATUS
Nursing home patients or hospitalized patients have higher risk due to increased *C. difficile* colonization.

# DIAGNOSIS

## DIFFERENTIAL DIAGNOSIS
### Gastrointestinal infection
The most common causes of diarrhea include viral enteritis and bacterial infections with *Escherichia coli*, and *Shigella*, *Salmonella*, *Campylobacter*, and *Yersinia* spp.

FEATURES
- Watery diarrhea, which may include blood and mucus
- Abdominal pain
- Fever
- Nausea and vomiting

### Inflammatory bowel disease
Distinguishing features of Crohn's disease and ulcerative colitis are as follows.

FEATURES
- Bloody diarrhea
- Abdominal pain
- Weight loss
- Extraintestinal features such as arthritis, ocular disease (especially ulcerative colitis), and perianal disease (Crohn's disease)

### Ischemic colitis
FEATURES
- Lower abdominal pain
- Bleeding per rectum or bloody diarrhea
- Pyrexia and leukocytosis
- Severe pain, peritonitis, and hypovolemic shock in acute gangrenous colitis
- Past history of postprandial abdominal cramping may be noted

### Diverticulitis
Diverticulitis implies microperforation of a diverticulum, with ensuing localized inflammation contained by pericolonic fat and mesentery.

FEATURES
- Abdominal pain
- Left lower quadrant tenderness, with or without guarding
- Low-grade fever
- Elevated leukocyte count
- Diarrhea or constipation may be present
- Anorexia, nausea, and vomiting are less common symptoms

## SIGNS & SYMPTOMS
### Signs
- Poor skin turgor, dry mucous membranes in patients with prolonged diarrhea
- Hypoalbuminemia
- Hypovolemia
- Abdominal tenderness, with possible guarding and rebound tenderness
- Fever (seen in <10% of cases)

### Symptoms
- Diarrhea (watery, green, foul-smelling, bloody)

- Abdominal tenderness (generalized or lower abdominal location)
- Abdominal cramps

## ASSOCIATED DISORDERS
- Surgery
- Peptic ulcer disease
- Intestinal obstruction
- Colon cancer
- Immunosuppression from chemotherapy

## KEY! DON'T MISS!
Fulminant pseudomembranous colitis with distended, compromised full-thickness bowel wall carries a dismal prognosis, even with surgical intervention.

## CONSIDER CONSULT
- Any signs of surgical abdomen require surgical referral, and patients with pseudomembranous colitis who demonstrate guarding or rebound tenderness should be referred to gastrointestinal or surgical consultant
- Refer to hospital if bowel perforation or toxic megacolon is suspected
- Excessive abdominal pain with bleeding may also warrant referral for gastrointestinal or surgical evaluation since other diagnoses may be missed

## INVESTIGATION OF THE PATIENT
### Direct questions to patient
**Q** Have you taken any antibiotics during the past 6 weeks? Nearly all antibiotics have been implicated in the occurrence of pseudomembranous colitis
**Q** Are you suffering from any other illness? For example, cancer or inflammatory bowel disease
**Q** Have you been hospitalized recently or discharged from a nursing home? This condition is frequently endemic in hospitals and nursing homes
**Q** Have you recently undergone surgery? Patients who have undergone abdominal surgery may be at greater risk

### Contributory or predisposing factors
**Q** Are you undergoing cancer chemotherapy? Fluorouracil, methotrexate, and combination regimens have been implicated in this condition
**Q** How old are you? The elderly are more susceptible to infection, and nursing homes may have endemic infectious populations
**Q** Do you have AIDS? The immunocompromised patient is more susceptible to *Clostridium difficile* infection

### Examination
- Does the patient have abdominal tenderness, pain, cramping upon palpation? If so, have the patient define the extent of pain, how long he or she has been experiencing the tenderness, and whether the discomfort migrates
- Does the patient have a fever? If not, does the patient report having had a fever over the past few days? Fever is seen in fewer than 10% of patients with pseudomembranous colitis

### Summary of investigative tests
- The presence of *C. difficile* toxin in a stool specimen can be detected using cytotoxin tissue-culture assay or enzyme-linked immunoassay
- A complete blood count should be performed; leukocytosis is usually present in *C. difficile*-associated colitis
- Fecal leukocytes (detected using microscopy or by lactoferrin assay) are generally present in stool specimens

- Flexible sigmoidoscopy with biopsy to identify plaques may be necessary when the clinical and laboratory diagnosis is inconclusive and diarrhea persists
- Abdominal film may help to rule out intestinal obstruction or further define cause of abdominal pain as well as rule out toxic megacolon
- Abdominal computed tomography scan is helpful in diagnosis in selected cases, particularly in evaluation of transmural involvement or of toxic dilated megacolon; such patients would normally be under the care of a specialist
- Endoscopy should be reserved for special situations, such as when a rapid diagnosis is needed, test results are delayed, stool is not available, or when other colonic diseases are included in the differential diagnosis

## DIAGNOSTIC DECISION

- The test of choice is stool cytotoxin assay
- Rapid results can also be obtained by rapid immunoassays for the exotoxins, which is now performed by many hospital laboratories, without the need for a tissue culture facility
- Pseudomembranous colitis can be diagnosed through confirmation of *C. difficile* infection by stool culture. Culture is very sensitive but not specific, taking several days, and many strains prove to be toxin negative

## CLINICAL PEARLS

- Marked leukocytosis may be a clue to diagnosis in patients with diarrhea
- In severely ill patients with gastrointestinal symptoms, the diagnosis may be suggested by findings of pseudomembranous colitis on computed tomography scan
- Use of antibiotics may antedate onset of symptoms by up to 6 weeks

## THE TESTS
### Body fluids
CLOSTRIDIUM DIFFICILE TOXIN ASSAY
*Description*
- A random stool specimen is collected and then refrigerated immediately
- Samples are tested using cytotoxin tissue-culture assay or enzyme-linked immunoassay
- Cytotoxin tissue-culture assay detects presence of *C. difficile* toxin, and enzyme-linked immunoassay detects specific *C. difficile* toxins (A and B)

*Advantages/Disadvantages*
Advantages:
- Simple sample collection procedure to confirm presence of *C. difficile* toxins
- Tissue culture assay and enzyme-linked immunoassay are highly sensitive (94–100% and 75%, respectively) and highly specific (99% and 99%, respectively)

Disadvantage: typically not done by primary care physician; requires off-site laboratory involvement.

*Normal*
Negative result.

*Abnormal*
- Positive result
- Keep in mind the small possibility of false-positive results

*Cause of abnormal result*
*Clostridium difficile* infection.

*Drugs, disorders and other factors that may alter results*
- Stool specimens from patients receiving barium, bismuth, oil, or antibiotics may not be satisfactory
- A high percentage of infants are normal carriers of *C. difficile* and are positive for toxin B without exhibiting symptoms of colitis
- False-negative results from tissue culture have been seen. These false-negative results are usually caused by inactivation of toxins during specimen storage or shipping to the laboratory, medications used by the patient, or dilution of stool specimens in the laboratory. A negative result for toxin B enzyme immunoassay in cell culture does not rule out *C. difficile* as the cause of the diarrhea

## MICROSCOPY FOR DETECTION OF FECAL LEUKOCYTES
*Description*
Stool sample is obtained and examined under the microscope for the presence of fecal leukocytes.

*Advantages/Disadvantages*
Advantages:
- Simple, cost-effective test
- Easily performed with fast result

Disadvantage: nonspecific.

*Normal*
Leukocytes not detected.

*Abnormal*
- Presence of fecal leukocytes
- Keep in mind the possibility of false-positive and false-negative results

*Cause of abnormal result*
Intestinal infection.

*Drugs, disorders and other factors that may alter results*
Result is also positive in other intestinal infections, diverticulitis, ischemic colitis, and inflammatory bowel disease.

## LACTOFERRIN ASSAY FOR DETECTION OF FECAL LEUKOCYTES
*Description*
A test for the detection of elevated levels of fecal lactoferrin, which is a marker for fecal leukocytes.

*Advantages/Disadvantages*
Advantages:
- Rapid result
- Easy to perform
- More sensitive than microscopy

*Abnormal*
- Detection of lactoferrin released from fecal leukocytes
- Keep in mind the possibility of false-positive and false-negative results

*Cause of abnormal result*
Presence of fecal leukocytes.

COMPLETE BLOOD COUNT
*Description*
Venous blood sample to look for leukocytosis.

*Advantages/Disadvantages*
- Advantage: simple test, inexpensive
- Disadvantage: nonspecific

*Normal*
Leukocytes 4.0–11.0x10$^9$/L.

*Abnormal*
- Result higher than normal reference range
- Keep in mind the possibility of false-positive and false-negative results

## Biopsy
FLEXIBLE SIGMOIDOSCOPY
*Description*
- The most rapid way to establish the diagnosis of pseudomembranous colitis is via endoscopy, with biopsy of suspicious lesions
- Flexible sigmoidoscopy has been found to be more effective than rigid endoscopy in detecting cases of pseudomembranous colitis
- Sigmoidoscopy should be performed without prior cleansing enema

*Advantages/Disadvantages*
- Advantage: fastest way to confirm diagnosis
- Disadvantage: increased risk of bowel perforation

*Abnormal*
- Raised, yellowish nodules or plaque-like pseudomembranes
- Nodules usually 2–10mm in diameter
- In advanced stages nodules are increased in number, enlarged, and coalesced to form plaques or membranes that cover large segments of inflamed mucosa
- Microscopic examination of lesions shows epithelial necrosis, goblet cells distended with mucus, edema, and infiltration of the lamina propria with leukocytes, epithelial cells, fibrin, and mucin
- Keep in mind the possibility of false-positive results (e.g. in infectious or ischemic colitis)

*Cause of abnormal result*
- Pseudomembranous colitis
- Nonspecific colitis or simple *C. difficile* colitis (if pseudomembranes not present at endoscopy)

*Drugs, disorders and other factors that may alter results*
Partially treated colitis may appear normal.

## Imaging
PLAIN ABDOMINAL X-RAY
*Advantages/Disadvantages*
- Advantage: useful in patients with generalized abdominal pain; helps to rule out intestinal obstruction
- Disadvantage: cannot confirm diagnosis of pseudomembranous colitis

*Abnormal*
- May observe loss of haustral markings, colonic distension
- Keep in mind the possibility of false-positive results

*Cause of abnormal result*
- Colonic infection
- Gastrointestinal obstruction
- Toxic dilation of the colon
- Perforation of the colon

## TREATMENT

### CONSIDER CONSULT
Refer to hospital in cases of severe dehydration, in order to allow for intravenous hydration.

### IMMEDIATE ACTION
- Discontinue antibiotic treatment
- Provide supportive therapy (intravenous rehydration therapy) until *Clostridium difficile*-associated diarrhea diagnosis is confirmed
- If diagnosis of *C. difficile* diarrhea is highly likely and patient is seriously ill, then metronidazole or vancomycin may be given empirically before the diagnosis is established

### PATIENT AND CAREGIVER ISSUES
#### Patient or caregiver request
Q Is this diarrhea caused by changes in my diet or recent foreign travel? Unless the patient was taking antibiotics while traveling, it is unlikely that *C. difficile*-associated diarrhea is related to diet or recent travel

Q Why do many antibiotics cause diarrhea? Antibiotic use is a common cause of diarrhea because the gut flora is often radically altered by antibiotic use. *C. difficile* is a more serious cause of antibiotic-related diarrhea and one that can be very dangerous

Q I think that I'm allergic or sensitive to milk products; could this be causing the diarrhea? It's unlikely that your recent diarrhea is from dairy products; however, it is best to avoid all milk products in any patient with diarrhea

#### Health-seeking behavior
Have you been self-medicating with over-the-counter or alternative medicines? If so, what medications have been used? Laxative abuse is a frequent cause of diarrhea.

### MANAGEMENT ISSUES
#### Goals
- Stop all antibiotics if possible!
- Replace fluids and electrolytes lost due to diarrhea
- Diphenoxylate and loperamide are not recommended in treatment of pseudomembranous colitis – they may reduce the frequency but not the duration of the diarrhea, and theoretically might predispose to ileus and megacolon by inhibiting colonic motility
- Reduce/resolve inflammation of colon
- Prevent further attacks

#### Management in special circumstances
COEXISTING DISEASE
Patients undergoing cancer chemotherapy are often immunocompromised and may have altered fecal flora, making them more susceptible to repeated *C. difficile* infection.

COEXISTING MEDICATION
For the patient whose triggering antibiotic cannot be discontinued, progression of the disease may continue despite treatment.

SPECIAL PATIENT GROUPS
- Pregnant women: pseudomembranous colitis is considered a serious complication. Most of the antimicrobial agents used to treat this condition should not be prescribed during pregnancy
- Children: this patient population can frequently be reinfected through nosocomial exposure or in childcare settings. A small proportion of patients develop multiple recurrences with short-lived responses to repeated treatment
- The elderly: this patient population has a higher mortality rate from pseudomembranous colitis,

often because of the greater severity of the condition or because of reinfection while in the nursing home or hospital setting
- Patients with AIDS: colitis due to *C. difficile* is common in this patient population, owing to the variety of antibiotic agents needed for prophylaxis and treatment in AIDS
- The hospitalized patient: patients receiving parenteral nutrition may also be in a debilitated condition that makes them more susceptible to reinfection

## SUMMARY OF THERAPEUTIC OPTIONS
### Choices
The first line of treatment is to stop the offending antibiotics. In many instances, this alone will stop the diarrhea. Alternatively:
- The recommended first-line therapy is oral metronidazole. Intravenous metronidazole has been used to treat patients with pseudomembranous colitis who are unable to take the medication orally
- Second-choice treatment is oral vancomycin, which is more often used for severe colitis and for colitis that fails to respond to standard oral metronidazole treatment. Owing to the side effect profile of oral metronidazole, vancomycin is often used to treat children under the age of 10 years and pregnant women in their first trimester
- In mild cases, treatment with nonabsorbable anion-binding resins (cholestyramine or colestipol) may be used to bind the *C. difficile* toxins for excretion into the feces
- Bacitracin may also be used to treat the underlying bacterial infection
- If all medical therapies are ineffective, colectomy may be the only treatment alternative in rare severe refractory cases

### Clinical pearls
If the patient is hospitalized with ileus or poor gut motility, consider switching from oral vancomycin or metronidazole to intravenous metronidazole.

### Never
Never use antidiarrheal agents, including loperamide and morphine derivatives, in patients with pseudomembranous colitis.

## FOLLOW UP
### Plan for review
- If the symptoms have worsened on follow up, consider re-evaluating the patient and possibly modifying treatment
- Review tolerability of treatment and patient compliance, as well as the treatment of any comorbid illnesses that may have worsened the patient's colitis. Review and revise all therapies if not effective

### Information for patient or caregiver
- Provide information to patient about treatment options, side effects of each therapy, and the relative costs (if patients have little or no prescription insurance plan)
- Provide patient with information about the possibility of recurrences or worsening of pseudomembranous colitis

## DRUGS AND OTHER THERAPIES: DETAILS
### Drugs
METRONIDAZOLE
For treatment of adults with *C. difficile* diarrhea, this is the first-line drug choice.

*Dose*
- Adult oral (off-label indication): 250–500mg, four times daily for 10–14 days; or 500–750mg, three times daily for 10–14 days

- Pediatric oral (off-label indication): 20–50mg/kg/day; total dose divided for administration every 6–8h
- Adult intravenous (off-label indication): 500–750mg infusion over 1h, three or four times daily for 10–14 days

*Efficacy*
- Effective in treating *C. difficile* infection, both mild and moderate-to-severe cases
- Useful in treating recurring *C. difficile* in patients originally treated with vancomycin

*Risks/benefits*
Risks:
- Nausea and vomiting likely if alcohol is taken
- Avoid in pregnancy and breast-feeding
- Use caution in hepatic and renal impairment, central nervous system disease, or history of seizures

Benefits:
- Cost of treatment is low
- Side effects are relatively minor
- Response rate is high

*Side effects and adverse reactions*
- Central nervous system: dizziness, headache, seizures, ataxia, peripheral neuropathy
- Gastrointestinal: nausea, vomiting, taste disturbance, diarrhea, abdominal pain, dry mouth, anorexia, constipation
- Genitourinary: urination difficulties, cystitis, vaginal dryness
- Hematologic: blood cell disorders
- Skin: rashes, itching, flushing

*Interactions (other drugs)*
- **Alcohol** - **Antiepileptics** - **Anticoagulants** - **Barbiturates** - **Carbamazepine** - **Cholestyramine** - **Cimetidine** - **Colestipol** - **Disulfiram** - **Fluorouracil** - **Lithium** - **Warfarin**

*Contraindications*
- **Pregnancy** - **Impaired hepatic or renal function** - **Blood dyscrasias**

*Acceptability to patient*
Acceptable; side effects may be a problem.

*Follow up plan*
- Monitor patient's complete blood count during treatment for evidence of neutropenia
- Monitor patient's compliance; side effects may be sufficient for patient to reduce dose or discontinue medication

*Patient and caregiver information*
- Patient should be aware that drinking any alcoholic beverage while taking oral metronidazole (including the first 24h after discontinuing treatment) will cause a disulfiram-like reaction
- Patients should be informed of the unpleasant metallic taste, darkening of the urine, and other side effects of taking oral metronidazole
- Patients who are breast-feeding and receiving single-dose treatment should be instructed to discontinue breast-feeding for 12–24h to allow excretion of the drug

## VANCOMYCIN

*Dose*
- Adults: 0.5–2g/day orally in three to four divided doses for 7–10 days
- Child: 40mg/kg/day in three to four divided doses for 7–10 days (not to exceed 2g/day)

*Efficacy*
Effective for severe disease and when metronidazole is not effective.

*Risks/benefits*
Risks:
- Use caution in renal disease and inflammatory bowel disease
- Use caution in neonates and the elderly

Benefits:
- Fewer side effects than metronidazole
- May be used in pregnant patients and in children

*Side effects and adverse reactions*
- Cardiovascular system: cardiac arrest, cardiovascular collapse, phlebitis
- Ears, eyes, nose, and throat: hearing disturbances, ototoxicity
- Gastrointestinal: nausea
- Genitourinary: renal damage
- Hematologic: neutropenia, eosinophilia, leukopenia
- Skin: rashes, chills, fever, 'red man's syndrome'

*Interactions (other drugs)*
- Aminoglycosides - Amphotericin B - Capreomycin - Cholestyramine, colestipol (oral vancomycin) - Cidofovir - Cisplatin - Cyclosporine - Ethacrynic acid - Indomethacin - Methotrexate - Neuromuscular blockers - Paromomycin - Pentamidine - Polymyxin B - Salicylates - Streptozocin - Surfactants

*Contraindications*
- Hearing deficit - Cidofovir (vancomycin should be discontinued 7 days before cidofovir treatment) - Intramuscular administration

*Acceptability to patient*
Generally acceptable.

*Follow up plan*
- Test renal function before and during treatment
- Follow up to ensure improvement of symptoms

*Patient and caregiver information*
- Inform physician if symptoms do not improve while on treatment
- Report any hearing difficulty or tinnitus

## CHOLESTYRAMINE
Nonabsorbable anion-binding resin.

*Dose*
- Adult: 4g anhydrous cholestyramine resin, one to two times daily. Not to exceed 32g/day
- Child: 240 mg/kg/day of anhydrous cholestyramine resin in two to three divided doses. Not to exceed 8g/day with dose titration based on response and tolerance

*Efficacy*
Useful as part of the treatment strategy for patients with recurrent colitis who have short-lived responses to repeated treatment.

*Risks/benefits*
Risks:
- Use caution in renal disease and inflammatory bowel disease
- Use caution in neonates and the elderly

*Side effects and adverse reactions*
- Cardiovascular system: cardiac arrest, cardiovascular collapse, phlebitis
- Eyes, ears, nose, and throat: hearing disturbances, ototoxicity
- Gastrointestinal: nausea
- Genitourinary: renal damage
- Hematologic: neutropenia, eosinophilia, leukopenia
- Skin: rashes, chills, fever, 'red man's syndrome'

*Interactions (other drugs)*
- Aminoglycosides
- Amphotericin B
- Capreomycin
- Colestipol (oral vancomycin)
- Cidofovir
- Cisplatin
- Cyclosporine
- Ethacrynic acid
- Indomethacin
- Methotrexate
- Neuromuscular blockers
- Paromomycin
- Pentamidine
- Polymyxin B
- Salicylates
- Streptozocin
- Surfactants

*Contraindications*
- Hearing deficit
- Cidofovir (vancomycin should be discontinued 7 days before cidofovir treatment)
- Intramuscular administration

*Acceptability to patient*
Generally acceptable.

*Patient and caregiver information*
- Give separately from other medications
- Mix drug with liquid before consumption

COLESTIPOL
Nonabsorbable anion-binding resin.

*Dose*
- Adult: tablets, 2–16g/day given once or in divided doses. The starting dose should be 2g once or twice daily. Increases of 2g, once or twice daily, should occur at one- or 2-month intervals
- Adult: suspension, one dose (one packet or one level teaspoon) contains 5g of colestipol HCl. One dose (one packet or one level scoopful) of flavored colestipol HCl is approximately 7.5g, which contains 5g of colestipol HCl
- The recommended daily adult dose is one to six packets or level scoopfuls given once or in divided doses. Treatment should be started with one dose once or twice daily with an increment of one dose/day at one- or 2-month intervals

*Efficacy*
These products are useful as part of the treatment strategy for patients with recurrent colitis who have short-lived responses to repeated treatment.

*Risks/benefits*
Risks:
- Poor absorption of other oral medications when taken with colestipol

- Chronic use of colestipol HCl may be associated with an increased bleeding tendency due to hypoprothrombinemia from vitamin K deficiency

Benefit: colestipol monotherapy has been demonstrated to retard the rate of progression and to increase the rate of regression of coronary atherosclerosis.

*Side effects and adverse reactions*
Gastrointestinal: constipation, moderate to severe impairment of bowel function, abdominal pain and cramping, bloating, flatulence, indigestion, heartburn, diarrhea, loose stools, nausea, vomiting, aggravation of hemorrhoids.

*Interactions (other drugs)*
- May delay or reduce the absorption of concomitant oral medication
- Reduced absorption of the following has been shown: tetracycline, furosemide, penicillin G, hydrochlorothiazide, gemfibrozil, chlorothiazide
- Patients should take other drugs at least 1h before or 4h after colestipol HCl to avoid impeding their absorption

*Contraindications*
- Complete biliary obstruction where bile is not secreted into the intestine
- Hypersensitivity to colestipol
- Active liver disease or unexplained persistent elevations of serum transaminases

*Acceptability to patient*
Generally acceptable.

*Patient and caregiver information*
Take other medications separately.

## BACITRACIN

*Dose*
25,000U four times daily for 10 days (orphan drug status).

*Efficacy*
Good symptomatic relief; less effective than other antibiotics at eradicating bacteria from intestine.

*Risks/benefits*
Risks:
- Use caution with pregnancy and nursing mothers
- Use caution in cutaneous tuberculosis
- Systemic absorption can occur if applied to denuded skin

*Side effects and adverse reactions*
- Eyes, ears, nose, and throat: poor corneal wound healing, visual disturbances
- Gastrointestinal: nausea, vomiting, diarrhea
- Genitourinary: tubular and glomerular necrosis leading to renal failure
- Skin: rashes

*Interactions (other drugs)*
- Aminoglycosides
- Amphotericin B
- Cisplatin
- Cyclosporine
- Foscarnet
- Loop diuretics
- Pentamidine
- Tacrolimus
- Vancomycin

*Contraindications*
- Severe renal disease
- Aminoglycoside hypersensitivity
- Neomycin hypersensitivity
- Fungal or viral infections
- Ocular application

*Acceptability to patient*
One of the side effects is diarrhea, which may limit acceptability.

*Follow up plan*
Follow up to ensure antibacterial is effective.

### Surgical therapy
COLECTOMY
Colectomy is the treatment of last resort, when all other therapies have failed.

*Efficacy*
Effective, since colon is removed.

*Risks/benefits*
Risks:
- General risks of surgery
- Long-term risks of ileostomy or anastomosis

*Acceptability to patient*
Generally not well accepted by patients.

*Follow up plan*
- Close postoperative follow up to monitor for complications
- Long-term follow up for complications related to ileostomy or anastomosis

*Patient and caregiver information*
Patients will need extensive pre- and postoperative counseling and education.

## OUTCOMES

### EFFICACY OF THERAPIES
- Most patients recover fully with suitable treatment, although relapse recurs in 20% of patients
- Mortality rate can be as high as 10% in untreated patients

### PROGNOSIS
If treated, patient's condition improves within 3 days. Virtually all treated patients recover, but relapses occur in 20%. If untreated, reports have documented a 10–30% mortality. Factors that contribute to poor prognosis include:
- Hypoalbuminemia
- Rapid fall in albumin
- Use of more than three antibiotics
- Persistence of *Clostridium difficile* toxin after 7 days of treatment

#### Clinical pearls
The recurrence of diarrhea after metronidazole therapy does not necessarily imply treatment failure. *C. difficile* is a known spore-former and the regermination of spores (since spores are drug-resistant) is the cause of the recurrent diarrhea. Retreatment with metronidazole often results in successful therapy.

#### Therapeutic failure
If all medical therapies are ineffective, colectomy may be the only treatment alternative.

#### Recurrence
- For relapsing disease, slow tapering courses of vancomycin are often tried first
- Use of the *Lactobacillus* GG strain has been effective in attempts to restore the colonization resistance of the fecal flora of patients with relapses
- Some patients who have relapsed have also received oral administration of *Saccharomyces boulardii* for about 4 weeks, beginning 4 days before the end of conventional antibiotic therapy (metronidazole or vancomycin) to treat the recurrence
- The use of intravenous immune globulin has been reported to be effective in prevention of recurrences, especially in children with various immunoglobulin deficiencies; however, these anecdotal reports have not been substantiated by clinical trial findings

#### Deterioration
If the patient continues to deteriorate despite treatment, consider referral to a gastroenterologist or hospital for evaluation of additional conditions or need for surgery.

### COMPLICATIONS
Possible complications include:
- Dehydration
- Hypovolemia
- Shock
- Electrolyte imbalance
- Hypoalbuminemia
- Ascites
- Toxic megacolon
- Bowel perforation
- Reactive arthritis
- Reiter's syndrome
- Death

## CONSIDER CONSULT
For patients who continue to deteriorate despite treatment, consider referral to gastroenterologist or hospital for evaluation of additional conditions or need for surgery.

# PREVENTION

Prevention of *Clostridium difficile* infection is the primary focus behind the prevention of pseudomembranous colitis.

## RISK FACTORS
**Nosocomial or child-care setting infections:** spores of the organism are resistant to drying and to some disinfectants, and frequently contaminate bathrooms and diaper-changing areas of hospital rooms or child-care areas.

## MODIFY RISK FACTORS
Modifying procedures to prevent exposure to *C. difficile* is the primary focus for people who do not have the disorder.

### Lifestyle and wellness
ENVIRONMENT
- Prevention of *C. difficile*-associated diarrhea requires meticulous hand washing and appropriate environmental cleaning (disinfection of objects contaminated with *C. difficile* with sodium hypochlorite, alkaline glutaraldehyde, or ethylene oxide)
- In the hospital, nursing home, or home-care setting, stool isolation precautions should be used for patients with *C. difficile* diarrhea, and gloves should be worn when contacting these patients or their surroundings. Medical, nursing, and other hospital staff members should be educated about the disease and its epidemiology

DRUG HISTORY
Causative antimicrobial therapy should be stopped if possible.

## SCREENING
Since many healthy people and patients without diarrhea carry *C. difficile* in their intestines, there is little reason to screen all people for this organism.

## PREVENT RECURRENCE
### Reassess coexisting disease
If patient has other conditions that require use of antibiotics, keep the course of treatment as brief as possible.

INTERACTION ALERT
Judicious use of antimicrobial agents, with restriction of the use of drugs that may lead to bacterial resistance, is important.

PATIENT SATISFACTION/LIFESTYLE PRIORITIES
Exposure to environments where infection is highly likely (hospitals, nursing homes, day-care settings) should be restricted if possible.

# RESOURCES

## ASSOCIATIONS

American College of Gastroenterology
4900 B South 31st Street
Arlington, VA 22206
Tel: (703) 820-7400
Fax: (703) 931-4520
http://www.acg.gi.org

American Gastroenterological Association
National Office
7910 Woodmont Avenue, 7th Floor
Bethesda, MD 20814
Tel: (301) 654-2055
Fax: (301) 652-3890
E-mail: webinfo@gastro.org
http://www.gastro.org

## KEY REFERENCES

- Fekety R. Guidelines for the diagnosis and management of *Clostridium difficile*-associated diarrhea and colitis. Am J Gastroenterol 1997;92:739–50
- Teasley DG, Gerding DN, Olson MM, et al. Prospective randomized trial of metronidazole versus vancomycin for *Clostridium difficile*-associated diarrhoea and colitis. Lancet 1983;2:1043–6
- Bartlett JG. Pseudomembranous colitis and antibiotic-associated colitis. In: Feldman M, Scharschmidt BF, Sleisenger MH, Klein S, eds. Sleisenger & Fordtran's gastrointestinal and liver disease, 6th edn. Philadelphia: WB Saunders, 1998
- Zimmerman MJ. Review article: treatment of *Clostridium difficile* infection. Aliment Pharmacol Ther 1997;11:1003–12
- Fischbach F. A manual of laboratory and diagnostic tests, 6th edn. Philadelphia: Lippincott, Williams & Wilkins, 2000

## CONTRIBUTORS

Fred F Ferri, MD, FACP
Lawrence S Friedman, MD
Braden Kuo, MD
J Adrian Lunn, MD

# PYLORIC STENOSIS

| | | |
|---|---|---|
| ■ | Summary Information | 530 |
| ■ | Background | 531 |
| ■ | Diagnosis | 533 |
| ■ | Treatment | 539 |
| ■ | Outcomes | 548 |
| ■ | Prevention | 549 |
| ■ | Resources | 550 |

## SUMMARY INFORMATION

### DESCRIPTION
- A form of gastric outlet obstruction
- Obstruction of the pyloric lumen due to pyloric muscular hypertrophy
- Most commonly found in infants, usually between 4 and 8 weeks. Rarely seen in adults
- A medical emergency and the most common reason for surgery in the first 6 months of life

### URGENT ACTION
- Intravenous hydration, electrolyte repletion
- If pyloric stenosis is suspected, obtain an abdominal ultrasound or an X-ray upper gastrointestinal study (barium swallow)

### KEY! DON'T MISS!
Delayed diagnosis may lead to repeated vomiting, dehydration, and hypochloremic metabolic alkalosis (from losses of hydrochloric acid).

## BACKGROUND

### ICD9 CODE
537.0 Acquired hypertrophic pyloric stenosis

### SYNONYMS
- Idiopathic hypertrophic pyloric stenosis
- Infantile hypertrophic pyloric stenosis
- HPS

### CARDINAL FEATURES
- Progressive nonbilious vomiting, weight loss, and dehydration in infants, usually presenting between 4 and 8 weeks of life
- Rarely seen at birth, the onset of vomiting may occur as early as the first week of life but occasionally may be delayed 4–5 months
- However, approx. 10–20% of babies become symptomatic shortly after birth. Another category of patients do well for the first few weeks of life but suddenly develop projectile vomiting, leading to dehydration within a few days
- Diffuse hypertrophy of the smooth muscle of the antrum of the stomach and the pylorus leads to a narrowing of the channel, which can then become obstructed easily. The antral region is elongated and thickened to as much as twice its normal size
- Abdominal distension is common and gastric peristaltic waves may be seen crossing the epigastrium from left to right
- With skilled palpation, a 'pyloric olive' can be felt in up to 80% of cases
- Occurs rarely in adults, sometimes as a result of an overlooked infantile case. Patients may complain of postprandial fullness and pain. Gastric cancer should be considered in the differential diagnosis when adults present with these symptoms

### CAUSES
#### Common causes
The causes are unclear but proposed theories include:
- Abnormal circular muscle innervation
- Immature ganglion cells
- Decreased nitric oxide stimulation of muscle fibers
- Abnormal levels of gastrin have been postulated as a possible cause. It is unclear whether the elevation of serum gastrin is primary or secondary to gastric distension caused by outlet obstruction
- Muscle and nerve abnormalities in the stomach region

Adult pyloric obstruction has various causes and is classified as either secondary or primary:
- Most reported cases have been secondary to local disease such as exuberant healing of a previous gastric or duodenal ulcer, gastric carcinoma, extrinsic postoperative adhesions, and bezoars
- Idiopathic adult hypertrophic pyloric stenosis is a much more rare condition. Etiology is obscure but some cases probably represent persistence of a mild form of the juvenile condition into adulthood. A single case report documents the presence of a congenital form as well as the adult form in one family

#### Rare causes
- Increased production of the hormone gastrin, which increases cell growth in the stomach muscles
- Chromosomal abnormalities. There are reports of associations of hypertrophic pyloric stenosis (HPS) with other congenital abnormalities such as esophageal atresia, Cornelia de Lange's syndrome, Hirchsprung's disease, phenylketonuria (PKU), and congenital rubella

### Contributory or predisposing factors
- Male relatives of affected females are at increased risk for developing HPS
- Other infants with increased incidence are first-born males, especially males who have high birthweights or are born to professional parents

## EPIDEMIOLOGY
### Incidence and prevalence
INCIDENCE
- Occurs in 2/1000 births
- HPS is seen in 2–3/1000 infants in North America

PREVALENCE
- The most common cause of gastrointestinal obstruction in infants
- Accounts for 30% of all patients presenting with nonbilious vomiting before age one year

FREQUENCY
- HPS is usually a disease of the full-term infant
- Only 3% of cases are found in premature infants

### Demographics
AGE
- HPS most commonly is seen in infants aged 3–6 weeks
- Very occasionally seen in older people, usually with chronic ulcer disease, though a small proportion could represent missed infantile cases

GENDER
Males are affected four to five times more often than females.

RACE
- Most common in Caucasians
- Seen less commonly in African-American infants or infants of Asian descent

GENETICS
- A genetic component exists, since an increased incidence is observed in families in which a sibling or parent has had the disease
- Associated with Cornelia de Lange's syndrome, Hirchsprung's disease, and PKU

GEOGRAPHY
International incidence of HPS is equal to that in North America.

# DIAGNOSIS

## DIFFERENTIAL DIAGNOSIS
### Bowel obstruction in the newborn
Bowel obstruction in the newborn is a medical emergency. Consider any infant or child with bilious vomiting to have a bowel obstruction until proven otherwise.

FEATURES
- Bilious vomiting
- Hypotension, metabolic acidosis, progressive respiratory failure, and thrombocytopenia
- Abdominal distension or tenderness, abdominal wall erythema, a palpable mass, or visible loop of bowel
- Careful perineal inspection will identify incarcerated hernia, an anterior ectopic anus, or imperforate anus

### Esophageal atresia
Esophageal atresia is a congenital disease of newborn infants caused by a discontinuity of the esophagus.

FEATURES
- Onset of gagging, nonbilious (saliva) vomiting within hours of birth
- Vomiting on feeding
- Bowel sounds may be reduced or absent
- Cyanosis and dyspnea may be observed
- Normal meconium stools

### Duodenal atresia
Duodenal atresia is a congenital disease of newborn infants caused by a discontinuity or occlusion of the duodenum.

FEATURES
- Intestine on either side of the defect may be in apposition (type I), separated by a fibrous cord (type II) or a gap (type III)
- Regardless of atresia severity, the proximal intestinal segment is always dilated and the distal segment empty
- Onset of vomiting within hours of birth
- Vomitus is most often bilious, but may be nonbilious
- Scaphoid abdomen: epigastric fullness from dilation of the stomach and proximal duodenum
- Passing meconium within the first 24h of life usually is not altered but bowel movements cease after 1–3 days
- Dehydration, weight loss, and electrolyte imbalance soon follow unless fluid and electrolyte losses are adequately replaced
- Often associated with Down syndrome

### Intestinal malrotation
Intestinal nonrotation or incomplete rotation around the superior mesenteric artery: malrotation is most commonly caused by incomplete rotation (<270° of counterclockwise rotation occurring between 5 and 12 weeks; predisposes to midgut volvulus, which can result in short-bowel syndrome or even death). Caused by disruption in the normal embryologic development of the bowel.

FEATURES
- The proximal small bowel (jejunum) is in the right upper quadrant
- The cecum is in the upper and/or left abdomen

- The large bowel is in the left abdomen
- Other associated anomalies are seen around the ampulla of Vater

### Acute midgut volvulus

A consequence of malrotation of the intestine. The malrotated bowel is prone to torsion, resulting in midgut volvulus.

FEATURES
- Abdominal distension frequently present
- The infant appears in acute pain
- As vascular compromise persists intraluminal bleeding may occur, which leads to blood per rectum, and sometimes hematemesis
- Abdominal guarding prevents palpation of intestinal loops
- As symptoms persist, the infant may develop signs of shock, including poor perfusion, decreased urine output, and hypotension
- Signs of peritonitis: abdominal tenderness and skin discoloration

### Gastroesophageal reflux (GERD)

Gastroesophageal reflux disease (GERD) occurs when there is incompetence of the lower esophageal sphincter, and stomach contents can leak back into the esophagus.

FEATURES
- Heartburn, with or without regurgitation of gastric contents into the mouth
- Esophagitis may cause odynophagia and even hemorrhage, which can be massive
- Peptic stricture causes a gradually progressive dysphagia for solid foods
- Peptic esophageal ulcers may cause the same type of pain as gastric or duodenal ulcers

### Gastroenteritis

Gastroenteritis is common, has a variety of causes and can be serious in infants.

FEATURES
- Diarrhea, which may vary in frequency, amount, and quality (bloody, watery, color, mucous threads)
- Vomiting, which may vary in frequency, amount, and quality (bilious, bloody, food content)
- Infant may appear pale, with mottled skin, sunken eyes, and dry mouth. Lethargy and irritability may also be signs of dehydration
- Abdominal pain, which may vary in frequency, location, quality, duration, and radiation
- Fever may or may not be present

### Gastric cancer

Gastric cancer should be considered, particularly in adult patients.

FEATURES
- Postprandial fullness
- Weight loss
- Nausea, emesis, and dyspepsia usually not relieved by antacids
- Epigastric discomfort, often lessened by fasting and increased by eating

### SIGNS & SYMPTOMS
#### Signs
In infants:
- Failure to gain weight or pronounced weight loss
- The infant is ravenously hungry and nurses avidly, though in the late stages of hypertrophic pyloric stenosis (HPS) the infant may lose interest in feeding

- Although vomiting may be infrequent initially, over several days it becomes more predictable, occurring at nearly every feeding
- Vomiting intensity also increases and projectile vomiting may occur
- Upper abdomen is distended, and gastric peristaltic waves can be seen in many cases, particularly in 'wasted' children and during feeding
- An olive-sized tumor, which may be felt to the right of the umbilicus in most of the patients, is usually more readily palpable immediately after the infant has vomited
- Dehydration: loss of skin turgor, fretfulness, apathy
- Slight hematemesis of either bright red flecks or a coffee-ground appearance
- Patient usually is not otherwise ill-appearing or febrile

In adults:
- Bouts of mild vomiting may occur

## Symptoms
In infants:
- Vomiting, often projectile – may be intermittent or may occur after each feeding
- Vomit may become blood-tinged
- Persistent hunger
- Weight loss
- Dehydration
- Lethargy
- Infrequent or absent bowel movements

In adults:
- Feelings of early satiety, dyspepsia, occasional episodes of mild vomiting, and postprandial pain

## ASSOCIATED DISORDERS
- Pyloric stenosis and esophageal atresia may coexist
- Other congenital defects including tracheoesophageal fistula
- Cornelia de Lange's syndrome
- Hirchsprung's disease
- Phenylketonuria (PKU)
- Congenital rubella

## KEY! DON'T MISS!
Delayed diagnosis may lead to repeated vomiting, dehydration, and hypochloremic metabolic alkalosis (from losses of hydrochloric acid).

## CONSIDER CONSULT
Refer urgently to gastroenterology and pediatric surgery for HPS and any of the differential diagnoses.

## INVESTIGATION OF THE PATIENT
### Direct questions to patient
Questions to parent/caregiver:
- **Q** For how long has your baby been vomiting? Usually since shortly after birth
- **Q** Does he/she vomit after feeding? Parents may describe vomiting with every feeding or intermittent vomiting that may be projectile
- **Q** Is it getting worse? Vomiting worsens over time
- **Q** When was he/she last sick? Establish history of progressive forceful vomiting
- **Q** Is the vomit clear, with bits of food in it, or is it brownish or yellowish in color? Bilious vomiting is rare

- **Q** Is he/she losing weight? Information about the duration and type of vomiting should be obtained as well as the infant's weight
- **Q** How old is your child? Infants tend to present between 4 and 8 weeks of life
- **Q** Do you know if you or anyone in the family had this problem or had an operation on the stomach when you/they were babies? A family history helps diagnosis
- **Q** Has there been any diarrhea? Eliminate other gastrointestinal problems such as gastroenteritis, which is very serious in infants
- **Q** Is he/she feverish? Check for fever

### Contributory or predisposing factors
Has your baby been given the antibiotic erythromycin recently? There is evidence of a link with administration of erythromycin.

### Family history
Do you know if you or other members of your family had a stomach operation as a child? Explain that the information will help diagnosis, as HPS may be hereditary.

### Examination
The first and most important step in patient work-up of suspected HPS is physical examination. Assess the pylorus:
- The patient must be calm and co-operative: a pacifier or small amount of dextrose water may help calm the infant
- If the stomach is distended aspiration using a nasogastric tube will be necessary
- Palpate the liver edge: with the infant supine and the examiner on the child's right side, gently palpate the liver edge near the xiphoid process
- Displace the liver superiorly: downward palpation should reveal the pyloric olive just on or to the right of the midline
- Location of the pyloric olive: an enlarged pylorus, classically described as an olive, can be palpated in the right upper quadrant or epigastrium of the abdomen
- Specificity: the pyloric olive, which represents the thickened and elongated pylorus, is said to be felt by skilled surgeons in up to 80% of patients
- Refer to surgery? If the pyloric olive is felt, some surgeons recommend the patient proceeds directly to surgery without imaging studies; however, most physicians will want to conduct further examinations, particularly ultrasound

### Summary of investigative tests
- Abdominal ultrasound is the preferred modality in the work-up of any vomiting infant and is recommended for all patients with clinical suspicion. Sensitivity and specificity of ultrasound are close to 100% for the diagnosis of HPS
- X-ray barium study of upper gastrointestinal (UGI) tract: if the vomiting infant is outside the usual age range for HPS or if clinical suspicion is low, an upper gastrointestinal study is recommended, since it may rule out other problems such as malrotation and gastroesophageal reflux
- Upper gastrointestinal endoscopy (UGIE): more useful in adult forms of gastric outlet obstruction when malignancy is high in the differential and tissue diagnosis is necessary. The upper gastrointestinal series is considered more cost effective than ultrasound examination because patients with normal results on ultrasound examination still require additional testing to determine the cause of vomiting. However, most clinicians prefer to avoid routine UGI study because of the risk of vomiting and aspiration of contrast material

### DIAGNOSTIC DECISION
- Ultrasonography is important in the diagnosis of HPS. Diagnosis is made by identifying the hypertrophied pyloric muscle by abdominal ultrasonography

- Diagnosis can be made by palpation of a discrete, 2–3cm (0.8–1.2 inches), firm, movable pyloric olive-like mass deep in the right side of the epigastrium
- If the diagnosis is uncertain, a barium swallow will show delayed gastric emptying and the typical 'string sign' of a markedly narrowed, elongated pyloric lumen
- Electrolyte picture is one of metabolic alkalosis accompanied by severe potassium depletion
- Up to 30% of patients will have an indirect reacting hyperbilirubinemia, which as yet remains unexplained
- Establishing an early diagnosis in the newborn or young infant with vomiting can sometimes be difficult. On the other hand, delayed diagnosis may lead to undernutrition, dehydration, aspiration pneumonia, and other complications

## CLINICAL PEARLS
- Hypertrophic pyloric stenosis should be the first diagnosis to consider in vomiting infants with failure to gain weight within the first 3 months of life
- The ultrasound examination should be directed to rule out a hypertrophied pylorus
- A normal ultrasound should be followed by an UGI series

## THE TESTS
### Imaging
ABDOMINAL ULTRASOUND
*Description*
- Ultrasonography is recommended in all patients whose disease is clinically suspicious
- Transverse images at the epigastrium identify the pylorus to the left of the gallbladder and anteromedial to the right kidney, giving the classic 'donut' sign
- A distended stomach displaces and distorts the pylorus

*Advantages/Disadvantages*
Advantages:
- The criterion standard imaging technique for diagnosing HPS
- Diagnostic accuracy of ultrasound for HPS is high – sensitivity and specificity approach 100%
- Reliable and easily performed
- The technique includes feeding glucose water to the baby, which often improves visualization of the pylorus but allows continuous observation of the gastroesophageal junction to diagnose reflux in the case of a negative study
- Positive ultrasound for HPS almost always indicates HPS

Disadvantages:
- Although most infants with presumed HPS can be readily diagnosed by ultrasound, there are cases of inconclusive ultrasound (false-negative ultrasound)
- In patients <5 weeks old and in those with a history of vomiting of <5 days, the sensitivity of ultrasound significantly decreases
- A negative ultrasound often leads to an UGIE to rule out other diagnoses that focused ultrasound does not detect

*Abnormal*
- Depicts the hypertrophied musculature as a hyperdense, broad ring (donut sign)
- Gastric aspirate of >5mL in a baby who has had nil by mouth for several hours indicates gastric outlet obstruction
- Failure of the channel to open during a minimum of 15min of scanning
- Retrograde or hyperperistaltic contractions
- A false-negative can occur in a patient seen early in the disease or in a younger patient whose muscle thickness is <3mm

*Drugs, disorders and other factors that may alter results*
False-negatives:
- Small infant or early presentation
- Excess gastric contents. Place a nasogastric tube and withdraw gastric secretions from any infant whose pylorus is not visualized on ultrasound
- Measuring the gastric contents of an infant who presents with nonbilious vomiting is appropriate before ordering additional tests
- Failure to identify the pylorus (inexperience in performing ultrasound for HPS). Small infant or early presentation

False-positives:
- Pylorospasm – the normal pylorus opens at least once in 15min
- The thickened muscle and elongated pylorus should be fixed

## UPPER GASTROINTESTINAL STUDY
*Description*
Barium X-ray of stomach.

*Advantages/Disadvantages*
Advantages:
- Useful because a negative ultrasound often leads to an UGI study to rule out other diagnoses that focused ultrasound does not detect
- A second test, such as ultrasound, rarely follows a negative UGI study for HPS
- An UGI series has high sensitivity (>90%) and lower specificity
- Can identify gastroesophageal reflux

Disadvantage: slight risk of vomiting and aspiration of barium. After UGI study it is advisable to irrigate and remove any residual barium from the stomach to avoid aspiration.

*Normal*
Normal appearance of pylorus and stomach.

*Abnormal*
- String sign: barium passing through the narrowed channel creating a single, markedly attenuated, and elongated track
- Abdominal radiographs may show a fluid-filled or air-distended stomach, suggesting gastric outlet obstruction
- A markedly dilated stomach with exaggerated incisura (caterpillar sign) may be seen, which represents increased gastric peristalsis in these patients

*Drugs, disorders and other factors that may alter results*
It is impossible to confirm an HPS diagnosis if barium does not leave the stomach.
False-positives/negatives:
- High intestinal obstruction can be seen with midgut volvulus, duodenal obstruction (from stenosis, duodenal web, annular pancreas), gastric outlet obstruction from focal foveolar hyperplasia, and eosinophilic gastroenteritis
- False-negative radiographs may be seen in a child who has vomited recently

## TREATMENT

### CONSIDER CONSULT
Early consults facilitate decisions for diagnostic studies, fluid resuscitation, and scheduling the operative procedure. This is especially important if the child requires transfer to another facility for surgical care.

### IMMEDIATE ACTION
- Preoperative management is directed at correcting the fluid deficiency and electrolyte imbalance
- Base fluid resuscitation on infant's degree of dehydration. Most infants can have their fluid status corrected within 24h; severely dehydrated children, however, sometimes require several days for correction
- If necessary, administer an initial fluid bolus of 10mL/kg with lactated Ringer's solution or normal saline. Continue intravenous therapy at an initial rate of 1.25 to two times the normal maintenance rate until adequate fluid status is achieved
- Adequate amounts of both chloride and potassium are necessary to correct metabolic acidosis. Unless renal insufficiency is a concern, initially add 2–4mEq (2–4mmol/L) of potassium chloride/100cm$^3$ of intravenous fluid. Adequate chloride for resuscitation usually can be provided by dextrose 5% normal saline. Avoid adding hypertonic chloride or ammonium chloride
- Urine output and serial electrolyte determinations are performed during resuscitation. Correction of serum chloride level to 90mEq/L (90mmol/L) or greater usually is adequate to proceed with surgical intervention

### PATIENT AND CAREGIVER ISSUES
#### Forensic and legal issues
- Failure to choose the best radiologic investigation for the vomiting infant
- A good physical examination performed by a surgeon with pediatric expertise is required. A child with a pyloric olive likely has hypertrophic pyloric stenosis (HPS). Imaging may be requested to confirm HPS. Ultrasonography is the preferred choice. Following rehydration, perform pyloromyotomy when the child is stable
- If clinical history suggests HPS, and the child is stable, perform ultrasonography to diagnose or rule out HPS. If ultrasonography is negative, perform an upper gastrointestinal (UGI) series to confirm or rule out other pathology
- If concern exists about malrotation, with or without volvulus (no olive is felt, patient is sick), an UGI series is necessary
- Failure to choose the best test, which is dictated by patient history, physical examination, and the surgeon's level of suspicion. Ultrasonography, while reliable in diagnosing HPS, may miss malrotation, which is the most serious cause of vomiting in infants. These children require upper gastrointestinal examination

#### Impact on career, dependants, family, friends
- Parents should be reassured that the condition is curable and that following surgery, feeding should be restored
- With earlier presentation, the incidences of dehydration, metabolic alkalosis, weight loss, and failure to thrive as manifestations of HPS have decreased dramatically

#### Health-seeking behavior
Parents often report trying several different baby formulas as they assume vomiting is due to intolerance.

## MANAGEMENT ISSUES
### Goals
- Reassure the parents that testing will likely determine the problem and that corrective surgery is available
- Make sure the child is rehydrated
- Arrange for urgent referral and tests

### Management in special circumstances
COEXISTING DISEASE
Infant may have other congenital abnormalities, but HPS requires immediate treatment in any case.

PATIENT SATISFACTION/LIFESTYLE PRIORITIES
Reassurance of parents and instructions on postoperative feeding.

## SUMMARY OF THERAPEUTIC OPTIONS
### Choices
- Surgery: the treatment of choice is a Ramstedt longitudinal pyloromyotomy, which leaves the mucosa intact and separates the incised muscle fibers. Postoperatively, the infant usually tolerates feedings within a few days
- Endoscopic balloon dilation is controversial. This treatment is not standard for HPS; endoscopy may be used for adult HPS only. Balloon catheter dilation through an endoscope. Rarely used in infants with persistent vomiting secondary to incomplete pyloromyotomy
- Vagotomy and pyloroplasty: performed on adult patients. Vagotomy cuts the vagus nerve that stimulates acid secretion in the stomach. However, this surgery may impair stomach emptying. Pyloroplasty enlarges the pyloric opening into the duodenum so that stomach contents can empty more easily
- Two classes of acid-suppressing medications currently in use are histamine $H_2$ receptor agonists and proton pump inhibitors (PPIs; inhibitors of the gastric $H^+$, $K^+$-ATPase (proton pump) enzyme system, the final step in gastric acid secretion). Both classes are available in intravenous or oral preparations. However, most gastroenterologists agree that oral PPIs are better than oral $H_2$ receptor agonists
- Acid suppression therapy for adult HPS caused by peptic ulcers. PPIs are the drugs of choice, e.g. esomeprazole, lansoprazole, omeprazole, pantoprazole, and rabeprazole

### Clinical pearls
- Nonoperative approaches are appropriate in adults where peptic disease may be causing reversible gastric outlet obstruction
- Acid suppression with a PPI is important even when there is no evidence of active ulcer disease. Suppressing acid secretion will reduce gastric volume and decrease the symptom of vomiting
- When successful, endoscopic balloon dilation can prevent the need for surgical resection. However, serial dilation is often required and there is a risk of perforation

### Never
- Never prescribe erythromycin if HPS is suspected
- Never fail to recognize dehydration or failure to gain weight in an infant

## FOLLOW UP
Postoperative management:
- Feeding can be resumed and advanced over a 24h period for most patients
- Premature infants sometimes require apnea monitoring if they have a history of apnea spells
- Postoperative analgesics are employed, as with any other surgical patient. Once feeding by mouth has resumed, acetaminophen usually suffices

- Narcotic pain medications should be avoided in the postoperative period as opioids may precipitate apnea in the alkalotic newborn
- Infants can be discharged from hospital care once they can remain hydrated and have adequate enteral intake
- Infants generally recover rapidly after operative correction of HPS. Parents will be advised to increase food volume in the days after discharge
- A single postoperative visit 1–2 weeks after surgery is often all that is necessary to document weight gain
- Long-term sequelae from pyloromyotomy are virtually unheard of
- Studies have documented normal function returns in months to years after surgery

### Plan for review
- Document weight gain during subsequent follow-up visits
- Persistent emesis after surgery suggests incomplete pyloromyotomy, gastritis, hiatal hernia, or another cause for obstruction
- Postoperative vomiting can be managed conservatively. However, if it persists longer than 5 days, radiologic evaluation should be performed
- The infant should be watched for other complications, e.g. postoperative duodenal perforation, small bowel obstruction secondary to adhesions

### Information for patient or caregiver
- Surgery can cure the disease
- The infant should have nothing to eat or drink before surgery and for 12–24h after surgery
- Feedings are usually resumed 6–8h after operation. In most instances, gradually increasing volume and strength of feedings is recommended

The surgery should be explained to the parents:
- This surgery spreads open the muscle around the pyloric valve of the stomach
- The incision is about one inch long either right around the belly button or on the right-hand side of the abdomen
- Stitches that dissolve are used, so they won't have to be removed later
- Feedings will start slowly. The nurse will advise when to start
- The amount of formula will be limited at first and will be increased with each feed
- A few episodes of vomiting shortly after surgery are not uncommon but should resolve quickly

In adults:
- Patient education involves discussion regarding avoidance of nonsteroidal anti-inflammatory drugs if possible
- Patients should be aware of the significance and appearance of melena stool and should be instructed to alert their physicians at once if melena is noted

## DRUGS AND OTHER THERAPIES: DETAILS
### Drugs
ESOMEPRAZOLE
For ulcer-related adult HPS only:
- PPIs: inhibitors of the gastric $H^+$, $K^+$-ATPase (proton pump) enzyme system, the final step in gastric acid secretion
- Two classes of acid-suppressing medications currently in use are histamine $H_2$ receptor agonists and PPIs. Both classes are available in intravenous or oral preparations. However, most gastroenterologists agree that oral PPIs are better than oral $H_2$ receptor agonists

*Dose*
Oral 20 or 40mg once daily.

*Efficacy*
Effective acid suppression for adult HPS caused by peptic ulcers.

*Risks/benefits*
Risks:
- Symptomatic response to therapy with esomeprazole magnesium does not preclude the presence of gastric malignancy
- Atrophic gastritis has been noted occasionally in gastric corpus biopsies from patients treated long-term with omeprazole, of which esomeprazole magnesium is an enantiomer

*Side effects and adverse reactions*
- Central nervous system: headache
- Gastrointestinal: diarrhea, nausea, flatulence, abdominal pain, constipation, dry mouth

*Interactions (other drugs)*
- Diazepam
- Drugs where gastric pH is an important determinant of bioavailability (e.g. ketoconazole, iron salts, and digoxin)

*Contraindications*
- Known hypersensitivity to any component of the formulation or to substituted benzimidazoles
- Safety and efficacy in pediatric patients have not been established
- Pregnancy category B
- Breast-feeding

*Acceptability to patient*
Generally well tolerated.

*Follow up plan*
Review after 4 weeks.

*Patient and caregiver information*
Patients should be aware of the significance and appearance of melena stool and should be instructed to alert their physician at once if melena is noted.

LANSOPRAZOLE
*Dose*
Oral 30mg once daily.

*Efficacy*
Effective acid suppression for adult HPS caused by peptic ulcers.

*Risks/benefits*
Risk: symptomatic response to therapy with lansoprazole does not preclude the presence of gastric malignancy.

*Side effects and adverse reactions*
- Gastrointestinal: nausea, vomiting
- Genitourinary: urinary retention
- Hematologic: agranulocytosis, aplastic anemia, hemolytic anemia, leukopenia, neutropenia, pancytopenia, thrombocytopenia, and thrombotic thrombocytopenic purpura
- Skin: Stevens–Johnson syndrome (rare)
- Other: pseudomembranous colitis (treat with vancomycin), anaphylaxis

*Interactions (other drugs)*
- Sulcralfate
- Lansoprazole may interfere with the absorption of drugs where gastric pH is an important determinant of bioavailability, such as: ketoconazole, ampicillin esters, iron salts, digoxin

*Contraindications*
- Pregnancy and breast-feeding
- Gastric carcinoma
- Hepatic impairment
- Safety and efficacy in pediatric patients have not been established

*Acceptability to patient*
Generally well tolerated.

*Follow up plan*
Review after 4 weeks.

*Patient and caregiver information*
Patients should be aware of the significance and appearance of melena stool and should be instructed to alert their physician at once if melena is noted.

OMEPRAZOLE
*Dose*
Oral 20mg once daily.

*Efficacy*
It has been shown that omeprazole decreases the need for emergency surgery, improves hemostasis, and decreases the incidence of rebleeding in peptic ulcer hemorrhage.

*Risks/benefits*
Risks:
- Use caution in the elderly and children
- Gastric malignancy may still be present even if symptoms lessen with treatment

*Side effects and adverse reactions*
- Central nervous system: headache, dizziness
- Gastrointestinal: nausea, vomiting, diarrhea, constipation, flatulence, abdominal pain, hepatitis, pancreatitis
- Genitourinary: interstitial nephritis, gynecomastia, urinary problems, urinary infections
- Hematologic: agranulocytosis, thrombocytopenia, anemia, neutropenia, and other blood cell disorders
- Hypersensitivity: angioedema, rashes, anaphylactoid reactions
- Skin: purpura, Stevens–Johnson syndrome, alopecia, erythema multiforme

*Interactions (other drugs)*
- Calcium channel antagonists (nifedipine, nimodipine, nisoldipine, nitrendipine)
- Carbamazepine
- Cefpodoxime, cefuroxime
- Clarithromycin
- Diazepam
- Digoxin
- Enoxacin
- Glipizide, glyburide
- Itraconazole, ketoconazole
- Methotrexate
- Phenytoin
- Sucralfate
- Tacrolimus
- Tolbutamide
- Warfarin

*Contraindications*
- Pregnancy and breast-feeding
- Gastric carcinoma
- Hepatic impairment

*Acceptability to patient*
Generally well tolerated.

*Follow up plan*
Review after 4 weeks.

*Patient and caregiver information*
Patients should be aware of the significance and appearance of melena stool and should be instructed to alert their physician at once if melena is noted.

## PANTOPRAZOLE
*Dose*
Oral 40mg once daily.

*Efficacy*
Effective acid suppression for adult HPS caused by peptic ulcers.

*Risks/benefits*
Risk: symptomatic response to therapy with pantoprazole does not preclude the presence of gastric malignancy.

*Side effects and adverse reactions*
- Central nervous system: headache, asthenia, back pain, chest pain, neck pain, influenza syndrome, infection, pain, migraine, insomnia, anxiety, dizziness, hypertonia
- Gastrointestinal: diarrhea, flatulence, abdominal pain, eructation, constipation, dyspepsia, gastroenteritis, gastrointestinal disorder, nausea, rectal disorder, vomiting
- Metabolic: hyperglycemia, hyperlipidemia
- Musculoskeletal: arthralgia
- Respiratory: bronchitis, increased cough, dyspnea, pharyngitis, rhinitis, sinusitis, upper respiratory tract infection
- Skin: rash

*Interactions (other drugs)*
- **Digoxin** ■ **Itraconzaole** ■ **Ketoconazole**

*Contraindications*
- Safety and efficacy in pediatric patients have not been established ■ Pregnancy and breast-feeding ■ Gastric carcinoma ■ Hepatic impairment

*Acceptability to patient*
Generally well tolerated.

*Follow up plan*
Review after 4 weeks.

*Patient and caregiver information*
Patients should be aware of the significance and appearance of melena stool and should be instructed to alert their physician at once if melena is noted.

## RABEPRAZOLE
*Dose*
Oral 20mg once daily.

*Efficacy*
Effective acid suppression for adult HPS caused by peptic ulcers.

*Risks/benefits*
Risks:
- Symptomatic response to therapy with rabeprazole does not preclude the presence of gastric malignancy
- Use caution in hepatic impairment

*Side effects and adverse reactions*
- Cardiovascular system: hypertension, myocardial infarction, abnormal electrocardiogram, syncope, angina pectoris, bundle branch block, palpitation, sinus bradycardia, tachycardia
- Central nervous system: insomnia, anxiety, dizziness, depression, nervousness, somnolence, hypertonia, neuralgia, vertigo, convulsion, abnormal dreams, decreased libido, neuropathy, migraine, paresthesia, tremor, asthenia, fever, allergic reaction, chills, malaise, substernal chest pain, neck rigidity, photosensitivity reaction
- Eyes, ears, nose, and throat: cataract, amblyopia, glaucoma, dry eyes, abnormal vision, tinnitus, otitis media
- Gastrointestinal: diarrhea, nausea, abdominal pain, vomiting, dyspepsia, flatulence, constipation, dry mouth, eructation, gastroenteritis, rectal hemorrhage, melena, anorexia, cholelithiasis, mouth ulceration, stomatitis, dysphagia, gingivitis, cholecystitis, increased appetite, abnormal stools, colitis, esophagitis, glossitis, pancreatitis, proctitis
- Genitourinary: cystitis, urinary frequency, dysmenorrhea, dysuria, kidney calculus, metrorrhagia, polyuria
- Hematologic: anemia, ecchymosis, lymphadenopathy, hypochromic anemia
- Musculoskeletal: myalgia, arthritis, leg cramps, bone pain, arthrosis, bursitis
- Respiratory: dyspnea, asthma, epistaxis, laryngitis, hiccups, hyperventilation
- Skin: rash, pruritus, sweating, urticaria, alopecia

*Interactions (other drugs)*
- Digoxin
- Itraconzaole
- Ketoconazole

*Contraindications*
- **Pregnancy and breast-feeding**
- The safety and efficacy of rabeprazole in pediatric patients have not been established
- Rabeprazole is contraindicated in patients with known hypersensitivity to rabeprazole, substituted benzimidazoles or to any component of the formulation

*Acceptability to patient*
Generally well tolerated.

*Follow up plan*
Review after 4 weeks.

*Patient and caregiver information*
Patients should be aware of the significance and appearance of melena stool and should be instructed to alert their physician at once if melena is noted.

## Surgical therapy
Surgical techniques are used to correct HPS in infants and adults with great success.

PYLOROMYOTOMY
In 1907, Ramstedt suggested splitting the pyloric muscle and leaving it open to heal secondarily. This procedure has been used to treat infantile HPS since that time. Pyloromyotomy is not an emergency procedure and should be carried out when the dehydration and electrolyte

abnormalities are corrected. Adult therapy consists of gastrojejunostomy with or without surgical resection of the pylorus.

*Efficacy*
The procedure is highly effective and there are rarely any long-term sequelae.

*Risks/benefits*
Risks:
- Persistent vomiting, which suggests an incomplete pyloromyotomy, gastritis, gastroesophageal reflux disease, or another cause of obstruction
- Usual risks with surgery but the procedure is usually straightforward. Mortality is 0–0.5%

Benefit: the procedure is highly effective. Most children can start eating 4–6h after surgery and go home in about 2 days.

*Follow up plan*
- Postoperative appearance: symptoms may take time to clear; therefore, so do the abnormalities on ultrasonography
- Ultrasonography may show HPS (thickened muscle) for up to 12 weeks following pyloromyotomy. In these cases, an UGI series may provide more information than ultrasonography to rule out incomplete myotomy
- Continue intravenous maintenance fluid until infant is able to tolerate enteral feedings. In most instances, feedings can begin within 8h following surgery. Graded feedings usually can be initiated on an every 3h schedule, starting with Pedialyte and progressing to full-strength formula
- Although schedules that advance the volume of feeds more quickly, or those that begin with ad lib feeds, are associated with more frequent episodes of vomiting, they do not increase morbidity and actually may decrease the time to hospital discharge
- Addition of a prokinetic agent can be beneficial sometimes
- Treat persistent vomiting expectantly as it usually will resolve within 1–2 days
- The temptation to repeat an ultrasound or UGI barium study should be avoided as these invariably will demonstrate a deformed pylorus and be difficult to interpret

*Patient and caregiver information*
The pyloromyotomy can be explained to the parents:
- An incision is made in the skin on the right side of the baby's abdomen
- The surgeon will split the thickened muscle to open it
- The incision is then closed with stitches placed under the skin. They are made of an absorbable material that will dissolve after the incision has healed
- The incision will be covered with steri-strips (a long tape that will stick on for 7–10 days)
- Most children eat 4–6h after surgery and go home in about 2 days
- Glucose and saline feedings can usually be started 4h after surgery and within 2 days most infants can be fed milk every 4h
- Postoperative vomiting is common; many infants for whom operation has been successful exhibit some vomiting for the first 24–48h. The persistence of severe vomiting beyond 5 days may indicate an inadequate division of the hypertrophied pylorus or adhesions around a so-called duodenal niche. In these cases reoperation may be necessary. There is no explanation for the continued vomiting of many infants surgically relieved of HPS

## VAGOTOMY
Performed as part of the treatment of ulcer-related adult pyloric obstruction. Involves resection of the vagus nerve, which eliminates the autonomic stimulation of the parietal cells. Historically, a truncal vagotomy was performed; however, this led to gastric atony and subsequent stasis in as

many as 20% of patients. Currently, selective vagotomies are the procedures of choice.

*Efficacy*
- Only a few cases cited, as rare in adults
- Selective vagotomy preserves the celiac and hepatic branches of the vagus nerve, thus decreasing the incidence of gastric atony
- However, a gastric drainage procedure (e.g. pyloroplasty) remains an essential component of this surgical approach. Highly selective vagotomy results in denervation of the parietal cells but preserves nerves supplying the pyloroantral region

*Acceptability to patient*
Will relieve patient of symptoms if acid suppression therapy fails.

## OUTCOMES

### EFFICACY OF THERAPIES
- Pyloromyotomy works by two mechanisms: initially, the pyloric channel widens as a result of incising the muscle; the procedure secondarily induces regression of muscle hypertrophy
- Adult cases of hypertrophic pyloric stenosis (HPS) as a result of ulcer disease or Crohn's disease may be successfully treated by partial (distal) gastrectomy or vagotomy and/or pyloroplasty
- Acid suppression therapy, particularly proton pump inhibitors (PPIs), are proven for adult patients with HPS related to duodenal or peptic ulcer disease

### Review period
A single postoperative visit 1–2 weeks after surgery often is all that is necessary to document weight gain.

### PROGNOSIS
The complete relief of symptoms occurs after adequate surgical repair and the child is able to feed properly.

### Clinical pearls
- Complete recovery without sequelae is the rule after pyloromyotomy
- Postoperative dumping symptoms do not occur after surgery for HPS
- Gastric stasis symptoms may persist after gastric resection for adult pyloric stenosis due to the chronic nature of the condition

### Therapeutic failure
Persistent vomiting:
- Incomplete pyloromyotomy is rare but complications can occur due to injury to the mucosa from injudicious spreading during the myotomy
- The persistence of severe vomiting beyond 5 days may indicate an inadequate division of the hypertrophied pylorus or adhesions around a so-called duodenal niche. In these cases reoperation may be necessary

### Recurrence
Occasionally, adult patients present with obstructive symptoms resulting from pyloric stenosis associated with muscular hypertrophy. This is rarely caused by persistence of a missed case of infantile pyloric stenosis. Most commonly, it is associated with juxtapyloric peptic ulceration.

### COMPLICATIONS
Failure to gain weight in the newborn period.

Risks associated with surgery:
- Undetected mucosal perforation: a search for mucosal transgressions should be made during surgery and the infant examined again before initiating feedings. Return to the operating theater if perforation is suspected
- Bleeding: in most instances, venous oozing from the myotomy site is self-limited and not a concern in the postoperative period. Reports of continued bleeding are exceedingly rare but can occur, especially in children with undetected coagulopathy

### CONSIDER CONSULT
Patients should be referred to a pediatric surgeon whenever the diagnosis is established, or to a pediatric gastroenterologist when the diagnosis is suspected but initial tests are negative.

## PREVENTION

Hypertrophic pyloric stenosis (HPS) probably cannot be prevented, as it is often a genetic disorder.

### RISK FACTORS
No established risk factors, but diet during pregnancy is often cited as a contributory factor.

### MODIFY RISK FACTORS
- Good nutrition just before and during pregnancy helps prevent the occurrence of certain abnormalities at the time of or following birth, including pyloric stenosis
- Women who are planning to become pregnant should be counseled about proper nutrition

#### Lifestyle and wellness
TOBACCO
Women should cease smoking during pregnancy.

ALCOHOL AND DRUGS
Ideally, women should not drink alcohol during pregnancy.

DIET
- Dietary habits and, in particular, folic acid intake are important
- Prenatal vitamins may also supply some of the vital nutrients that the body needs just before conception and during pregnancy
- Because up to 50% of pregnancies are not planned, all women of child-bearing age, especially women who are thinking of getting pregnant, should take folic acid supplements
- Synthetic folic acid, which is a monoglutamate, is preferable to folate that occurs naturally because it is absorbed faster
- Avoiding foods that may cause allergies could also benefit newborns prior to developing HPS by decreasing the possibility of stomach upset and colic
- Nonbreast-fed infants may do better on a soy formula or a hydrosylate formula because these formulas are easier to digest

FAMILY HISTORY
Parents may need advice, either before becoming pregnant or afterwards, if there is a family history of HPS.

DRUG HISTORY
Erythromycin may be associated with HPS.

### PREVENT RECURRENCE
Corrective surgical procedures should prevent recurrence.

# RESOURCES

## ASSOCIATIONS

**American Pediatric Surgical Association**
60 Revere Drive, Suite 500
Northbrook, IL 60062
Tel: (847) 480-9576
Fax: (847) 480-9282
E-mail: mepel@eapsa.org
http://www.eapsa.org

**American Academy of Family Physicians**
11400 Tomahawk Creek Parkway
Leawood, KS 66211-2672
Tel: (913) 906-6000
E-mail: fp@aafp.org
http://www.aafp.org

## KEY REFERENCES

- Silverman A, Roy CC. Clinical pediatric gastroenterology. Philadelphia, PA: Mosby, 1983, p162–5
- Ravitch MM, Welch KJ, et al. Pediatric surgery, 3rd edn. Chicago: Year Book, 1979, p891– 5
- Graadt van Roggen JF, van Krieken JH. Adult hypertrophic pyloric stenosis: case report and review. J Clin Pathol 1998;51:479–80
- Khullar SK, DiSario JA. Gastric outlet obstruction. Gastrointestinal Endosc Clin North Am 1996;6:585–603
- Hulka F, Campbell JR, Harrison MW. Cost-effectiveness in diagnosing infantile hypertrophic pyloric stenosis. J Pediatr Surg 1997;32:1604–8
- Hulka F, Campbell TJ, Campbell JR. Evolution in the recognition of infantile hypertrophic pyloric stenosis. Pediatrics 1997;100:E9
- Teele RL, Smith EH. Ultrasound in the diagnosis of idiopathic hypertrophic pyloric stenosis. N Engl J Med 1977;296:1149–50

## FAQS

### Question 1
What symptoms are the most specific for the diagnosis of hypertrophic pyloric stenosis (HPS)?

### ANSWER 1
The combination of forceful or projectile vomiting and either weight loss or the failure to gain weight are most suggestive of HPS.

### Question 2
What should be done if the ultrasound is negative?

### ANSWER 2
A careful upper gastrointestinal X-ray to identify pyloric narrowing, a string sign, should be performed, and if this is also negative endoscopy should be considered.

### Question 3
Do all patients with adult pyloric stenosis require surgery?

### ANSWER 3
No, it is worthwhile to attempt to manage the condition with a combination of medication and dilation. If peptic disease is the cause, the appropriate medication is a proton pump inhibitor; for Crohn's disease, corticosteroids are the treatment of choice.

## Question 4
Is dilation safe?

ANSWER 4
Dilation of the pylorus can be more risky than esophageal dilation. With an esophageal stricture, the lumen distal to the stricture is large, i.e. the stomach. But with pyloric strictures, one encounters a less voluminous and curved structure, the duodenum. This area is at risk for perforation during pyloric dilation.

## CONTRIBUTORS
Dennis F Saver, MD
Andrew F Ippoliti, MD
Jaime Oviedo, MD

# RECTAL MALIGNANCY

| | | |
|---|---|---|
| ■ | Summary Information | 554 |
| ■ | Background | 555 |
| ■ | Diagnosis | 558 |
| ■ | Treatment | 572 |
| ■ | Outcomes | 581 |
| ■ | Prevention | 584 |
| ■ | Resources | 587 |

## SUMMARY INFORMATION

### DESCRIPTION
- Colorectal adenocarcinoma; two-thirds of cases arise in rectum or sigmoid colon
- Fourth most common cancer: approx. 130,000 new cases each year with approx. 60,000 deaths annually
- Early clinical course usually asymptomatic, diagnosis primarily through colonoscopy with biopsy
- Treatment goal is curative surgical resection, radiotherapy, and chemotherapy when indicated
- Overall 5-year survival is 50%; prognosis depends on tumor-node-metastases (TNM) stage

### URGENT ACTION
- Evidence of bowel perforation or obstruction demands emergency surgical consultation/intervention
- Evidence of life-threatening colorectal hemorrhage mandates immediate endoscopic or surgical intervention
- Evidence of deep vein thrombosis requires anticoagulation

### KEY! DON'T MISS!
- Do not mistake the nonspecific abdominal complaints of rectal cancer (e.g. pain, bleeding) as hemorrhoids, irritable bowel syndrome, or diverticulosis
- Do not mistake anemia as anemia of chronic disease, especially in the elderly or those with multiple medical problems
- Colorectal cancer should be suspected in any patient who presents with rectal bleeding/microcytic hypochromic anemia, and is over the age of 40 or has risk factors (e.g. polyposis syndrome)
- Evidence of life-threatening colorectal hemorrhage mandates immediate endoscopic or surgical intervention
- Evidence of deep vein thrombosis requires anticoagulation
- Individuals with colorectal cancer are at increased risk for synchronous and metachronous carcinoma

## BACKGROUND

### ICD9 CODE
- 154.0 Colorectal cancer
- 154.1 Primary neoplasm of rectum (ampulla)
- 154.8 Primary neoplasm of contiguous sites with anus or rectum

### SYNONYMS
- Rectal adenocarcinoma
- Rectal carcinoma
- Rectal cancer
- Colorectal adenocarcinoma
- Colorectal carcinoma

### CARDINAL FEATURES
- Colorectal adenocarcinoma; two-thirds of cases arise in rectum or sigmoid colon
- Anatomically, rectal cancers are located distal to the rectosigmoid junction
- Distribution: 20% rectum, 10% rectosigmoid, 25% sigmoid, 5% descending colon, 15% transverse colon, 25% ascending colon/cecum
- Approx. 6% of Americans will develop colorectal cancer
- Lifetime mortality risk: 2.6%
- Can be hereditary (i.e. hereditary nonpolyposis colorectal cancer) or sporadic
- Probably results from a complex interplay of environmental and genetic factors
- Genetic predisposition is emerging as an increasingly important risk factor for colorectal cancer not associated with an inherited neoplastic syndrome (i.e. familial adenomatous polyposis)
- Most arise from colorectal adenomas/polyps with risk related to number and size of adenomas/polyps
- Adenomas/polyps that exhibit atypia/dysplasia, villous architecture or are large (>1cm) have an increased risk of malignant transformation
- Estimated annual malignant transformation for adenomas/polyps: 3% for those >1cm; 17% for those with villous architecture; and 37% for those exhibiting atypia/dysplasia
- Early clinical course is usually asymptomatic; bleeding and change in bowel habits are common presenting symptoms
- Definitive diagnosis requires colonoscopy with biopsy. Laboratory testing (i.e. complete blood count, carcinoembryonic antigen) and radiographic procedures (i.e. barium studies, computed tomography) may also be used
- Screening should be a part of routine care for all adults over the age of 50 years, especially those with first-degree relatives with colorectal cancer. Established screening guidelines are available, usually employing fecal occult blood testing, sigmoidoscopy, and colonoscopy
- Improved survival rates are probably secondary to screening and ability to identify premalignant and early neoplastic disease
- Only half of all colorectal lesions can be seen through a flexible sigmoidoscope
- Advanced disease results from local extension or hematogenous/lymphatic spread
- Most commonly metastasize to liver and lung; however, lumbar/thoracic vertebral metastases can occur
- Treatment options include curative surgical resection, radiotherapy, and chemotherapy when indicated
- Overall 5-year survival is 50%; prognosis depends on tumor-node mestastases (TNM) stage

### CAUSES
#### Common causes
Definitive etiology unknown; however, it is generally believed that neoplasia results from a complex interplay of genetic and environmental insults.

### Rare causes
- There are groups that have a high incidence of colorectal cancer, including those with hereditary conditions, such as familial polyposis, hereditary nonpolyposis colon cancer (HNPCC), Lynch I syndrome and Lynch II syndrome. Together they account for 10–15% of colorectal cancers
- Crohn's disease and ulcerative colitis also increase risk

### Contributory or predisposing factors
Increased risk seen with:
- Diet: high fat, low fiber/bulk, heterocyclin amines (from fried and charbroiled food), beer/ale, and poor selenium
- Occupational: automotive industry mold-makers
- Polyposis syndromes: familial juvenile polyposis, familial polyposis, Gardner's syndrome, Muir-Torre syndrome, Peutz–Jeghers syndrome, and Turcot's syndrome
- Inflammatory bowel disease: Crohn's disease and ulcerative colitis
- More common conditions with an increased risk for this disease include: a personal history of colorectal cancer or adenomas, first-degree family history of colorectal cancer or adenomas, and a personal history of ovarian, endometrial, or breast cancer. These high-risk groups account for 23% of all colorectal cancers
- Family history: patients with a first-degree relative who has a history of colorectal cancer, especially if cancer occurred prior to age 50, have a 2- to 3-fold increased risk; increased risk also seen with HNPCC

## EPIDEMIOLOGY
### Incidence and prevalence
- Geographical frequency varies considerably
- Geographical variation is more pronounced for colon cancer

INCIDENCE
- Overall incidence is 135,000 new cases/year in US
- Third most common cancer in men and the second in women
- Colorectal cancer is the fourth leading cause of cancer mortality because it has a better prognosis than more common cancers
- Incidence of rectal cancer in Caucasian populations has been stable for approx. 50 years, but it is increasing in non-Caucasian populations

### Demographics
AGE
- Risk increases sharply after age 50
- Most common from 60–80 years of age

GENDER
- More common in men
- Mortality rates have decreased for Caucasian women, but increased for non-Caucasian men and women
- Male incidence rates, adjusted for age and race, appear greater than female rates for both proximal and distal cancers (odds ratio (OR), 1.32 for proximal cancers and 1.68 for distal cancers, respectively)

RACE
More common in Caucasian males than African-American males.

## GENETICS
- It is estimated that 80% of cases are sporadic and not associated with any known hereditary mutations
- Probably results from a complex interplay of genetic and environmental factors, with genetics playing an increasingly appreciated role
- Cumulative effect of multiple hereditary and acquired genetic insults appears to be playing an ever-increasing role in pathogenesis
- Genetic predisposition is emerging as an increasingly important risk factor for colorectal cancer not associated with an inherited neoplastic syndrome; the nature of these genetic lesions is presently undergoing active investigation
- Individuals with first-degree relatives who have a history of colorectal cancer have a 2- to 3-fold increased risk

## GEOGRAPHY
- The incidence is higher in developed countries than in developing countries
- Fewer than one-third of these cancers occur in developing countries
- The lifetime risk of developing colorectal cancer in developed countries appears to be 4.6% in men and 3.2% in women
- Sharp increases in incidence have been seen in eastern Europe and Japan
- The geographic differences in incidence appear to be due to differences in diet and environment, imposed on a background of genetic susceptibility
- Immigration from a low-incidence to a high-incidence environment will increase the risk
- Incidence varies in the US: higher in northeast and north central states, lower in western and southern states; however, regional differences are becoming less pronounced
- More prevalent in urban areas
- The frequency can vary from a low of 2.5–13/100,000 in Asia and Africa to a high of 32–38/100,000 population in the UK and the US

## SOCIOECONOMIC STATUS
There is no established association between colorectal cancer and socioeconomic status.

## DIAGNOSIS

## DIFFERENTIAL DIAGNOSIS
The vast majority of rectal cancers are adenocarcinomas; other tumors constitute approx. 5% of rectal neoplasias.

### Colorectal non-neoplastic polyps
- It is estimated that 2–5% of sporadic polyps will develop into an invasive carcinoma
- Morphologically may be sessile or pedunculated
- Tend to result from mucosal inflammation or abnormal maturation (e.g. hyperplastic polyp)
- Inflammatory polyps are especially common in ulcerative colitis and Crohn's disease

FEATURES
Like rectal cancer:
- Can present as a mass lesion with variable morphology
- Diagnosed through sigmoidoscopy or colonoscopy with biopsy
- Slow growing, and often asymptomatic

Unlike rectal cancer:
- Sessile or pedunculated
- Snare polypectomy or removal with biopsy forceps is treatment of choice

### Colorectal adenomas
- In the general population, the risk of development of a colorectal adenoma is approx. 19%
- Benign, premalignant, or malignant colorectal adenomas which range from sessile or pedunculated lesions to premalignant adenomas with variable architecture
- Histologically tubular, villous, or tubulovillous, and can harbor dysplasia that ranges from mild to carcinoma in situ
- Believed to be colorectal carcinoma precursors with risk of malignant transformation related to size, architecture, and severity of dysplasia

FEATURES
Like rectal cancer:
- More common with advanced age
- Can present as a mass lesion with variable morphology
- Slow growing and often asymptomatic
- Can cause bleeding and anemia
- Diagnosed through sigmoidoscopy or colonoscopy with biopsy

Unlike rectal cancer:
- Usually sessile or pedunculated
- Treatment is primarily endoscopic using snare polypectomy; however, adenomas with invasive carcinoma usually require extensive surgical resection

### Carcinoid tumors
- Carcinoid tumors originate from enterochromaffin-like cells, predominantly found in the appendix and small bowel but can occur throughout the gastrointestinal tract
- Most common in the fifth decade of life, and constitute <2% of colorectal tumors
- Better prognosis than colorectal cancer (overall 5-year survival: 90%); widespread disease and hepatic metastases confer a worse prognosis

FEATURES
Like rectal cancer:
- Have metastatic potential; however, while rectal carcinoids have low metastatic potential they

- tend to display aggressive local behavior
- Colonic carcinoids can display local/lymphatic invasion and distant metastasis (e.g. liver)
- Can be asymptomatic or can cause obstruction and diarrhea
- Diagnosed through sigmoidoscopy or colonoscopy with biopsy
- Can appear as single or multiple tumors
- Treatment is primarily surgical

Unlike rectal cancer:
- Patient may present with carcinoid syndrome

## Gastrointestinal lymphoma
- Gastrointestinal lymphoma constitutes 1–4% of all gastrointestinal malignancies, and the gastrointestinal tract is the most common site of extranodal lymphoma
- There are several subtypes: sporadic (Western), sprue associated, and Mediterranean
- 10–15% present in the proximal colon, 10% in the distal colon

### FEATURES
Like rectal cancer:
- Can present as a mass lesion
- Can be asymptomatic or cause anemia, bleeding, obstruction, and weight loss
- Diagnosed through sigmoidoscopy or colonoscopy with biopsy

Unlike rectal cancer:
- Colonic lymphomas may be initially treated nonsurgically with chemotherapy

## Metastatic disease
- Breast, lung, prostate, and stomach cancer can, rarely, metastasize to the gastrointestinal tract
- Lymphoma, leiomyosarcoma, and malignant melanoma may also metastasize to the gastrointestinal tract

### FEATURES
Like rectal cancer:
- Can present as a mass lesion with bleeding and ulceration
- Can be asymptomatic
- Diagnosed through sigmoidoscopy or colonoscopy with biopsy

Unlike rectal cancer:
- Arise in distant organs/sites, and metastasize to gastrointestinal tract

## Mesenchymal tumors
- Rare colorectal tumors that are benign or malignant, and include leiomyomas, leiomyosarcoma, Kaposi's sarcoma, and lipoma
- 5-year survival is variable

### FEATURES
Like rectal cancer:
- Can present as a mass lesion
- Can be asymptomatic or can cause bleeding
- Diagnosed through sigmoidoscopy or colonoscopy with biopsy
- Treatment is primarily surgical

## Miscellaneous rare colorectal tumors
Rare colorectal neoplasms, including cloacogenic (transitional cell carcinoma) and melanocarcinomas.

### FEATURES
- Like rectal cancer: diagnosed through sigmoidoscopy or colonoscopy with biopsy
- Unlike rectal cancer: cloacogenic and melanocarcinomas tend to arise at the anorectal junction

### Squamous cell carcinoma
Squamous cell carcinoma involving the anus or anorectal junction.

### FEATURES
- Like rectal cancer: diagnosed through sigmoidoscopy with biopsy
- Unlike colorectal adenocarcinoma: tends to arise at the anorectal junction

## SIGNS & SYMPTOMS
### Signs
- Abdominal mass
- Anemia, microcytic hypochromic (i.e. iron deficiency)
- Fistula (e.g. bladder, vagina)
- Per rectum mass
- Signs consistent with obstruction or perforation of the bowel
- Rectal bleeding

### Symptoms
Because of slow growth, many rectal cancers are clinically silent and are usually well advanced when symptomatic.
- Abdominal pain/discomfort
- Bloody stools/hematochezia
- Changes in bowel habit (often alternating constipation and diarrhea)
- Perineal pain
- Rectal bleeding
- Tenesmus
- Dyspnea, from anemia
- Fatigue, from anemia
- Angina, from anemia
- Back/spine/sacral pain

## ASSOCIATED DISORDERS
- Several familial polyposis syndromes are associated with rectal cancer, including: Turcot's syndrome, Muir–Torre syndrome, Peutz–Jeghers syndrome, familial juvenile polyposis, Gardner's syndrome, and familial adenomatous polyposis
- Almost every patient with familial adenomatous polyposis and Gardner's syndrome will develop colorectal carcinoma. Many of these individuals undergo prophylactic colectomy
- Hereditary nonpolyposis colon cancer (HNPCC) is autosomal dominant and associated with rectal cancer
- Ulcerative colitis, Crohn's disease, and acromegaly (high prevalence rates of 6.3–25% for colon cancer and 14–35% for adenomatous polyps were observed in acromegalics) are also associated with colorectal cancer
- Ulcerative colitis carries a 6.6–30% risk of colorectal cancer; risk depends on disease duration, with disease of <10 years' duration having minimal risk
- Crohn's disease increases colorectal cancer risk by 4- to 20-fold

## KEY! DON'T MISS!
- Do not mistake the nonspecific abdominal complaints of rectal cancer (e.g. pain, bleeding) as hemorrhoids, irritable bowel syndrome, or diverticulosis

- Do not mistake anemia as anemia of chronic disease, especially in the elderly or those with multiple medical problems
- Colorectal cancer should be suspected in any patient who presents with rectal bleeding/microcytic hypochromic anemia, and is over the age of 40 or has risk factors (e.g. polyposis syndrome)
- Evidence of life-threatening colorectal hemorrhage mandates immediate endoscopic or surgical intervention
- Evidence of deep vein thrombosis requires anticoagulation
- Individuals with colorectal cancer are at increased risk for synchronous and metachronous carcinoma

## CONSIDER CONSULT
- Refer to a gastroenterologist for colonoscopy with biopsy
- Major hemorrhage mandates emergency surgical or gastroenterologic referral
- Refer to an oncologist after histologic diagnosis

## INVESTIGATION OF THE PATIENT
### Direct questions to patient
**Q** Have you passed any blood from your anus or noticed your stool streaked with blood? Colorectal cancer can cause bright red blood per rectum and hematochezia, especially lesions of the distal colon and rectum

**Q** Are you tired or fatigued? Rectal cancers can cause anemia and fatigue

**Q** Are you short of breath? Rectal cancers can cause anemia that results in dyspnea

**Q** Do you have chest pain with exertion or at rest? Rectal cancers can cause severe anemia that can result in angina

**Q** Have you had diarrhea? Rectal cancers can cause diarrhea

**Q** Do you feel that after a bowel movement you still have not completely emptied your bowel? Rectal cancers can cause tenesmus

**Q** Do you have abdominal pain? Colorectal cancer can cause abdominal pain; however, this is usually a late finding

**Q** Do you have pain in your lower back or between your legs? Neural invasion is an uncommon and late complication of colorectal cancer

**Q** Have you passed stool from your penis or vagina? Urogenital fistula is an uncommon complication of colorectal cancer

**Q** Have you noticed a change in your bowel habits or a change in the caliber of your stool? Change of bowel habits and stool caliber can result from partially obstructive colorectal lesions

**Q** Are you constipated? Constipation can result from obstructive bowel lesions

**Q** Have you noticed that you are having more frequent bowel movements? Increased bowel movement frequency may result when small amounts of retained stool pass beyond an obstructive lesion

**Q** Have you noticed one leg getting bigger than the other or any sudden shortness of breath? Deep vein thrombosis complicated by pulmonary embolism is a recognized complication of malignancy

### Contributory or predisposing factors
**Q** Do you have a history of a bowel problems or colorectal cancer? Many inherited polyposis and nonpolyposis syndromes increase colorectal cancer risk

**Q** Do you have a history of Crohn's disease or ulcerative colitis? Inflammatory bowel disease increases colorectal cancer risk

### Family history
**Q** Does anyone in your family have a history of bowel problems or colorectal cancer? Having a first-degree relative with colorectal cancer increases risk, as can several inherited polyposis and nonpolyposis syndromes

**Q Has anyone in your family been diagnosed with colorectal cancer before age 40?** Several inherited polyposis/colorectal cancer syndromes are characterized by early-onset colorectal cancer

## Examination
- **Does the patient have a palpable rectal mass?** Some rectal cancers may be palpable on digital rectal examination
- **Does the patient have a palpable abdominal mass?** Rectal cancers can grow large prior to becoming symptomatic, and may produce a palpable abdominal mass
- **Is the patient's stool positive for occult blood?** Rectal cancers can cause bleeding; the amount of bleeding is related to tumor size and degree of ulceration
- **Does the patient appear anemic?** Microcytic hypochromic anemia (i.e. iron-deficiency anemia) is a common complication of colorectal cancer
- **Is there evidence of large bowel obstruction?** Obstruction of the large bowel is an uncommon complication of colorectal cancer, and most commonly involves the descending and sigmoid colon
- **Is there rebound tenderness or evidence of peritonitis?** Bowel perforation is an uncommon complication of colorectal cancer
- **Is there unilateral leg swelling?** Deep vein thrombosis is a recognized complication of cancer

## Summary of investigative tests
Initial studies to document disease include:
- Colonoscopy is the initial test of choice to demonstrate a colorectal lesion
- If colonoscopy cannot be performed, air-contrast barium enema is the second choice, preferably followed by sigmoidoscopy as tumors below the rectosigmoid junction cannot be diagnosed by barium enema
- Colorectal cancers can appear grossly as a bulky tumor mass, polypoid mass, 'apple core' (i.e. 'napkin ring') lesion or a flat intramural lesion, all with variable degrees of ulceration, hemorrhage, and necrosis
- Once a colorectal lesion is identified, biopsy is performed concurrently with colonoscopy or sigmoidoscopy
- Definitive diagnosis requires biopsy; mucosal dysplasia/atypia should heighten suspicion for coexisting carcinoma
- Histologically classified as well, moderately or poorly differentiated adenocarcinomas
- Colonoscopy with biopsy is indicated if colorectal lesion is identified on air-contrast barium enema
- Colonoscopy should be performed if carcinoma is found on sigmoidoscopy as approximately half of these patients will have synchronous lesions
- Fecal occult blood testing (FOBT) is not sensitive or specific for colorectal cancer. If clinical suspicion of colorectal cancer is high despite negative FOBT, colonoscopy should be performed

Once a rectal malignancy is confirmed, the following tests are used to further evaluate and stage the cancer:
- Computed tomography (CT) scan may be indicated for staging and can be used to evaluate liver for metastasis, resection or hepatic artery chemotherapeutic infusion
- Chest X-ray to rule out lung metastasis
- CT scan of the chest may be indicated if lung lesion is suspected
- Hemoglobin, hematocrit, and iron studies should be reviewed to evaluate anemia from possible colorectal bleed
- Carcinoembryonic antigen (CEA) is used to evaluate disease progression (although it should not be used alone for this purpose) and recurrence
- Liver function tests (LFTs): alanine aminotransferase (ALT), aspartate aminotransferase (AST), and alkaline phosphatase (ALP) are measured to evaluate hepatic metastasis (ALP most sensitive to presence of liver metastases, though none is particularly specific)

- Transrectal ultrasound is under investigation for preoperative staging (normally performed by a specialist)

Screening for colorectal malignancies:
- The American Cancer Society recommends annual FOBT and flexible sigmoidoscopy every 3–5 years for asymptomatic individuals of average risk (i.e. over age 50). Colonoscopy every 10 years is an acceptable alternative screening option to flexible sigmoidoscopy (The American Cancer Society guidelines on screening and surveillance for early detection of adenomatous polyps and cancer – update 2001. In: American Cancer Society guidelines for the early detection of cancer [1]
- The US Preventive Services Task Force recommends annual FOBT and/or sigmoidoscopy for all individuals age 50 and older (The United States Preventive Services Task Force. Screening for colorectal cancer [2]

## DIAGNOSTIC DECISION
- Colorectal cancer should be suspected in any individual who presents with rectal bleeding/microcytic hypochromic anemia and is over 40 years of age or has risk factors (any male who presents with microcytic anemia at any age and is found to be iron deficient by iron studies should have a colonoscopy; actively menstruating women should also be considered for colonoscopy unless uterine bleeding is particularly heavy)
- A lower age threshold for colonoscopy may be appropriate for those with alarm symptoms (e.g. anemia, bleeding, rectal mass) or those from high-risk populations (e.g. family history, inherited polyposis syndrome)
- Clinical suspicion often results from screening test outcomes or the investigation of individuals who present with signs and symptoms suggestive of rectal cancer
- Don't mistake the vague nonspecific symptoms of rectal cancer with hemorrhoids, irritable bowel syndrome or diverticulosis
- Clinical presentation is often vague and does not suggest neoplastic disease
- Early diagnosis is difficult; many patients present with advanced disease
- Always consider the possibility of malignancy in patients with gastrointestinal complaints; clinical index of suspicion heightened by age and other risk factors
- If clinical index of suspicion for rectal pathology is high, the first test is usually colonoscopy; if colorectal lesion is identified, biopsy is indicated
- CT of the abdomen and pelvis may be used to determine resectability and stage
- Chest X-ray is used for staging followed by CT of the chest if indicated
- CEA is not sensitive or specific for rectal cancer; however, once carcinoma is identified, CEA may be useful to evaluate postoperative recurrence
- Elevated liver aminotransferases are indicative of hepatic involvement but are not diagnostic
- Anemia can result from gastrointestinal blood loss but is not sensitive or specific for rectal malignancy, check complete blood count (CBC) for severe anemia
- Laboratory testing cannot establish or exclude a diagnosis of rectal cancer
- Definitive diagnosis of rectal cancer requires biopsy

### Guidelines
The American Society of Clinical Oncology. 2000 update of recommendations for the use of tumor markers in breast and colorectal cancer: clinical practice guidelines of the American Society of Clinical Oncology [3]

## CLINICAL PEARLS
The treatment should not be decided based only on age; studies have shown that patients older than 80 years submitted for curative surgery have similar operative mortality when compared with patients in their 50s to 70s.

## THE TESTS
### Body fluids
#### HEMATOCRIT

*Description*
Venous blood, 5–7mL in a lavender-top tube.

*Advantages/Disadvantages*
Advantages:
- Decreased hematocrit may be indicative of rectal blood loss
- Routine part of complete blood count (CBC)
- Safe, simple, and inexpensive
- Minimal risk of infection

Disadvantages:
- Abnormal red blood cell size may alter results
- Not sensitive or specific for rectal cancer

*Normal*
- Male: 42–52%
- Female: 37–47%
- Elderly may have slightly lower values

*Abnormal*
- Decreased hematocrit from bleeding caused by rectal cancer
- Markedly elevated white blood count may alter results
- May not accurately reflect blood loss immediately after acute hemorrhage
- Keep in mind the possibility of a false-positive result

*Cause of abnormal result*
Decreased hematocrit may result from bleeding secondary to a rectal lesion, but anemia is not diagnostic for rectal carcinoma.

*Drugs, disorders and other factors that may alter results*
- Drugs that may decrease hematocrit: chloramphenicol, penicillin
- Conditions that may increase hematocrit: burns, chronic high altitude, congestive heart disease, diarrhea, eclampsia, erythrocytosis, dehydration, polycythemia vera, shock
- Conditions that may decrease hematocrit: anemia, bone marrow failure, cancer, chronic disease, cirrhosis, gastrointestinal bleed, hemodilution, hemolysis, hemorrhage, hyperthyroidism, malnutrition, pregnancy, renal disease, rheumatoid arthritis, surgery, trauma

#### HEMOGLOBIN

*Description*
Venous blood, 5–7mL in a lavender-top tube.

*Advantages/Disadvantages*
Advantages:
- Decreased hemoglobin may be indicative of rectal bleeding
- Routine part of CBC
- Safe, simple, and inexpensive
- Minimal risk of infection

Disadvantages:
- Abnormal red blood cell size may alter results
- Not sensitive or specific for rectal cancer

*Normal*
- Male: 14–18g/dL (8.7–11.2mmol/L)
- Female: 12–16g/dL (7.4–9.9mmol/L)
- Elderly may have slightly lower values

*Abnormal*
- Result below normal reference range
- May not accurately reflect blood loss immediately after acute hemorrhage
- Keep in mind the possibility of a false-positive result

*Cause of abnormal result*
Decreased hemoglobin may result from bleeding secondary to a rectal lesion, but anemia is not diagnostic for rectal carcinoma.

*Drugs, disorders and other factors that may alter results*
- Drugs that may decrease hemoglobin: antibiotics, antineoplastic agents, aspirin, indometacin, rifampin, sulfonamides
- Drugs that may increase hemoglobin: gentamicin, methyldopa
- Conditions that may increase hemoglobin: burns, chronic high altitude, chronic obstructive pulmonary disease, congenital heart disease, congestive heart disease, dehydration, diarrhea, erythrocytosis, polycythemia vera
- Conditions that may decrease hemoglobin: anemia, bone marrow failure, cancer, chronic disease, gastrointestinal bleed, hemodilution, hemolysis, hemorrhage, hyperthyroidism, malnutrition, pregnancy, rheumatoid arthritis, renal disease, surgery, trauma

## IRON STUDIES
*Description*
Venous blood sample.

*Advantages/Disadvantages*
Advantages:
- Simple test
- Inexpensive

*Normal*
- Serum iron: male 81–175mcg/dL (14–31mcmol/L); female 64–173mcg/dL (11–30mcmol/L)
- Total iron-binding capacity: 300–417mcg/dL (54–75mcmol/L)
- Serum ferritin: 12–200ng/mL (12–200mcg/L)
- Transferrin: 139.6–279.3mcg/dL (25–50mcmol/L)
- Transferrin saturation: 10–55%

*Abnormal*
- Serum iron, ferritin, and transferrin below normal reference range
- Raised total iron-binding capacity
- Keep in mind the possibility of a false-positive result

*Cause of abnormal result*
Chronic blood loss from an ulcerated tumor depletes iron stores.

*Drugs, disorders and other factors that may alter results*
Poor iron intake or decreased absorption, or the administration of oral iron supplements may alter the results.

## CARCINOEMBRYONIC ANTIGEN

*Description*
Venous blood. Collection tube depends on commercial laboratory performing test.

*Advantages/Disadvantages*
Advantages:
- Approx. 70% of colorectal cancers express CEA
- May have prognostic value for Duke's C carcinomas with four or more involved lymph nodes
- May be used for preoperative staging and postoperative evaluation of recurrence
- Elevated levels may indicate neoplastic disease
- Safe, simple, and inexpensive
- Minimal risk of infection

Disadvantage: not sensitive or specific for rectal cancer, should not be used for screening.

*Normal*
<5ng/mL (<5mcg/L).

*Abnormal*
- Elevated levels can be found with rectal cancer
- Keep in mind the possibility of a false-positive result

*Cause of abnormal result*
- Levels >20ng/mL (>20mcg/L) are highly suggestive of colorectal malignancy
- Levels may rise more rapidly with metastatic disease than with local recurrence

*Drugs, disorders and other factors that may alter results*
CEA may be raised due to:
- Smoking
- Inflammatory disease (e.g. colitis, pancreatitis, diverticulitis, liver disease)
- Breast cancer
- Cirrhosis
- Gastric cancer
- Hepatobiliary cancer
- Lung cancer
- Pancreatic cancer
- Sarcomas

## LIVER FUNCTION TESTS

*Description*
Venous blood, 7–10mL in a red-top tube.

*Advantages/Disadvantages*
Advantages:
- Elevated ALP, ALT, and AST may indicate liver metastasis
- Safe, simple, and inexpensive
- Minimal risk of infection

Disadvantage: not sensitive or specific for rectal cancer.

*Normal*
- AST: 5–40mU/mL (5–40 IU/L)
- ALT: 5–40mU/mL (5–35 IU/L)
- ALP: 30–110mU/mL (30–110 IU/L)

*Abnormal*
- Elevated levels found with liver metastasis
- AST/ALT ratio often >1.0 in liver metastasis
- Keep in mind the possibility of a false-positive result

*Cause of abnormal result*
ALP, ALT, and AST may be elevated from hepatic metastasis, but are not diagnostic of rectal cancer.

*Drugs, disorders and other factors that may alter results*
- Many medications can affect LFTs
- Alcohol abuse can cause abnormal LFTs

## Biopsy
### COLONOSCOPY WITH BIOPSY
*Description*
- Examination of the entire rectum and colon using a flexible colonoscope
- Rectal/colonic tissue obtained for histologic review using endoscopically guided forceps or snare polypectomy
- Patients suspected of having rectal cancer should undergo colonoscopy; if lesion is identified, biopsy is indicated

*Advantages/Disadvantages*
Advantages:
- Invasive diagnostic procedure of choice
- Detection rate for colorectal carcinoma: 95%
- False-negative rate: 5%
- Provides tissue for definitive diagnosis of rectal malignancy

Disadvantages:
- Complications include bleeding and perforation
- Some may refuse colonoscopy, necessitating an alternative diagnostic evaluation
- Some patients may find the procedure uncomfortable and conscious sedation is usually necessary

*Normal*
- No colorectal lesion identified
- No abnormal histology

*Abnormal*
- Colorectal lesion identified
- Abnormal histology

*Cause of abnormal result*
Colorectal cancer can appear grossly as a bulky tumor mass, polypoid mass, 'apple core' (i.e. 'napkin ring') lesion, or a flat intramural lesion, all with variable degrees of ulceration, hemorrhage, and necrosis

Other lesions that can cause abnormal result:
- Colorectal non-neoplastic polyps
- Adenomas
- Carcinoid tumors
- Lymphoma

- Metastatic disease
- Mesenchymal tumors
- Squamous cell carcinoma

*Drugs, disorders and other factors that may alter results*
- Inadequate bowel preparation or heavy bleeding may interfere with endoscopist's ability to visualize and biopsy colon and rectum
- Previous bowel resection/surgery can make colonoscopy technically difficult
- Severe obstruction may prevent passage of colonoscope beyond lesion

## SIGMOIDOSCOPY WITH BIOPSY
*Description*
- Examination of the rectum and sigmoid colon using a flexible fiberoptic sigmoidoscope with biopsy when indicated
- Rectal/colonic tissue is frequently obtained for histologic review using endoscopically guided forceps or snare polypectomy
- Patients found to have a rectal or sigmoid lesion on sigmoidoscopy should undergo complete colonoscopy

*Advantages/Disadvantages*
Advantages:
- Approx. 50% of all colorectal lesions can be identified by a 60cm sigmoidoscope
- Provides tissue for histologic diagnosis

Disadvantages:
- False-negative rate: approx. 15%
- Some patients may find the procedure uncomfortable

*Normal*
- No colorectal lesion identified
- No abnormal histology

*Abnormal*
- Colorectal lesion identified
- Abnormal histology
- Because of the risk for synchronous lesions, full colonoscopy should be performed if a colorectal carcinoma is identified by sigmoidoscopy

*Cause of abnormal result*
Colorectal cancers can appear grossly as a bulky tumor mass, polypoid mass, 'apple core' (i.e. 'napkin ring') lesion, or a flat intramural lesion, all with variable degrees of ulceration, hemorrhage, and necrosis

Other lesions that can cause abnormal result:
- Colorectal non-neoplastic polyps
- Adenomas
- Carcinoid tumors
- Lymphoma
- Metastatic disease
- Mesenchymal tumors
- Squamous cell carcinoma

*Drugs, disorders and other factors that may alter results*
- Inadequate bowel preparation or heavy bleeding may interfere with endoscopist's ability to visualize and biopsy colon and rectum
- Previous bowel resection/surgery can make sigmoidoscopy technically difficult
- Severe obstruction may prevent passage of sigmoidoscope beyond lesion

## Imaging
### AIR-CONTRAST BARIUM ENEMA
*Description*
- Patients should have a total colon examination by either a combination of flexible sigmoidoscopy and barium enema, or by a colonoscopy
- Barium enema may miss a distal cancer and should not be used alone
- Radiographic visualization of the rectum and colon using air and barium as contrast

*Advantages/Disadvantages*
Advantages:
- Detection rate of air-contrast barium enema for colorectal carcinoma: 92% (detection rate of single-column barium enema for colorectal carcinoma: 85%)
- A properly performed air-contrast barium enema examination can have a sensitivity of 85–95% for detecting colorectal polyps

Disadvantages:
- Common sources of error include inadequate cleaning of the colon, which contributes to the 5–10% false-positive rate, and diagnostic difficulty caused by the presence of diverticulosis or redundant bowel, which results in a 10% false-negative rate
- Rectosigmoid lesions may be difficult to visualize with air-contrast barium enema, hence proctosigmoidoscopy should be performed
- Some patients may find the procedure uncomfortable

*Normal*
No lesions identified.

*Abnormal*
Lesion identified.

*Cause of abnormal result*
Colorectal cancers can appear as a bulky mass, polypoid mass, 'apple core' (i.e. 'napkin ring') lesion, or a flat intramural lesion.

Other lesions that can cause abnormal result:
- Colorectal non-neoplastic polyps
- Adenomas
- Carcinoid tumors
- Lymphoma
- Metastatic disease
- Mesenchymal tumors
- Squamous cell carcinoma

*Drugs, disorders and other factors that may alter results*
Inadequate bowel preparation may interfere with radiologist's ability to visualize colon and rectum.

## COMPUTED TOMOGRAPHY SCAN
*Description*
- CT of the abdomen or pelvis to evaluate primary tumor (i.e. staging), recurrence, or metastasis
- Chest CT may be indicated if lung lesion is identified on chest X-ray

*Advantages/Disadvantages*
Advantages:
- Can identify colorectal lesions and extent of local invasion
- Can identify metastatic disease or evidence of recurrence
- Can determine feasibility of hepatic resection for liver metastasis
- Occasionally used to evaluate hepatic artery for chemotherapeutic infusion
- Painless procedure

Disadvantage: significant radiation exposure.

*Abnormal*
Lesion(s) identified.

*Cause of abnormal result*
Primary colorectal tumor with or without metastatic disease.

## CHEST X-RAY
*Description*
X-ray of chest to evaluate presence of pulmonary lesion(s) or evidence of cardiopulmonary disease.

*Advantages/Disadvantages*
Advantages:
- Evaluates presence of neoplastic lesion or evidence of cardiopulmonary disease
- Routine test for preoperative evaluation and cancer staging

Disadvantage: may be contraindicated in pregnant patients.

*Abnormal*
Pulmonary lesion(s) identified.

*Cause of abnormal result*
Rectal cancer can metastasize to the lung, resulting in a pulmonary lesion.

*Drugs, disorders and other factors that may alter results*
- Severe shortness of breath may prevent patient from taking and holding a deep breath
- Severe pain may prevent patient from holding still, or from taking and holding a deep breath

## Other tests
### FECAL OCCULT BLOOD TESTING
*Description*
Testing stool for hemoglobin by placing stool on guaiac-impregnated paper, applying hydrogen peroxide and observing for a positive reaction (i.e. change of color).

*Advantages/Disadvantages*
Advantages:
- Can detect bleeding from colorectal cancer, even early stage disease
- Approx. 2mL of blood will produce a positive reaction

- False-positive rate: 2%
- Safe, simple, convenient, and inexpensive
- Minimal risk of infection

Disadvantages:
- False-negative rate: 40%
- Can be falsely negative as a result of heterogenous distribution of blood in feces, ascorbic acid, and other antioxidants that interfere with test reagents, and extended delay before testing stool samples
- The reported positive predictive value among asymptomatic persons aged 50 and older is about 2–11% for carcinoma and about 20–30% for adenomas
- Multiple samples should be obtained to limit false-negative result
- Recommended sampling: two samples a day for 3 days
- Storage conditions, fecal hydration, and location of tumor may influence results
- Not specific for rectal cancer
- Amount of fecal hydration increases sensitivity, but decreases specificity
- The relatively high rate of false-positive results for fecal occult blood testing can be expected to lead to unnecessary colonoscopies and double-contrast barium studies, with attendant risk for colonic perforation of 1/500–3000 and 1/5000–10,000 examinations, respectively

Detailed recommendations regarding performance and interpretation of FOBT are available at the National Guideline Clearinghouse: American College of Physicians. Suggested technique for fecal occult blood testing and interpretation in colorectal cancer screening [4]

*Normal*
No colored reaction.

*Abnormal*
- Colored reaction
- Keep in mind the possibility of a false-positive result

*Cause of abnormal result*
- Bleeding rectal cancers release hemoglobin, yielding a positive reaction
- Hemoglobin from dietary sources or gastrointestinal bleed

*Drugs, disorders and other factors that may alter results*
- Drugs that may cause false-positive results: aspirin, iron supplements, nonsteroidal anti-inflammatory medications
- False-positive can be caused by: red meat, raw fruit (e.g. cantaloupes), raw vegetables (e.g. broccoli, cauliflower), topical iodine, and excessive rehydration
- False-negative can be caused by: ascorbic acid (vitamin C), stool sampling errors

# TREATMENT

## CONSIDER CONSULT
- Multidisciplinary team approach enhances patient satisfaction and may improve survival
- Refer to an experienced colorectal surgeon for resection
- The need for referral to an oncologist or radiation oncologist is case-specific. Patients presenting with stage IV disease may be referred directly to an oncologist. Patients with localized disease may require referral, depending on the extent of invasion. The surgeon and primary care provider should decide together whether referral is required for adjuvant chemoradiation therapy
- Refer to dietitian for nutritional support
- Referral to a clinical trial may be appropriate

## IMMEDIATE ACTION
- Evidence of bowel perforation or obstruction demands hospital admission and emergency surgical consultation/intervention
- Evidence of life-threatening colorectal hemorrhage mandates immediate endoscopic or surgical intervention
- Evidence of deep vein thrombosis requires anticoagulation

## PATIENT AND CAREGIVER ISSUES
### Forensic and legal issues
- Most patients will be able to consent for treatment
- If patient cannot give consent, determine who has authority to consent
- With the exception of life-threatening hemorrhage, or other life-threatening emergency, rectal cancer treatment can be delayed until consent is obtained

### Impact on career, dependants, family, friends
- If lesion is resectable/curable, many patients can return to work after postoperative recovery
- In advanced disease some patients may be able to return to work, depending on their overall health status
- Those with advanced disease and poor prognosis will have to deal with end-of-life issues that often involve family and friends
- Psychologic impact of cancer diagnosis is profound, with patient, family, and friends experiencing a variety of emotions including, but not limited to, anger, anxiety, bereavement, denial, depression, and grief
- Potential significant impact on career given physical and psychologic demands of diagnosis/treatment and potential poor prognosis

### Patient or caregiver request
- Association with Barrett's esophagus, prior cholecystectomy, and subtotal gastrectomy not established
- Assure patient that most people will not need a colostomy

## MANAGEMENT ISSUES
### Goals
- Primary goal is curative surgical resection
- To initiate evaluation for surgery and chemoradiotherapy
- To achieve complete curative resection
- To preserve bowel function without colostomy
- To prevent spread of disease
- To enhance survival and quality of life
- To achieve adequate pain control
- To evaluate social support

- To determine desire for resuscitation
- To prepare patient to return to a normal or near normal lifestyle
- To determine attitudes toward hospice if disease is terminal
- To prepare patient for end of life if disease is terminal

## Management in special circumstances
### COEXISTING DISEASE
- Some patients with hereditary polyposis syndromes may elect to have prophylactic colectomy
- Those with severe medical conditions or severe cardiopulmonary disease may not be surgical candidates
- Those with terminal disease from colorectal cancer or another disorder are usually not considered appropriate surgical candidates

### PATIENT SATISFACTION/LIFESTYLE PRIORITIES
- Patients will have questions regarding treatment and prognosis
- Patients with a good prognosis will be especially concerned with returning to work and a normal lifestyle
- Patients with a poor prognosis will be concerned with pain control, quality-of-life, and end-of-life issues
- Patients will be concerned, and have questions, about bowel habits, the need for colostomy, and their chances for return to normal bowel function
- Patients with advanced disease will need assistance with end-of-life issues
- Side effects of chemoradiotherapy may negatively impact quality of life
- Severe disability with terminal disease

## SUMMARY OF THERAPEUTIC OPTIONS
### Choices
- First choice is complete macroscopic and microscopic rectal resection with regional lymphadenectomy, with hepatic metastases resection and adjuvant chemoradiotherapy when indicated
- Adjuvant chemoradiotherapy usually indicated for stage II and III disease
- Surgical technique depends on surgeon, tumor location, and extent of disease
- Second choice for unresectable or advanced disease is palliative surgical resection/debulking with chemotherapy and radiation therapy if indicated
- Third choice for unresectable disease is palliative endoscopic therapy to maintain bowel lumen patency
- Adjuvant chemotherapy can delay recurrence and enhance survival
- Most common chemotherapeutic combination is 5-fluorouracil (5-FU) with levamisole
- Multiple chemotherapeutic regimens are under investigation
- Radiotherapy is primarily used to treat rectal and rectosigmoid carcinoma
- Laser therapy used primarily to recanalize the rectum in advanced disease or poor surgical candidates
- Immunotherapy, immunostimulant therapy, and immunotargeted therapy are under investigation
- Treatment decision must take into consideration overall health along with tumor size, location, histologic differentiation, and stage
- For patients with limited (three or less) hepatic metastases, resection may be considered with 5-year survival rates of 20–40%
- For those patients with hepatic metastases deemed unresectable (due to factors such as location, distribution, excessive number), cryosurgical ablation has been associated with long-term tumor control
- Prognostic variables that predict a favorable outcome for cryotherapy are similar to those for hepatic resection and include low preoperative carcinoembryonic antigen level, absence of extrahepatic disease, negative margin, and lymph node negative primary

## Guidelines
- National Comprehensive Cancer Network Practice Guidelines for colorectal cancer, Version 2000 [5]

The following guidelines are available at the National Guideline Clearinghouse:
- Practice parameters for the treatment of rectal carcinoma [6]
- Cancer Care Ontario Practice Guidelines Initiative. Postoperative adjuvant radiotherapy and/or chemotherapy for resected stage II or III rectal cancer [7]
- The Society for Surgery of the Alimentary Tract. Surgical treatment of cancer of the colon or rectum [8]

## Clinical pearls
- Rectal cancer patients benefit from perioperative irradiation more than colon cancer patients, due to an increased tendency for first failure in locoregional sites only
- Both preoperative and postoperative radiation therapy decrease local failure, but alone they will not improve survival
- Patients with resected stage II or III rectal cancer should be offered adjuvant therapy with the combination of radiotherapy and chemotherapy

## Never
Never initiate treatment without obtaining a definitive tissue diagnosis.

## FOLLOW UP
- Follow-up includes evaluation of treatment efficacy, recurrence/spread, and management of surgery or chemoradiotherapy-related complications
- Patients with colostomy will need evaluation for discontinuation of colostomy

## Plan for review
- Evaluate for symptom relief and recurrence/spread
- Evaluate for signs and symptoms of postoperative complications, chemotherapy and radiotherapy toxicity
- Successfully treated patients require physical examination, with fecal occult blood testing (FOBT), complete blood count (CBC), and serum chemistries every 3 months for 2 years, and every 6 months for 5 years
- If carcinoembryonic antigen (CEA) was elevated at diagnosis or within one week of colectomy, repeat CEA every 6 months for 2 years and then annually for 5 years
- Colonoscopy should be performed within one year of the surgery. If there are no symptoms or polyps, investigation is recommended once every 3 years

## Information for patient or caregiver
- Patients need to know that rectal cancer has variable morbidity and mortality and that the only hope for cure is curative resection
- Patients with a poor prognosis will have to decide on end-of-life issues, and be educated regarding options
- Appropriate hospice, skilled nursing facility or home healthcare referral may be needed depending on patient's medical condition, personal preference, and social/financial support
- Patients with colostomy will need to be educated regarding colostomy care

## DRUGS AND OTHER THERAPIES: DETAILS
### Surgical therapy
- All surgical candidates should have a colonoscopy, as findings will result in a modified operative approach in approx. 10% of cases
- Complete tumor resection/lymphadenectomy with adequate and negative resection margins is

the treatment of choice and offers the only hope for cure
- Adequate resection margins are usually more difficult to achieve for rectal cancer when compared with colon carcinoma
- Total pelvic extirpation is often necessary for rectal cancer
- Goal of surgical intervention is curative resection and resumption of normal bowel function

## RECTAL RESECTION WITH LYMPHADENECTOMY
- Standard surgical approach includes complete wide resection of involved rectum with draining lymphadenectomy
- Only hope for cure is complete surgical resection with macroscopic and microscopic negative resection margins
- Approx. 80% of people with colorectal cancer have surgery with curative intent
- Sphincter-preserving resection, and thus avoidance of a colostomy, is the preferred treatment where possible (low anterior resection)
- Resection of rectosigmoid and upper rectal lesions can usually be done with a low anterior abdominal resection/lymphadenectomy with primary anastomosis
- Total mesorectal excision/lymphadenectomy with coloanal anastomosis or temporary colostomy is also used
- Abdominoperineal resection is indicated for bulky lesions, inadequate distal resection margin, poorly differentiated grade, and extensive local disease
- Minimum resection margin is 5cm on both sides of tumor, wider resection margin may be indicated given local blood supply
- Primary tumor should be resected regardless of metastatic disease to prevent bleeding or obstruction
- Fulguration of rectal lesions may be indicated for poor surgical candidates or those with advanced disease
- Hartmann's procedure may be indicated for patients who present with obstruction or perforated carcinoma, and for patients in whom colorectal anastomosis is clinically inadvisable

### Efficacy
- Surgery is the definitive treatment for rectal carcinoma
- Total mesorectal resection may reduce local recurrence
- Super-radical resection/lymphadenectomy does not appear to offer a survival advantage when compared with segmental resection

### Risks/benefits
Risks:
- Complications include anastomotic leak, bleeding, fecal frequency/urgency, fistula, infection, wound infection
- Total mesorectal resection may reduce local recurrence; however, this can be at the expense of more complications (i.e. fecal frequency, anastomotic leak)
- Rectal abdominoperineal resection necessitates permanent sigmoid colostomy
- Age, comorbidities, poor performance status, and obstructive lesions increase risk of perioperative morbidity and mortality

Benefit: advanced age is not a contraindication to surgery.

### Evidence
- Surgery is the preferred treatment for colorectal cancer. Primary surgical resection is indicated in nearly all patients with newly diagnosed colorectal cancer, unless survival is unlikely, or life expectancy is very short [8] *Level C*
- If curative surgery is not possible, palliative surgery should be performed to prevent obstruction and further bleeding [8] *Level C*

- Abdominoperineal resection is generally indicated for tumors of the lower one-third of the rectum, or for higher lesions when tumor characteristics and anatomic factors favor such a resection [6] *Level C*
- Sphincter-preserving resection is possible for most patients with rectal carcinoma [6] *Level C*

*Acceptability to patient*
- Rectal resection is usually accomplished without colostomy or with temporary colostomy; this is acceptable to most patients
- Permanent colostomy may be unacceptable to some patients

*Follow up plan*
- Recommendations vary regarding appropriate follow up
- Routine follow up includes history and physical examination, FOBT, CEA, and liver function tests every 3 months for 2 years, then every 6 months for 5 years
- Postresection colonoscopy should be performed within 6–12 months, then annually for 2 years, then every 3 years
- Follow up may also include chest X-ray and computed tomography (CT) of the liver
- Colonoscopy is useful for detecting synchronous and metachronous lesions
- Pelvic CT may be indicated, especially postresection of a rectosigmoid tumor
- CEA is used to evaluate recurrence and guide decisions regarding 'second-look' laparotomy for colorectal cancer and hepatic metastases
- Restoration of bowel continuity is of primary importance; most patients will not need permanent colostomy
- Ensure adequate postoperative pain control
- Observe for bleeding, wound infection, and other postoperative complications

*Patient and caregiver information*
- Patients and caregivers need to be able to recognize major postoperative complications such as bleeding and wound infection
- Patients and caregivers need to be able to change and maintain colostomy bag

## HEPATIC METASTASES RESECTION
- Liver is the most common site of colorectal metastasis
- 10–25% of patients have liver metastasis at presentation
- 70–80% of hepatic metastases present within 2 years of initial resection
- Unresected hepatic metastases portend a poor prognosis
- Patients without evidence of extrahepatic spread who have had or are scheduled to undergo curative resection should have hepatic lesions resected
- 4.5–11% of hepatic metastases are resectable
- Resection is usually not indicated if four or more hepatic lesions are present

*Efficacy*
- 5-year survival: 20–34%
- Bilobar involvement increases risk of recurrent hepatic metastases

*Risks/benefits*
Risks:
- Perioperative mortality: 2%
- Mortality and morbidity is in part dependent on surgical expertise

*Follow up plan*
- In approx. 35% of patients who are postresection of hepatic metastases, the liver is the initial site of postresection recurrence

- Resection of hepatic recurrence may be indicated if lesion is solitary
- Resection of pulmonary metastatic disease may also be indicated

*Patient and caregiver information*
Patients and caregivers need to be able to recognize major postoperative complications such as bleeding and wound infection.

## Radiation therapy
Radiation therapy used as an adjunct to curative resection.

### EXTERNAL-BEAM RADIATION THERAPY
- Radiotherapy is primarily used to treat rectal and rectosigmoid carcinomas
- Preoperative and/or postoperative radiotherapy are used for Dukes' B2 and C rectal or rectosigmoid cancer and can reduce local recurrence risk
- Radiotherapy can be used preoperatively to enhance or achieve resectability
- Adjuvant chemoradiotherapy should be considered for Dukes' B2 or C (stage II or III) rectal cancer, and may reduce recurrence and enhance survival
- Occasionally used to palliate pain and bleeding from advanced disease

*Efficacy*
- Preoperative radiotherapy may increase postoperative morbidity and mortality
- Postoperative radiotherapy usually used for high recurrence risk
- Radiotherapy has no significant impact on systemic recurrence
- When compared with preoperative radiotherapy, postoperative radiotherapy may result in an increased risk of anastomotic breakdown and stricture formation
- Postoperative chemoradiotherapy may reduce overall mortality by 29% in patients with stage II or III rectal cancer
- Recurrence rate for lesions treated by surgery alone: 40–50%
- Recurrence rate for lesions treated with surgery and postoperative radiotherapy: 6–16%

*Risks/benefits*
Risks:
- While radiation therapy can modestly enhance survival and reduce recurrence risk, this benefit must be weighed against increased morbidity
- Some authors believe that preoperative radiotherapy 'is unlikely to provide much absolute benefit' for T1 and T2 rectal cancers
- Complications of radiation therapy include anastomotic breakdown, cardiac events, damage to surrounding structures (e.g. small bowel), diarrhea, fecal frequency/urgency, hip fracture, intestinal obstruction, pain, radiation proctitis, stricture formation, venous thrombosis/embolism, and wound breakdown/infection
- Complications result from radiation damage to surrounding organs
- Radiation therapy can double incidence of certain postoperative complications (e.g. wound infection/breakdown 20 vs 10%)
- Approx. 30% of those treated with preoperative radiation therapy will experience fecal urgency and frequency
- Anastomotic complications are more common with postoperative radiation therapy
- Preoperative radiation therapy can delay surgery and distort tumor architecture, making accurate staging difficult

Benefits:
- Preoperative radiation therapy may improve survival
- Preoperative and/or postoperative radiation therapy can reduce local recurrence

*Evidence*
- A systematic review found that preoperative radiation therapy plus surgery was superior to surgery alone in the treatment of rectal adenocarcinoma. There was a significant reduction in overall mortality after 5 years with combination therapy, and local recurrence rate was also reduced. There was no significant reduction in the risk of distant metastases [9] *Level M*
- A randomized controlled trial (RCT) compared preoperative and postoperative radiotherapy in patients with Dukes' B or C rectal cancer. There was no significant difference in overall survival at 5 years between the groups, but there was a significant reduction in local recurrences in the preoperative radiation therapy group [10] *Level P*
- Approximately one-third of patients will suffer from impairment of bowel function as a result of radiation therapy [11]

*Acceptability to patient*
- Aggressively manage nausea, vomiting, and diarrhea that can limit patient compliance
- Profound fatigue is common during radiation therapy; instruct the patient to get adequate rest
- Warn patient about potential skin irritation over radiated site

*Follow up plan*
Evaluate patient for evidence of disease recurrence/spread or radiation-induced complications.

*Patient and caregiver information*
- Advise patient to receive adequate rest to limit profound fatigue
- Warn patient that radiation therapy may cause nausea, vomiting, and diarrhea; however, emphasize that these side effects can be managed
- Warn patient about potential skin irritation over radiated site

## Chemotherapy
- Standard chemotherapy is 5-FU with levamisole
- Levamisole is not effective when used alone
- Standard chemotherapy for metastatic disease is 5-FU with leucovorin (5-FU + LV)
- Chemotherapy can delay recurrence and enhance survival
- Chemotherapy is best initiated within 8 weeks of primary surgery
- Consider entry into clinical trial, especially for palliative chemotherapy
- Other chemotherapeutic agents are under investigation
- Portal vein chemotherapy infusion is under active investigation
- Adjuvant chemoradiotherapy should be considered in Dukes' B2 or C (stage II or III) rectal cancer
- Chemotherapy results are disappointing for advanced disease, with any response lasting approx. 4–5 months with no significant impact on survival
- For hepatic metastasis, direct arterial infusion of several chemotherapy agents can be used; floxuridine response rate is 54–83%
- Irinotecan is under investigation for patients with metastatic colorectal cancer who have failed 5-FU + LV

### 5-FLUOROURACIL (5-FU)
5-FU is the most common chemotherapy agent for colorectal cancer.

*Efficacy*
- Adjuvant chemotherapy can improve survival in 9% of Dukes' B or C rectal carcinoma
- One study reported a 42% recurrence risk reduction and a 33% reduction in overall mortality with 5-FU/levamisole/surgery vs surgery alone in patients with Dukes' C, stage III colon cancer
- 5-FU/levamisole may enhance disease-free survival for Dukes' B and C colon cancer
- Postoperative chemoradiotherapy may reduce overall mortality by 29% with recurrence/metastasis in patients with stage II or III rectal cancer

- Response rate to 5-FU and other agents for advanced disease is 12–20%
- Several studies suggest response rates to 5-FU and high-dose leucovorin is 30–48%; however, there is no survival advantage and toxicity is increased. Low-dose leucovorin is usually better tolerated

*Risks/benefits*
Risks:
- Specialist advice must be followed
- Will cause bone marrow suppression
- Use caution with impaired hepatic or renal function
- High-dose pelvic irradiation
- Previous use of alkylating agents
- Discontinue as soon as signs of toxicity appear (diarrhea, watery stools, frequent bowel movements, gastrointestinal ulceration and bleeding, hemorrhage, leukopenia, stomatitis or esophagopharyngitis, thrombocytopenia, vomiting)
- 5-FU can increase dermatologic toxicity of radiotherapy
- Catheter-related complications include catheter leak, hemorrhage, infection, thrombosis, and catheter migration into receiving artery
- 5-FU toxicity is related to dose and route of administration
- Severe vomiting or diarrhea can be complicated by dehydration and hypotension

*Side effects and adverse reactions*
- Cardiovascular system: angina, myocardial ischemia
- Central nervous system: headache, nystagmus, acute cerebellar syndrome
- Eyes: photophobia
- Gastrointestinal: stomatitis, esophagopharyngitis, diarrhea, emesis, nausea, vomiting
- Hematologic: bone marrow suppression, leukopenia, thrombocytopenia, agranulosis, pancytopenia, anemia
- Skin: alopecia, dermatitis, photosensitivity

*Interactions (other drugs)*
- **Leucovorin calcium** ■ **Cimetidine** ■ **Filgrastim** ■ **Metronidazole**

*Contraindications*
- **Hypersensitivity to fluorouracil** ■ **Severe hematologic toxicity** ■ **Gastrointestinal hemorrhage** ■ **Depressed bone marrow** ■ **Poor nutritional state** ■ **Serious infections**

*Evidence*
- A systematic review compared adjuvant systemic chemotherapy with no adjuvant chemotherapy in patients with Dukes' C colon cancer, and Dukes' B or C rectal cancer. There was a small but significant improvement in overall survival in patients receiving chemotherapy (5% for colon; 9% for rectal). The results were less clear with Dukes' B tumors [12] *Level M*
- Another systematic review compared one week of continuing portal vein infusion chemotherapy (5-FU) commenced within 5–7 days of surgery vs no additional treatment after surgery, in patients with Dukes' A, B, and C colorectal tumors. A significant survival advantage was seen at 6 years in the chemotherapy group. The benefit was only seen for patients with colon cancer [13] *Level M*
- A RCT compared adjuvant levamisole with placebo in patients with colorectal carcinoma and no evidence of residual disease. There was no significant difference in recurrence or survival at 3 years in patients treated with levamisole [14] *Level P*
- A systematic review found that palliative chemotherapy was effective for prolonging time to disease progression in patients with advanced colorectal cancer. An absolute improvement in survival of 16% was seen at 6 and 12 months [15] *Level M*

*Acceptability to patient*
- Nausea, vomiting, diarrhea, gastrointestinal ulceration, and neurologic toxicity manifesting as ataxia and somnolence may limit compliance
- Warn patient about possibility of alopecia and skin rash

*Follow up plan*
- Pay particular attention to complete blood count as myelosuppression manifesting as granulocytopenia and thrombocytopenia are major toxicities occurring 2–4 weeks post-treatment
- Aggressively manage nausea, vomiting, and diarrhea
- Diarrhea should be managed with adequate hydration and loperamide. Octreotide has been used for severe diarrhea
- Nausea can usually be controlled with standard antiemetics
- Monitor fluid status in patient with profound diarrhea/vomiting

*Patient and caregiver information*
Warn patient of high side effect profile while reassuring that side effects can be managed.

### Endoscopic therapy
Endoscopic therapy is primarily used for palliation and to relieve bowel obstruction.

LASER THERAPY
- Nd:YAG laser used primarily for palliation for advanced disease or poor surgical risk; used to recanalize the rectum
- Electrofulguration and photodynamic therapy have also been used

*Efficacy*
Rectal patency is usually achieved, but may be compromised by tumor growth.

*Risks/benefits*
Risks: complications include bleeding and perforation.

*Acceptability to patient*
Given palliative role, usually accepted by patient.

*Follow up plan*
- Evaluate for evidence of reobstruction
- Evaluate for bleeding or perforation

## OUTCOMES

### EFFICACY OF THERAPIES
- Surgical therapy with adjuvant chemoradiotherapy (when indicated) often has a favorable outcome for resectable disease; a significant percentage of patients achieve cure
- For advanced or metastatic disease, surgery with chemoradiotherapy has a less favorable outcome than curative resection with chemoradiotherapy, but can enhance survival
- Chemotherapy or radiotherapy without surgery offer no benefit and do not affect outcome
- Endoscopic therapy is used only for palliation and does not affect outcome

### Evidence
- Preoperative radiotherapy plus surgery has been shown to be superior to surgery alone in the treatment of rectal adenocarcinoma. There was a significant reduction in overall mortality after 5 years with combination therapy, and local recurrence rate was also reduced. There was no significant reduction in the risk of distant metastases [9] *Level M*
- Adjuvant systemic chemotherapy has been shown to significantly improve overall survival compared with no adjuvant chemotherapy in patients with Dukes' C colon cancer, and Dukes' B or C rectal cancer. The results were less clear with Dukes' B tumors [12] *Level M*
- A significant survival advantage was seen at 6 years in patients treated with one week of continuing portal vein infusion chemotherapy (5-FU) commenced within 5–7 days of surgery vs no additional treatment after surgery in patients with Dukes' A, B, and C colorectal tumors. The benefit was only seen for patients with colon cancer [13] *Level M*
- A systematic review found that palliative chemotherapy was effective for prolonging time to disease progression in patients with advanced colorectal cancer. An absolute improvement in survival of 16% was seen at 6 and 12 months [15] *Level M*

### PROGNOSIS
- 5-year survival for Dukes' A, tumor-node-metastases (TNM) stage I (T1N0M0): >90%
- 5-year survival for Dukes' B1, TNM stage I (T2N0M0): 85%
- 5-year survival for Dukes' B2, TNM stage II (T3N0M0): 70–80%
- 5-year survival for Dukes' C, TNM stage III (TxN1M0): 35–65%
- 5-year survival for Dukes' D, TNM stage IV (TxNxM1): 5%
- Prognosis is related to stage, morphology, and histology
- Prognosis is most dependent on extent of lymph node invasion and tumor penetration, both of which are highly inter-related (i.e. tumor penetration is often related to number of involved lymph nodes)
- 5-year survival for patients with symptoms: 49%
- 5-year survival for patients without symptoms: 71%
- Tumor location may influence prognosis, postoperative disease-free survival is 2–14% greater for left-sided cancers than right-sided colonic neoplasms
- Several studies indicate that colon cancer has a better outcome than rectal cancer
- Disease-specific mortality has recently declined for unknown reasons
- Colorectal carcinoma increases risk of synchronous and metachronous carcinoma
- Synchronous carcinoma frequency: 2–6%
- Prognosis for synchronous carcinoma depends on stage

Multiple classification systems are in use. The preferred staging system is TNM classification that has five stages (0–IV).

#### TNM classification
Stage 0:
- Tis, N0, M0: carcinoma in situ

Stage I:
- T1, N0, M0: invades submucosa
- T2, N0, M0: invades muscularis propria

Stage II:
- T3, N0, M0: invades muscularis propria into subserosa or perirectal tissue, or nonperitonealized pericolic tissue
- T4, N0, M0: perforates visceral peritoneum or directly invades adjacent organs or structures

Stage III:
- Includes any bowel perforation with regional lymph node metastasis
- N1: one to three pericolic or perirectal lymph nodes
- N2: four or more pericolic or perirectal lymph nodes
- N3: metastasis to any lymph node along a named vascular trunk
- Any T, N1, M0
- Any T, N2, N3, M0

Stage IV:
- Invasion of bowel wall with evidence of distant metastasis with or without lymph node metastasis
- Any T, any N, M1

### Dukes' classification system
Dukes' A:
- Tumor limited to mucosa

Dukes' B:
- Tumor invades bowel wall
- B1: tumor extends, but not through, muscularis propria
- B2: tumor penetrates bowel wall, but without lymph node involvement

Dukes' C:
- Tumor with regional lymph node involvement
- C1: same as B1, but with regional lymph node involvement
- C2: same as B2, but with regional lymph node involvement

Dukes' D:
- Distant metastases (bone, liver, lung)

All of the following are negative prognostic indicators:
- Age less than 30, especially with ulcerative colitis or familial adenomatous polyposis
- Aneuploidy/nondiploid
- Carcinoembryonic antigen (CEA) level elevated
- Colonic obstruction/perforation
- Histology: mucinous, poorly differentiated, scirrhous, and signet ring
- Invasion: perineural, vascular or lymphatic, increased tumor depth
- Metastases: liver, lung, bone
- Lymph nodes: more than four
- Morphology: ulcerating or infiltrating

All of the following confer a better prognosis:
- Rectal bleeding at presentation
- Inflammation

- Lymph nodes: four or fewer involved lymph nodes
- Morphology: exophytic and polypoid

### Clinical pearls
- The skill of the surgeon has an important bearing on outcome for rectal cancer patients. Studies found a significant local recurrence and survival advantage in patients of surgeons with colorectal surgery fellowship training and surgeons with a higher caseload
- A greater rate of sphincter preservation for low rectal cancer also was found to be associated with higher case loads
- Other studies suggest that hospital volume, hospital type (university vs community), and surgeon experience improve survival and recurrence outcomes

### Therapeutic failure
- Consider entry into clinical trial
- Pain control and quality of life should be a priority

### Recurrence
- Recurrence occurs in approx. 50% of patients
- Number of involved lymph nodes and serosal penetration correlate with recurrence risk
- Local recurrence is related to depth of primary transmural tumor invasion
- One to four positive nodes: 35% recur
- More than four positive nodes: 61% recur
- Perineural and venous invasion increase local recurrence risk as do perforating or obstructing lesions
- Elevated CEA indicates increased recurrence risk, and shortens recurrence interval
- Local recurrence rate for stage II rectal cancer: 25–30%
- Local recurrence rate for stage III rectal cancer: over 50%
- Colorectal carcinoma increases risk of metachronous carcinoma
- Metachronous carcinoma usually presents distant from initial site; can occur up to 23 years after primary lesion
- Incidence of metachronous carcinoma: 1.1–4.7%
- Approx. 50% of metachronous colorectal cancers present within 5–7 years

### Deterioration
- Entry into a clinical trail should be strongly considered
- Pain control and quality of life should be a priority

### Terminal illness
- Pain control and quality of life should be a priority
- Assist patient and family in dealing with end-of-life issues
- Have patient evaluated for hospice or home healthcare

## COMPLICATIONS
- Ulceration and vascular compromise can result in significant hemorrhage
- Pain may be severe and should be managed aggressively
- Deep vein thrombosis is a recognized complication of malignancy

## CONSIDER CONSULT
- Consider referral to an academic/university center for clinical trial entry
- Refer to hospice for treatment failure, clinical deterioration, or terminal disease
- Refer to a psychiatrist/psychologist for emotional support and insight
- Refer to a pain specialist for intractable pain

# PREVENTION

## RISK FACTORS

- Some authorities recommend prophylactic colectomy for ulcerative colitis of over 10 years' duration
- Prophylactic colectomy may be indicated for several inherited polyposis syndromes

## MODIFY RISK FACTORS

There is no evidence documenting that risk factor modification can reduce the incidence of rectal cancer.

### Lifestyle and wellness

ALCOHOL AND DRUGS
Aspirin and nonsteroidal anti-inflammatory drugs may reduce the risk of rectal cancer.

DIET
- High-fiber diet may protect against rectal cancer
- Diets high in yellow-green vegetables, calcium, and vitamins A, C, and E may decrease risk

PHYSICAL ACTIVITY
Regular exercise may reduce the risk of rectal cancer.

## SCREENING

- Screening programs are intended either to identify and remove adenomas prior to malignant transformation or to identify colorectal carcinoma, preferably in an early stage
- Tumors diagnosed in asymptomatic individuals tend to be less advanced; this may confer a survival advantage
- Screening for colorectal cancer can reduce mortality; however, adherence to routine screening is needed to achieve this benefit
- Screening recommendations are based on degree of risk, and include average, increased, and high risk
- Multiple screening recommendations are available; those from the American Cancer Society and the US Preventive Services Task Force are representative

Average risk:
- Most screening programs for average-risk individuals start at age 50 and include annual digital rectal examination with fecal occult blood testing (FOBT) with periodic (every 3–5 years) sigmoidoscopy and/or colonoscopy
- The American Cancer Society recommends annual FOBT and flexible sigmoidoscopy every 3–5 years for asymptomatic individuals of average risk (i.e. over age 50). Colonoscopy every 10 years is an acceptable screening alternative option to flexible sigmoidoscopy
- The US Preventive Services Task Force recommend annual FOBT and/or sigmoidoscopy for all individuals age 50 and older

Increased risk (according to the American Cancer Society):
- Increased risk includes individuals with adenomas, a history of colorectal cancer status postcurative resection and those with first-degree relatives who, prior to age 60, had a history of adenomas or colorectal cancer
- Colonoscopy is the screening procedure of choice for individuals at high risk
- Adenomas, low risk: colonoscopy recommended 3–6 years after polypectomy for single adenoma <1cm
- Adenomas, high risk: colonoscopy recommended within 3 years after polypectomy for people with adenomas >1cm, multiple adenomas, villous adenomas or adenomas with high-grade dysplasia

- Personal history: colonoscopy recommended within one year after curative resection of colorectal cancer
- Family history: colonoscopy recommended at age 40 or 10 years prior to the youngest index case for individuals who have a family history of a first-degree relative with adenomas or colorectal cancer prior to age 60, or in two or more first-degree relatives regardless of age of index case

High risk:
- High-risk individuals require more intensive monitoring/screening, and include those with: personal or family history of familial adenomatous polyposis (FAP), hereditary nonpolyposis colon cancer, female genital tract cancer, Gardner's syndrome, Crohn's disease, and ulcerative colitis (long standing)
- Screening for those with FAP or Gardner's syndrome usually begins at puberty, and includes genetic counseling and annual or biannual flexible sigmoidoscopy/colonoscopy
- Screening for those with 'cancer family syndrome' or those with hereditary nonpolyposis colorectal cancer usually begins at age 21 or 5 years prior to youngest index case, and includes genetic counseling and annual FOBT with colonoscopy every 2–3 years
- Screening for those with ulcerative colitis begins after 7–8 years of pancolitis or 15 years of left-sided colitis, and includes colonoscopy with multiple biopsies annually or biannually
- Screening recommendations for Crohn's disease have not been established; however, colonoscopy is periodically indicated and may be needed every 3–6 months, should low-grade dysplasia or active inflammation be described
- Colectomy is usually indicated for high-grade dysplasia or frank lesion in Crohn's disease; some advocate colectomy for low-grade dysplasia
- Several serologic tumor markers are under investigation; however, none is presently recommended for routine screening
- Several genetic tests are under investigation; however, with the exception of testing for APC gene alteration in patients with a family history of FAP, no genetic tests are presently recommended for routine screening
- Air-contrast barium enema is not considered a cost-effective screening modality

## Screening guidelines

The following guidelines are available at the National Guideline Clearinghouse:
- The American Cancer Society guidelines on screening and surveillance for early detection of adenomatous polyps and cancer - update 2001. In: American Cancer Society guidelines for the early detection of cancer [1]
- The United States Preventive Services Task Force. Screening for colorectal cancer [2]
- Colorectal cancer screening [16]
- The American Gastroenterological Association. Colorectal cancer screening: clinical guidelines and rationale [17]

## FECAL OCCULT BLOOD TESTING (FOBT)

- Testing of stool for presence of blood, applying hydrogen peroxide in denatured alcohol on stool placed on guaiac-impregnated paper and observing for a positive reaction (i.e. change of color)
- Usually performed annually
- Several commercial tests are available, including: Hemoccult, Hemoccult SENSA, HemoQuant, and HemeSelect

### Cost/efficacy
- Several studies report that annual FOBT can reduce colorectal cancer-related mortality from 15–43%
- Can detect early carcinoma, usually Dukes' A or B

- Colorectal cancers prevented: 22.5%
- Considered to be the most cost-effective screening modality
- Cost per prevented death: $225,000
- Approximate cost per procedure: $16.00
- Compliance rate: 15–80%
- Compliance poor among minorities and elderly
- Efficacy is directly related to compliance

### FLEXIBLE SIGMOIDOSCOPY
Direct examination of the rectum and sigmoid colon with a flexible fiberoptic sigmoidoscope.

*Cost/efficacy*
- Approx. 50% of all colorectal lesions can be identified by a 60cm sigmoidoscope
- Can reduce colorectal cancer mortality for lesions within range of sigmoidoscopy from 70–80%
- Colorectal cancers prevented: 50%
- Cost per prevented death: $250,000
- Approx. cost per procedure: $160–205
- Efficacy is directly related to compliance

### COLONOSCOPY
- Direct examination of the entire rectum and colon with a flexible fiberoptic colonoscope
- Postoperative colonoscopy is recommended every 3–5 years
- Surveillance endoscopy with biopsy recommended for patients with long-standing (e.g. longer than 7 years) ulcerative colitis
- Carcinoma is found in approx. 25% of colons with high-grade/severe dysplasia

*Cost/efficacy*
- Colonoscopy screening has significant impact on colorectal mortality
- Colorectal cancers prevented: 68%
- Cost per prevented death: $274,000
- Approximate cost per procedure: $745
- Surveillance colonoscopy with biopsy may increase life expectancy for patients with ulcerative colitis
- Efficacy is directly related to compliance

### COMPUTED TOMOGRAPHY OF LIVER
Some authorities advocate postoperative computed tomography of the liver every 3–5 years.

## PREVENT RECURRENCE
Recurrence can be prevented/delayed by choosing appropriate surgical candidates, multimode therapy, and ensuring macroscopic-/microscopic-free resection margins.

### Reassess coexisting disease
PATIENT SATISFACTION/LIFESTYLE PRIORITIES
- Most patients with recurrence will be concerned with quality-of-life and end-of-life issues
- Pain control and patient comfort should be a priority

# RESOURCES

## ASSOCIATIONS

**American Association for Cancer Research**
Public Ledger Building, Suite 826
150 South Independence Mall West
Philadelphia, PA 19106-3483
Tel: (215) 440-9300
Fax: (215) 440-9313
http://www.aacr.org

**American Cancer Society**
1599 Clifton Road NE
Atlanta, GA 30329
Tel: (800) 227-2345 (800-ACS-2345)
http://www.cancer.org

**American Society of Clinical Oncology**
1900 Duke Street, Suite 200
Alexandria, VA 22314
Tel: (703) 299-0150
Fax: (703) 299-1044
E-mail: asco@asco.org
http://www.asco.org

**National Cancer Institute**
Public Inquires Office
Building 31, Room 10A03
31 Center Drive, MSC 2580
Bethesda, MD
Tel: (800) 422-6237 (800-4-CANCER)
E-mail: cancermail@cips.nci.nih.gov
http://www.cancer.gov

**National Comprehensive Cancer Network**
50 Huntington Pike, Suite 200
Rockledge, PA 19046
Tel: (215) 728-3877 or (888) 909-6226 (888-909-NCCN)
E-mail: information@nccn.org
http://www.nccn.org

## KEY REFERENCES

- DeVita VT, Hellman S, Rosenberg SA, eds. Cancer: principles and practice of oncology, 6th edn. New York: Lippincott-Raven, 2001
- Holm T, Singnomklao T, Rutqvist LE, et al. Adjuvant preoperative radiotherapy in patients with rectal carcinoma. Adverse effects during long term follow-up of two randomized trials. Cancer 1996;78:968–76
- Kievit J. Colorectal cancer follow up: a reassessment of empirical evidence on effectiveness. Eur J Surg Oncol 2000;26:322–8
- Krook JE, Moertel CG, Gunderson LL, et al. Effective surgical adjuvant therapy for high-risk rectal carcinoma. N Engl J Med 1991;324:709–15
- Ooi BS, Tjandra JJ, Green MD. Morbidities of adjuvant chemotherapy and radiotherapy for resectable rectal cancer: an overview. Dis Colon Rectum 1999;42:403–18

### Evidence references and guidelines

1. The American Cancer Society guidelines on screening and surveillance for early detection of adenomatous polyps and cancer – update 2001. In: American Cancer Society guidelines for the early detection of cancer. CA Cancer J Clin 2001;51:44–54. Available at the National Guideline Clearinghouse
2. The United States Preventive Services Task Force. Screening for colorectal cancer. In: Guide to clinical preventive services, 2nd edn. Baltimore, MD: Williams and Wilkins, 1996. Available at the National Guideline Clearinghouse
3. The American Society of Clinical Oncology. 2000 update of recommendations for the use of tumor markers in breast and colorectal cancer: clinical practice guidelines of the American Society of Clinical Oncology. J Clin Oncol 2001;19:1865–78. Available at the National Guideline Clearinghouse
4. American College of Physicians. Suggested technique for fecal occult blood testing and interpretation in colorectal cancer screening. Ann Intern Med 1997;126(10):808–10. Available at the National Guideline Clearinghouse
5. National Comprehensive Cancer Network Practice Guidelines for colorectal cancer, Version 2000
6. Practice parameters for the treatment of rectal carcinoma. Arlington Heights, IL: American Society of Colon and Rectal Surgeons, 1998–1999. Available at the National Guideline Clearinghouse
7. Cancer Care Ontario Practice Guidelines Initiative. Postoperative adjuvant radiotherapy and/or chemotherapy for resected stage II or III rectal cancer. Curr Oncol 2000;7:37–51. Available at the National Guideline Clearinghouse
8. The Society for Surgery of the Alimentary Tract. Surgical treatment of cancer of the colon or rectum. Manchester, MA: Society for Surgery of the Alimentary Tract, 2000. Available at the National Guideline Clearinghouse
9. Camma C, Giunta M, Pagliaro L. Preoperative radiotherapy for resectable rectal cancer. A meta analysis. JAMA 2000;284:1008–15. Reviewed in: Clinical Evidence 2001;6:344–50
10. Jansson Frykholm G, Glimelius B, Pahlman L. Preoperative or postoperative irradiation in adenocarcinoma of the rectum. Final treatment results of a randomized trial and an evaluation of late secondary effects. Dis Colon Rectum 1993;36:564–72. Reviewed in: Clinical Evidence 2001;6:344–50
11. Scholefield J. Colorectal cancer: Digestive system disorders. In: Clinical Evidence 2001;6:344–50. London: BMJ Publishing Group
12. Dube D, Heyen F, Jenicek M. Adjuvant chemotherapy in colorectal carcinoma. Results of a meta analysis. Dis Colon Rectum 1997;40:35–41. Reviewed in: Clinical Evidence 2001;6:344–50
13. Liver Infusion Meta-analysis Group. Portal vein chemotherapy for colorectal cancer: a meta-analysis of 4000 patients in 10 studies. J Natl Cancer Inst 1997;89:497–505. Reviewed in: Clinical Evidence 2001;6:344–50
14. QUASAR Collaborative Group. Comparison of fluorouracil with additional levamisole, higher dose folinic acid or both as adjuvant chemotherapy for colorectal cancer: a randomised trial. Lancet 2000;355:1588–96. Reviewed in: Clinical Evidence 2001;6:344–50
15. Best L, Simmonds P, Baughan C, et al. Palliative chemotherapy for advanced or metastatic colorectal cancer (Cochrane Review). In: The Cochrane Library, 1, 2002. Oxford: Update Software.
16. Colorectal cancer screening. Bloomington, MN: Institute for Clinical Systems Improvement (ICSI), 2001. Available at the National Guideline Clearinghouse
17. American Gastroenterological Association. Colorectal cancer screening: clinical guidelines and rationale. Gastroenterology 1997;112:594–642. Available at the National Guideline Clearinghouse

## FAQS
### Question 1
Is preoperative radiation therapy effective in preventing death and recurrence?

ANSWER 1
Preoperative radiation therapy (at biologically effective doses greater than or equal to 30Gy) reduces the risk of local recurrence and death from rectal cancer. If safety can be improved without compromising effectiveness, then overall survival would be moderately improved by use of preoperative radiation therapy, especially for young, high-risk patients.

### Question 2
Is it really necessary to recommend dietary restriction prior to fecal occult blood tests (FOBT) for rectal cancer screening?

ANSWER 2
A new piece of information, provided by a meta-analysis, may change the usual recommendations of dietary restrictions before testing. Dietary restriction is often recommended during FOBT as a

means of increasing test accuracy, but concern surrounds whether such restriction also reduces the chance that patients will complete the test. Available data suggest that advice to perform modest dietary restriction during nonrehydrated FOBT does not affect the completion rate, but more severe restrictions may. Dietary restriction also does not appear to affect positivity rates. On the basis of these data, physicians do not need to advise patients to restrict their diet for nonrehydrated FOBTs.

## Question 3
Does chemotherapy improve survival in patients with metastatic disease?

ANSWER 3
Chemotherapy is effective in prolonging time to disease progression and survival in patients with advanced colorectal cancer. It was associated with a 35% reduction in the risk of death, which translates into an absolute improvement in survival of 16% at both 6 and 12 months and an improvement in median survival of 3.7 months.

## CONTRIBUTORS
Fred F Ferri, MD, FACP
Luciana G O Clark, MD
Laura Targownik, MD, FRCP(C)

# ULCERATIVE COLITIS

- Summary Information — 592
- Background — 593
- Diagnosis — 595
- Treatment — 608
- Outcomes — 619
- Prevention — 621
- Resources — 622

## SUMMARY INFORMATION

### DESCRIPTION

- Ulcerative colitis is characterized by inflammation of the gastrointestinal tract
- It invariably involves the rectum and almost always extends proximally in a continuous fashion to involve part or all of the colon
- Ulcerative colitis is a chronic, recurrent condition marked by remissions and exacerbations
- Ulcerative colitis causes a diffuse pattern of inflammation of the mucosal surface
- Mainstays of therapy include 5-aminosalicylic acid derivatives, corticosteroids, and other immunosuppressive therapies

### KEY! DON'T MISS!

- Symptoms should not be ascribed to irritable bowel syndrome, if there is evidence of loss of mucosal integrity (rectal bleeding) or an inflammatory disorder (fever, weight loss)
- Bleeding that has been attributed to hemorrhoids: flexible sigmoidoscopy should be considered in all patients with hemorrhoidal bleeding. This more comprehensive evaluation to exclude inflammatory bowel disease may be warranted

# BACKGROUND

## ICD9 CODE
556.9 Ulcerative colitis

## SYNONYMS
Chronic idiopathic inflammatory bowel disease

## CARDINAL FEATURES
- Often abrupt onset, although patients may present with more chronic symptoms
- Bloody diarrhea is the hallmark feature, often associated with lower abdominal cramps and pain on defecation
- Typically symptoms of bowel urgency and frequency are the most disabling
- Anemia and low serum albumin are frequently seen on laboratory tests
- Negative stool cultures (although infection with *Clostridium difficile* must be ruled out – secondary infection sometimes occurs)
- Usually characterized by periods of symptomatic flare-ups and remissions
- Sigmoidoscopy is the key to diagnosis: mucosal appearance is characterized by edema, friability, and confluent ulceration
- Inflammation is localized primarily in the mucosa and involves the rectum, extending proximally to involve part or all of the large bowel
- Ulcerative proctitis refers to disease limited to the rectum
- Left-sided colitis refers to disease that does not extend past the splenic flexure
- Colonic inflammation extending past the splenic flexure is referred to as pancolitis, even if it does not extend all the way to the cecum

## CAUSES
### Common causes
- Precise cause is still a subject of ongoing research. Likely to be multifactorial and with both genetic and environmental influences
- Stress can exacerbate symptoms and may be involved in pathogenesis
- 20% of patients with ulcerative colitis have an affected relative, suggesting a genetic predisposition in some individuals

### Contributory or predisposing factors
- The chance of developing inflammatory bowel disease if a family member is affected is 10–15%
- If a young adult has inflammatory bowel disease, the likelihood of a sibling or parent being afflicted by ulcerative colitis is 1–3%
- The risk to a child of a parent with inflammatory bowel disease is about 2%
- In identical twins, if one twin is affected, the risk to the other is approximately 40%
- Cigarette smoking appears to protect against ulcerative colitis but is associated with Crohn's disease. Often, ulcerative colitis flares after a 'predisposed' person stops smoking (usually within the first 2 years)

## EPIDEMIOLOGY
### Incidence and prevalence
- Ulcerative colitis occurs among all age groups, but has a peak incidence in the second and third decades, with a smaller second peak at 55–75 years
- Inflammatory bowel disease is predominantly found in the US, northern and western Europe, and Australia
- Ulcerative colitis is approximately three times more common than Crohn's disease

- Approximately 20% of ulcerative colitis patients first manifest the disease when they are <20 years of age

### INCIDENCE
- Ulcerative colitis: 5–10/100,000 population
- Crohn's disease: 2–6/100,000 population

### PREVALENCE
- Ulcerative colitis: 50–80/100,000 population
- Crohn's disease: 30–50/100,000 population
- Combined prevalence: 1/1000

## Demographics
### AGE
- Two peak ages of incidence: 15–35 and 55–75 years
- Ulcerative colitis may be seen as early as infancy, whereas Crohn's disease is rare before the age of 10 years

### GENDER
Males slightly more disposed to develop ulcerative colitis.

### RACE
- Seen in all ethnic groups
- Higher prevalence in Jews who have immigrated from northern Europe (not in Sephardic Jews of Mediterranean or Middle Eastern origin)
- Less common in African-Americans

### GENETICS
Inflammatory bowel disease has a strong genetic component.

### GEOGRAPHY
- More common in urban areas
- More common in northern Europe and North America than elsewhere

### SOCIOECONOMIC STATUS
- May be linked to a high standard of living: the incidence in Japan and southern Europe has risen as standards of living have increased
- Within a specific region, the incidence does not vary between socioeconomic groups

# DIAGNOSIS

## DIFFERENTIAL DIAGNOSIS
- Ulcerative colitis most often confused with Crohn's disease, infectious colitis, acute ischemic colitis, and acute self-limited colitis
- Other conditions that may be included in the differential diagnosis include irritable bowel syndrome, diverticulitis, hemorrhoids, radiation colitis, and *Clostridium difficile* infection
- Other infectious agents should be considered (including *Chlamydia trachomatis*, *Neisseria gonorrhoeae*, *Cryptosporidium* spp., herpes simplex virus, cytomegalovirus, *Isospora belli*, and *Mycobacterium tuberculosis*) in patients who are immunocompromised or who engage in high-risk sexual behavior

## Crohn's disease
Crohn's disease is an inflammatory disease of the bowel, most commonly involving the terminal ileum, colon, or both.

### FEATURES
- Variable presentation depending on site of lesion(s)
- Abdominal pain with diarrhea and fever may be present
- Diarrhea usually less severe than in ulcerative colitis
- Bloody diarrhea with pus and/or mucus is less commonly a feature than with ulcerative colitis
- Any part of the gastrointestinal tract from mouth to anus may be involved
- 10–20% of patients with inflammatory bowel disease have an indistinguishable form of colitis termed 'indeterminate colitis'

## Irritable bowel syndrome
Irritable bowel syndrome is a chronic functional disorder of the intestine of unknown etiology, occurring in approximately 20% of the population of industrialized countries.

### FEATURES
- Commonly there is a long duration of symptoms, usually not severe, with chronic, cramping abdominal pain, bloating, and intermittent loose stool
- Typically variable bowel habit with some normal days, possibly with some fluctuation between constipation and diarrhea
- No rectal bleeding and no weight loss or systemic features
- X-rays and endoscopic studies (both macroscopically and histologically) are normal

## Hemorrhoids
Hemorrhoids involve veins around the anus or lower rectum being swollen and inflamed.

### FEATURES
- Bright red rectal bleeding on the paper or pan rather than mixed in with the stool
- Pruritus
- Pain may occur if there are thrombosed hemorrhoids
- Constipation is more of a factor than diarrhea

## Yersinia enterocolitica enteritis
*Y. enterocolitica* is a small rod-shaped, Gram-negative bacterium. There are three pathogenic species in the genus *Yersinia*, but only *Y. enterocolitica* and *Y. pseudotuberculosis* cause gastroenteritis.

### FEATURES
- Acute onset with persisting symptoms beyond one week
- Fever

- Right lower quadrant pain
- Rare and tends to occur in epidemics
- Typically with systemic features such as polyarthritis, sacroiliitis, Reiter's syndrome, and osteomyelitis
- Diagnosed by positive stool culture or serology

### Colorectal carcinoma

Colorectal carcinoma remains a leading cause of cancer death among adults in the US.

FEATURES
- Bleeding per rectum
- Constipation if distal lesion; high-grade lesions may lead to overflow diarrhea
- Anemia
- Tenesmus
- Abdominal pain

### Diverticulitis with abscess formation

Diverticulitis is the most common complication of diverticulosis and occurs when increased intraluminal pressure and inspissated food particles lead to inflammation and focal necrosis.

FEATURES
- Bloody diarrhea generally not a feature of acute diverticulitis
- Fever and systemic malaise
- Left lower quadrant pain
- Nausea and vomiting
- Elevated white blood cell count
- Acute abdomen
- Left lower quadrant mass

### Acute ischemic colitis

Ischemic colitis involves inflammation of the colon resulting from restriction of the colonic blood supply.

FEATURES
- Often associated with risk factors for cardiovascular disease, most commonly type 2 diabetes and smoking
- Usually precipitated by a systemic low blood flow state, less often secondary to embolic disease
- May present with symptoms identical to ulcerative colitis, with fever, abdominal pain, and bloody diarrhea
- Abdominal pain generally more severe than in ulcerative colitis
- Generally older age at presentation (age over 50 years)
- Colonoscopy usually shows ulceration in transverse, descending, and sigmoid colon, with most intense involvement around splenic flexure
- Self-limited in 90% cases and resolves without specific therapy; may be recurrent or lead to chronic stricture in less than 10% of cases

### Viral gastroenteritis

FEATURES
- Typically lasts only 1–4 days and is self-limiting
- No rectal bleeding with negative stool culture

## Bacterial/amoebal gastroenteritis
### FEATURES
- Most bacterial pathogens produce self-limited disease lasting 7–14 days or less
- Rectal bleeding, fever, fecal leukocytes, and mucosal appearance may be indistinguishable from ulcerative colitis or Crohn's disease in acute phase
- Positive cultures obtained in approximately 40% of cases
- *Shigella, Salmonella, Escherichia coli, Campylobacter,* and *Entamoeba histolytica* are the main causative organisms
- HSV and chlamydial and gonorrheal proctitis should be considered in patients with recent, unprotected anal intercourse

## Clostridium difficile infection
Infection with *Clostridium difficile* is associated with antibiotic therapy, and causes pseudomembranous colitis.

### FEATURES
- Symptoms and endoscopic appearance can mimic those of ulcerative colitis or Crohn's disease
- Stool culture for enteric pathogens and studies for *C. difficile* toxin should be obtained, especially if the patient has recently been taking antibiotics
- Often found in hospital patients, the immunocompromised, and the elderly

## Radiation colitis
### FEATURES
- Associated with previous exposure to abdominal or pelvic radiotherapy
- Can present both acutely during radiation therapy or chronically months to years after
- Nausea and vomiting
- Diarrhea (with or without blood) and cramping pain
- Obstruction secondary to stricture formation may occur
- Perforation and fistula formation may rarely occur in chronic radiation colitis

## Acute self-limited colitis
This condition has the same clinical picture as ulcerative colitis with bleeding and diarrhea.

### FEATURES
- Stool cultures are negative
- The sigmoidoscopy findings are the same as ulcerative colitis or Crohn's colitis
- The histology shows acute inflammation without evidence of chronic changes
- It will resolve spontaneously and is not recurrent

## SIGNS & SYMPTOMS
### Signs
- Tenderness on abdominal examination
- Abdominal distension
- Fever
- Signs of anemia
- Obvious weight loss
- Signs of hypovolemia or dehydration in severe disease episode or presentation
- 25% of cases are associated with extraintestinal manifestations: erythema nodosum, pyoderma gangrenosum (up to 12% of patients ), episcleritis, oligoarticular nondeforming arthritis, iritis, and uveitis

## Symptoms

- Diagnosis is often difficult because presenting symptoms are frequently nonspecific, and they vary according to the extent of disease, the severity of inflammation, and the presence of complications
- About 5–10% of patients who have had a diagnosis of either Crohn's disease or ulcerative colitis change diagnostic category over time
- Diarrhea – more than 70% of patients with ulcerative colitis present with diarrhea that is usually progressive with many episodes of bloody diarrhea, that gradually become more numerous or severe
- Nearly all patients present with rectal bleeding
- Lower abdominal cramping
- Frequent bowel movements with fecal urgency, incomplete emptying, and tenesmus (resulting from the rectal involvement that is characteristic of ulcerative colitis)
- At presentation, most patients have mild to moderate disease. Severe disease occurs in one-third or less. Physical findings may be absent in mild disease
- Ulcerative colitis may be classified by severity – mild, moderate, severe, or fulminant
- Mild disease: fewer than four stools daily with or without bleeding, no systemic signs of toxicity, and a normal erythrocyte sedimentation rate (ESR)
- Moderate disease: more than four stools daily with or without bleeding, and minimal signs of toxicity
- Severe disease: more than six bloody stools daily and evidence of toxicity (e.g. fever, tachycardia, anemia, or an elevated ESR)
- Fulminant disease (a subset of severe disease): characterized by rapidly worsening symptoms with signs of toxicity, toxic megacolon

## ASSOCIATED DISORDERS

The inflammatory bowel diseases are associated with a number of extraintestinal manifestations, which can serve as markers for disease. Approx. 10% of patients present with these extraintestinal manifestations and they are more commonly associated with ulcerative colitis than with Crohn's disease:

- Ankylosing spondylitis and seronegative arthritis are the most common extraintestinal manifestation of ulcerative colitis
- Migratory, often involving the hip, ankle, wrist, or elbow
- Usually monoarticular and asymmetric, with no synovial destruction
- Course of the arthritis parallels the course of the colitis
- Sclerosing cholangitis may be seen in 5% of patients, which often progresses to cirrhosis
- Carcinoma of the biliary tract may also be seen with more frequency than in the general population, as a complication of primary sclerosing cholangitis
- Conjunctivitis
- Iritis, which tends to follow a course that is independent of the course of the bowel disease
- Episcleritis, which often parallels the activity of the bowel disease
- Uveitis (when patients are HLA-B27 positive)
- Anemia, leukocytosis, and thrombocytosis
- Elevated erythrocyte sedimentation rate
- Pyoderma gangrenosum
- Erythema nodosum

## KEY! DON'T MISS!

- Symptoms should not be ascribed to irritable bowel syndrome if there is evidence of loss of mucosal integrity (rectal bleeding) or an inflammatory disorder (fever, weight loss)
- Bleeding that has been attributed to hemorrhoids: flexible sigmoidoscopy should be considered in all patients with hemorrhoidal bleeding. This more comprehensive evaluation to exclude inflammatory bowel disease may be warranted

## CONSIDER CONSULT

All patients with suspected ulcerative colitis should be referred to a gastroenterologist to confirm the diagnosis, determine the extent of the disease by colonoscopy, and rule out other causes. Urgent referral to a gastroenterologist and admittance to the hospital are necessary if patients present with any of the following:

- Fulminant ulcerative colitis (up to10% of patients with ulcerative colitis). Presents with severe diarrhea, abdominal pain, hemorrhage, fever, sepsis, and signs and symptoms of dehydration or shock. Requires aggressive therapy including hospitalization, resuscitation, correction of electrolyte abnormalities, and treatment with intravenous corticosteroids
- Toxic megacolon (up to 2% and usually as sequel to acute episode of colitis). Development of an acute abdomen that requires emergency surgery (otherwise perforation will occur); toxic megacolon and perforation are suggested by absent bowel sounds, distended abdomen, and peritonitis
- Bowel obstruction, perforation, or signs of other abdominal complications
- Anemia from chronic blood loss, dehydration, or hypovolemia from acute bleeding (suggested on clinical examination by tachycardia and orthostatic hypotension)
- Severe gastrointestinal bleeding, a medical emergency for which surgery is the definitive treatment
- Patients with evidence of extracolonic soft-tissue disease (erythema nodosum, pyoderma gangrenosum, primary sclerosing cholangitis) should be referred urgently to a dermatologist or rheumatologist
- Patients with ophthalmologic symptoms should be promptly referred to an ophthalmologist

## INVESTIGATION OF THE PATIENT
### Direct questions to patient

**Q** Do you have abdominal pain? Where is it located and what is its quality? Location and quality of pain may help in differential diagnosis. Pain of active ulcerative colitis is generally constant, mild to moderate in severity, located diffusely throughout the abdomen, and worsened immediately prior to a bowel movement

**Q** How many bowel movements are you having each day? Are they loose and watery? Frequency of bowel movements can help determine severity of disease. However, loose bowel movements are characteristic of many gastrointestinal disorders

**Q** Have you had any rectal bleeding? Has there been blood in your bowel movements? Is it mixed with the stool, or streaking the outside of hard stool? Bloody bowel movements are characteristic of ulcerative colitis but sometimes patients can mistake bleeding from hemorrhoids, especially when constipated. Thus blood mixed in with stool is more likely to be an indicator of ulcerative colitis. Bloody diarrhea may also be found in ischemic colitis, infectious colitis secondary to bacterial or ameobal pathogens, and radiation colitis

**Q** Have you had any fever recently? Are the episodes of increasing abdominal pain associated with fever or myalgia? Frequently flares of ulcerative colitis will be associated with constitutional symptoms such as fever and myalgia

**Q** Does the abdominal pain or diarrhea wake you from sleep? Symptoms of irritable bowel syndrome seldom wake patients from sleep. Helps to differentiate irritable bowel syndrome from ulcerative colitis

**Q** Do you have pain on defecation and tenesmus? Rectal symptoms are common in ulcerative colitis and proctitis

**Q** Do you have arthritis or red nodules on the skin that sometimes come and go? These extraintestinal manifestations are characteristic of ulcerative colitis and are sometimes found in the absence of gastrointestinal symptoms. Colonoscopy should be considered for patients with classic extraintestinal manifestations of inflammatory bowel disease to rule out occult gastrointestinal disease

### Contributory or predisposing factors

- **Q** **Do you smoke? Have you recently quit smoking?** Cigarette smoking appears to protect against ulcerative colitis. Often, ulcerative colitis begins after a 'predisposed' person stops smoking
- **Q** **Do you have any risk factors for atherosclerotic disease? Are you on antihypertensives?** The presence of atherosclerotic disease or antihypertensive use may predispose to acute ischemic colitis, which has similar symptoms to those of ulcerative colitis
- **Q** **Have you participated in any unprotected anal intercourse?** This may predispose patients to proctitis secondary to herpes simplex virus, gonorrhea, or chlamydia, which can present with symptoms similar to those of ulcerative colitis
- **Q** **Any recent travel to underdeveloped areas or ingestion of potentially unclean water?** Drinking on unpurified water may lead to infection with *E. histolytica*, which can result in a dysenteric syndrome similar to that of ulcerative colitis
- **Q** **Have you been on antibiotics in the last 2 months?** This may a risk factor for development of pseudomembranous colitis secondary to *C. difficile*
- **Q** **Have you ever been treated for radiation therapy, particularly for uterine or prostatic malignancy?** Radiation proctitis and colitis may occur during therapy, immediately following therapy, or months to years following completion of radiation
- **Q** **Do you have HIV or risk factors for HIV? Are you immunosuppressed due to another condition, such as organ or post-bone marrow transplant?** Immunosuppressed patients are at risk for diarrhea secondary to cytomegalovirus, which can present with symptoms similar to ulcerative colitis
- **Q** **Have you been taking aspirin or nonsteroidal anti-inflammatory drugs?** These agents can cause flare of colitis

### Family history

- **Q** **Is there a family history of Crohn's disease or ulcerative colitis in your family?** Patients with a family history of inflammatory bowel disease have a predisposition to developing the disease themselves
- **Q** **Does anyone in your family have problems with an 'irritable bowel' or other chronic and nonspecific gastrointestinal complaints that have never been firmly diagnosed?** Patients may have a family member with inflammatory bowel disease that was never diagnosed

### Examination

- **Record the vital signs.** Tachycardia, hypotension fever, reduced capillary refill, pallor, or dry mucous membranes are suggestive of dehydration, sepsis, or shock
- **Perform a general inspection.** Patients with inflammatory bowel disease are usually thin and look generally unwell prior to treatment, though patients with mild disease may appear well overall
- **Inspect for clinical evidence of anemia.** This may be the result of acute or chronic blood loss
- **Check for signs of peritoneal inflammation, including rebound tenderness and involuntary guarding.** This could indicate an acute abdomen associated with bowel perforation, as well as toxic megacolon with obstructive colitis
- **Check for blood in the stool and tenderness on rectal examination.** Proctitis is common in ulcerative colitis
- **Examine for any sign of extraintestinal disease; check for arthritis, skin lesions, clubbing of the fingers, uveitis, and episcleritis.** Ankylosing spondylitis, erythema nodosum, pyoderma gangrenosum, clubbing, and ocular lesions are all associated with ulcerative colitis

### Summary of investigative tests

- **Sigmoidoscopy** is the diagnostic test of choice and will usually confirm or exclude the diagnosis of inflammatory bowel disease. The pattern of affected bowel may give an indication of whether the disease is Crohn's or ulcerative colitis. The abnormal mucosa should be biopsied at sigmoidoscopy to confirm the diagnosis histologically. Histology cannot usually

- distinguish between Crohn's disease and ulcerative colitis but can be useful in differentiating from infections or ischemic colitis
- Colonoscopy. May be used to determine the extent of colonic involvement in ulcerative colitis and screen for cancer in long-standing disease. Normally performed by a specialist
- Laboratory stool examination. Can be used to exclude infection. Should check for common stool bacterial pathogens, ova, and parasites if amoebal disease is suspected, and toxin for *C. difficile* if pseudomembranous colitis is suspected
- Abdominal plain film (obstructive series). Used to evaluate an acute abdomen. Will demonstrate perforation (air under the diaphragm in an upright patient) and colonic dilation in patients who have signs and symptoms of toxicity, such as fever, tachycardia, or leukocytosis, or signs of peritoneal irritation on physical examination
- Serum laboratory tests (including complete blood count, erythrocyte sedimentation rate (ESR), liver function tests, and serum electrolytes). Findings such as leukocytosis, an elevated ESR, hypoalbuminemia, and electrolyte abnormalities may indicate inflammatory bowel disease. Increased alkaline phosphatase or transaminase levels may indicate hepatobiliary involvement

## DIAGNOSTIC DECISION

The definitive diagnosis can be obtained histologically by biopsy of the abnormal mucosa. Severity of the disease can be assessed clinically and by endoscopic and radiologic tests. Clinical criteria for assessment of severity are as follows:
- Mild disease includes three or fewer bowel movements/day, minimal rectal bleeding, pyrexia, absence of tachycardia, and normal hemoglobin and ESR
- Moderate disease includes four to six bowel movements/day, moderate rectal bleeding, low grade fever, mild tachycardia, and hemoglobin above 10.5g/dL
- Severe disease includes six or more bowel movements/day, significant rectal bleeding, fever (intermittent or constant), tachycardia below 90 beats/min, hemoglobin below 10.5g/dL, and ESR above 30mm/h

## CLINICAL PEARLS

- Importance of sigmoidoscopy in patients with rectal bleeding
- Initial examination of rectosigmoid prior to initiation of treatment is the most helpful in distinguishing ulcerative colitis from Crohn's colitis because once treatment is initiated healing can occur in a patchy distribution and patchiness is a feature of Crohn's disease
- Thrombocytosis is more likely to be found in patients with inflammatory bowel disease than in those with an infectious colitis
- Rectosigmoid biopsy is the only test to identify patients with acute self-limited colitis
- While bleeding is an important sign of severity and a great patient concern it may be the last feature to resolve

## THE TESTS
### Body fluids
COMPLETE BLOOD COUNT
*Description*
Venous blood sample.

*Advantages/Disadvantages*
Advantages:
- Inexpensive
- Easy to perform
- Indices serve as important markers for disease activity

Disadvantage: nonspecific.

*Normal*
Normal values depend on the accepted standards of a particular laboratory or institution.
- Hemoglobin: 13.6–17.7g/dL (men); 12.0–15.0g/dL (women)
- White cell count: 3200–9800/mm$^3$
- Platelet count: 130,000–300,000/mm$^3$

*Abnormal*
Results outside normal reference range.

*Cause of abnormal result*
- Anemia can be caused by blood loss, chronic illness, and malabsorption
- Infection or inflammatory conditions cause leukocytosis and thrombocytosis

ERYTHROCYTE SEDIMENTATION RATE
*Description*
Venous blood sample.

*Advantages/Disadvantages*
Advantages:
- Inexpensive
- Easy to perform
- Indices serve as important markers for disease activity but are only helpful if they are abnormal

Disadvantage: normal value does not exclude active disease.

*Normal*
- Males: 0–15mm/h
- Females: 0–20mm/h

*Abnormal*
Results above normal reference range.

*Cause of abnormal result*
Elevated sedimentation rate is a marker of active inflammation and is associated with disease severity.

*Drugs, disorders and other factors that may alter results*
- Anemia will give a falsely high erythrocyte sedimentation rate
- ESR can be elevated in many other inflammatory, infectious, or malignant process; may also be mildly elevated in the elderly

LIVER FUNCTION TESTS
*Description*
Venous blood sample.

*Advantages/Disadvantages*
Advantages:
- Inexpensive
- Easy to perform
- May indicate disease severity or complications

Disadvantage: may be useful indicator of primary sclerosing cholangitis but also can be abnormal in patients with active ulcerative colitis; does not reflect chronic liver injury, i.e. can be misleading.

*Normal*
- Bilirubin (direct): 0–0.2mg/dL
- Bilirubin (indirect): 0–1.0mg/dL
- Alanine aminotransferase (ALT): 0–35U/L
- Aspartate aminotransferase (AST): 0–35U/L
- Alkaline phosphatase (ALP): 30–120U/L
- Serum albumin: 4–6g/dL
- Prothrombin time (PT): 10–12s

*Abnormal*
Results outside normal reference range.

*Cause of abnormal result*
- Hypoalbuminemia may be secondary to active or chronic disease or protein losing enteropathy
- Abnormal liver function, especially alkaline phosphatase, may indicate associated liver disease (e.g. sclerosing cholangitis)
- More common are elevations of transaminase, which reflect active ulcerative colitis not active liver disease

*Drugs, disorders and other factors that may alter results*
- Low albumin is also caused by cirrhosis, nephrotic syndrome, chronic illness, or malignancy
- Many drugs and disorders cause abnormal liver function tests

## SERUM ELECTROLYTES
*Description*
Venous blood sample.

*Advantages/Disadvantages*
Advantages:
- Inexpensive
- Easy to perform

Disadvantage: nonspecific.

*Normal*
- Sodium: 135–145mmol/L (135–145mEq/L)
- Potassium: 3.5–5.0mmol/L (3.5–5.0mEq/L)
- Urea: 2.5–6.5mmol/L (8–18mg/dL)

*Abnormal*
- Results outside normal reference range
- Hypokalemia may be seen with severe diarrhea
- Hypernatremia and raised urea are seen with dehydration

*Cause of abnormal result*
Acute or chronic diarrhea may cause dehydration and electrolyte abnormalities.

## LABORATORY STOOL EXAMINATION
*Description*
Fresh stool sample to identify presence of infection, cysts, or ova.

*Advantages/Disadvantages*
Advantages:
- Useful if positive; a negative result does not rule out infection
- Cheap and easy to perform

*Normal*
Absence of pathogenic organisms.

*Abnormal*
Presence of noncommensal gut organisms such as *Salmonella, Shigella, Campylobacter*, cysts, and ova.

*Cause of abnormal result*
Infection.

*Drugs, disorders and other factors that may alter results*
Antibiotic use may affect result.

### STOOL FOR CLOSTRIDIUM DIFFICILE TOXIN
*Description*
- Assay of stool to assess for presence of toxin produced by *C. difficile*
- Test may check for toxin A, toxin B, or both, depending on the laboratory

*Advantages/Disadvantages*
Advantages:
- Useful if positive; a negative result does not rule out infection
- Cheap and easy to perform

*Normal*
Absence of *C. difficile* toxin.

*Abnormal*
Presence of *C. difficile* toxin.

*Cause of abnormal result*
Presence of toxin-producing strain of *C. difficile*.

## Biopsy
### BIOPSY AT SIGMOIDOSCOPY OR COLONOSCOPY
*Description*
Biopsy generally obtained at time of sigmoidoscopy or colonoscopy by biopsy forceps passed through the instrument channel of the endoscope.

*Advantages/Disadvantages*
Advantages:
- Allows for histologic confirmation of disease and ruling out other causes of bloody diarrhea
- No findings are pathognomonic of ulcerative colitis, though may be highly suggestive in the correct clinical context

Disadvantage: architectural distortion is an important sign of chronicity seen in inflammatory bowel disease but not acute self-limited colitis.

*Abnormal*
- Most common finding in acute colitis: crypt abscess (neutrophil aggregate in crypts)
- Inflammation is generally confined to the mucosa and submucosa
- Chronically, there may be chronic lymphocytic infiltration, crypt shortening, crypt branching, and overall decrease in the number of crypts

*Cause of abnormal result*
- Inflammatory bowel disease
- Ischemic colitis
- Radiation colitis

*Drugs, disorders and other factors that may alter results*
- Nonsteroidal anti-inflammatory drugs
- *C. difficile* colitis

## Imaging
### ABDOMINAL PLAIN FILM (OBSTRUCTIVE SERIES)
*Description*
- An obstructive series includes a supine and erect (or lateral decubitus in an acutely ill or weak patient) abdominal film. It can evaluate for free air under the diaphragm, a marker for bowel perforation, as well as air fluid levels
- A series of films taken on consecutive days can be used for comparison to identify response to therapy or continued deterioration

*Advantages/Disadvantages*
- Advantages: simple, quick, and relatively safe investigation
- Disadvantage: involves a small dose of radiation

*Abnormal*
- Often demonstrates a tubular, ahaustral segment of the colon in the presence of distal ulcerative colitis with fecal matter proximal to diseased mucosa (known as lead-pipe colon)
- Intestinal edema, ulceration, or thumbprinting may give a gross estimate of disease activity
- Diagnosis of toxic megacolon, a complication of ulcerative colitis, can be made when the colon is dilated to a diameter of 10cm or more, measured radiographically at the midtransverse colon

*Cause of abnormal result*
Generally normal in mild-moderate colitis, but thumbprinting or dilation indicates severe colitis.

## Special tests
### SIGMOIDOSCOPY
*Description*
- In acute ulcerative colitis, the diagnosis is readily established by sigmoidoscopy, which reveals the presence and pattern of distal colonic inflammation
- The absence of rectal disease excludes the diagnosis of ulcerative colitis (but not Crohn's disease), with the caveat that patients who have already initiated treatment may have decreased distal findings. This is seen particularly with enema or suppository therapy
- When a diagnosis of ulcerative colitis is suspected, sigmoidoscopy and rectal biopsy should be performed at the first available opportunity because effective management can then be started with a minimum of delay. These tests can make a diagnosis of ulcerative colitis as this disease always involves the rectum

- After patients have been on therapy and the acute symptoms have improved, colonoscopy is performed to accurately determine the extent and pattern of the disease

*Advantages/Disadvantages*
- Advantage: in ulcerative colitis, the extent and severity of the disease are best assessed by sigmoidoscopy, with biopsies taken for histology from each part of the colon
- Disadvantage: sigmoidoscopy should be performed with caution in patients with severe, active disease because of the risk of bowel perforation

*Abnormal*
Despite clues offered by pathology, at least 10% of patients are not easily classified as having either Crohn's disease or ulcerative colitis and are said to have indeterminate colitis:
- Edematous, friable rectal mucosa in a continuous pattern on sigmoidoscopy is the key to diagnosis of ulcerative colitis
- Sigmoidoscopy may reveal a narrowed and straightened lumen, with loss of haustral folds
- Edema, bleeding, friability, mucosal granularity, and erosions are indicative of colitis
- Loss of normal vascular pattern with granular mucosal appearance
- Histologic examination may show distorted crypt architecture and acute and chronic inflammation of the lamina propria

*Cause of abnormal result*
Inflammation and ulceration of the mucosa of the colon.

*Drugs, disorders and other factors that may alter results*
- Some laxatives, particularly sodium triphosphate solution, used to prepare the bowel for sigmoidoscopy can also lead to minute bowel erosions that might be mistaken for colitis, hence the value of examining the unprepped patient
- Ischemic colitis, Crohn's disease, *C. difficile* colitis, and infectious colitides can present with similar or identical endoscopic findings

COLONOSCOPY
*Description*
Endoscopic examination of the entire colon to the terminal ileum is possible.

*Advantages/Disadvantages*
Advantages:
- May be used to determine the extent of colonic involvement in either ulcerative colitis or Crohn's disease
- May be used to screen for cancer in long-standing ulcerative colitis
- Can distinguish Crohn's disease from ulcerative colitis

Disadvantages:
- More uncomfortable for patient in setting of acute inflammation
- Carries with it a higher risk of perforation
- Patient is sedated to decrease discomfort

*Abnormal*
- In acute colitis, the mucosal appearance is characterized by edema, bleeding, friability, mucosal granularity, and erosions
- Degree of mucosal injury can be graded as mild, moderate, or severe
- In patients with mild disease, the endoscopic findings can be subtle, with only mucosal edema and loss of the normal vascular pattern and erythema

- Moderate ulcerative colitis is characterized by diffusely edematous and erythematous mucosa with loss of the normal vascular pattern and superficial erosions
- In severe ulcerative colitis, frank ulceration and spontaneous bleeding uniformly occur over the involved areas
- In chronic or resolving colitis, the mucosa loses its characteristic normal appearance and a diagnosis can be readily established on biopsy of the involved mucosa
- Ulcerative colitis typically begins in the rectum and extends proximally in a uniform, circumferential manner
- At presentation, 40% of patients have only rectal disease, 40% have disease up to the hepatic flexure, and 10–20% have pancolitis
- The inflammation involves the mucosal surface but is not transmural
- The endoscopic appearance of infectious colitis and ischemic colitis can appear endoscopically similar
- The terminal ileum is not involved in ulcerative colitis; its presence is highly suggestive of Crohn's disease or infectious ileitis
- Patchy involvement of the colon can occur in ulcerative colitis after treatment

*Cause of abnormal result*
Inflammation of the mucosa of the large intestine.

*Drugs, disorders and other factors that may alter results*
- Some laxatives used to prepare the bowel for colonoscopy can also lead to minute bowel erosions that might be mistaken for colitis. However, biopsy of these lesions will be essentially normal
- Ischemic colitis, Crohn's disease, *C. difficile* colitis, and infectious colitides can present with similar or identical endoscopic findings

# TREATMENT

## CONSIDER CONSULT

- Disease refractory to first-line management should be referred at the earliest opportunity to a specialist center for both medical and surgical management and follow up
- Difficulty in maintaining remission is the most common reason for further specialist referral

## IMMEDIATE ACTION

- In the presence of fulminant disease, obstruction, or toxic megacolon, refer patient to hospital immediately
- Intravenous fluids for volume resuscitation will be started as early as possible
- Intravenous steroids will be given if fulminant disease, obstruction, or toxic megacolon is suspected
- Antibiotics will be considered
- Surgery may be necessary

## PATIENT AND CAREGIVER ISSUES
### Patient or caregiver request

Q Will I lose my colon as a result of this disease? About 10% of people with ulcerative colitis develop a severe form of the disease that requires an operation to remove the large bowel. Also, colectomy may be considered in the future if you develop colon cancer or to prevent colon cancer if advanced precancerous lesions (dysplasia) are found

Q Does this disease increase my risk of colon cancer? If pancolitis is present, the risk of cancer increases starting at 8 years after diagnosis. From this point, the risk of cancer increases about 1% per year. The risk of colorectal cancer after 20 years of disease is around 30%. Regular screening colonoscopy with random surveillance biopsies will be necessary every 1–2 years to detect precancerous (dysplasia) or cancerous changes that sometimes develop after long periods of inflammation as a result of active disease. This should start 8 years after initial presentation if pancolitis is present and 15 years from initial presentation if only left-sided colitis is present. If only proctitis is present, then specialized dysplasia screening is not required, although patient should still have standard colorectal cancer screening. (Risk of cancer increases about 1% for each year of active disease after first 8 years.) The risk of colon cancer in patients with proctitis only is same as that in general population

## MANAGEMENT ISSUES
### Goals

- To achieve remission, defined by the Food and Drug Administration Gastrointestinal Advisory Panel as the absence of inflammatory symptoms (rectal bleeding or diarrhea), in conjunction with evidence of mucosal healing (absence of ulceration, significant granularity, or friability), when off steroids
- Adoption of a regimen of maintenance therapy to prevent a recurrence of clinical or endoscopic signs of active disease

### Management in special circumstances
SPECIAL PATIENT GROUPS

- Pregnant patients with active disease may be more likely to have a miscarriage, premature delivery, or low-birthweight baby
- Investigation with X-rays and endoscopy should be avoided
- Medical management is usually effective during pregnancy and is less harmful than untreated disease. Sulfasalazine and corticosteroids are safe. Immunosuppressants should be avoided where possible, as should metronidazole

## SUMMARY OF THERAPEUTIC OPTIONS
### Choices
Guidelines for the management of ulcerative colitis are published by the American Academy of Family Physicians 1998:
- Severe ulcerative colitis should be treated with an oral corticosteroid (prednisone) treatment, with or without an oral 5-aminosalicylic acid (5-ASA) (sulfasalazine, olsalazine, and mesalamine)
- Consideration should be given to urgent referral, depending on the patient's condition and response to treatment
- Admission for intravenous corticosteroids and pain control can be considered if patient appears severely ill
- Fluid resuscitation is required if hypovolemic or septic
- Mild to moderate ulcerative colitis should be treated with an oral 5-ASA (sulfasalazine, olsalazine, and mesalamine)
- Consider addition of an oral corticosteroid (prednisone) if the patient fails to make a rapid improvement (resolution within 2 weeks) or if deterioration occurs
- Mild ulcerative colitis should be confined to the distal colon or rectum – local treatment with corticosteroid enemas is reasonable
- Mesalamine enemas are a good alternative choice in mild disease
- Treatment should be escalated to systemic therapy if symptoms have not resolved within a couple of weeks
- An oral 5-ASA (sulfasalazine, olsalazine, and mesalamine) is the generally preferred maintenance therapy
- 6-Mercaptopurine/azathioprine are established in the management of Crohn's disease and ulcerative colitis. These therapies are usually prescribed by specialists. They are generally used for disease that is recurrent despite maintenance therapy with sulfasalazine or 5-ASA compounds. They may also be used as steroid-sparing agents for patients who are unable to fully taper their steroid dose without recurrence of symptoms
- Corticosteroids are no longer recommended for use as maintenance therapy
- Loperamide may be used to treat chronic diarrhea without active disease
- Surgery may be the required treatment for complications and should be performed by an experienced surgeon
- Acute complications of ulcerative colitis include toxic megacolon and bowel perforation
- Chronic complications of ulcerative colitis include the development of dysplasia or adenocarcinoma
- Surgery would also be considered for failed medical therapy. This includes acute medical failure (severe disease that is not responsive to 7–10 days of intravenous corticosteroids), as well as chronic disease that is troubling to the patient, as colectomy can provide the only cure for ulcerative colitis
- Colectomy with temporary ileostomy and ileoanal pouch construction is the usual option; however, proctocolectomy and permanent ileostomy may be preferred in some cases
- Lifestyle changes may include dietary supplements and modifications and may be beneficial for phases of acute inflammation and while in remission

### Clinical pearls
- For flares of ulcerative colitis refractory to treatment consider the possibility of a concurrent infection with *Clostridium difficile*, *Salmonella/Shigella*, or cytomegalovirus. Cytomegalovirus is likely to be seen in immunosuppressed ulcerative colitis patients
- Absence of systemic signs of steroid side effects at high doses is a typical finding in patients refractory to the therapeutic effect and should not suggest noncompliance

### Never
- Corticosteroids and other immunosuppressive agents should generally be prescribed only with advice from a gastroenterologist

- Never delay treatment and referral in both acute and chronic disease as both can be more effectively treated at an early stage
- In the presence of fulminant disease and/or toxic megacolon, anticholinergic or antidiarrhea drugs should never be used since they can precipitate or aggravate toxic megacolon
- During an acute flare, colonoscopy should be avoided as there is an increased risk of complications, especially perforation

## FOLLOW UP
### Plan for review
- As inflammatory bowel disease is a relapsing and remitting illness, it is accepted that patients with quiescent disease or maintained remission do not need to be followed up regularly
- Review relapses at the first opportunity
- Regularly review, as part of the treatment plan, patients with active, complex, or refractory disease
- Drug toxicity needs regular monitoring including the use of steroids, 5-ASA, and 6-mercaptopurine/azathioprine
- Patients on corticosteroids for over 3 months require calcium and vitamin D supplementation. A bone mineral densitometry should be considered, and bisphosphonate therapy should be instituted if the z-score is more than two standard deviations below normal
- Annual bone mineral densitometry should be considered for patients on chronic corticosteroids
- Patients with pancolitis require screening for dysplasia and colorectal cancer after 8 years
- Patients with left-sided colitis require screening for dysplasia and colorectal cancer after 15 years
- Follow up should be shared between the primary care physician (PCP) and gastroenterologist

### Information for patient or caregiver
- You have an illness that can affect you throughout your life and as yet has no known cause or cure
- There will be times when the activity of the disease settles down and you will be free of symptoms. This is called remission and the aim of treatment is to keep you at this stage
- You may need to take medication periodically or for longer periods of time in order to control the symptoms and the inflammation. This will help get you into remission as well as prevent relapses. You may need to take medication indefinitely to control symptoms and prevent relapses
- It is difficult to predict the course of your illness. You may get better and stay that way for years but you could also get rapidly worse and need to be admitted to hospital. Most people fall somewhere in between

## DRUGS AND OTHER THERAPIES: DETAILS
### Drugs
SULFASALAZINE
- Sulfasalazine is a compound of sulfapyridine and 5-aminosalicylic acid (5-ASA) molecules
- Sulfasalazine is the oldest and cheapest 5-ASA
- The risk of agranulocytosis and Stevens–Johnson syndrome is very low but still significant; this has led most gastroenterologists to prescribe instead the newer 5-ASA (mesalamine and olsalazine), which have improved side effect profiles

*Dose*
- For patients with active ulcerative colitis, the recommended starting dosage is 0.5g orally twice daily, slowly enhancing, as tolerated, to 0.5–1.0g orally four times daily
- The usual maintenance dose is 1g orally twice daily

*Efficacy*
In ulcerative colitis it is useful for the treatment of mild to moderate acute exacerbations and as maintenance therapy.

*Risks/benefits*
Benefit: concomitant relief of symptoms of coexisting gastrointestinal inflammatory disease.

*Side effects and adverse reactions*
- Cardiovascular system: pericarditis, allergic myocarditis
- Central nervous system: dizziness, drowsiness, headache, seizures
- Eyes, ears, nose, and throat: blurred vision, tinnitus
- Gastrointestinal: abdominal pain, diarrhoea, hepatotoxicity, melena, vomiting
- Genitourinary: renal failure, urinary retention
- Hematologic: blood cell disorders
- Musculoskeletal: arthralgia, myalgia, osteoporosis
- Skin: Stevens–Johnson syndrome

*Interactions (other drugs)*
- Digoxin
- Methenamine
- Phenytoin
- Tolbutamide
- Warfarin

*Contraindications*
- Contraindicated in porphyria and gastrointestinal or urinary tract obstruction
- Cross-hypersensitivity with salicylates
- Caution required in patients with renal or hepatic impairment and glucose-6-phosphate deficiency

*Acceptability to patient*
- Well tolerated by 80% of patients
- Use with caution in pregnancy and breast-feeding

*Follow up plan*
- Patients remaining in remission should be continued on these drugs at maintenance dose. Stopping increases the risk of relapse
- The evidence for maintained remission is valid for about 4 years (the length of the longer trials of continued use)
- Therefore some gastroenterologists advocate stopping the drugs after a period of 4 years without any evidence of relapse
- Obviously, if the patient subsequently relapses they need to be restarted

*Patient and caregiver information*
Oral medications should be taken with food if there are significant gastrointestinal side effects.

## MESALAMINE
- Mesalamine is a 5-aminosalicylic acid (5-ASA) that lacks the sulfa moiety of sulfasalazine and is associated with fewer side effects
- Can be used in many patients who are intolerant of sulfasalazine
- Mesalamine is also available in suppository and enema forms: systemic absorption is poor and the side effect profile for topical treatment is good

*Dose*
- In active disease, the recommended dosage is 2.4–4.8g/day for Asacol
- Standard maintenance dose is 1g/day for Pentasa
- The dosage recommendation for mesalamine suppositories is 250mg or 500mg rectally twice daily and for enemas 1–2g once daily
- Clinical experience shows that the higher 4.8g dosage of oral mesalamine produces significantly better results than the 2.4g dosage
- Disease that has not responded to smaller amounts of mesalamine often goes into remission with the 4.8g dosage

- Once the disease is in remission (usually after an 8-week course), these oral dosages can be tapered to 400mg three times daily (or occasionally 800mg three times daily) of mesalamine. The higher dosage can be reinstituted if the patient has recurrences at these levels
- When disease is confined to the rectum, effective treatment may be mesalamine suppositories in a dosage of 500mg twice daily
- When disease extends above the rectum but not past the splenic flexure, a mesalamine or hydrocortisone enema proves most effective. Use of an enema with 4g of mesalamine at night has demonstrated efficacy
- The 4g mesalamine enemas prove most effective for inducing and maintaining remission of distal ulcerative colitis. Continue topical therapy long enough for patients to benefit (normal bowel movements without blood or urgency). More than 6 weeks are usually needed to achieve remission
- To maintain remission of proctitis, gradually taper the mesalamine suppositories, switching to a 1g mesalamine enema every third night for maintenance

*Efficacy*
Patients usually have a gradual response to this medication.

*Risks/benefits*
Benefits:
- In left-sided colitis and proctitis, topical therapy is appropriate and has an excellent side effect profile
- There is less risk of immunosuppression or bone marrow suppression with mesalamine than with sulfasalazine

*Side effects and adverse reactions*
Common side effects include headache, abdominal pain, nausea, fever, rash, dyspepsia, diarrhea, hepatitis, and occasionally bone marrow suppression. Interstitial nephritis occurs in up to 1 in 300 patients. These can occur with both oral and topical therapies.

*Interactions (other drugs)*
**Absorption of digoxin is possibly reduced.**

*Contraindications*
**History of allergy or intolerance to aspirin.**

*Acceptability to patient*
The benefits of mesalamine must be weighed against the considerably lower cost of sulfasalazine.

*Follow up plan*
Patients need to be followed closely by a specialist. If this first-line agent does not quell disease activity, addition of corticosteroid may be required.

*Patient and caregiver information*
- Patients should be instructed to take oral medication as whole tablets
- Patients should lie on their left side while administering an enema
- Patients need to be inactive for 30min after administering a suppository or enema

## OLSALAZINE
- Olsalazine is a 5-ASA, which lacks the sulfa moiety of sulfasalazine and is associated with fewer side effects
- Can be used in many patients who are intolerant of sulfasalazine

*Dose*
- 250mg tablets
- In active disease, the recommended dosage is 1g/day
- Standard maintenance dose is 1g/day

*Efficacy*
Patients usually have a gradual response to this medication.

*Risks/benefits*
Risks: use caution in renal disease, children, breast-feeding, and pregnancy.

*Side effects and adverse reactions*
- Central nervous system: fever, depression, dizziness, headache
- Gastrointestinal: nausea, vomiting, diarrhea, abdominal pain, anorexia, bloating, raised liver enzymes, hepatitis
- Hematologic: blood cell dyscrasias
- Musculoskeletal: arthralgia
- Skin: rash, pruritus

*Interactions (other drugs)*
**Digoxin.**

*Contraindications*
- **Hypersenstivity to salicylates** ■ **Severe renal impairment**

*Follow up plan*
- Patients need to be followed closely by a specialist
- If this first-line agent does not quell disease activity, addition of corticosteroid may be required

## PREDNISONE
- Oral corticosteroids such as prednisone are beneficial in patients with acute episodes of moderate and severe ulcerative colitis and may be given in conjunction with 5-ASA
- Some extracolonic manifestations of ulcerative colitis also generally respond to prednisone, such as erythema nodosum, and arthritis
- Other extracolonic disease, most notably sclerosing cholangitis and pyoderma gangrenosum, do not respond to steroid therapy

*Dose*
- 20–40mg/day, for several weeks
- When symptoms lessen and improvement is noted on proctoscopic examination, prednisone can be tapered over 2–3 months and then discontinued. Improvement in endoscopic findings often lag behind clinical improvement
- A typical course consists of 40mg daily for 2 weeks, followed by 30mg for 1–2 weeks, followed by a tapering dose by 5mg every 1–2 weeks according to severity and response. This should give an 8–14-week course
- If there is failure to respond to steroids then specialist help should be sought for consideration of steroid-sparing therapy with 6-mercaptopurine, azathioprine, or other experimental therapy

*Efficacy*
- Oral corticosteroids are indicated only for the treatment of acute exacerbations and should not be used for long-term maintenance
- It is important to start the oral corticosteroid at the recommended dosage. A common mistake is to give suboptimal amounts hoping to avoid side effects

- At lower dosages, patients still risk getting side effects without ever getting the benefits of an appropriately high dosage

### Risks/benefits
Risks:
- Use caution in congestive heart failure, diabetes mellitus, glaucoma, renal disease, ulcerative colitis, and peptic ulcer
- Use caution in elderly
- Prednisone taken in doses higher than 7.5mg for a period of 3 weeks or longer may lead to clinically relevant suppression of the pituitary-adrenal axis

### Side effects and adverse reactions
- Side-effects are minimized by short duration of therapy
- Cardiovascular system: hypertension, thromboembolism
- Central nervous system: insomnia, euphoria, depression, psychosis, seizures
- Endocrine: adrenal suppression, impaired glucose tolerance, growth suppression in children
- Eyes, ears, nose, and throat: cataract, glaucoma, blurred vision
- Gastrointestinal: dyspepsia, peptic ulceration, oesophagitis, oral candidiasis
- Musculoskeletal: proximal myopathy, osteoporosis
- Skin: delayed healing, acne, striae, fragile skin

### Interactions (other drugs)
- **Aminoglutethimide (increased clearance of prednisone)** ■ **Antidiabetics (hypoglycemic effect inhibited)** ■ **Antihypertensives (effects inhibited)** ■ **Barbiturates (increased clearance of prednisone)** ■ **Cardiac glycosides (toxicity increased)** ■ **Cholestyramine, colestipol (reduced absorption of corticosteroids)** ■ **Clarithromycin, erythromycin, troleandomycin (may enhance steroid effect)** ■ **Cyclosporine (may increase levels of both drugs; may cause seizures)** ■ **Diuretics (effects inhibited)** ■ **Isoniazid (reduced plasma levels of isoniazid)** ■ **Ketoconazole** ■ **Nonsteroidal anti-inflammatory drugs (increased risk of bleeeding)** ■ **Oral contraceptives (enhanced effects of corticosteroids)** ■ **Rifampin (may inhibit hepatic clearance of prednisone)** ■ **Salicylates (increased clearance of salicylates)** ■ **Warfarin (alters clotting time)**

### Contraindications
- **Systemic infection** ■ **Avoid live virus vaccines in those receiving immunosuppressive doses** ■ **History of tuberculosis** ■ **Cushing's syndrome** ■ **Recent myocardial infarction**

### Acceptability to patient
- Systemic corticosteroids have an extensive side effect profile
- Acute effects include acne and severe mood changes, which are particularly common in young patients
- Other changes include edema and fat distribution to the abdomen and upper back, as well as facial changes (moon facies), all of which can be troubling to patients

### Follow up plan
- Patients on steroids need to be closely monitored by a physician and need to have their steroid doses carefully tapered
- Patients should not be left on treatment with long-term steroids
- Patients who require long-tem (>3 months) steroids should be placed on calcium and vitamin D replacement for osteoporosis prophylaxis. Annual bone mineral densitometry should be considered. Patients who fall more than two standard deviations below the mean should be considered for bisphosphonate therapy

*Patient and caregiver information*
- Patients should be cautioned regarding the side effects of steroid therapy but that the potential benefit outweighs these risks in the short term
- Patients on prolonged treatment should carry a 'steroid card' and ensure that treatment does not stop abruptly

CORTICOSTEROID ENEMA
- Corticosteroid enemas are recommended as adjunctive therapy in patients with colitis confined to the left-sided colon and rectum
- In patients who fail to respond rapidly to mesalamine or who are unable to tolerate mesalamine, it is appropriate to use corticosteroid enemas in the short term
- Corticosteroid enemas are not recommended as maintenance therapy for ulcerative colitis

*Dose*
- Left-sided colitis/ulcerative proctitis: 100mg/day of hydrocortisone
- Short-term use (less than 2 weeks) is preferred
- If therapy continues for more than 2 weeks, gradual withdrawal from treatment is advised
- 10% hydrocortisone foam at night or twice daily (containing 20mg prednisolone)

*Efficacy*
- Topical corticosteroids are less effective than 5-ASA enemas and may result in adrenal suppression on long-term use
- When disease extends above the rectum but not past the splenic flexure, a hydrocortisone enema proves most effective
- In comparison to mesalamine, hydrocortisone is not effective for maintaining remission
- Use of an enema with 100mg of hydrocortisone at night has demonstrated efficacy

*Risks/benefits*
Risks:
- Dependency on corticosteroids is often encountered in patients with inflammatory bowel disease
- In many cases, the dose of corticosteroids cannot be tapered without an increase in disease activity

*Side effects and adverse reactions*
Toxic effects of corticosteroids are related to the dose and duration of therapy and include:
- Acne, striae
- Weight gain, moon-like face
- Growth retardation
- Osteoporosis
- Diabetes mellitus
- Hypertension

*Interactions (other drugs)*
**Cyclosporine.**

*Contraindications*
**Long-term use of corticosteroids is associated with serious, potentially irreversible side effects and should be avoided.**

*Acceptability to patient*
- Patients may be resistant to using enemas initially
- There may be some systemic effects from the use of topical corticosteroids

*Follow up plan*
- Steroid enemas do not require dose tapering prior to discontinuation
- Patients should not be left on treatment with long-term steroids

*Patient and caregiver information*
- Most patients have heard of the bad side effects of steroids. However, steroids are still very good and safe when given as a treatment for acute attacks of the disease
- Patients should lie on their left side while administering an enema

## LOPERAMIDE
Loperamide is an anticholinergic agent that increases both colonic water absorption and internal sphincter function.

*Dose*
2mg orally initially, then 2mg after each unformed stool, to a maximum of 16mg/day.

*Efficacy*
- Loperamide can afford symptomatic relief for patients who do not have systemic symptoms but who continue to have diarrhea despite adequate primary therapy for both extensive and distal ulcerative colitis disease
- Loperamide is preferred for its safety and efficacy

*Risks/benefits*
Risks:
- Use caution in liver disease, dehydration, and severe ulcerative colitis
- Not recommmended in children

*Side effects and adverse reactions*
- Central nervous system: fatigue, dizziness, drowsiness
- Gastrointestinal: nausea, constipation, toxic megacolon, abdominal cramps and bloating, paralytic ileus, vomiting
- Genitourinary: nephrotoxicity
- Respiratory: respiratory depression
- Skin: rash

*Interactions (other drugs)*
- Bethanechol - Cholestyramine - Cisapride - Metoclopramide - Erythromycin

*Contraindications*
- Development of abdominal distension or inhibition of peristalsis - Acute diarrhea due to infectious organisms such as *Escherichia coli*, *Salmonella*, *Shigella* - Pseudomembranous colitis associated with broad-spectrum antibiotics - Acute dysentery

*Acceptability to patient*
Generally acceptable for symptomatic treatment.

*Patient and caregiver information*
Patients should not take this medication if they experience severe or different symptoms, and should see their PCP.

## 6-MERCAPTOPURINE/AZATHIOPRINE
6-Mercaptopurine (6-MP) and its prodrug, azathioprine, are immunomodulatory agents used as steroid-sparing therapy for ulcerative colitis and to help retain remission of ulcerative colitis.

*Dose*
- Generally starting at 50–75mg, can be increased to maximum of 200mg/day. The dose of azathioprine is generally twice that of 6-MP
- Patients should be screened first for TMTT enzyme activity. Roughly 10% of the population lack this enzyme, which is necessary for 6-MP and azathioprine to be converted to its active metabolite. Patients lacking this enzyme invariably develop severe though reversible hematologic toxicity with these agents. 6-MP metabolite levels can be monitored and serial complete blood count (CBC) and blood chemistries can be checked
- Should generally be prescribed initially by a gastroenterologist trained in the treatment of inflammatory bowel disease

*Efficacy*
- 6-MP and azathioprine have been shown to be effective at maintaining remission of ulcerative colitis in 60% and 70% of patients, respectively
- It may take 3–6 months to reach full effect, other therapy is generally necessary during this 'bridge' period

*Risks/benefits*
Risks: among the major risks are bone marrow suppression, hepatotoxicity, and pancreatitis.

*Side effects and adverse reactions*
- Major side-effects include bone marrow suppression and pancreatitis.
- Other side-effects include diarrhea, fever, weakness, oral lesions, nausea, vomiting, abdominal pain, and anorexia. Bone marrow suppression, particularly neutropenia, is dose-dependent
- Pancreatitis develops in 3–15% of patients. It typically develops after several weeks of therapy and resolves spontaneously after the drug has been discontinued. It rapidly recurs if the drug is given again

*Interactions (other drugs)*
- Bactrim (increases risk of bone marrow suppression with mercaptopurine) - Cyclosporine: (azathioprine decreases the concentration of cyclosporine)

*Contraindications*
Safety and efficacy are not established in children under 12 years.

*Acceptability to patient*
- Generally acceptable for symptomatic treatment
- May need to be discontinued if there is development of toxic side effects
- Development of leukopenia or thrombocytopenia may necessitate a dose reduction

*Follow up plan*
- Measurement of the active 6-thioguanine metabolite of 6-MP and azathioprine allows gastroenterologists to better titrate the effect and avoid hematologic toxicity
- Patients should have a CBC monthly after starting 6-MP or azathioprine
- Once dose is stable, CBC can be followed periodically

*Patient and caregiver information*
Patients should not take this medication if they experience severe or different symptoms, and should see their PCP.

## Surgical therapy
TOTAL COLECTOMY
- In ulcerative colitis, surgical removal of the colon should be considered in patients who have failed medical management, are having toxic side effects from medical therapy, or have severe

complications, including toxic megacolon, severe gastrointestinal bleeding, bowel perforation, dysplasia, or cancer
- A variation on this surgery is ileal pouch anal anastomosis, also known as an ileoanal pull-through. This procedure allows patients to maintain anal function and continence. However, pouchitis, an inflammatory process involving the ileal pouch, is a long-term problem of this method that affects 30–50% of patients

*Efficacy*
- Ulcerative colitis is a surgically curable disease if the entire colorectal mucosa is removed
- For this reason, total proctocolectomy with permanent end ileostomy has been the operation of choice for many years
- More recently, the preferred operation is total proctocolectomy with an ileoanal pull-through. This generally allows preservation of bowel defecatory function, although patients will have frequent loose bowel movements
- Ileostomy is generally only required now for emergency colectomy or when the ileoanal pull-through fails

*Risks/benefits*
Risks: includes the risks of anesthesia and infection and complications associated with any major surgery, as well as the possibility that the anastomosis might fail and precipitate the need for additional surgeries for revision of the initial procedure.

*Acceptability to patient*
Acceptable if medical therapy is not controlling symptoms.

*Follow up plan*
- Patients are routinely followed up postoperatively at 4–8 weeks
- Surgical follow up is required

*Patient and caregiver information*
Patients should be educated and counseled before and after the surgery regarding the extent of the surgery and the effect it will have on their lifestyle.

## LIFESTYLE
- There are no known dietary agents that have been linked to ulcerative colitis or to worsening of the existing condition
- Folic acid supplements may be necessary for patients taking sulfasalazine, as absorption is affected
- Oral iron may prevent anemia

### RISKS/BENEFITS
Benefits:
- May improve symptoms
- Exacerbations may be avoided
- Effective treatment of deficiencies

### ACCEPTABILITY TO PATIENT
Patients may be unwilling to change their diet.

### PATIENT AND CAREGIVER INFORMATION
If the intake of milk does not affect the nature of the disease, it does not need to be avoided.

## OUTCOMES

### EFFICACY OF THERAPIES
- Generally, physicians will increase therapy with immunosuppressive agents, until either remission is induced, or chronic, active disease is brought under control
- The newer 5-ASA medications (mesalamine and olsalazine) have been shown to be slightly more efficacious than sulfasalazine in inducing remission, but are less cost-effective
- Sulfasalazine remains the most effective medication for maintaining remission
- Corticosteroids are effective in the treatment of active disease but are not recommended for maintenance therapy
- Total colectomy is curative for patients with ulcerative colitis but is usually only considered if there is failure of medical therapy, dysplasia, or cancer

### Review period
6 months.

### PROGNOSIS
- Response to treatment is highly variable
- Remission may be achieved in most patients with ulcerative colitis
- The prognosis is worse when there is involvement of the entire colon
- Relapse is common
- Colectomy is required in approx. 20–25% of patients

### Clinical pearls
- Combination of oral and topical therapy is common during disease flares
- Frequent low-volume bowel movements suggest proctitic symptoms and respond best to suppositories even in patients with pancolitis
- Corticosteroid tapering is highly individualized. Gradual tapering is always preferable and dose should not be reduced if symptoms are active
- Sigmoidoscopy during treatment is helpful when the patient is not responding clinically in order to confirm the severity and extent of activity
- Topical therapy can be used with rectosigmoid disease
- Immunomodulators such as 6-mercaptopurine (6-MP) and azathioprine are not helpful during the acute disease because of delayed onset of action
- Cyclosporine can be used in the severely ill patient because it works promptly

### Therapeutic failure
- Generally, physicians will increase immunosuppressive agents until remission is induced or chronic, active disease is brought under control
- Azathioprine and mercaptopurine should be prescribed by specialists
- Surgery should be considered when medical management has failed

### Deterioration
- Corticosteroids should be added to 5-ASA treatment if an acute attack fails to respond to 5-ASA
- Surgical treatment is reserved for the most resistant cases

### COMPLICATIONS
- Toxic megacolon is severe colitis with dilation of the transverse colon of more than 10cm. Perforation may occur with or without dilation. Peritonitis indicates perforation and requires immediate surgical referral
- Fistula formation, stricture formation, or abscess formation are less common in ulcerative colitis than in Crohn's disease

- Fulminant ulcerative colitis when disease is severe and refractory to medical management
- Severe bleeding
- Anemia may be secondary to blood loss or chronic disease
- Ulcerative colitis is a risk factor for colorectal carcinoma, and the cumulative risk begins to rise after 8–15 years of having the disease. Patients should be screened for colorectal carcinoma

## CONSIDER CONSULT
Patients with signs of systemic infection should be referred to a specialist for immediate antimicrobial therapy.

## PREVENTION

### RISK FACTORS
Some studies suggest that certain foods, notably milk or lactose, may act as secondary triggers for ulcerative colitis, but these findings are not widely accepted.

### SCREENING
In the absence of characteristic symptoms, screening is not effective.

### PREVENT RECURRENCE
- Treatment aims to maximize duration of remissions; depending on the severity of the disease, different drugs may be taken for extended periods of time to induce and extend remissions
- As the drugs are toxic and regimens have to be tailored, it is generally recommended that a gastroenterologist be consulted

# RESOURCES

## ASSOCIATIONS

American College of Gastroenterology
7910 Woodmont Avenue
7th Floor
Bethesda, MD 20814
Tel: (703) 820-7400
Fax: (703) 931-4520
http://www.acg.gi.org/

Crohn's and Colitis Foundation of America
241 Forsegate Drive
Suite 104
Jamesburg, NJ 08831
Tel: (732) 656-1244
http://www.ccfa.org/

## KEY REFERENCES

- Hanauer SB. Drug therapy: inflammatory bowel disease. N Engl J Med 1996;334:841–8
- Allan RN, Keighley MRB, Rhodes JM, et al, eds. Inflammatory bowel disease, 3rd edn. New York: Churchill Livingstone, 1996
- Sandborn WJ. A review of immune modifier therapy for inflammatory bowel disease: azathioprine, 6-mercaptopurine, cyclosporine, and methotrexate. Am J Gastroenterol 1996;91:423–33
- Stenson WF. Inflammatory bowel disease. In: Yamada T, ed. Textbook of gastroenterology, 2nd edn. Vol 2. Philadelphia: Lippincott, 1995, p1748–1805
- Sutherland L, Roth D, Beck P, et al. 5-aminosalicylic acid for inducing remission in ulcerative colitis (Cochrane Review). In: The Cochrane Library, 1, 2001. Oxford: Update Software
- Sutherland L, Roth D, Beck P, May G, Makiyama K. Oral 5-aminosalicyclic acid for maintaining remission in ulcerative colitis (Cochrane Review). In: The Cochrane Library, 1, 2001. Oxford: Update Software

## FAQS

### Question 1
When should sigmoidoscopy be done in a patient with bloody diarrhea?

ANSWER 1
- In a patient with negative cultures
- In a patient not responding to antibiotics
- In a patient who is not improving after 3–4 days
- Prior to initiating treatment for ulcerative colitis

### Question 2
When should colonoscopy be done in a patient recently diagnosed with ulcerative colitis?

ANSWER 2
Once the acute flare has resolved and the patient is stable, colonoscopy should be done to determine disease extent and exlude Crohn's disease, if possible, by biopsy and examination of the terminal ileum.

### Question 3
When should steroids be started?

## ANSWER 3
With both 5-ASAs and steroids the clinical response is rapid. Improvement should be seen within a week with a standard dose of Asacol, 3.6–4.8g/day. If there is no improvement, start steroid treatment.

## Question 4
When should hospitalization be recommended?

## ANSWER 4
In patients not responding to high-dose oral steroids +/- 5-ASA, short-term hospitalization is often beneficial. Patients receive intravenous steroid, bowel and bed rest, and correction of fluid, electrolyte, and protein deficiencies, if needed, as well as transfusions. Within 5–7 days patients usually go into remission.

## Question 5
What should be done when an adenomatous polyp is found on colonoscopy in a patient with chronic ulcerative colitis?

## ANSWER 5
For patients in their 40s and over, this can be handled as a sporadic adenomatous polyp with endoscopic removal, if the polyps are not numerous and there is no dysplasia without polyp formation elsewhere in the colon. These patients should be followed closely.

## CONTRIBUTORS
Russell C Jones, MD, MPH
Andrew F Ippoliti, MD
Laura Targownik, MD, FRCP(C)

# Index

**Acute appendicitis** — *1*
- Summary Information — *2*
- Background — *3*
- Diagnosis — *5*
- Treatment — *11*
- Outcomes — *12*
- Prevention — *13*
- Resources — *14*

**Budd-Chiari syndrome** — *15*
- Summary Information — *16*
- Background — *17*
- Diagnosis — *19*
- Treatment — *32*
- Outcomes — *39*
- Prevention — *40*
- Resources — *41*

**Celiac disease** — *43*
- Summary Information — *44*
- Background — *45*
- Diagnosis — *47*
- Treatment — *57*
- Outcomes — *67*
- Prevention — *69*
- Resources — *70*

**Cholecystitis** — *73*
- Summary Information — *74*
- Background — *75*
- Diagnosis — *77*
- Treatment — *88*
- Outcomes — *95*
- Prevention — *97*
- Resources — *99*

**Cirrhosis** — *101*
- Summary Information — *102*
- Background — *103*
- Diagnosis — *105*
- Treatment — *117*
- Outcomes — *125*
- Prevention — *127*
- Resources — *128*

**Crohn's disease** — *131*
- Summary Information — *132*
- Background — *133*
- Diagnosis — *135*
- Treatment — *148*
- Outcomes — *161*
- Prevention — *163*
- Resources — *164*

**Diverticular disease** — *167*
- Summary Information — *168*
- Background — *169*
- Diagnosis — *171*
- Treatment — *179*
- Outcomes — *186*
- Prevention — *188*
- Resources — *189*

**Gastroesophageal reflux disease in adults** — *193*
- Summary Information — *194*
- Background — *195*
- Diagnosis — *198*
- Treatment — *208*
- Outcomes — *221*
- Prevention — *223*
- Resources — *224*

**Hemorrhoids** — *229*
- Summary Information — *230*
- Background — *231*
- Diagnosis — *233*
- Treatment — *238*
- Outcomes — *253*
- Prevention — *255*
- Resources — *256*

**Alcoholic hepatitis** — *257*
- Summary Information — *258*
- Background — *259*
- Diagnosis — *261*
- Treatment — *276*
- Outcomes — *288*
- Prevention — *290*
- Resources — *292*

**Viral hepatitis** — *295*
- Summary Information — *296*
- Background — *297*
- Diagnosis — *299*
- Treatment — *310*
- Outcomes — *314*
- Prevention — *316*
- Resources — *318*

**Femoral and inguinal hernia** — *321*
- Summary Information — *322*
- Background — *323*
- Diagnosis — *325*
- Treatment — *329*
- Outcomes — *334*
- Prevention — *335*
- Resources — *337*

**Irritable bowel syndrome** — *339*
- Summary Information — *340*
- Background — *341*
- Diagnosis — *343*
- Treatment — *352*
- Outcomes — *364*
- Prevention — *365*
- Resources — *366*

**Lactose intolerance** — *369*
- Summary Information — *370*
- Background — *371*
- Diagnosis — *373*
- Treatment — *379*
- Outcomes — *383*
- Prevention — *384*
- Resources — *385*

**Mallory-Weiss syndrome** — *387*
- Summary Information — *388*
- Background — *389*
- Diagnosis — *391*
- Treatment — *397*
- Outcomes — *402*
- Prevention — *404*
- Resources — *405*

**Pancreatitis** — *407*
- Summary Information — *408*
- Background — *409*
- Diagnosis — *411*
- Treatment — *422*
- Outcomes — *426*
- Prevention — *428*
- Resources — *430*

**Peptic ulcer** — *433*
- Summary Information — *434*
- Background — *435*
- Diagnosis — *438*
- Treatment — *447*
- Outcomes — *458*
- Prevention — *460*
- Resources — *462*

**Acute peritonitis** — *465*
- Summary Information — *466*
- Background — *467*
- Diagnosis — *468*
- Treatment — *477*

# Index

- Outcomes — *486*
- Prevention — *487*
- Resources — *488*

**Proctitis** — ***489***
- Summary Information — *490*
- Background — *491*
- Diagnosis — *493*
- Treatment — *498*
- Outcomes — *505*
- Prevention — *506*
- Resources — *507*

**Pseudomembranous colitis** — ***509***
- Summary Information — *510*
- Background — *511*
- Diagnosis — *512*
- Treatment — *518*
- Outcomes — *525*
- Prevention — *527*
- Resources — *528*

**Pyloric stenosis** — ***529***
- Summary Information — *530*
- Background — *531*
- Diagnosis — *533*
- Treatment — *539*
- Outcomes — *548*
- Prevention — *549*
- Resources — *550*

**Rectal malignancy** — ***553***
- Summary Information — *554*
- Background — *555*
- Diagnosis — *558*
- Treatment — *572*
- Outcomes — *581*
- Prevention — *584*
- Resources — *587*

**Ulcerative colitis** — ***591***
- Summary Information — *592*
- Background — *593*
- Diagnosis — *595*
- Treatment — *608*
- Outcomes — *619*
- Prevention — *621*
- Resources — *622*

**Ulcerative colitis** — ***591***
- Summary Information — *592*
- Background — *593*
- Diagnosis — *595*
- Treatment — *608*
- Outcomes — *619*
- Prevention — *621*
- Resources — *622*